# Cochrane Handbook for Systematic Reviews of Interventions

# Cochrane Handbook for Systematic Reviews of Interventions

Cochrane Book Series

**Edited by**

**Julian PT Higgins and Sally Green**

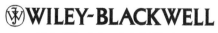

A John Wiley & Sons, Ltd., Publication

THE COCHRANE
COLLABORATION®

This work is a co-publication between The Cochrane Collaboration and John Wiley & Sons Ltd.

Published by John Wiley & Sons Ltd, The Atrium, Southern Gate, Chichester, West Sussex PO19 8SQ, England
Telephone (+44) 1243 779777

Email (for orders and customer service enquiries): cs-books@wiley.co.uk
Visit our Home Page on www.wiley.com

Reprinted with corrections April 2009
Reprinted July, September 2009, October 2010, August 2011, August 2012

*Other Wiley Editorial Offices*

John Wiley & Sons Inc., 111 River Street, Hoboken, NJ 07030, USA

Jossey-Bass, 989 Market Street, San Francisco, CA 94103-1741, USA

Wiley-VCH Verlag GmbH, Boschstr. 12, D-69469, Weinheim, Germany

John Wiley & Sons Australia Ltd, 42 McDougall Street, Milton, Queensland 4064, Australia

John Wiley & Sons (Asia) Pte Ltd, 2 Clementi Loop #02-01, Jin Xing Distripark, Singapore 129809

John Wiley & Sons Canada Ltd, 6045 Freemont Blvd, Mississauga, Ontario, L5R 4J3, Canada

Wiley also publishes its books in a variety of electronic formats. Some content that appears in print may not be available in electronic books.

*Library of Congress Cataloging-in-Publication Data*

Cochrane handbook for systematic reviews of interventions / edited by Julian Higgins and Sally Green.
     p. ; cm.—(Cochrane book series)
  Includes bibliographical references and index.
  ISBN 978-0-470-69951-5 (alk. paper)—ISBN 978-0-470-05796-4 (alk. paper)
  1. Evidence-based medicine—Methodology.  2. Medicine—Research—Evaluation.  3. Outcome assessment (Medical care)  4. Meta-analysis.  I. Higgins, Julian.  II. Green, Sally, Prof.  III. Cochrane Collaboration.  IV. Series.
    [DNLM:  1. Outcome and Process Assessment (Health Care)  2. Evidence-Based Medicine—methods.
3. Meta-Analysis as Topic.  4. Review Literature as Topic. WA 84.1 C663 2008]
    R723.7.C63 2008
    610.72—dc22

                      2008022132

*British Library Cataloguing in Publication Data*

A catalogue record for this book is available from the British Library

ISBN 978-0-470-69951-5 (H/B)

Typeset in 10.5/12.5pt Times by Aptara Inc., New Delhi, India
Printed and bound by CPI Group (UK) Ltd, Croydon, CR0 4YY

# Contents

## 4  Guide to the contents of a Cochrane protocol and review          **51**

*Edited by Julian PT Higgins and Sally Green*

## Part 2   GENERAL METHODS FOR COCHRANE REVIEWS          **81**

## 5  Defining the review question and developing criteria for including studies          **83**

*Edited by Denise O'Connor, Sally Green and Julian PT Higgins*

## 6  Searching for studies          **95**

*Carol Lefebvre, Eric Manheimer and Julie Glanville on behalf of the Cochrane Information Retrieval Methods Group*

## 14 Adverse effects 433

*Yoon K Loke, Deirdre Price and Andrew Herxheimer on behalf of the Cochrane Adverse Effects Methods Group*

## 15 Incorporating economics evidence 449

*Ian Shemilt, Miranda Mugford, Sarah Byford, Michael Drummond, Eric Eisenstein, Martin Knapp, Jacqueline Mallender, David McDaid, Luke Vale and Damian Walker on behalf of the Campbell and Cochrane Economics Methods Group*

## 16 Special topics in statistics 481

*Edited by Julian PT Higgins, Jonathan J Deeks and Douglas G Altman on behalf of the Cochrane Statistical Methods Group*

# Preface

The *Cochrane Handbook for Systematic Reviews of Interventions* (the *Handbook*) provides guidance to authors for the preparation of Cochrane Intervention reviews (including Cochrane Overviews of reviews). The *Handbook* is a long-standing document and is updated regularly to reflect advances in systematic review methodology and in response to feedback from users. This book coincides with version 5.0.1 of the online publication of the *Handbook*.

## Keeping up to date

Please refer to the following web site for the most recent version, for interim updates to the guidance and for details of previous versions of the *Handbook*.

www.cochrane.org/resources/handbook

Users of the *Handbook* are encouraged to send feedback and corrections to the *Handbook* editors; contact details are available on the web site.

## Central sources of support

### Present sources of support

The Cochrane Collaboration

Medical Research Council, United Kingdom

Department of Health and Ageing, Australia

Monash University, Australia

## Previous sources of support

National Health Service Research and Development Programme, United Kingdom

Health Research Board, Ireland

National Institute of Public Health, Norway

Copenhagen Hospital Corporation, Denmark

Health Services Research and Development Service and the University of Texas Health Science Center, San Antonio, USA

US Veterans Health Administration, USA

Oxford Regional Health Authority, UK

Nuffield Provincial Hospitals Trust, UK

LW Frohlich Fund, USA

Norwegian Ministry of Health and Social Affairs, Norway

Norwegian Research Council, Norway

Glaxo Wellcome, Norway

# Acknowledgements

We are grateful to all past and current members of the Handbook Advisory Group for discussions and feedback, and would particularly like to thank Doug Altman, Chris Cates, Mike Clarke, Jon Deeks, Donna Gillies, Andrew Herxheimer, Harriet MacLehose, Philippa Middleton, Ruth Mitchell, David Moher, Donald Patrick, Ian Shemilt, Lesley Stewart, Jessica Thomas, Jane Tierney and Danielle Wheeler.

Many contributed constructive and timely peer review. We thank Phil Alderson, Claire Allen, Judith Anzures, Chris Cates, Jonathan Craig, Miranda Cumpston, Chris Del Mar, Kay Dickersin, Christian Gluud, Peter Gøtzsche, Frans Helmerhorst, Jini Hetherington, Sophie Hill, Sally Hopewell, Steve McDonald, David Moher, Ann Møller, Duncan Mortimer, Karen New, Denise O'Connor, Jordi Pardo, Rob Scholten, Simon Thompson, Jan Vandenbroucke, Janet Wale, Phil Wiffen, Hywel Williams, Paula Williamson, Jim Wright and Diana Wyatt.

Specific administrative support for this version of the *Handbook* was provided by Jane Lane. In addition, skilled and generous administrative and technical support provided by Claire Allen, Dave Booker, Jini Hetherington, Monica Kjeldstrøm, Cindy Manukonga, Rasmus Moustgaard, Jane Predl and Jacob Riis has contributed greatly to the preparation and co-ordination of this *Handbook*. We would like to thank Lucy Sayer, Fiona Woods, Laura Mellor and Jon Peacock at Wiley-Blackwell for their patience, support and advice, and also Neil Manley for providing an index and Wendy Langford for proof-reading.

This major revision of the *Handbook* would not have been possible without the generous support provided to the editors by colleagues at the MRC Biostatistics Unit and the Institute of Public Health in Cambridge, UK and at the Australasian Cochrane Centre, Monash University, Australia.

# The *Handbook* editors

Julian Higgins is a Senior Statistician at the MRC Biostatistics Unit, Institute of Public Health, University of Cambridge and a Visiting Fellow at the UK Cochrane Centre, Oxford, UK.

Sally Green is a Professorial Fellow at the Institute of Health Services Research at Monash University, Melbourne, Australia and Director of the Australasian Cochrane Centre.

# Major contributors

**Acquadro, Catherine**
MAPI Research Institute, Lyon, France

**Alderson, Philip**
National Institute for Health and Clinical Excellence, London/Manchester, United Kingdom

**Altman, Douglas G**
Centre for Statistics in Medicine, University of Oxford, Oxford, United Kingdom

**Armstrong, Rebecca**
The McCaughey Centre: VicHealth Centre for the Promotion of Mental Health and Community Wellbeing, University of Melbourne, Melbourne, Australia

**Askie, Lisa M**
NHMRC Clinical Trials Centre, University of Sydney, Camperdown, Australia

**Becker, Lorne A**
Department of Family Medicine, SUNY Upstate Medical University, Syracuse, NY, United States of America

**Berlin, Jesse A**
Pharmacoepidemiology, Johnson & Johnson Pharmaceutical Research and Development Titusville, NJ, USA

**Booth, Andrew**
School of Health and Related Research, University of Sheffield, Sheffield, United Kingdom

**Byford, Sarah**
Centre for the Economics of Mental Health, Institute of Psychiatry, King's College, London, United Kingdom

**Clarke, Mike**
UK Cochrane Centre, National Institute for Health Research, Oxford, United Kingdom

**Deeks, Jonathan J**
Department of Public Health and Epidemiology, University of Birmingham, Birmingham, United Kingdom

**Doyle, Jodie**
The McCaughey Centre: VicHealth Centre for the Promotion of Mental Health and Community Wellbeing, University of Melbourne, Melbourne, Australia

**Drummond, Michael**
Centre for Health Economics, University of York, York, United Kingdom

**Egger, Matthias**
Institute of Social and Preventive Medicine, University of Bern, Bern, Switzerland

**Eisenstein, Eric**
Duke Clinical Research Center, Duke University, Durham, NC, United States of America

**Ghersi, Davina**
Department of Research Policy and Cooperation, World Health Organization, Geneva, Switzerland

**Glanville, Julie**
Centre for Reviews and Dissemination, University of York, York, United Kingdom

**Glasziou, Paul P**
Department of Primary Health Care, University of Oxford, Oxford, United Kingdom

**Green, Sally**
Australasian Cochrane Centre, Monash University, Melbourne, Australia

**Guyatt, Gordon H**
Departments of Clinical Epidemiology and Biostatics, McMaster University, Ontario, Canada

**Hannes, Karin**
Belgian Centre for Evidence-Based Medicine, Leuven, Belgium

**Herxheimer, Andrew**
Co-founder, DIPEx; Emeritus Fellow, UK Cochrane Centre, London, United Kingdom

**Higgins, Julian PT**
MRC Biostatistics Unit, Cambridge, United Kingdom

**Knapp, Martin**
Institute of Psychiatry, King's College London, and London School of Economics, London, United Kingdom

**Lefebvre, Carol**
UK Cochrane Centre, National Institute for Health Research, Oxford, United Kingdom

**Loke, Yoon K**
School of Medicine, Health Policy and Practice, University of East Anglia, Norwich, United Kingdom

**Mallender, Jacqueline**
Matrix Knowledge Group Ltd., London, United Kingdom

**Manheimer, Eric**
Center for Integrative Medicine, University of Maryland School of Medicine, Baltimore, MA, United States of America

**McDaid, David**
Personal Social Services Research Unit, London School of Economics and Political Science, London, United Kingdom

**Moher, David**
Chalmers Research Group, Children's Hospital of Eastern Ontario Research Institute; Department of Epidemiology and Community Medicine, University of Ottawa, Ottawa, Canada

**Mugford, Miranda**
Health Economics Group, School of Medicine, Health Policy and Practice, University of East Anglia, Norwich, United Kingdom

**Noyes, Jane**
Centre for Health-Related Research, School of Healthcare Sciences, Bangor University, Bangor, Wales, United Kingdom

**O'Connor, Denise**
Australasian Cochrane Centre, Monash University, Melbourne, Australia

**Oxman, Andrew D**
Preventive and International Health Care Unit, Norwegian Knowledge Centre for the Health Services, Oslo, Norway

**Patrick, Donald L**
Department of Health Services and Seattle Quality of Life Group, University of Washington, Seattle, WA, United States of America

**Pearson, Alan**
Joanna Briggs Institute, University of Adelaide, Adelaide, Australia

**Popay, Jennie**
Institute for Health Research, Lancaster
University, Lancaster,
United Kingdom

**Price, Deirdre**
Department of Clinical Pharmacology,
University of Oxford, Oxford,
United Kingdom

**Reeves, Barnaby**
Bristol Heart Institute,
University of Bristol,
Bristol, United Kingdom

**Scholten, Rob**
Dutch Cochrane Centre, Academic
Medical Center, Amsterdam, The
Netherlands

**Schünemann, Holger J**
INFORMA/CLARITY Research/
Department of Epidemiology, National
Cancer Institute Regina Elena,
Rome, Italy

**Shemilt, Ian**
Health Economics Group, School of
Medicine, Health Policy and Practice,
University of East Anglia, Norwich,
United Kingdom

**Sterne, Jonathan AC**
Department of Social Medicine,
University of Bristol, Bristol,
United Kingdom

**Stewart, Lesley A**
Centre for Reviews and Dissemination,
University of York, York, United Kingdom

**Tierney, Jayne F**
MRC Clinical Trials Unit, London, United
Kingdom

**Vale, Luke**
Health Economics Research Unit,
University of Aberdeen, Aberdeen, United
Kingdom

**Vist, Gunn E**
Preventive and International Health Care
Unit, Norwegian Knowledge Centre for the
Health Services, Oslo, Norway

**Walker, Damian**
Health Systems Program, Department of
International Health, Johns Hopkins
Bloomberg School of Public Health,
Baltimore, MA, United States of America

**Waters, Elizabeth**
The McCaughey Centre: VicHealth Centre
for the Promotion of Mental Health and
Community Wellbeing, University of
Melbourne, Melbourne, Australia

**Wells, George A**
Department of Epidemiology and
Community Medicine, University of
Ottawa, Ottawa, Ontario, Canada

# PART 1: Cochrane reviews

# 1 Introduction

**Sally Green, Julian PT Higgins, Philip Alderson, Mike Clarke, Cynthia D Mulrow and Andrew D Oxman**

## Key Points

- Systematic reviews seek to collate all evidence that fits pre-specified eligibility criteria in order to address a specific research question.

- Systematic reviews aim to minimize bias by using explicit, systematic methods.

- The Cochrane Collaboration prepares, maintains and promotes systematic reviews to inform healthcare decisions (Cochrane reviews).

- Cochrane reviews are published in the *Cochrane Database of Systematic Reviews* in *The Cochrane Library*.

- The *Cochrane Handbook for Systematic Reviews of Interventions* contains methodological guidance for the preparation and maintenance of Cochrane Intervention reviews and Cochrane Overviews of reviews.

## 1.1 The Cochrane Collaboration

### 1.1.1 Introduction

The Cochrane Collaboration (www.cochrane.org) is an international organization whose primary aim is to help people make well-informed decisions about health care by preparing, maintaining and promoting the accessibility of systematic reviews of the evidence that underpins them. By providing a reliable synthesis of the available evidence on a given topic, systematic reviews adhere to the principle that science is cumulative and facilitate decisions considering all the evidence on the effect of an intervention. Since it was founded in 1993, The Cochrane Collaboration has grown to include over 15,000 contributors from more than 100 countries, easily making it the largest organization involved in this kind of work (Allen 2006, Allen 2007). The international Collaboration was launched one year after the establishment of the Cochrane Centre in Oxford (now the UK Cochrane Centre) founded by Sir Iain Chalmers and colleagues, and named after British epidemiologist Archie Cochrane. The Cochrane Collaboration is now an internationally renowned initiative (Clarke 2005, Green 2005).

The work of The Cochrane Collaboration is underpinned by a set of 10 key principles, listed in Box 1.1.a.

---

**Box 1.1.a   The principles of The Cochrane Collaboration**

1. Collaboration, by internally and externally fostering good communications, open decision-making and teamwork.
2. Building on the enthusiasm of individuals, by involving and supporting people of different skills and backgrounds.
3. Avoiding duplication by good management and co-ordination to maximize economy of effort.
4. Minimizing bias, through a variety of approaches such as scientific rigour, ensuring broad participation, and avoiding conflicts of interest.
5. Keeping up to date, by a commitment to ensure that Cochrane reviews are maintained through identification and incorporation of new evidence.
6. Striving for relevance, by promoting the assessment of healthcare interventions using outcomes that matter to people making choices in health care.
7. Promoting access, by wide dissemination of the outputs of the Collaboration, taking advantage of strategic alliances, and by promoting appropriate prices, content and media to meet the needs of users worldwide.
8. Ensuring quality, by being open and responsive to criticism, applying advances in methodology, and developing systems for quality improvement.
9. Continuity, by ensuring that responsibility for reviews, editorial processes and key functions is maintained and renewed.
10. Enabling wide participation in the work of the Collaboration by reducing barriers to contributing and by encouraging diversity.

---

## 1.1.2   Structure of The Cochrane Collaboration

The work of The Cochrane Collaboration revolves around 52 Cochrane Review Groups (CRGs), responsible for preparing and maintaining reviews within specific areas of health care. The members of these groups include researchers, healthcare professionals and people using healthcare services (consumers), all of whom share a common enthusiasm for generating reliable, up-to-date evidence relevant to the prevention and treatment of specific health problems or groups of problems.

Cochrane Review Groups are supported in review preparation by Methods Groups, Centres and Fields. Cochrane Methods Groups provide a forum for methodologists to discuss development, evaluation and application of methods used to prepare Cochrane reviews. They play a major role in the production of the *Cochrane Handbook for Systematic Reviews of Interventions* (the *Handbook*) and, where appropriate, chapters contain information about the relevant Methods Group. Cochrane Centres are located in different countries and together they represent all regions and provide training and support for review authors and CRGs in addition to advocacy and promotion of access to Cochrane reviews. Cochrane Fields focus on broad dimensions of health care, such as the setting of care (e.g. primary care), the type of consumer (e.g. children), or the type of intervention (e.g. vaccines). People associated with Fields help to ensure that priorities and perspectives in their sphere of interest are reflected in the work of CRGs.

## 1.1.3 Publication of Cochrane reviews

Cochrane reviews are published in full online in the *Cochrane Database of Systematic Reviews (CDSR)*, which is a core component of *The Cochrane Library*. *The Cochrane Library* is published by Wiley-Blackwell on the internet (www.thecochranelibrary.com) and on CD-ROM, and is available free at the point of use in some countries thanks to national licences and free access provided by Wiley-Blackwell in the most resource-poor settings. Elsewhere it is subscription based, or pay-per-view. In addition to *CDSR*, *The Cochrane Library* contains several other sources of knowledge, listed in Box 1.1.b.

---

**Box 1.1.b  Databases published in *The Cochrane Library***

- The *Cochrane Database of Systematic Reviews* (*CDSR*) contains the full text (including methods, results and conclusions) for Cochrane reviews and protocols.
- The *Database of Abstracts of Reviews of Effects* (*DARE*), assembled and maintained by the Centre for Reviews and Dissemination in York, UK, contains critical assessments and structured abstracts of other systematic reviews, conforming to explicit quality criteria.
- The *Cochrane Central Register of Controlled Trials* (*CENTRAL*) contains bibliographic information on hundreds of thousands of studies, including those published in conference proceedings and many other sources not currently listed in other bibliographic databases.
- The *Cochrane Methodology Register* (*CMR*) contains bibliographic information on articles and books on the science of reviewing research, and a prospective register of methodological studies.
- The Cochrane Collaboration section contains contact details and other information about CRGs and the other contributing groups within The Cochrane Collaboration.

---

*CDSR* is published four times a year, each time with new reviews and updates of existing reviews. Issue 1, 2008 of *CDSR* contained more than 3000 Cochrane reviews and over 1700 protocols for reviews in progress.

## 1.2 Systematic reviews

### 1.2.1 The need for systematic reviews

Healthcare providers, consumers, researchers, and policy makers are inundated with unmanageable amounts of information, including evidence from healthcare research. It is unlikely that all will have the time, skills and resources to find, appraise and interpret this evidence and to incorporate it into healthcare decisions. Cochrane reviews respond to this challenge by identifying, appraising and synthesizing research-based evidence and presenting it in an accessible format (Mulrow 1994).

### 1.2.2 What is a systematic review?

A systematic review attempts to collate all empirical evidence that fits pre-specified eligibility criteria in order to answer a specific research question. It uses explicit, systematic methods that are selected with a view to minimizing bias, thus providing more reliable findings from which conclusions can be drawn and decisions made (Antman 1992, Oxman 1993). The key characteristics of a systematic review are:

- a clearly stated set of objectives with pre-defined eligibility criteria for studies;

- an explicit, reproducible methodology;

- a systematic search that attempts to identify all studies that would meet the eligibility criteria;

- an assessment of the validity of the findings of the included studies, for example through the assessment of risk of bias; and

- a systematic presentation, and synthesis, of the characteristics and findings of the included studies;

Many systematic reviews contain meta-analyses. Meta-analysis is the use of statistical methods to summarize the results of independent studies (Glass 1976). By combining information from all relevant studies, meta-analyses can provide more precise estimates of the effects of health care than those derived from the individual studies included within a review (see Chapter 9, Section 9.1.3). They also facilitate investigations of the consistency of evidence across studies, and the exploration of differences across studies.

## 1.3 About this *Handbook*

The science of research synthesis is rapidly evolving; hence the methods employed in the conduct of Cochrane reviews have developed over time. The aim of the *Cochrane Handbook for Systematic Reviews of Interventions* (the *Handbook*) is to help Cochrane review authors make appropriate decisions about the methods they use, rather than to dictate arbitrary standards. Wherever possible, recommendations are informed by empirical evidence. The guidance provided here is intended to help review authors to be systematic, informed and explicit (but not mechanistic) about the questions they pose and how they derive answers to those questions. Interpretation and implementation of this guidance requires judgement and should be done in conjunction with editorial bases of CRGs.

This *Handbook* focuses on systematic reviews of the effects of interventions. Most of the advice contained within it is oriented to the synthesis of clinical trials, and of randomized trials in particular because they provide more reliable evidence than other study designs on the relative effects of healthcare interventions (Kunz 2007). Some chapters, however, provide advice on including other types of evidence, particularly in forms of care where randomized trials may not be possible or appropriate and in considerations of safety or adverse effects. In 2003, The Cochrane Collaboration expanded its scope to include Cochrane Diagnostic test accuracy reviews. Guidance for the conduct of these reviews is contained in a separate document: the *Cochrane Handbook for Systematic Reviews of Diagnostic Test Accuracy*.

This *Handbook* has 22 chapters organized into three parts. Part 1 introduces Cochrane reviews, covering their planning and preparation, and their maintenance and updating, and ends with a guide to the contents of a Cochrane review or protocol. Part 2 provides general methodological guidance relevant to all Cochrane reviews, covering question development, eligibility criteria, searching, collecting data, within-study bias, analysing data, reporting bias, presenting and interpreting results. Part 3 addresses special topics that will be relevant to some, but not all, Cochrane reviews, including particular considerations in addressing adverse effects, meta-analysis with non-standard study designs and using individual patient data. This part has chapters on incorporating economic evaluations, non-randomized studies, qualitative research, patient-reported outcomes in reviews, prospective meta-analysis and reviews in health promotion and public health. A final chapter describes the new review type, Overviews of reviews.

Each chapter contains a list of key points to summarize the information and draw out the main messages for review authors.

The *Handbook* is largely prepared by The Cochrane Collaboration's Methods Groups, whose members conduct much of the methodological and empirical research that informs the guidance.

Although the main intended audience for the *Handbook* is authors of Cochrane Intervention reviews, many of the principles and methods are applicable to systematic reviews applied to other types of research and to systematic reviews of interventions undertaken by others (Moher 2007).

## 1.4   Contributors to the *Handbook*

"If I have seen further, it is by standing on the shoulders of Giants"
                                                          – Isaac Newton

This *Cochrane Handbook for Systematic Reviews of Interventions* (Version 5) is a major revision of a document that has evolved over time since the early days of The Cochrane Collaboration. Many chapters build on previous versions of the *Handbook*, and others are newly authored for Version 5. It is a truly collaborative effort, reflecting the principles of The Cochrane Collaboration. Many people have contributed directly to this revision, as chapter authors, chapter editors, peer reviewers, members of the Cochrane Handbook Advisory Group, and in numerous other ways. The *Handbook* also reflects the invaluable contributions of previous editors, past and present members of Cochrane Methods Groups, review authors, Cochrane Review Groups, the RevMan Advisory Group, Cochrane Centres and Cochrane Fields.

The initial methodological guidance for Cochrane review authors was developed by Andy Oxman, Iain Chalmers, Mike Clarke, Murray Enkin, Ken Schulz, Mark Starr, Kay Dickersin, Andrew Herxheimer and Chris Silagy, with administrative support from Sally Hunt. It was published in March 1994 as *Section VI: Preparing and maintaining systematic reviews ('The Cochrane Collaboration Tool Kit')* of a comprehensive handbook for the Collaboration. It described the original structured format of a Cochrane review, which was developed by Mike Clarke, Murray Enkin, Chris Silagy and Mark Starr, with input from many others. The guidance became a stand-alone document in October 1996 as the *Cochrane Collaboration Handbook* (Version 3), under the editorship of Andy Oxman and Cynthia Mulrow, supported by the newly formed Handbook Advisory Group. Version 4, named the *Cochrane Reviewers' Handbook*, was released in 1999 to coincide with the launch of RevMan 4 and was edited by Mike Clarke and Andy Oxman from 1999 until December 2003, when Phil Alderson, Julian Higgins and Sally Green became editors (from Version 4.2.1). The introduction of Cochrane Diagnostic test accuracy reviews and the need for a new handbook specific to those reviews prompted, from Version 4.2.4 in March 2005, the change in title to the *Cochrane Handbook for Systematic Reviews of Interventions,* edited by Julian Higgins and Sally Green.

The current *Handbook* editors are supported by advice from the Handbook Advisory Group. The current membership of the Handbook Advisory Group is: Lisa Askie, Chris Cates, Jon Deeks, Matthias Egger, Davina Ghersi, Donna Gillies, Paul Glasziou, Sally Green (Co-Convenor), Andrew Herxheimer, Julian Higgins (Co-Convenor), Jane Lane (Administration), Carol Lefebvre, Harriet MacLehose, Philippa Middleton, Ruth Mitchell, David Moher, Miranda Mugford, Jane Noyes, Donald Patrick, Jennie Popay, Barney Reeves, Jacob Riis, Ian Shemilt, Jonathan Sterne, Lesley Stewart, Jessica Thomas, Jayne Tierney and Danielle Wheeler.

In addition to the previous editors, named above, the following have made substantial contributions to previous versions of the *Handbook*: Christina Aguilar, Doug Altman, Bob Badgett, Hilda Bastian, Lisa Bero, Michael Brand, Joe Cavellero, Mildred Cho, Kay Dickersin, Lelia Duley, Frances Fairman, Jeremy Grimshaw, Gord Guyatt, Peter Gøtzsche, Jeph Herrin, Nicki Jackson, Monica Kjeldstrøm, Jos Kleijnen,

Kristen Larson, Valerie Lawrence, Eric Manheimer, Rasmus Moustgaard, Melissa Ober, Drummond Rennie, Dave Sackett, Mark Starr, Nicola Thornton, Luke Vale and Veronica Yank.

## 1.5 Chapter information

**Authors:** Sally Green, Julian PT Higgins, Philip Alderson, Mike Clarke, Cynthia D Mulrow and Andrew D Oxman.

**This chapter should be cited as:** Green S, Higgins JPT, Alderson P, Clarke M, Mulrow CD, Oxman AD. Chapter 1: Introduction. In: Higgins JPT, Green S (editors), *Cochrane Handbook for Systematic Reviews of Interventions*. Chichester (UK): John Wiley & Sons, 2008.

## 1.6 References

**Allen 2006**
  Allen C, Clarke M. International activity in Cochrane Review Groups with particular reference to China. *Chinese Journal of Evidence-based Medicine* 2006; 6: 541–545.
**Allen 2007**
  Allen C, Clarke M, Tharyan P. International activity in Cochrane Review Groups with particular reference to India. *National Medical Journal of India* 2007; 20: 250–255.
**Antman 1992**
  Antman EM, Lau J, Kupelnick B, Mosteller F, Chalmers TC. A comparison of results of meta-analyses of randomized control trials and recommendations of clinical experts: Treatments for myocardial infarction. *JAMA* 1992; 268: 240–248.
**Clarke 2005**
  Clarke M. Cochrane Collaboration. In: Armitage P, Colton T (editors). *Encyclopedia of Biostatistics* (2nd edition). Chichester (UK): John Wiley & Sons, 2005.
**Glass 1976**
  Glass GV. Primary, secondary and meta-analysis of research. *Educational Researcher* 1976; 5: 3–8.
**Green 2005**
  Green S, McDonald S. The Cochrane Collaboration: More than systematic reviews? *Internal Medicine Journal* 2005; 35: 4–5.
**Kunz 2007**
  Kunz R, Vist G, Oxman AD. Randomisation to protect against selection bias in healthcare trials. *Cochrane Database of Systematic Reviews* 2007, Issue 2. Art No: MR000012.
**Moher 2007**
  Moher D, Tetzlaff J, Tricco AC, Sampson M, Altman DG. Epidemiology and reporting characteristics of systematic reviews. *PLoS Medicine* 2007; 4: e78.
**Mulrow 1994**
  Mulrow CD. Rationale for systematic reviews. *BMJ* 1994; 309: 597–599.
**Oxman 1993**
  Oxman AD, Guyatt GH. The science of reviewing research. *Annals of the New York Academy of Sciences* 1993; 703: 125–133.

# 2 Preparing a Cochrane review

**Edited by Sally Green and Julian PT Higgins**

## Key Points

- The publication of protocols for Cochrane reviews in the *Cochrane Database of Systematic Reviews (CDSR)* prior to publication of the Cochrane review reduces the impact of authors' biases, promotes transparency of methods and processes, reduces the potential for duplication, and allows peer review of the planned methods.

- Cochrane reviews, and protocols for reviews, are prepared in the Cochrane Collaboration's Review Manager (RevMan) software and have a uniform format.

- An outline of a Cochrane Intervention review is provided in this chapter.

- Titles for Cochrane Intervention reviews are agreed by and registered with Cochrane Review Groups (CRGs), who then manage the editorial process of publishing protocols and reviews.

- Cochrane reviews are prepared by teams.

- There are guidelines for co-publication of Cochrane reviews in other journals.

- The Cochrane Collaboration has a code of conduct for avoiding potential financial conflicts of interest.

## 2.1 Rationale for protocols

Preparing a Cochrane review is complex and involves many judgements. In order to minimize the potential for bias in the review process, these judgements should be made in ways that do not depend on the findings of the studies included in the review. Review authors' prior knowledge of the results of a potentially eligible study may, for example, influence the definition of a systematic review question, the subsequent criteria for study eligibility, the choice of intervention comparisons to analyse, or the outcomes to be reported in the review. Since Cochrane reviews are by their nature retrospective (one exception being prospective meta-analyses, as described in Chapter 19), it is important that the methods to be used should be established and documented in advance. Publication of a protocol for a review prior to knowledge of the available studies reduces the impact of review authors' biases, promotes transparency of methods and processes, reduces the potential for duplication, and allows peer review of the planned methods (Light 1984).

While the intention should be that a review will adhere to the published protocol, changes in a review protocol are sometimes necessary. This is similarly the case for a protocol for a randomized trial, which must sometimes be changed to adapt to unanticipated circumstances such as problems with participant recruitment, data collection or unexpected event rates. While every effort should be made to adhere to a predetermined protocol, this is not always possible or appropriate. It is important, however, that changes in the protocol should not be made on the basis of how they affect the outcome of the research study. *Post hoc* decisions made when the impact on the results of the research is known, such as excluding selected studies from a systematic review, are highly susceptible to bias and should be avoided.

Protocols for Cochrane reviews are published before the completed systematic review in the *Cochrane Database of Systematic Reviews (CDSR)*. Changes in the protocol should be documented and reported in the 'Differences between protocol and review' section of the completed review, and sensitivity analyses (see Chapter 9, Section 9.7) exploring the impact of deviations from the protocol should be undertaken when possible.

## 2.2 Format of a Cochrane review

### 2.2.1 Rationale for the format of a Cochrane review

All Cochrane reviews of interventions have the same format. Benefits of this uniform format include:

1. helping readers find the results of research quickly and to assess the validity, applicability and implications of those results;

2. guiding review authors to report their work explicitly and concisely, and minimizing the effort required to do this;

3. facilitating electronic publication and maintenance of reviews; and

4. enabling the development of derivative products (e.g. Overviews of reviews, see Chapter 22) and empirical research studies based on multiple systematic reviews.

The format is flexible enough to fit different types of reviews, including those making a single comparison, those making multiple comparisons and those prepared using individual patient data. Standard headings and tables embedded in RevMan guide review authors when preparing their report and make it easier for readers to identify information that is of particular interest to them. The headings within RevMan are listed in Sections 2.2.2 and 2.2.3. A detailed guide to the content that should follow each heading is provided in Chapter 4.

### 2.2.2    Outline of a protocol for a Cochrane review

Box 2.2.a lists the elements that define a complete protocol for a Cochrane review, and indicate how the protocol is likely to appear in the *CDSR* (which may not be the same as in RevMan). If any of the sections marked with an asterisk (*) are empty, the protocol will not be published until something has been added to the section, that is they are 'mandatory fields'.

### 2.2.3    Detailed outline of a Cochrane review

Box 2.2.b lists the elements that define a complete Cochrane review, and indicate how the review is likely to appear in the *CDSR* (which may not be the same as in RevMan). If any of the sections marked with an asterisk (*) are empty, the review will not be published until something has been added to the section, that is they are 'mandatory fields'.

## 2.3    Logistics of doing a review

### 2.3.1    Motivation for undertaking a review

A number of factors may motivate authors to undertake a systematic review. For example, reviews can be conducted in an effort to resolve conflicting evidence, to address questions where clinical practice is uncertain, to explore variations in practice, to confirm the appropriateness of current practice or to highlight a need for future research. The overarching aim of Cochrane reviews should be to summarize and help people to understand the evidence. They should help people make practical decisions about health care. This aim has important implications for deciding whether or not to undertake a Cochrane review, how to formulate the question that a review will address, how to develop eligibility criteria to guide study inclusion based on the review question, how to develop the protocol and how to present the results of the review.

### 2.3.2    Planning the topic and scope of a review

Some important points to consider when planning a review and developing a protocol are as follows:

- review questions should address the choices (practical options) people face when deciding about health care;

## Box 2.2.a   Sections of a protocol for a Cochrane review

**Title***
**Protocol information**:
  Authors*
  Contact person*
  Dates
  What's new
  History
**The protocol:**
  Background*
  Objectives*
  Methods:
    Criteria for selecting studies for this review:
      Types of studies*
      Types of participants*
      Types of interventions*
      Types of outcome measures*
    Search methods for identification of studies*
    Data collection and analysis*
  Acknowledgements
  References:
    Other references:
      Additional references
      Other published versions of this review
  Tables and figures:
    Additional tables
    Figures
**Supplementary information**:
  Appendices
  Feedback:
    Title
    Summary
    Reply
    Contributors
**About the article**:
  Contributions of authors
  Declarations of interest*
  Sources of support:
    Internal sources
    External sources
  Published notes

## Box 2.2.b   Sections of a Cochrane review

**Title***
**Review information**:
  Authors*
  Contact person*
  Dates*
  What's new
  History
**Abstract:**
  Background*
  Objectives*
  Search methods*
  Data collection and analysis*
  Results*
  Authors' conclusions*
**Plain language summary:**
  Plain language title*
  Summary text*
**The review:**
  Background*
  Objectives*
  Methods:
    Criteria for selecting studies for this review:
      Types of studies*
      Types of participants*
      Types of interventions*
      Types of outcome measures*
    Search methods for identification of studies*
    Data collection and analysis*
  Results:
    Description of studies*
    Risk of bias in included studies*
    Effects of interventions*
  Discussion*
  Authors' conclusions:
    Implication for practice*
    Implication for research*
  Acknowledgements
  References:
    References to studies:
      Included studies
      Excluded studies
      Studies awaiting classification
      Ongoing studies

Other references:
   Additional references
   Other published versions of this review
  Tables and figures:
   Characteristics of studies:
    Characteristics of included studies (*includes 'Risk of bias' tables*)
    Characteristics of excluded studies
    Characteristics of studies awaiting assessment
    Characteristics of ongoing studies
   'Summary of findings' tables
   Additional tables
   Figures
**Supplementary information**:
  Data and analyses
  Appendices
  Feedback:
   Title
   Summary
   Reply
   Contributors
**About the article**:
  Contributions of authors
  Declarations of interest*
  Differences between protocol and review
  Sources of support:
   Internal sources
   External sources
  Published notes

- reviews should address outcomes that are meaningful to people making decisions about health care;

- review authors should describe how they will address adverse effects as well as beneficial effects;

- the methods used in a review should be selected to optimize the likelihood that the results will provide the best current evidence upon which to base decisions, and should be described in sufficient detail in the protocol for the readers to fully understand the planned steps;

- it is important to let people know when there is no reliable evidence, or no evidence about particular outcomes that are likely to be important to decision makers. No evidence of effect should not be confused with evidence of no effect;

- it is not helpful to include evidence for which there is a high risk of bias in a review, even if there is no better evidence. See Chapter 8 for a more detailed discussion of bias;

- similarly, it is not helpful to focus on trivial outcomes simply because those are what researchers have chosen to measure in the individual studies (see Chapter 5); and

- so far as is possible, it is important to take an international perspective. The evidence collected should not be restricted by nationality or language without good reason, background information such as prevalence and morbidity should where possible take a global view, and some attempt should be made to put the results of the review in a broad context.

## 2.3.3   Registering a protocol

The first step in the review process is to agree on a review topic with a Cochrane Review Group (CRG), The topics covered by each of the 52 CRGs are described in their scope, published in the *CDSR*. Many CRGs will have developed priorities for reviews of importance, and will require the completion of a 'title registration form'. A title will be registered, possibly after discussion among the CRG editors, and the review authors will be invited to submit a protocol. Once a protocol has been completed it will be sent to the CRG for editors and staff at the editorial base to peer review. When they are satisfied with the protocol (this may take several iterations) they will include it in the CRG's module for publication and dissemination in the *CDSR*. Editors and authors should not include a protocol in a module unless there is a firm commitment to complete the review within a reasonable time frame and to keep it up to date once it is completed.

It is Cochrane Collaboration policy that protocols that have not been converted into full reviews within two years should generally be withdrawn from the *CDSR*. If a protocol is withdrawn for any reason other than it being superseded by a review, a withdrawal notice should be published in *CDSR* for one issue. Thereafter, information on the withdrawal of the protocol should be noted in the CRG's module.

## 2.3.4   The review team

### 2.3.4.1   *The importance of a team*

It is essential that Cochrane reviews be undertaken by more than one person. This ensures that tasks such as selection of studies for eligibility and data extraction can be performed by at least two people independently, increasing the likelihood that errors are detected. If more than one team expresses an interest in undertaking a review on the same topic, it is likely that a CRG will encourage them to work together.

Review teams must include expertise in the topic area being reviewed and include, or have access to, expertise in systematic review methodology (including statistical expertise). First-time review authors are encouraged to work with others who are experienced in the process of systematic reviews and to attend training events organized by the Collaboration (see Section 2.3.6). The Cochrane Collaboration is committed to user-involvement in principle (the tenth principle of the Collaboration is enabling wide participation, see Chapter 1, Box 1.1a) and encourages review authors to seek and incorporate the views of users, including consumers, clinicians and those from varying regions and settings in the development of protocols and reviews. Where a review topic is of particular relevance in a region or setting (for example reviews of malaria in the developing world), involvement of people from that setting is encouraged.

### 2.3.4.2   *Consumer involvement*

The Cochrane Collaboration encourages the involvement of healthcare consumers, either as part of the review team or in the editorial process. Consumer involvement helps ensure that reviews:

- address questions that are important to people;

- take account of outcomes that are important to those affected;

- are accessible to people making decisions; and

- adequately reflect variability in the values and conditions of people, and the circumstances of health care in different countries.

Relatively little is known about the effectiveness of various means of involving consumers in the review process or, more generally, in healthcare research (Nilsen 2006). However, the Collaboration supports consumer involvement in principle. This is based on our principles, good logic, and evidence that the views and perspectives of consumers often differ greatly from those of healthcare providers and researchers (Bastian 1998).

Consumers are participating in the development of protocols and reviews in the following ways:

- supporting CRGs to establish priority lists for reviews;

- co-authoring reviews;

- contributing to a consumer consultation during protocol and review development; and

- peer reviewing protocols and reviews.

Whenever consumers (or others) are consulted during the development of a protocol or review, their contribution should be acknowledged in the Acknowledgements section of the protocol or review. Where input to the review is more substantive formal inclusion in the list of review authors for citation may also be appropriate, as it is for other contributors (see Chapter 4, Section 4.2.2).

### 2.3.4.3    Advisory groups

Systematic reviews are likely to be more relevant to the end user and of higher quality if they are informed by advice from people with a range of experiences, in terms of both the topic and the methodology (Khan 2001, Rees 2004, Thomas 2004). As the priorities of decision makers and consumers may be different from those of authors, it is important that authors address the questions of importance to stakeholders and include relevant interventions, outcomes and populations. It may be useful to form an advisory group of people, including representation of relevant stakeholders, with relevant interests, skills and commitment. This may be of greater importance in reviews anticipated to be of high impact or for reviews of complex interventions relevant to diverse settings. Box 2.3.a outlines an example of where an advisory group was used to benefit a review.

The input of the advisory group will need to be coordinated by the review team to inform key review decisions. The Effective Public Health Practice Project, Canada, has found that six members can cover all areas and is manageable for public health reviews (Effective Public Health Practice Project 2007). However, the broader the review, the broader the experience required of advisory group members.

It is important to consider the needs of resource-poor countries in the review process. To increase the relevance of systematic reviews, authors could also consult people in developing countries to identify priority topics on which reviews should be conducted (Richards 2004). It may also be important to include vulnerable and marginalized people in the advisory group (Steel 2001) in order to ensure that the conclusions regarding the value of the interventions are well informed and applicable to all groups in society.

Terms of reference, job descriptions or person specifications for an advisory group may be developed to ensure there is clarity about the task(s) required. Examples are provided in briefing notes for researchers (Hanley 2000) or at the INVOLVE web site (www.invo.org.uk). Advisory group members may be involved in one or more of the following tasks:

- making and refining decisions about the interventions of interest, the populations to be included, priorities for outcomes and, possibly, subgroup analyses;

- providing or suggesting important background material that elucidates the issues from different perspectives;

- helping to interpret the findings of the review; and

- designing a dissemination plan and assisting with dissemination to relevant groups.

---

**Box 2.3.a   An example of the benefits of using an advisory group in the planning process**

A review of HIV prevention for men who have sex with men (Rees 2004) employed explicit consensus methods to shape the review with the help of practitioners, commissioners and researchers. An advisory group was convened of people from research/academic, policy and service organizations and representatives from charities and organizations that have emerged from and speak on behalf of people living with, or affected by, HIV/AIDS. The group met three times over the course of the review.

The group was presented with background information about the proposed review: its scope, conceptual basis, aims, research questions, stages and methods. Discussion focused on the policy relevance and political background/context to the review; the eligibility criteria for studies (interventions, outcomes, subgroups of men); dissemination strategies; and timescales. Two rounds of voting identified and prioritized outcomes for analysis. Open discussion identified subgroups of vulnerable men. A framework for characterizing interventions of interest was refined through advisory group discussions.

The review followed this guidance by adopting the identified interventions, populations and outcomes to refine the inclusion criteria, performing a meta-analysis as well as subgroup analyses. The subsequent product included synthesized evidence directly related to health inequalities.

---

### 2.3.5   Cochrane software for review authors and editorial bases of Cochrane Review Groups

To support the preparation and editorial oversight of Cochrane reviews, The Cochrane Collaboration uses the Cochrane Information Management System (IMS). The IMS consists of two main components, the review writing software, Review Manager (RevMan) and a central server for managing documents and contact details, Archie. The IMS functions as the electronic infrastructure of The Cochrane Collaboration and facilitates efficient collaboration between staff at editorial bases of CRGs and their author teams, often working in different continents.

RevMan is a mandatory tool for Cochrane authors to use when preparing and maintaining protocols and reviews in the format described in Section 2.2. The software is developed through a continuing process of consultation with its users and Cochrane methodologists, to support standards and guidelines for Cochrane reviews, and provides improved analytic methods, 'online' help and error checking mechanisms.

As well as supporting the preparation of a Cochrane Intervention review, RevMan supports the preparation of Cochrane Methodology reviews, Cochrane Diagnostic test accuracy reviews, and Overviews of reviews (see Chapter 22).

RevMan is free to use for authors preparing a Cochrane review and by academic institutions. Commercial companies may use the software if they purchase a license. Technical support is only provided to Cochrane authors who have registered their reviews with a CRG.

While RevMan is used for preparing and editing reviews, Archie is used for storing drafts and published versions of reviews. Storing all relevant versions of a review centrally, the system facilitates access to the latest published version of a review when it is due for an update. Through Archie, authors can also view previous versions of a review, and compare two versions of the same review to identify changes introduced from one version to the next. In addition, authors maintain their contact details and access the contact details of their co-authors and their editorial base. Cochrane review authors can get access to Archie by contacting the editorial base of their CRG.

The IMS is developed and maintained by the Nordic Cochrane Centre. The ongoing development of the IMS is overseen by the Cochrane Information Management System Group with guidance from the relevant advisory groups. More information about The Cochrane Collaboration's software, such as the latest versions and planned developments, is available at the IMS web site: www.cc-ims.net.

## 2.3.6 Training

It is important to ensure that those contributing to the work of the Collaboration have the knowledge, skills and support that they need to do a good job. Training may be needed by review authors, editors, criticism editors, peer reviewers, CRG Co-ordinators and Trials Search Co-ordinators, hand-searchers, trainers and users of Cochrane reviews. We focus here on the training needs of review authors and editors to help them to prepare and maintain high quality reviews.

While some review authors who join a CRG have training and experience in conducting a systematic review, many do not. In addition to the training materials and support to authors provided by many CRGs, Cochrane Centres are responsible for working with Methods Groups to develop training materials based on the *Handbook* and for organizing training workshops for members of CRGs. Each CRG is responsible for ensuring that review authors have adequate training and methodological support. Training materials and opportunities for training are continually developed and updated to reflect the evolving needs of the Collaboration and its standards and guidelines.

Training for review authors is delivered in many countries by Cochrane Centres, Methods Groups and CRGs. Training timetables are listed on The Cochrane Collaboration's training web site (www.cochrane.org/resources/training.htm), along with various training resources, including The Cochrane Collaboration's Open Learning Material. Details of Cochrane Centres can be found on www.cochrane.org.

## 2.3.7 Editorial procedures of a Cochrane Review Group

The editorial team of the CRG is ultimately responsible for the decision to publish a Cochrane review on their module. This decision will be made following peer review and appropriate revisions by the review authors. This may take several iterations.

The editorial team of each CRG is responsible for maintaining a module, which includes information about the Group, including their editorial processes. Any specific methods used by the CRG, beyond the standard methods specified in the *Handbook*, should be documented in their module, including:

- methods used to review protocols;

- standard eligibility criteria for considering studies for inclusion in reviews;

- search methods and specific search strategies used to develop and maintain the Specialized Register used by the CRG, and method of distributing potentially relevant citations or full-text reports to authors;

- additional search methods that authors are instructed to use routinely;

- standard methods used to select studies for reviews and any templates for inclusion assessment forms;

- standard criteria or methods beyond the 'Risk of bias' table used to appraise the included studies; and

- standard methods used for data collection and any templates for data extraction forms.

Descriptions of specific additional methods used by each CRG are published as part of the group's module in *The Cochrane Library*. Authors should familiarize themselves with the contents of their Group's module.

## 2.3.8    Resources for a systematic review

Individual Cochrane reviews are prepared by authors working within CRGs. Each CRG has an editorial team responsible for producing a module of edited reviews for dissemination through the *CDSR* in *The Cochrane Library*.

Because The Cochrane Collaboration is built around CRGs, it is important that each author is linked with one from the beginning of the process. Besides ensuring that Cochrane reviews are carried out appropriately, this structure reduces the burden placed on individual authors since the editorial teams are responsible for providing most or all of the following types of support:

- conducting systematic searches for relevant studies and coordinating the distribution of potentially relevant studies to authors;

- establishing specific standards and procedures for the CRG; and

- ensuring that authors receive the methodological support they need.

The main resource required by authors is their own time. The majority of authors will contribute their time free of charge because it will be viewed as part of their existing efforts to keep up to date in their areas of interest. In some cases, authors may need additional resources or, at least, be able to justify the amount of time required for a systematic review to colleagues who do not yet understand either what systematic reviews entail, or their importance.

The amount of time required will vary, depending on the topic of the review, the number of studies, the methods used (e.g. the extent of efforts to obtain unpublished information), the experience of the authors, and the types of support provided by the editorial team. The workload associated with undertaking a review is thus very variable. However, consideration of the tasks involved and the time required for each of these might help authors to estimate the amount of time that will be required. These tasks include training, meetings, protocol development, searching for studies, assessing citations and full-text reports of studies for eligibility, assessing the risk of bias of included studies, collecting data, pursuing missing data and unpublished studies, analyzing the data, interpreting the results and writing the review, keeping the review up to date.

A time chart with target dates for accomplishing key tasks can help with scheduling the time needed to complete a review. Such targets may vary widely from review to review. Authors, together with the editorial team for the CRG, must determine an appropriate time frame for a specific review. An example of a time chart with target dates can be found in Box 2.3.b.

Resources that might be required for these tasks, in addition to the authors' time, include:

- searching (identifying studies is primarily the responsibility of the editorial team of the CRG; however, authors may share this responsibility and it may be appropriate to search additional databases for a specific review);

- help for library work, interlibrary loans and photocopying;

- a second author, to assess studies for inclusion, assess the 'risk of bias' of included studies, obtain data and check data entry and analyses;

- statistical support for synthesizing (if appropriate) the results of the included studies;

- equipment (e.g. computing hardware and software);

- supplies and services (long distance telephone charges, internet connection, facsimiles, paper, printing, photocopying, audio-visual and computer supplies);

- office space for support staff; and

- travel funds.

---

**Box 2.3.b  Timeline for a Cochrane review**

| Month | Activity |
|---|---|
| 1–2 | Preparation of protocol. |
| 3–8 | Searches for published and unpublished studies. |
| 2–3 | Pilot test of eligibility criteria. |
| 3–8 | Inclusion assessments. |
| 3 | Pilot test of 'Risk of bias' assessment. |
| 3–10 | Validity assessments. |
| 3 | Pilot test of data collection. |
| 3–10 | Data collection. |
| 3–10 | Data entry. |
| 5–11 | Follow up of missing information. |
| 8–10 | Analysis. |
| 1–11 | Preparation of review report. |
| 12– | Keeping the review up to date. |

---

### 2.3.9  Seeking funding

Many organizations currently provide funding for priority systematic reviews. These include research funding agencies, those organizations that provide or fund healthcare services, those responsible for health technology assessment and those involved in the development of clinical practice guidelines.

The Collaboration has a policy that neither the preparation of Cochrane reviews nor infrastructure costs of CRGs can be funded through a commercial source or agency with a vested interest in the review (see Section 2.6).

## 2.4  Publication of Cochrane reviews in print journals and books

Authors may wish to seek co-publication of Cochrane reviews in peer-reviewed health-care journals, particularly in those journals that have expressed enthusiasm for co-publication of Cochrane reviews. For The Cochrane Collaboration, there is one essential condition of co-publication: Cochrane reviews must remain free for dissemination in any and all media, without restriction from any of them. To ensure this, Cochrane authors grant the Collaboration worldwide licences for these activities, and do not sign over exclusive copyright to any journal or other publisher. A journal is free to request a non-exclusive copyright that permits it to publish and re-publish a review, but this cannot restrict the publication of the review by The Cochrane Collaboration in whatever form the Collaboration feels appropriate. To republish material published in the *CDSR* elsewhere, most particularly in print journals, authors must complete a 'permission to publish' form available in the Cochrane Manual (www.cochrane.org/admin/manual.htm), along with an explanation of the procedures to follow.

Authors are strongly discouraged from publishing Cochrane reviews in journals before they are ready for publication in *CDSR*. This applies particularly to Centre directors and editors of CRGs. However, journals will sometimes insist that the publication of the review in *CDSR* should not precede publication in print. When this is the case, authors should submit a review for publication in the journal after agreement from their CRG editor and before publication in *CDSR*. Publication in print should not be subject to lengthy production times, and authors should not unduly delay publication of a Cochrane review either because of delays from a journal or in order to resubmit their review to another journal.

Journals can also request revision of a review for editorial or content reasons. External peer review provided by journals may enhance the value of the review and should be welcomed. Journals generally require shorter reviews than those published in *CDSR*. Selective shortening of reviews may be appropriate, but there should not be any substantive differences between the review as published in the journal and *CDSR*. If a review is published in a journal, it should be noted that a fuller and maintained version of the review is available in *CDSR*. Typically, this should be done by including a statement such as the following in the introduction: 'A more detailed review will be published and updated in the *Cochrane Database of Systematic Reviews*'. The reference should be to the protocol for the review published in *CDSR*. A similar statement should be included in the introduction if a review is published in *CDSR* prior to publishing a version of the review in a journal. After a version of a Cochrane review has been published in a journal, a reference to the journal publication must be added under the heading 'Other published versions of this review'. Authors are also encouraged to add the following statement to versions of Cochrane reviews that are published in journals:

*'This paper is based on a Cochrane review first published [or most recently substantively amended, as appropriate] in The Cochrane Library YYYY, Issue X (see http://www.thecochranelibrary.com/ for information). Cochrane reviews are regularly updated as new evidence emerges and in response to feedback, and The Cochrane Library should be consulted for the most recent version of the review.'*

The following modification of the disclaimer published in *The Cochrane Library* should be added to Cochrane reviews published in journals.

*'The results of a Cochrane review can be interpreted differently, depending on people's perspectives and circumstances. Please consider the conclusions presented carefully. They are the opinions of review authors, and are not necessarily shared by The Cochrane Collaboration.'*

The passage below can be provided to journal editors upon submission of a review for publication, and the letter of submission should be copied to the CRG editorial base for information. This policy and procedure may be new to some journal editors and may require direct discussion with the journal editor. The CRG editorial base should be informed of any problems encountered in this process. The following passage is suggested for inclusion in letters of submission to journal editors:

*'This systematic review has been prepared under the aegis of The Cochrane Collaboration, an international organization that aims to help people make well-informed decisions about healthcare by preparing, maintaining and promoting the accessibility of systematic reviews of the effects of healthcare interventions. The Collaboration's publication policy permits journals to publish reviews, with priority if required, but permits The Cochrane Collaboration also to publish and disseminate such reviews. Cochrane reviews cannot be subject to the exclusive copyright requested by some journals.'*


## 2.5   Publication of previously published reviews as Cochrane reviews

Most reviews that have been conducted by authors outside of The Cochrane Collaboration (referred to as 'previously published reviews' here) require substantial additional work before they can be published as a Cochrane review in *CDSR*. In light of this additional work and substantial differences from the previously published review, the Cochrane review can be considered a new publication. The previously published version of the review must be referenced in the Cochrane review under the heading 'Other published versions of this review'. However, it is generally not necessary to seek permission from the publisher of the previously published review.

Occasionally a Cochrane review will be similar enough to a previously published review that the only change is in the formatting of the review. In these cases authors should obtain permission from the publisher of the previously published review prior to publishing the review in *CDSR*. If authors are in doubt about whether they should request permission, they are encouraged to do so. This is unlikely to present a problem, provided it is done well in advance of the planned submission to *CDSR*. If it is known in advance that there is interest in publishing in *CDSR* a version of a review already published in a journal, authors should not assign exclusive copyright to the journal (see Section 2.4). The Cochrane Collaboration does not require exclusive copyright. It is therefore not a problem to publish a version of a Cochrane review in a journal after it has been published in *CDSR*, provided it is not called a Cochrane review and that it is acknowledged that it is based on a Cochrane review (see Section 2.4).


## 2.6   Declaration of interest and commercial sponsorship

Cochrane reviews should be free of any real or perceived bias introduced by the receipt of any benefit in cash or in kind, any hospitality, or any subsidy derived from any source that may have or be perceived to have an interest in the outcome of the review.

There should be a clear barrier between the production of Cochrane reviews and any funding from commercial sources with financial interests in the conclusions of Cochrane reviews. Thus, sponsorship of a Cochrane review by any commercial source or sources (as defined above) is prohibited. Other sponsorship is allowed, but a sponsor should not be allowed to delay or prevent publication of a Cochrane review and a sponsor should not be able to interfere with the independence of the authors of reviews in regard to the conduct of their reviews. The protocol for a Cochrane review should specifically mention that a sponsor cannot prevent certain outcome measures being assessed in the review.

These rules also apply to 'derivative products' (containing Cochrane reviews) so that commercial sponsors cannot prevent or influence what would be included in such products. Receipt of benefits from any source of sponsored research must be acknowledged and conflicts of interest must be disclosed in *CDSR* and other publications that emanate from the Collaboration.

The Cochrane Collaboration code of conduct for avoiding potential financial conflicts of interest appears in Box 2.6.a. If a proposal for undertaking a review raises a question of serious conflict of interest, this should be forwarded to the Collaboration's funding arbiter (fundingarbiter@cochrane.org) for review. It is not mandatory to send funding proposals to the local Cochrane Centre or Steering Group prior to accepting them. However, this would be desirable in the cases of restricted donations, or any donation that appears to conflict with the general principle noted above.

It is impossible to abolish conflict of interest, since the only person who does not have some vested interest in a subject is somebody who knows nothing about it (Smith 1994). Financial conflicts of interest cause the most concern, can and should be avoided, but must be disclosed if there are any. Any secondary interest (such as personal conflicts) that might unduly influence judgements made in a review (concerning, for example, the inclusion or exclusion of studies, assessments of the risk of bias in included studies or the interpretation of results) should be disclosed. A common example occurs when a review author is also an author of a potentially eligible study. This should be disclosed in the review and, where possible, there should be an independent assessment of eligibility and risk of bias by a second author with no conflict of interest.

Disclosing a conflict of interest does not necessarily reduce the worth of a review and it does not imply dishonesty. However, conflicts of interest can influence judgements in subtle ways. Authors should let the editors of their Cochrane Review Group know of potential conflicts even when they are confident that their judgements were not or will not be influenced. Editors may decide that disclosure is not warranted or they may decide that readers should know about such a conflict of interest so that they can make up their own minds about how important it is. Decisions about whether or not to publish such information should be made jointly by authors and editors.

To help ensure the integrity and perceived integrity of Cochrane reviews, all authors must sign the relevant statements in the form giving The Cochrane Collaboration permission to publish their review in addition to declarations of interest, and the editorial team of each CRG must also disclose any potential conflict of interest that they might have, both on their module and within relevant reviews.

## Box 2.6.a    The Cochrane Collaboration Code of Conduct for Avoiding Potential Financial Conflicts of Interest

### General Principle

The essential activity of The Cochrane Collaboration is co-ordinating the preparation and maintenance of systematic reviews of the effects of healthcare interventions performed by individual authors according to procedures specified by The Cochrane Collaboration. The performance of the review must be free of any real or perceived bias introduced by receipt of any benefit in cash or kind, any hospitality, or any subsidy derived from any source that may have or be perceived to have an interest in the outcome of the review. All entities that constitute The Cochrane Collaboration must accept this General Principle as a condition of participation in the organization.

### Policy

(i) Receipt of benefits from any source of sponsored research must be acknowledged and conflicts of interest must be disclosed in the Cochrane Database of Systematic Reviews and other publications that emanate from The Cochrane Collaboration.

(ii) If an author is involved in a study included in his/her review, this must be acknowledged, as it could be perceived as a potential conflict of interest.

(iii) If a proposal raises a question of serious conflict of interest, this should be forwarded to the local Cochrane Centre for review (and the Steering Group notified accordingly). If the issue involves a Cochrane Centre, the issue should be referred to the Steering Group.

(iv) It is not mandatory to send funding proposals to the local Cochrane Centre or Steering Group prior to accepting them. However, such reviews would be desirable in cases of restricted donations, or any donation that appears to conflict with the General Principle.

(v) The Steering Group should receive (and review at least annually) information about all external funds accepted by Cochrane entities. The Steering Group will use this information to prepare and distribute an annual report on the potential conflicts of interest attendant on The Cochrane Collaboration's solicitation and use of external funds.

(vi) The Steering Group is considering constituting an Ethics Subgroup to view potential conflicts of interest, to offer recommendations for their resolution, and to consider appropriate sanctions to redress violations of the General Principle.

## 2.7 Chapter information

**Editors:** Sally Green and Julian PT Higgins.

**This chapter should be cited as:** Green S, Higgins JPT (editors). Chapter 2: Preparing a Cochrane review. In: Higgins JPT, Green S (editors). *Cochrane Handbook for Systematic Reviews of Interventions*. Chichester (UK): John Wiley & Sons, 2008.

**Contributing authors** (since Mar 2005): Ginny Brunton, Sally Green, Julian Higgins, Monica Kjeldstrøm, Nicki Jackson and Sandy Oliver.

**Acknowledgements:** This section builds on earlier versions of the *Handbook*. For details of previous authors and editors of the *Handbook*, see Chapter 1 (Section 1.4). We thank Chris Cates, Carol Lefebvre, Philippa Middleton, Denise O'Connor and Lesley Stewart for comments on drafts since March 2005.

## 2.8 References

**Bastian 1998**
Bastian H. Speaking up for ourselves: the evolution of consumer advocacy in health care. *International Journal of Technology Assessment in Health Care* 1998; 14: 3–23.

**Effective Public Health Practice Project 2007**
Effective Public Health Practice Project. Effective Public Health Practice Project [Updated 25 October 2007]. Available from: http://www.city.hamilton.on.ca/PHCS/EPHPP (accessed 1 January 2008).

**Hanley 2000**
Hanley B, Bradburn J, Gorin S, Barnes M, Goodare H, Kelson M, Kent A, Oliver S, Wallcraft J. *Involving Consumers in Research and Development in the NHS: Briefing Notes for Researchers*. Winchester (UK): Help for Health Trust, 2000. Available from www.hfht.org/ConsumersinNHSResearch/pdf/involving_consumers_in_rd.pdf.

**Khan 2001**
Khan KS, ter Riet G, Glanville J, Sowden AJ, Kleijnen J (editors). *Undertaking Systematic Reviews of Research on Effectiveness: CRD's Guidance for those Carrying Out or Commissioning Reviews (CRD Report Number 4)* (2nd edition). York (UK): NHS Centre for Reviews and Dissemination, University of York, 2001.

**Light 1984**
Light RJ, Pillemer DB. *Summing Up: The Science of Reviewing Research*. Cambridge (MA): Harvard University Press, 1984.

**Nilsen 2006**
Nilsen ES, Myrhaug HT, Johansen M, Oliver S, Oxman AD. Methods of consumer involvement in developing healthcare policy and research, clinical practice guidelines and patient information material. *Cochrane Database of Systematic Reviews* 2006, Issue 3. Art No: CD004563.

**Rees 2004**

Rees R, Kavanagh J, Burchett H, Shepherd J, Brunton G, Harden A, Thomas S, Oakley A. *HIV Health Promotion and Men who have Sex with Men (MSM): A Systematic Review of Research Relevant to the Development and Implementation of Effective and Appropriate Interventions.* London (UK): EPPI-Centre, Social Science Research Unit, Institute of Education, University of London, 2004.

**Richards 2004**

Richards T. Poor countries lack relevant health information, says Cochrane editor. *BMJ* 2004; 328: 310.

**Smith 1994**

Smith R. Conflict of interest and the BMJ. *BMJ* 1994; 308: 4–5.

**Steel 2001**

Steel R. Involving marginalised and vulnerable groups in research: a discussion document. Consumers in NHS research [2001]. Available from: http://www.invo.org.uk/pdf/Involving_Marginalised_Groups_in_Research.pdf (accessed 1 January 2008).

**Thomas 2004**

Thomas BH, Ciliska D, Dobbins M, Micucci S. A process for systematically reviewing the literature: providing the research evidence for public health nursing interventions. *Worldviews on Evidence-Based Nursing* 2004; 1: 165–184.

# 3 Maintaining reviews: updates, amendments and feedback

## Julian PT Higgins, Sally Green and Rob JPM Scholten

### Key Points

- Systematic reviews that are not maintained may become out of date or misleading.

- The Cochrane Collaboration policy is that Cochrane Intervention reviews should either be updated within two years or include a commentary to explain why this is not the case.

- Any change to a Cochrane review is either an update or an amendment. Updates involve a search for new studies, any other change is an amendment.

- Cochrane reviews have a citation version. This chapter includes a list of criteria for determining when a new citation version is appropriate.

- In addition to a search for new studies, updating a Cochrane review may involve revision of the review question and incorporation of new methods.

- Feedback on Cochrane reviews informs the updating and maintaining process.

- The 'Date review assessed as up to date' is entered by review authors and is published at the beginning of a review. The criteria for assessing a review as up to date are given in this chapter.

## 3.1 Introduction

### 3.1.1 Why maintain a review?

The main aim of a Cochrane review is to provide the 'best available' and most up-to-date evidence on the effects of interventions for use by consumers, clinicians and policy makers to inform healthcare decisions. Since evidence on a given subject is generally dynamic and continually evolving, incorporating additional studies as they become available can change the results of a systematic review (Chalmers 1994). Therefore, systematic reviews that are not maintained run the risk of becoming out of date and even misleading. An important feature of Cochrane reviews is that review authors are committed not only to preparing systematic reviews of evidence, but also to maintaining (and updating) these reviews on a regular basis.

### 3.1.2    How frequently should a review be revisited?

To date, there is little empirical evidence available to allow informed decisions about what is a reasonable and efficient approach to revisiting evidence in Cochrane reviews, although some guidelines do exist (Moher 2007, Shojania 2007a, Shojania 2007b). The Cochrane Collaboration policy is that reviews should either be updated within two years or include a commentary to explain why this is not the case. We define the term 'update' in Section 3.2.2. The two-year period starts from the date on which the review was assessed as being up to date (see Section 3.3.2).

In addition to the potential availability of new evidence, other developments may result in the need to revise a review. For example, within the clinical field, better tools or markers for characterizing sub-groups may have been developed, new treatment regimens may be available, or new outcome measures (or refined measurement methods of existing outcomes) may be in use. Furthermore, advances in the methods for conducting a Cochrane review may produce the need to revisit a review.

While conducting a review, authors may be able to judge if relevant research is being published frequently, and therefore may be able to predict and suggest the need for more frequent updating of the review. Alternatively, in some topic areas new data emerge slowly or are unlikely to emerge, and a review prepared many years earlier is still current and valuable. In these cases updating a review every two years may be unnecessary and wasteful (Chapman 2002). Review authors are advised to discuss with their Cochrane Review Group (CRG) if it is felt that their review does not need to be updated at least every two years. The reason why the review is not being updated in line with the Collaboration policy should be stated in the 'Published notes' section of the review.

## 3.2    Some important definitions

### 3.2.1    Introduction

Here we introduce and explain some important definitions used by The Cochrane Collaboration relevant to maintaining reviews, and their application to the publication of reviews. Section 3.3 deals specifically with the definitions and use of dates in describing events associated with the review. While much of this detailed information is technical, authors will need an understanding of these issues to ensure correct use of terms and dates in their review, and when completing the relevant fields in RevMan.

## 3.2.2 Updates and amendments

Any change to a Cochrane review is either an **update** or an **amendment**.

An **update** *must* involve a search for new studies. If any new studies are found, these must be added to the relevant section of the review as included, excluded or ongoing studies (or 'Studies awaiting classification' if all reasonable efforts to classify it one of these ways have failed) before labelling the revised review as an update (see Section 3.2.5.1).

Any other change to a Cochrane review, and any change to a protocol, is an **amendment**, which could involve a little or a lot of work. These terms, and when to apply them, are described in more detail in Section 3.2.4.

## 3.2.3 Citation versions of Cochrane reviews and protocols

Each publication of a Cochrane review or protocol has a current **citation version**. For *reviews*, citation versions are considered to be major new publications and result in entries in reference databases such as MEDLINE and Science Citation Index (SCI). *Protocols* do not have citations in MEDLINE or SCI. Events triggering the creation of a citation version are listed in Box 3.2.a.

---

**Box 3.2.a Events leading to the creation of a citation version of a Cochrane protocol or review**

1. A protocol is first published.
2. A protocol is re-published after declaring it to be a new citation version.
3. A review is first published (i.e. on conversion from a protocol to a review).
4. A review is re-published (amended or updated) after declaring it to be a new citation version.
5. A review is re-published after it has been withdrawn; or a review is created by splitting an existing protocol or review; or a review is created by merging existing protocols or reviews.

---

Some reviews undergo important changes (updates or amendments) that warrant new citations in the *Cochrane Database of Systematic Reviews* (*CDSR*) and new MEDLINE and SCI records (e.g. changes to conclusions, authors or correcting serious errors).

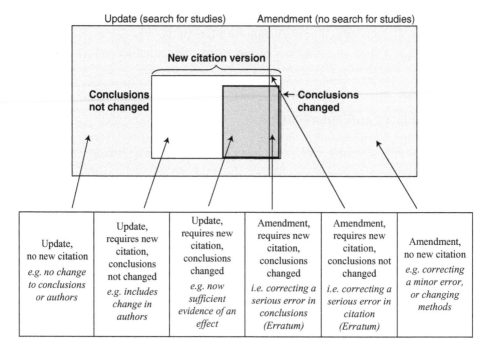

| Update, no new citation e.g. no change to conclusions or authors | Update, requires new citation, conclusions not changed e.g. includes change in authors | Update, requires new citation, conclusions changed e.g. now sufficient evidence of an effect | Amendment, requires new citation, conclusions changed i.e. correcting a serious error in conclusions (Erratum) | Amendment, requires new citation, conclusions not changed i.e. correcting a serious error in citation (Erratum) | Amendment, no new citation e.g. correcting a minor error, or changing methods |
|---|---|---|---|---|---|

**Figure 3.2.a**  Summary of changes to Cochrane reviews

We call these **new citation versions**. In addition, some new citation versions warrant additional highlighting in the *CDSR* (e.g. using a flag) – in particular, those that change their conclusions such that they should be read again. We refer to this special subset of new citation versions as reviews with **conclusions changed.** As all updated reviews are very important, even if they do not meet the criteria for a new citation version, all updated reviews should be highlighted as updated reviews in the *CDSR* (using a 'New search' flag).

Protocols that undergo important changes (e.g. to authors or eligibility criteria) warrant a **new citation version**. Protocols are not listed in databases such as MEDLINE and SCI, so this affects only the citation quoted within *CDSR*. Protocols that change in such a way that they should be re-read by interested users warrant highlighting in the *CDSR* (e.g. using a flag). We call these protocols with a **major change**.

Figure 3.2.a summarizes these various types of changes to a Cochrane review, and Figure 3.2.b the types of changes to a Cochrane protocol.

## 3.2.4   Application of terms to Cochrane protocols

### 3.2.4.1   *Amendments to protocols*

Any modification or edit (including withdrawal) of a published protocol gives the protocol the status of amended. It is not possible to 'update' a protocol. Amended protocols are re-published on the *CDSR*. A protocol may receive an amendment at any

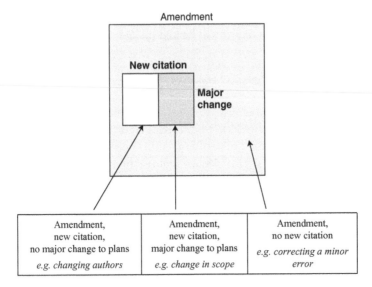

**Figure 3.2.b**    Summary of changes to Cochrane protocols

time. An amendment can involve much or little work, and result in big or small changes to the document.

### 3.2.4.2   New citation versions of protocols

An amended protocol may, at the discretion of the CRG, be published as a new citation version using the criteria in Box 3.2.b. This changes the formal citation of the document within *CDSR*, although citations for protocols are not included in MEDLINE or SCI.

---

**Box 3.2.b   Criteria for a new citation version of a Cochrane protocol**

**Criteria for a new citation version of a protocol: Major change**

A protocol should be classified as a new citation version with major change if there has been an important change to the objectives or scope of the proposed review, usually through a change to the criteria for including studies. Such protocols will be highlighted as 'Major change' in the *CDSR* upon next publication.

**Criteria for a new citation version of a protocol: No major change**

A protocol should be classified as a new citation version with no major change if there has been an important change to the review team. Such protocols will not be highlighted in the *CDSR*.

---

New citation versions of protocols are further classified as having a major change or not. A protocol with a major change will be highlighted on *CDSR*.

### 3.2.4.3   Examples of changes to protocols that do not indicate a new citation version

The following amendments should not typically lead to a protocol being classed as a new citation version, unless the protocol also fulfils one or both of the two criteria in Box 3.2.b. Such changes will result in an amendment to the published protocol, but the existing citation will be maintained.

- Changes to the text of the protocol (e.g. the Background section).

- Changes in planned methodology.

- Changes to the order of existing authors (other than a change in the first author), or deletion of authors.

- Corrections.

## 3.2.5   Application of terms to Cochrane reviews

### 3.2.5.1   Updates of reviews

An update to a Cochrane review is defined as any modification to the published document that includes the findings (including that of no new studies) from a more recent search for additional included studies than the previous published review. The review is said to be have been updated. Updated reviews are highlighted as 'New search' in the CDSR. Any newly identified studies must be incorporated into the updated review (and not left among 'Studies awaiting classification' unless all reasonable efforts have been made to classify it as Included, Excluded or Ongoing). A review is still considered to be updated if a new and thorough search did not identify any additional studies.

This definition draws on a definition for an update of a systematic review as "a discrete event with the aim to search for and identify new evidence to incorporate into a previously completed systematic review" (Moher 2006). An update to a Cochrane review may involve much or little work, depending on the search results, and should in principle be undertaken at least every two years (see Section 3.1.2).

### 3.2.5.2   Amendments to reviews

An amendment to a Cochrane review is any modification or edit (including withdrawal) that does not include an update. The review is then said to have been amended. Examples of amendments include any or all of the following in the absence of a new search for studies: (i) a change in methodology; (ii) the correction of a spelling error; (iii) the re-writing of a Background section; (iv) the full inclusion of a study that was previously 'awaiting classification'; or (v) the changing of conclusions on discovery of a major coding error. A Cochrane review may receive an amendment at any time. An amendment can involve much or little work, and result in big or small changes to the review.

### 3.2.5.3 New citation versions of reviews

A Cochrane review may be re-published as a new citation version. Only an update or an amendment can be given this status. Authors and CRGs jointly decide whether a review should be classified as a new citation version. There are six explicit criteria for classifying a review as a new citation version, and these are described in Box 3.2.c. With three specific exceptions (essential corrections to conclusions, urgent incorporation of new information and essential changes to the citation of the review), only updated reviews are eligible to be new citation versions.

---

**Box 3.2.c   Criteria for a new citation version of a Cochrane review**

**Criteria for a new citation version of a review: Conclusions changed**

1. Change in conclusions on an update
A review must be classified as a new citation version with conclusions changed if the Authors' Conclusions change during an update to the extent that users of the review are recommended to re-read the review.

These conclusions may change as a result of adding (or removing) studies, changes in methodology, or important changes to the scope of the review (for example, new outcomes, comparisons, types of participants or developments in the intervention or its delivery). Changes in conclusions will almost invariably apply to implications for practice regarding the effects of the studied intervention(s). However, sometimes there will be an important change to the implications for research (for example, if newly included data have resolved uncertainties that were highlighted as needing further research in the previous version of the review). All important changes to conclusions in a 'conclusions changed' review must warrant reporting (and be reported) in the abstract of the review.

2. Change in conclusions on correction of a serious error (Erratum)
A review must be classified as a new citation version with conclusions changed if the Authors' Conclusions change upon correction of a serious error to the extent that users of the review are recommended to re-read the review. Such changes are the sort that would warrant a published erratum in a traditional paper journal.

3. Change in conclusions on urgent incorporation of new information about the effects of an intervention

---

A review must be classified as a new citation version with conclusions changed if the Authors' Conclusions change upon urgent incorporation of new information on the effects of an intervention to the extent that users of the review are recommended to re-read the review.

### Criteria for a new citation version of a review: Conclusions not changed

4. New authorship

An updated review may be considered to be a new citation version with conclusions not changed, at the joint discretion of the CRG and the authors, if a substantial amount of new information has been added, or if there have been important changes to the methodology, or if the review has undergone extensive replication or re-writing (not affecting the conclusions), AND there has been an important change to the list of authors for citation (including a change in the first author, but usually not including re-ordering of other authors or deletion of authors), and all authors meet criteria for authorship as outlined in Chapter 4, Section 4.2.2.

The commitment that Cochrane review authors make to maintain their review may require extensive work to update a review, and this may not change the conclusions. Substantial amounts of work by the same review team should not lead to a new citation version if the conclusions do not change (as the review team already has the citation). However, when the review team changes through addition or replacement of authors, the review may be declared to be a new citation version to give appropriate credit to the new authors.

5. Accumulation of changes

An updated review may be considered to be a new citation version with conclusions not changed, at the joint discretion of the CRG and the authors, if the citation version dates from more than five years ago AND the review now looks substantially different from the citation version, irrespective of any changes to the conclusions or authors. A review may look different, for example, due to rewriting, the addition of numerous studies, or due to a substantial modification of the methodology, which has accumulated over time.

Note that every review should include a date on which it was last assessed as being up to date. Therefore this criterion for declaring a review to be a new citation version should be used only for triggering a new citation for the review in reference databases such as MEDLINE and SCI, and not for determining the date on which events or changes occurred.

6. Correction of serious error in citation (Erratum)

A review may be classified as a new citation version with conclusions not changed if a serious error in the citation record needs to be corrected. Such changes (e.g. to spelling of an author's name) are the sort that would warrant a published erratum in a traditional paper journal. An update is not necessary for an erratum. Critical errors that affect conclusions are covered under criterion 2 above.

New citation versions are further classified as 'conclusions changed' or 'conclusions not changed'. Reviews marked as 'conclusions changed' are highlighted in the *CDSR*.

Reviews may be updated or amended between publications of new citation versions, and these updated or amended reviews will be published in the *CDSR* without triggering a new citation. Thus it is critical that the extent to which a review is up to date is reflected in the 'Date review assessed as being up to date' field within the review (see Section 3.3.2).

### 3.2.5.4 *Examples of changes to reviews that do not indicate a new citation version*

The following changes should not typically lead to a review being classed as a new citation version unless the review also fulfils one or more of the six criteria in Box 3.2.c. Such changes will result in either an update or an amendment to the review, but the existing citation will be maintained.

- Addition of new studies.

- Changes in results of analyses (e.g. in effect estimates or confidence intervals), without a change of conclusions.

- Changes to the text of the review (e.g. the Background or Discussion sections).

- Changes in methodology.

- Changes to the order of existing authors (other than a change in the first author), or deletion of authors.

- Corrections.

## 3.3  Important dates associated with Cochrane reviews

### 3.3.1  Introduction

There are several dates associated with a Cochrane review. Some of these are automatically generated by RevMan, and some need to be entered by the review author. These dates are important both to inform readers of the review and to facilitate management of review publication. It is essential that authors apply these definitions when entering dates into relevant fields during an update or amendment to a review.

## 3.3.2    Date review assessed as up to date

Entered by review authors (reviews only, not protocols). On publication, this date is reproduced in a prominent place in the review to inform readers of how recently the review has been assessed as up to date. The criteria for assessing a review as up to date are listed in Box 3.3.a.

---

### Box 3.3.a    Guidance for declaring a review as being up to date

The date a review is assessed as being up to date must be chosen so that the review (new, updated or amended) meets the following key criterion:

1. The evidence is up to date on the effects of the intervention(s)

The list of included studies should include all available evidence, and should result from a most recent search typically being within six months of the date on which the review is assessed as being up to date.

In addition, it is highly desirable, but not mandatory, that:

2. The methods of the review are up to date

All mandatory methods for Cochrane reviews (as described in the current version of the Cochrane Handbook for Systematic Reviews of Interventions) should be incorporated.

3. Factual statements are correct

Factual statements, for example, in the Background and Discussion, should not be unreasonably out-dated.

---

A review might be considered to be up to date even if it has received only minimal edits for many years, for example if a recent search for studies identifies no new evidence since the review was published. All reviews submitted for publication must include a date on which the review was last assessed as being up to date. The date should be entered by the authors, and will often coincide with the date on which the authors submit the review for consideration to be published in the *CDSR*. It may be appropriate to amend the date on approval of the review for publication.

## 3.3.3    Date of search

This date is entered by review authors (for reviews only, not protocols). 'Search' here refers to the searches of all the databases searched for the review. If different databases were searched on different dates, the most recent date of the search for each database should be given within the text of the review and the earliest of the dates should be put in this field. For example, if the most recent searches of the following databases were on the following dates (MEDLINE 5 June 2007, EMBASE 12 June 2007, CRG's Specialized Register 26 June 2007 and CENTRAL 28 June 2007) the 'Date of search' would be 5 June 2007.

### 3.3.4   Date next stage expected

Entered by review authors as:

- for protocols: the date on which the full review is expected; and

- for reviews: the date on which the next update is expected.

### 3.3.5   Date of last edit

This is recorded automatically in RevMan, based on any modification to the review, and will not be published. It will be used to determine the date on which the current published review first appeared exactly as it is.

### 3.3.6   Date declared review no longer needs to be updated

This date applies to very few reviews and should be employed with caution and in consultation with the Cochrane Review Group (CRG). A review that is no longer being updated is one that is highly likely to maintain its current relevance for the foreseeable future (measured in years rather than months). Such reviews are the exception rather than the rule, and the decision to stop updating a review should be negotiated with the CRG, and reviewed periodically. Situations in which a review may be declared to be no longer updated include:

- the intervention is superseded (bearing in mind that Cochrane reviews should be internationally relevant); and

- the conclusion is so certain that the addition of new information will not change it, and there are no foreseeable adverse effects of the intervention.

The review remains 'no longer updated' as long as the most recent 'What's new' entry is a declaration of a 'no longer updated' review. If a subsequent 'What's new' entry is added, the review is considered to be in line for updating as for other Cochrane reviews.

# 3.4    Considerations when updating a Cochrane review

## 3.4.1    Where to start

Few methodological studies have been conducted to inform decisions about how and when to update systematic reviews (Moher 2008), however this is a rapidly evolving area and the guidance contained in this chapter will be regularly updated in line with new knowledge from methodological research. An update to a Cochrane review should usually occur every two years and must involve a search for new studies. If new studies are identified, they must be assessed for inclusion and, if eligible, incorporated into the review. While preparing an update to a review, additional issues may be considered, for example:

1. any need for a change in research question and selection criteria of the review: e.g. addition of a new outcome or comparison, adding a newly specified subgroup analysis following improved methods for categorizing the condition; and

2. change to methodology: e.g. inclusion of 'Risk of bias' assessment of currently-included studies (Chapter 8) or the addition of a 'Summary of findings' table (Chapter 11).

## 3.4.2    Updating a review with an unchanged review question

### 3.4.2.1    Re-executing the search

When there are no changes to the review question and selection criteria, searching for new studies is the first, and defining, step of the updating process. For CRGs with sufficient resources, the periodic identification of potentially relevant studies and forwarding of citations to review authors is an ongoing function of the editorial team (usually the role of the Trials Search Co-ordinator). In other instances, review authors will need to execute the search themselves. At a minimum, strategies to identify new studies for a review update should include re-executing the search strategy, forward from the 'Date of search' of the last update (see Chapter 6, Section 6.4.12).

Where there have been advances in search methods or the authors believe the search strategy from the original review could be improved, the new search will need to be executed for the period from the date of last search, and the additional or modified search terms applied to the search period covered in the original review.

### 3.4.2.2    Updating reviews when no new studies are found

When no new studies meeting the selection criteria are found, the review update will simply require that this finding be recorded in the relevant sections of the review. Revision of the text of the review may be required in the following sections:

1. search methods (to ensure the appropriate 'Date of search' is recorded);

2. description of studies in the Results section (to revise numbers of identified, screened and excluded studies if relevant);

3. results (to ensure any dates are appropriate);

4. authors' conclusions (particularly if there is an ongoing need for further research); and

5. Abstract and Plain Language Summary.

In addition to revision of the text of the review, authors will need to ensure that the relevant date fields are correct and reflect the updated status of the review (see Section 3.3), and the 'What's new' table is completed (see Section 3.5).

In order to alert readers of the review to the fact that they are reading an updated version, a sentence can be added to the Background section of the Abstract stating that this is an update of a Cochrane review (with the earlier version cited) and including the year the review was originally published and the dates of any previous updates. In the Background section of the review itself, this sentence can be expanded to include discussion of the findings of the original review.

Finally, it is important to check that nothing else in the review is out of date (e.g. references to other Cochrane reviews which may have been updated, information about prevalence or incidence of the condition of interest, statements like 'recently, in 1998, it was shown that ...', 'next year, in 2002, there will be ...'). If there are changes or additions to the Acknowledgements and 'Declarations of interest' sections of the review these should be revised.

### 3.4.2.3   Updating reviews when new studies are found

If new, potentially relevant, studies are found, they need to be assessed for inclusion in the review using the same process (and study selection form) as the original review (for information about study selection, see Chapter 5).

If new studies are to be included in the updated review, citations should be entered into RevMan, data collected (see Chapter 7), and risk of bias assessed (see Chapter 8). Data collected from the newly identified and included studies should be entered into RevMan and, if sensible, a (new) meta-analysis performed (Chapter 9). Where possible the methods employed in the review update should mimic those of the original review, unless explicitly altered (for example through developments in systematic review methods such as use of 'Risk of bias' tables or inclusion of 'Summary of findings' tables). In cases where methods differ from those of the original review, these differences and their justification should be documented in the 'Differences between review and protocol' section of the review.

The amount of revision required to the text of an updated review including new studies will depend on the influence of the new data on the results of the review. Examples range from the addition of small studies bringing about no change in the results or conclusions of the review (and so requiring very little revision of the text beyond that described in Section 3.4.2.2) through to increased certainty of pre-existing results and conclusions (requiring some modification of the text) and, in some cases, a change in the conclusion of a review (with the subsequent need for a major rewrite of the Results, Discussion, Conclusion, 'Summary of findings' table, Abstract and Plain Language Summary). In addition, the statements in the Abstract and Background sections of the review alerting readers to the fact that this is an update of an earlier review (see Section 3.4.2.2) should be included.

Authors will need to ensure that the relevant date fields are correct and reflect the updated status of the review (see Section 3.3.2), and the 'What's new' table is completed (see Section 3.5). Finally, authors should check that nothing else in the review is out of date (e.g. references to other Cochrane reviews which may have been updated, information about prevalence or incidence of the condition of interest, statements like 'recently, in 1998, it was shown that ... ', 'next year, in 2002, there will be ... '). If there are changes or additions to the Acknowledgements and 'Declarations of interest' sections of the review these should be revised.

### 3.4.3    Revising review questions and selection criteria

There may be occasions when, in addition to re-executing the search, an update to a review also involves a change to the review question, the study selection criteria, or both. For example, evolving technology may lead to the inclusion of a new comparison; or a category of patients (e.g. children in addition to adults) or an important outcome (e.g. adverse effects) may not have been adequately addressed in the original review. If this is the case, the proposed changes and additions to the original protocol should be documented and justified in the 'Differences between protocol and review' section, explained in the text of the review (Background, Objectives and Methods sections) and highlighted in the 'What's new' table.

In addition, the search methods may need to be altered and re-executed to cover not only the period since the 'Date of search' of the previous version of the review, but also the period covered by the original review with the addition of new search terms relevant to any additional selection criteria. In some cases it may be sufficient to go back to the original search results and apply the updated selection criteria for inclusion of studies.

If a new comparison or a new outcome has been added to the review, it will be necessary to go back to the original included studies and check that they did not include any information relevant to this new outcome or comparison. The original data collection forms may need to be altered or extended, and piloted again, and new comparisons or outcomes may have to be added to the analyses.

Finally, the addition of new comparisons, populations or outcomes will result in the need for alteration of the text of the review (Background, Methods) and, if additional studies are identified and included, also to the Results, Conclusions, Plain Language Summary and 'Summary of findings' table.

### 3.4.4    Splitting reviews

In some instances, a review may become too large and it may be desirable to split the review into two or more new reviews. Splitting reviews into more narrowly defined review topics, with potentially fewer studies, may ease updating and allow for sharing of the updating burden between several review teams.

Splitting a review implies creating at least one new citation version of a review, and the formal link with previous versions of the review may be lost. Splitting a review sometimes involves withdrawing the original review. A decision to split a review should not be made lightly and always in consultation with the CRG's editorial board.

Cochrane Overviews of reviews (see Chapter 22) may facilitate the splitting of reviews, with the possibility of several more narrowly defined reviews (for example of single interventions for a particular condition) being combined in an Overview of all interventions for that particular healthcare condition.

### 3.4.5  Amending the methodology of a review

In addition to searching for new studies and revising the review question or study selection criteria, maintenance of a review may include amendment of the methodology of the review (Shea 2006). Methodological advances in systematic review conduct since publication of the original review may result in a need to revise or extend the methods of a review during an update. Review authors may decide to include a new analysis strategy in their updated review (for example, using statistical methods not previously available in RevMan). The introduction of 'Risk of bias' (Chapter 8) and 'Summary of findings' (Chapter 11) tables with RevMan 5, while not mandatory, provides the opportunity for reviews to be updated to include these new methods. Where a 'Risk of bias' table is to be added to a review, authors should decide whether to revisit the critical appraisal of studies included in previous versions of the review, updating all assessments of risk of bias, or whether to apply these new methods only to studies added in the update. In the published version of the review, a 'Risk of bias' table should be generated including only those studies where data are entered (i.e. without blank rows).

As part of a review update, authors may wish to include a 'Summary of findings' table (Chapter 11). Outcomes selected for presentation in the 'Summary of findings' table should be those of importance to people making decisions about health care (usually the primary outcomes of the review), and should be selected prior to commencement of the update to reduce the risk of selectively reporting outcomes with significant results rather than those of importance.

Changes to methodology may imply changes to the original protocol of the review. These changes, and their justifications, must be explicitly provided in the 'Differences between protocol and review' section and the 'What's new' table.

### 3.4.6  Other changes to the review

If there is a change in lead author, new authors have joined the team, or a new review team has updated the review, the by-line (list of authors) may need to be changed. The decision regarding who is named in the by-line of an updated review, and in what order, should relate to the historical contributions to the updated review coupled with approval of the final updated document. If an author is no longer able to approve an updated review, this author should not be listed in the by-line, but be mentioned in the Acknowledgements. The contributions of all authors to both the update and earlier versions of the review should be described in the 'Contributions of authors' section.

Changing authors of a review may have implications for awarding the review a new citation version (see Section 3.2.5.3).

### 3.4.7 Editorial process

After completion of the updating process, the review should be submitted to the editorial team for further processing. There is variation across CRGs in policies regarding when and if updated reviews go through the process of full editorial review. If an update involves no further analysis or change of result, it may not need to be refereed, however if there are new analyses, inclusion of new methods or changes to conclusion, the same pre-publication process as that of the original review is likely to be repeated.

On rare occasions a review needs to be withdrawn from the *CDSR*. This may be temporary (e.g. because the review is severely out of date, or contains a major error) or permanent (e.g. because the review has been split into a series of smaller reviews). The withdrawal of the review should be noted in the 'Published notes' section of the review. The review containing this withdrawal notice should be submitted for publication in each issue of the *CDSR*. If the withdrawal is temporary, the review may be re-instated when the content is judged to be satisfactory by the review authors and their CRG. If a review is withdrawn because its content has been merged with another review, a notice should be included in the 'Published notes' section to explain that it has been withdrawn for this reason.

## 3.5 'What's new' and History tables

### 3.5.1 'What's new' events

All updated and amended reviews and protocols should have a completed 'What's new' table, so that readers can quickly and clearly identify what has changed. The events added to the 'What's new' table determine what status the protocol or review has in the *CDSR* including the use of flags or other devices to highlight them, and the assigning of a new citation version.

### 3.5.2 Completing the 'What's new' table

Each row in a 'What's new' or History table comprises:

• the date on which the event was undertaken or recorded;

**Table 3.5.a**    Available 'What's new' events for protocols

| Type of event | Definition or discussion | Implication for published protocol |
|---|---|---|
| Amended. | See 3.2.2 and 3.2.4.1. | None. |
| Feedback incorporated. | See 3.6. | Protocol highlighted as 'Comment'. |
| New citation: no major change. | See 3.2.4.2. | New citation. |
| New citation: major change. | See 3.2.4.2. | New citation. Protocol highlighted as 'Major change'. |

**Table 3.5.b**    Available 'What's new' events for reviews

| Type of event | Definition or discussion | Implication for published review |
|---|---|---|
| Amended. | See 3.2.2 and 3.2.5.2. | None. |
| Updated. | See 3.2.2 and 3.2.5.1. | Review highlighted as 'New search'. |
| Feedback incorporated. | See 3.6. | Review highlighted as 'Comment'. |
| New citation: conclusions not changed. | See 3.2.3 and 3.2.5.3. | New citation (e.g. MEDLINE record); re-sets impact factor counter. |
| New citation: conclusions changed. | See 3.2.3 and 3.2.5.3. | Review highlighted as 'Conclusions changed'. New citation (e.g. MEDLINE record); re-sets impact factor counter. |
| No longer updated. | See 3.3.6. | None. |

- the type of event; and

- a brief description of what changes were made.

Table 3.5.a and Table 3.5.b list the available 'What's new' events for protocols and reviews, respectively. Authors should refer to the referenced section to select the appropriate event for inclusion in the 'What's new' table. Withdrawal of a review should be associated with an 'Amended' event.

While it is technically possible to enter several events into the 'What's new' table, authors should be aware that the table should include information only about the changes since the last version. Importantly the table must not have more than one new citation entry or more than one update entry (previous events should be moved to the History table).

## 3.5.3  History table

Entries in the 'What's new' table should be moved to the History table when they no longer apply to the latest version of the protocol or review. In addition, the History table will include the following information, which should be completed automatically by the Collaboration's information management system:

- year and issue protocol first published;
- year and issue review first published; and
- year and issue of each new citation version.

## 3.6 Incorporating and addressing feedback in a Cochrane review

There is a formal mechanism on *The Cochrane Library* to facilitate and manage feedback from users of reviews. Feedback, formerly called Comments and Criticisms, is designed to "... amend reviews in the light of new evidence... to reflect the emergence of new data, valid feedback, solicited or unsolicited, from whatever source" (Chalmers 1994).

Feedback on a review can be received at any time after publication and will be sent to the Feedback editor of the responsible CRG. This editor will ensure that the feedback and language is appropriate and then will pass it on to review authors for response (usually required within one month of sending). When responding to feedback, authors are asked to:

- confine the response to the points made in the feedback;

- reply to every substantive point, explicitly stating whether the author agrees or disagrees with the feedback and providing supporting evidence where necessary;

- describe any changes made to the review in response to the feedback; and

- reply in clear and plain language.

Updating a review provides the opportunity to incorporate feedback into the review, addressing valid concerns and adding any additional studies identified through the feedback mechanism.

## 3.7 Chapter information

**Authors:** Julian PT Higgins, Sally Green and Rob JPM Scholten.

**This chapter should be cited as:** Higgins JPT, Green S, Scholten RJPM. Chapter 3: Maintaining reviews: updates, amendments and feedback. In: Higgins JPT, Green

S (editors). *Cochrane Handbook for Systematic Reviews of Interventions.* Chichester (UK): John Wiley & Sons, 2008.

**Acknowledgements:** The Cochrane Collaboration Updating Working Group (members Mike Clarke, Mark Davies, Davina Ghersi, Sally Green, Sonja Henderson, Harriet MacLehose, Jessie McGowan, David Moher, Rob Scholten (convenor) and Phil Wiffen) provided comments on drafts.

# 3.8 References

**Chalmers 1994**
Chalmers I, Haynes B. Reporting, updating, and correcting systematic reviews of the effects of health care. *BMJ* 1994; 309: 862–865.

**Chapman 2002**
Chapman A, Middleton P, Maddern G. Early updates of systematic reviews – a waster of resources? *Pushing the Boundaries: Fourth Symposium on Systematic Reviews*, Oxford, 2002.

**Moher 2006**
Moher D, Tsertsvadze A. Systematic reviews: when is an update an update? *The Lancet* 2006; 367: 881–883.

**Moher 2007**
Moher D, Tsertsvadze A, Tricco AC, Eccles M, Grimshaw J, Sampson M, Barrowman N. A systematic review identified few methods and strategies describing when and how to update systematic reviews. *Journal of Clinical Epidemiology* 2007; 60: 1095–1104.

**Moher 2008**
Moher D, Tsertsvadze A, Tricco AC, Eccles M, Grimshaw J, Sampson M, Barrowman N. When and how to update systematic reviews. *Cochrane Database of Systematic Reviews* 2008, Issue 1. Art No: MR000023.

**Shea 2006**
Shea B, Boers M, Grimshaw JM, Hamel C, Bouter LM. Does updating improve the methodological and reporting quality of systematic reviews? *BMC Medical Research Methodology* 2006; 6: 27.

**Shojania 2007a**
Shojania KG, Sampson M, Ansari MT, Ji J, Doucette S, Moher D. How quickly do systematic reviews go out of date? A survival analysis. *Annals of Internal Medicine* 2007; 147: 224–233.

**Shojania 2007b**
Shojania KG, Sampson M, Ansari MT, Ji J, Garritty C, Rader T, Moher D. *Updating Systematic Reviews. Technical Review No 16 (Prepared by the University of Ottawa Evidence-based Practice Center under Contract No 290-02-0017).* Rockville (MD): Agency for Healthcare Research and Quality, 2007.

# 4 Guide to the contents of a Cochrane protocol and review

**Edited by Julian PT Higgins and Sally Green**

## Key Points

- Cochrane reviews have a highly structured format, and compliance with this format is facilitated by the use of RevMan. This chapter describes what an author is expected to include, and what a reader may expect to find, in each component of a Cochrane protocol or review.

- The chapter also serves as a guide to much of the *Handbook*, containing links to other chapters where further discussion of the methodological issues can be found.

- A 'Review information' (or 'Protocol information') section includes details of authors and important dates associated with maintaining and updating the review.

- The main text should be succinct and readable, so that someone who is not an expert in the area can understand it. The text of a protocol ends after the Methods section.

- A 'Studies and references' section provides a framework for classifying included, excluded and ongoing studies, as well as those for which insufficient information is available, and other references.

- Tables of characteristics of studies allow the systematic presentation of key descriptors of the studies considered for the review.

- A 'Data and analyses' section has a hierarchical structure, allowing data from included studies to be placed within particular subgroups of studies, which are in turn within meta-analyses of particular outcomes, which are in turn within particular intervention comparisons. For each meta-analysis, forest plots and funnel plots can be generated within RevMan.

- Further tables, figures and appendices can be included to supplement the inbuilt tables.

## 4.1    Introduction

Cochrane Intervention reviews all have the same format, and the preparation of a review with the required format is facilitated by the use of Review Manager (RevMan) software. In this chapter we discuss the content of the entire review (or protocol) and outline what should appear in each section. Extensive references to other chapters in the *Handbook* are included to signpost advice relevant to each section. Guidance on *using* the RevMan software itself is available in the help system within the software.

## 4.2    Title and review information (or protocol information)

### 4.2.1    Title

The title succinctly states the intervention(s) reviewed and the problem at which the intervention is directed. Explicit guidance for structuring titles of Cochrane reviews is provided in Table 4.2.a.

### 4.2.2    Authors

Authorship of all scientific papers (including Cochrane protocols and reviews) establishes accountability, responsibility and credit (Rennie 1997, Flanagin 1998, Rennie 1998). When deciding who should appear in the by-line of a Cochrane review, it is important to distinguish individuals who have made a substantial contribution to the review (and who should be listed) and those who have helped in other ways, which should be noted in the Acknowledgements section. Authorship should be based on substantial contributions to all of the following three steps, based on the 'Uniform requirements for manuscripts submitted to biomedical journals' (International Committee of Medical Journal Editors 2006). Authors must sign a 'License for Publication' form that affirms the following three contributions.

- Conception and design of study, or analysis and interpretation of data.
- Drafting the review or commenting on it critically for intellectual content.
- Final approval of the document to be published.

**Table 4.2.a**  Structure for Cochrane review titles

| Scenario | Structure | Example |
|---|---|---|
| Basic structure. | [Intervention] for [health problem]. | Antibiotics for acute bronchitis. |
| Comparing two active interventions. | [Intervention A] versus [intervention B] for [health problem]. | Immediate versus delayed treatment for cervical intraepithelial neoplasia. |
| Type of people being studied or location of intervention mentioned explicitly. | [Intervention] for [health problem] in [participant group/location]. | Inhaled nitric oxide for respiratory failure in preterm infants. |
| Not specifying a particular 'health problem' (e.g. 'Home versus hospital birth'), or if the intervention intends to influence a variety of problems (e.g. 'Prophylactic synthetic surfactant in preterm infants'). | [Intervention] in OR for [participant group/location]. | Restricted versus liberal water intake in preterm infants. |
| Sometimes it is necessary to specify that the intervention is for preventing, treating, or preventing and treating the health problem(s): If necessary, the word 'for' is followed by 'preventing', 'treating', or 'preventing and treating'. This is better than using 'for the prevention of' etc. | | Pool fencing for preventing drowning in children; Amodiaquine for treating malaria; Vitamin C for preventing and treating the common cold. |

The specific contributions should be listed under the section 'Contributions of authors' (see below). The list of authors can be the name of an individual, several individuals, a collaborative group (for example, 'Advanced Bladder Cancer Overview Collaboration') or a combination of one or more authors and a collaborative group. Ideally, the order of authors should relate to their relative contributions to the review. The person who contributed most should be listed first.

## 4.2.3  Contact person

Contact details should be provided for the person to whom correspondence about the review should be addressed, and who has agreed to take responsibility for maintaining and developing the review. Most usually, this person would (i) be responsible for developing and organizing the review team; (ii) communicate with the editorial base; (iii) ensure that the review is prepared within agreed timescales; (iv) submit the review to the editorial base; (v) communicate feedback to co-authors; and (vi) ensure that the updates are prepared.

The contact person need not be the first listed author, and the choice of contact person will not affect the citation for the review. If an existing contact person no longer wishes to be responsible for a published review and another member of the review team does not wish to take responsibility for it, then contact details for the Review Group Co-ordinator (RGC) should be listed here. The contact person for a review need not be listed as an author.

### 4.2.4   Dates

#### 4.2.4.1   *Assessed as up to date*

The date on which the review was last assessed as being up to date will often coincide with the date on which the authors submit the review for consideration to be published in the *Cochrane Database of Systematic Reviews* (*CDSR*). Specific criteria for describing a review as up to date appear in Chapter 3 (Section 3.2).

#### 4.2.4.2   *Date of search*

This date is used to help determine whether a review has been updated, and to inform the date on which the review is assessed as being up to date. It will not be published in the *CDSR*. Specific criteria for specifying the date of search appear in Chapter 3 (Section 3.3.3). Search methods are discussed in detail in Chapter 6 (Section 6.3).

#### 4.2.4.3   *Next stage expected*

A date for internal use only (it will not be published in the *CDSR*) indicating when the completed review (for protocols) or the next review update (for reviews) is due. Policies for updating reviews are described in Chapter 3 (Section 3.1).

#### 4.2.4.4   *Protocol first published*

The issue of the *CDSR* in which the protocol was first published (for example, Issue 2, 2004). The date cannot be edited in RevMan.

#### 4.2.4.5   *Review first published*

The issue of the *CDSR* in which the full review was first published (for example, Issue 1, 2005). The date cannot be edited in RevMan.

#### *4.2.4.6   Last citation issue*

The issue of the *CDSR* in which the current citation version of the review was first published (for example, Issue 1, 2007). The date cannot be edited in RevMan. Citation versions are discussed in detail in Chapter 3 (Section 3.2)

### 4.2.5   What's new and History

The 'What's new' section should describe the changes to the protocol or review since it was last published in the *CDSR*. At each update or amendment of a review, at least one 'What's new' event should be recorded, containing the type of event, the date of the change and a description of what was changed. This description might be, for example, a brief summary of how much new information has been added to the review (for example, number of studies, participants or extra analyses) and any important changes to the conclusions, results or methods of the review. Entries from the 'What's new' table that do not relate to the current citation version of the review should be listed in the 'History' table. 'What's new' table events are discussed in detail in Chapter 3 (Section 3.5).

## 4.3   Abstract

All full reviews must include an abstract of 400 words or fewer. The abstract should be brief without sacrificing important content. Abstracts to Cochrane reviews are published in MEDLINE and the Science Citation Index, and are made freely available on the internet. It is therefore important that they can be read as stand-alone documents. Guidance for the content of an abstract is provided in Chapter 11 (Section 11.8).

## 4.4   Plain language summary

The plain language summary (formerly called the 'synopsis') aims to summarize the review in a straightforward style that can be understood by consumers of health care. Plain language summaries are made freely available on the internet, so will often be read as stand-alone documents. Plain language summaries have two parts: a plain language title (a restatement of the review's title using plain language terms) and a summary text of not more than 400 words. Guidance for the content of a plain language summary is provided in Chapter 11 (Section 11.9).

## 4.5   Main text

The text of the review should be succinct and readable. Although there is no formal word limit for Cochrane reviews, review authors should consider 10,000 words an absolute maximum unless there is special reason to write a longer review. Most reviews should be substantially shorter than this. A review should be written so that someone who is not an expert in the area can understand it, in light of the following policy statement, stated in the Cochrane Manual (www.cochrane.org/admin/manual.htm):

> "The target audience for Cochrane reviews is people making decisions about health care. This includes healthcare professionals, consumers and policy makers with a basic understanding of the underlying disease or problem.
>
> It is a part of the mission and a basic principle of The Cochrane Collaboration to promote the accessibility of systematic reviews of the effects of healthcare interventions to anyone wanting to make a decision about health care. However, this does not mean that Cochrane reviews must be understandable to anyone, regardless of their background. This is not possible, any more than it would be possible for Cochrane reviews to be written in a single language that is understandable to everyone in the world.
>
> Cochrane reviews should be written so that they are easy to read and understand by someone with a basic sense of the topic who may not necessarily be an expert in the area. Some explanation of terms and concepts is likely to be helpful, and perhaps even essential. However, too much explanation can detract from the readability of a review. Simplicity and clarity are also vital to readability. The readability of Cochrane reviews should be comparable to that of a well written article in a general medical journal."

The text of a Cochrane review contains a number of fixed headings and subheadings that are embedded in RevMan. Additional subheadings may be added by the author at any point. Certain specific subheadings are **recommended** for use by all authors (and can be activated or deactivated in RevMan). However, these are not mandatory and should be avoided if they make individual sections needlessly short. Further, **optional** subheadings that may or may not be relevant to a particular review are also discussed below. Review authors who wish to mix recommended with optional subheadings should ensure that they are all displayed in appropriately consistent styles, which may require deactivating all of the recommended headings embedded in RevMan and creating them manually.

The following fixed headings are followed by fixed subheadings and can have no free text immediately after them: 'Methods', 'Criteria for including studies', 'Results', and 'Authors' conclusions'.

# Background

Well-formulated review questions occur in the context of an already-formed body of knowledge. The background should address this context, help set the rationale for the review, and explain why the questions being asked are important. It should be concise (generally around one page when printed) and be understandable to the users of the intervention under investigation. All sources of information should be cited.

## Description of the condition

The review should begin with a brief description of the condition being addressed and its significance. It may include information about the biology, diagnosis, prognosis and public health importance (including prevalence or incidence).

## Description of the intervention

A description of the experimental intervention(s) should place it in the context of any standard, or alternative interventions. The role of the comparator intervention(s) in standard practice should be made clear. For drugs, basic information on clinical pharmacology should be presented where available. This information might include dose range, metabolism, selective effects, half-life, duration and any known interactions with other drugs. For more complex interventions, a description of the main components should be provided.

## How the intervention might work

This section might describe the theoretical reasoning why the interventions under review may have an impact on potential recipients, for example, by relating a drug intervention to the biology of the condition. Authors may refer to a body of empirical evidence such as similar interventions having an impact or identical interventions having an impact on other populations. Authors may also refer to a body of literature that justifies the possibility of effectiveness.

## Why it is important to do this review

The background should clearly state the rationale for the review and should explain why the questions being asked are important. It might also mention why this review was undertaken and how it might relate to a wider review of a general problem. If this version of the review is an update of an earlier one, it is helpful to state this by writing, for example, "This is an update of a Cochrane review first published in YEAR, and previously updated in YEAR". This may be supplemented with a brief description of the main findings of the earlier versions, with a statement of any specific reasons there may be for updating the review.

# Objectives

This should begin with a precise statement of the primary objective of the review, ideally in a single sentence. Where possible the style should be of the form "To assess the effects of *[intervention or comparison]* for*[health problem]* for/in*[types of people, disease or* *problem and setting if specified]*". This might be followed by a series of specific ob-jectives relating to different participant groups, different comparisons of interventions or different outcome measures. It is not necessary to state specific hypotheses.

# Methods

The Methods section in a protocol should be written in the future tense. Because Cochrane reviews are updated as new evidence accumulates, methods outlined in the protocol should generally be written as if a suitably large number of studies will be identified to allow the objectives to be met (even if it is known this is not the case at the time of writing).

The Methods section in a review should be written in the past tense, and should describe what was done to obtain the *results and conclusions of the current review*. Review authors are encouraged to cite their protocol to make it clear that there was one. Often a review is unable to implement all of the methods outlined in the protocol, usually because there is insufficient evidence. In such circumstances, it is recommended that the methods that were not implemented be outlined in the section headed 'Differences between protocol and review' (see below), so that it serves as a protocol for future updates of the review.

## Criteria for considering studies for this review

### Types of studies

Eligible study designs should be stated here, along with any thresholds for inclusion based on the conduct of the studies or their risk of bias. For example, 'All randomized controlled comparisons' or 'All randomized controlled trials with blind assessment of outcome'. Exclusion of particular types of randomized studies (for example, cross-over trials) should be justified. Eligibility criteria for types of study designs are discussed in Chapter 5 (Section 5.5).

### Types of participants

The diseases or conditions of interest should be described here, including any restric-tions such as diagnoses, age groups and settings. Subgroup analyses should not be listed here (see 'Subgroup analysis and investigation of heterogeneity' under 'Methods'). El-igibility criteria for types of participants are discussed in Chapter 5 (Section 5.2).

### Types of interventions

Experimental and comparator interventions should be defined here, under separate subheadings if appropriate. It should be made clear which comparisons are of interest.

Restrictions on dose, frequency, intensity or duration should be stated. Subgroup analyses should not be listed here (see 'Subgroup analysis and investigation of heterogeneity' under 'Methods'). Eligibility criteria for types of interventions are discussed in Chapter 5 (Section 5.3).

### *Types of outcome measures*

Note that outcome measures do not always form part of the criteria for including studies in a review. If they do not, then this should be made clear. Outcome measures of interest should be listed in this section whether or not they form part of the eligibility criteria. Types of outcomes are discussed in Chapter 5 (Section 5.4). The importance of addressing patient-relevant outcomes is discussed further in Chapter 11 (Section 11.5.2); see also an extended discussion of patient-reported outcomes in Chapter 17.

***Primary outcomes*** The review's primary outcomes should normally reflect at least one potential benefit and at least one potential area of harm, and should be as few as possible. It is normally expected that the review should be able to analyse these outcomes if eligible studies are identified, and that the conclusions of the review will be based in large part on the effects of the interventions on these outcomes.

***Secondary outcomes*** Non-primary outcomes should be listed here. The total number of outcomes addressed should be kept as small as possible.

The following *optional* (level 4) headings may be helpful, as supplements or replacements for the headings above:

### *Main outcomes for 'Summary of findings' table*

### *Timing of outcome assessment*

### *Adverse outcomes*

### *Economic data*

## Search methods for identification of studies

The methods used to identify studies should be summarized. The following headings are recommended. Before starting to develop this section, authors should contact their Cochrane Review Group (CRG) for guidance. Search methods are discussed in detail in Chapter 6 (Sections 6.3).

*Electronic searches*

The bibliographic databases searched, the dates and periods searched and any constraints such as language should be stated. The full search strategies for each database should be listed in an appendix to the review. If a CRG has developed a specialized register of studies and this is searched for the review, a standard description of this register can be referred to but information should be included on when and how the specialized register was most recently searched for the current version of the review and the search terms used should be listed. Search strategies are discussed in detail in Chapter 6 (Section 6.4).

*Searching other resources*

List grey literature sources, such as internal reports and conference proceedings. If journals are specifically handsearched for the review, this should be noted but handsearching done by the authors to help build the specialized register of the CRG should not be listed because this is covered in the standardized description of the register. List people (e.g. trialists or topic specialists) and organizations who were contacted. List any other sources used, which may include, for example, reference lists, the World Wide Web or personal collections of articles.

The following *optional* headings may be used, either in place of 'Searching other resources' (in which case they would be level 3 headings) or as subheadings (level 4).

*Grey literature*

*Handsearching*

*Reference lists*

*Correspondence*

Other search resources are discussed in Chapter 6 (Section 6.2).

## Data collection and analysis

This should describe the methods for data collection and analysis.

*Selection of studies*

The method used to apply the selection criteria. Whether they are applied independently by more than one author should be stated, along with how any disagreements are resolved. Study selection is discussed in Chapter 7 (Section 7.2).

### *Data extraction and management*

The method used to extract or obtain data from published reports or from the original researchers (for example, using a data collection form). Whether data are extracted independently by more than one author should be stated, along with how any disagreements are resolved. If relevant, methods for processing data in preparation for analysis should be described. Data collection is discussed in Chapter 7, including which data to collect (Section 7.3), sources of data (Section 7.4), data collection forms (Section 7.5) and extracting data from reports (Section 7.6)

### *Assessment of risk of bias in included studies*

The method used to assess risk of bias (or methodological quality). Whether methods are applied independently by more than one author should be stated, along with how any disagreements are resolved. The tool(s) used should be described or referenced, with an indication of how the results are incorporated into the interpretation of the results. The recommended tool for assessing risk of bias is described in Chapter 8 (Section 8.5).

### *Measures of treatment effect*

The effect measures of choice should be stated. For example, odds ratio (OR), risk ratio (RR) or risk difference (RD) for dichotomous data; mean difference (MD) or standardized mean difference (SMD) for continuous data. The following *optional* headings may be used, either in place of 'Measures of treatment effect' (in which case they would be level 3 headings) or as subheadings (level 4):

#### *Dichotomous data*

#### *Continuous data*

#### *Time-to-event data*

Types of data and effect measures are discussed in Chapter 9 (Section 9.2).

### *Unit of analysis issues*

Special issues in the analysis of studies with non-standard designs, such as cross-over trials and cluster-randomized trials, should be described. Alternatively, *optional* (level 3) headings specific to the types of studies may be used, such as:

#### *Cluster-randomised trials*

#### *Cross-over trials*

### Studies with multiple treatment groups

Unit of analysis issues are discussed in Chapter 9 (Section 9.3). Some non-standard designs are discussed in detail in Chapter 16, including cluster-randomized trials (Section 16.3), cross-over trials (Section 16.4), and studies with multiple intervention groups (Section 16.5). Non-randomized studies are discussed in Chapter 13.

### Dealing with missing data

Strategies for dealing with missing data should be described. This will principally include missing participants due to drop-out (and whether an intention-to-treat analysis will be conducted), and missing statistics (such as standard deviations or correlation coefficients). Issues relevant to missing data are discussed in Chapter 16 (Sections 16.1) and intention-to-treat issues in Chapter 16 (Section 16.2).

### Assessment of heterogeneity

Approaches to addressing clinical heterogeneity should be described, along with how the authors will determine whether a meta-analysis is considered appropriate. Methods for identifying statistical heterogeneity should be stated (e.g. visually, using $I^2$, using a chi-squared test). Assessment of heterogeneity is discussed in Chapter 9 (Section 9.5).

### Assessment of reporting biases

This section should describe how publication bias and other reporting biases are addressed (for example, funnel plots, statistical tests, imputation). Authors should remember that asymmetric funnel plots are not necessarily caused by publication bias (and that publication bias does not necessarily cause asymmetry in a funnel plot). Reporting biases are discussed in Chapter 10.

### Data synthesis

The choice of meta-analysis method should be stated, including whether a fixed-effect or a random-effects model is used. If meta-analyses are not undertaken, systematic approaches to synthesizing the findings of multiple studies should be described. Meta-analysis and data synthesis are discussed in Chapter 9 (Section 9.4).

### Subgroup analysis and investigation of heterogeneity

All planned subgroup analyses should be listed (or independent variables for meta-regression). Any other methods for investigating heterogeneity of effects should be described. Investigating heterogeneity is discussed in Chapter 9 (Section 9.6).

*Sensitivity analysis*

This should describe analyses aimed at determining whether conclusions are robust to decisions made during the review process, such as inclusion/exclusion of particular studies from a meta-analysis, imputing missing data or choice of a method for analysis. Sensitivity analysis is discussed in Chapter 9 (Section 9.7).

The following further, *optional* (level 3) headings for the Methods section may be helpful:

*Economics issues*

*Methods for future updates*

Authors seeking to cover economics aspects of interventions in a review will need to consider economics issues from the earliest stages of developing a protocol. Economics issues are discussed in Chapter 15. Issues in updating reviews are discussed in Chapter 3.

# Results

## Description of studies

*Results of the search*

The results sections should start with a summary of the results of the search (for example, how many references were retrieved by the electronic searches, and how many were considered as potentially eligible after screening). Presentation of search findings is discussed in Chapter 6 (Section 6.6).

*Included studies*

It is essential that the number of included studies is clearly stated. This section should comprise a succinct summary of the information contained in the 'Characteristics of included studies' table. An explicit reference to this table should be included. Key characteristics of the included studies should be described, including the study participants, location (e.g. country), setting (if important), interventions, comparisons and outcome measures in the included studies and any important differences among the studies. The sex and age range of participants should be stated here except where their nature is obvious (for example, if all the participants are pregnant). Important details of specific interventions used should be provided (for radiotherapy, for example, this might summarize the total dose, the number of fractions and type of radiation used; for drugs, this might summarize preparation, route of administration, dose and frequency). Authors should note any other characteristics of the studies that they regard as important for readers of the review to know. The following *optional* (level 4) subheadings may be helpful:

*Design*

*Sample sizes*

*Setting*

*Participants*

*Interventions*

*Outcomes*

The 'Characteristics of included studies' table is discussed in detail in Section 4.6.1.

### Excluded studies

This should refer to the information contained in the 'Characteristics of excluded studies' table. An explicit reference to this table should be included. A succinct summary of why studies were excluded from the review should be provided. The 'Characteristics of excluded studies' table is discussed in detail in Section 4.6.3.

The following *optional* (level 3) headings may be used in the 'Description of studies' section:

### Ongoing studies

### Studies awaiting classification

### New studies found at this update

## Risk of bias in included studies

This should summarize the general risk of bias in results of the included studies, its variability across studies and any important flaws in individual studies. The criteria that were used to assess the risk of bias should be described or referenced under 'Methods' and not here. How each study was rated on each criterion should be reported in a 'Risk of bias' table and not described in detail in the text, which should be a concise summary. Presentation of 'Risk of bias' assessments is addressed in Chapter 8 (Section 8.6).

For large reviews, aspects of the assessment of risk of bias may be summarized for the primary outcomes under the following headings.

*Allocation*

A summary of how allocation sequences were generated and attempts to conceal allocation of intervention assignment should be summarized briefly here, along with any judgements concerning the risk of bias that may arise from the methods used.

*Blinding*

A brief summary of who was blinded or masked during the conduct and analysis of the studies should be reported here. Implications of blinding of outcome assessment may be different for different outcomes, so these may need to be addressed separately. Judgements concerning the risk of bias associated with blinding should be summarized.

*Incomplete outcome data*

The completeness of data should be summarized briefly here for each of the main outcomes. Concerns of the review authors over exclusion of participants and excessive (or differential) drop-out should be reported.

*Selective reporting*

Concerns over the selective availability of data may be summarized briefly here, including evidence of selective reporting of outcomes, time-points, subgroups or analyses.

*Other potential sources of bias*

Any other potential concerns should be summarized here.

## Effects of interventions

This should be a summary of the main findings on the effects of the interventions studied in the review. The section should directly address the objectives of the review rather than list the findings of the included studies in turn. The results of individual studies, and any statistical summary of these, should be included in 'Data and analysis' tables. Outcomes should normally be addressed in the order in which they are listed under 'Types of outcome measures'. Subheadings are encouraged if they make understanding easier (for example, for each different participant group, comparison or outcome measure if a review addresses more than one). Any sensitivity analyses that were undertaken should be reported.

Authors should avoid making inferences in this section. A common mistake to avoid (both in describing the results and in drawing conclusions) is the confusion of 'no evidence of an effect' with 'evidence of no effect'. When there is inconclusive evidence, it is wrong to claim that it shows that an intervention has 'no effect' or is 'no different' from the control intervention. In this situation, it is safer to report the data, with a confidence interval, as being compatible with either a reduction or an increase in the outcome.

Presentation of results is addressed in Chapter 11 (Section 11.7). Interpretation of numerical results is discussed in Chapter 12 (Sections 12.4, 12.5 and 12.6).

## Discussion

A structured discussion can aid the consideration of the implications of the review (Docherty 1999). Interpretation of results is discussed in Chapter 12.

### Summary of main results

Summarize the main findings (without repeating the 'Effects of interventions' section) and outstanding uncertainties, balancing important benefits against important harms. Refer explicitly to any 'Summary of findings' tables.

### Overall completeness and applicability of evidence

Describe the relevance of the evidence to the review question. This should lead to an overall judgement of the external validity of the review. Are the studies identified sufficient to address all of the objectives of the review? Have all relevant types of participants, interventions and outcomes been investigated? Comments on how the results of the review fit into the context of current practice might be included here, although authors should bear in mind that current practice might vary internationally.

### Quality of the evidence

Does the body of evidence identified allow a robust conclusion regarding the objective(s) of the review? Summarize the amount of evidence that has been included (numbers of studies, numbers of participants), state key methodological limitations of the studies, and reiterate the consistency or inconsistency of their results. This should lead to an overall judgement of the internal validity of the results of the review.

### Potential biases in the review process

State the strengths and limitations of the review with regard to preventing bias. These may be factors within, or outside, the control of the review authors. The discussion might include the likelihood that all relevant studies were identified, whether all relevant data could be obtained, or whether the methods used (for example, searching, study selection, data collection, analysis) could have introduced bias.

## Agreements and disagreements with other studies or reviews

Comments on how the included studies fit into the context of other evidence might be included here, stating clearly whether the other evidence was systematically reviewed.

# Authors' conclusions

The primary purpose of the review should be to present information, rather than to offer advice. Conclusions of the authors are divided into two sections:

## Implications for practice

The implications for practice should be as practical and unambiguous as possible. They should not go beyond the evidence that was reviewed and be justifiable by the data presented in the review. 'No evidence of effect' should not be confused with 'evidence of no effect'.

## Implications for research

This section of Cochrane reviews is used increasingly often by people making decisions about future research, and authors should try to write something that will be useful for this purpose. As with the 'Implications for practice', the content should be based on the available evidence and should avoid the use of information that was not included or discussed within the review.

In preparing this section, authors should consider the different aspects of research, perhaps using types of study, participant, intervention and outcome as a framework. Implications for *how* research might be done and reported should be distinguished from *what* future research should be done. For example, the need for randomized trials rather than other types of study, for better descriptions of studies in the particular topic of the review, or for the routine collection of specific outcomes should be distinguished from the lack of a continuing need for a comparison with placebo if there is an effective and appropriate active treatment, or for the need for comparisons of specific named interventions, or for research in specific types of people.

It is important that this section is as clear and explicit as possible. General statements that contain little or no specific information, such as "Future research should be better conducted" or "More research is needed" are of little use to people making decisions, and should be avoided. Guidance on formulating conclusions is provided in Chapter 12 (Section 12.7).

## Acknowledgements

This section should be used to acknowledge any people or organizations that the authors wish to acknowledge, including people who are not listed among the authors. This would include any previous authors of the Cochrane review or previous sources of support to the review, and might include the contributions of the editorial team of the CRG. Permission should be obtained from persons acknowledged.

## Contributions of authors

The contributions of the current co-authors to the protocol or review should be described in this section. One author should be identified as the guarantor of the review. All authors should discuss and agree on their respective descriptions of contribution before the review is submitted for publication on the *CDSR*. When the review is updated, this section should be checked and revised as necessary to ensure that it is accurate and up to date.

The following potential contributions have been adapted from Yank et al. (Yank 1999). This is a suggested scheme and the section should describe what people did, rather than attempt to identify which of these categories someone's contribution falls within. Ideally, the authors should describe their contribution in their own words.

- Conceiving the review.
- Designing the review.
- Coordinating the review.
- Data collection for the review.
  - Designing search strategies.
  - Undertaking searches.
  - Screening search results.
  - Organizing retrieval of papers.
  - Screening retrieved papers against eligibility criteria.
  - Appraising quality of papers.
  - Extracting data from papers.
  - Writing to authors of papers for additional information.
  - Providing additional data about papers.
  - Obtaining and screening data on unpublished studies.
- Data management for the review.
  - Entering data into RevMan.

- Analysis of data.
- Interpretation of data.
  - Providing a methodological perspective.
  - Providing a clinical perspective.
  - Providing a policy perspective.
  - Providing a consumer perspective.
- Writing the review (or protocol).
- Providing general advice on the review.
- Securing funding for the review.
- Performing previous work that was the foundation of the current review.

## Declarations of interest

Authors should report any present or past affiliations or other involvement in any organization or entity with an interest in the review that might lead to a real or perceived conflict of interest. Situations that might be perceived by others as being capable of influencing a review author's judgements include personal, political, academic and other possible conflicts, as well as financial conflicts. Authors must state if they have been involved in a study included in the review. A summary of the Collaboration's policy on conflicts of interest appears in Chapter 2 (Section 2.6).

Financial conflicts of interest cause the most concern, and should be avoided, but must be reported if there are any. Any secondary interest (such as personal conflicts) that might unduly influence judgements made in a review (concerning, for example, the inclusion or exclusion of studies, assessments of the validity of included studies or the interpretation of results) should be reported.

If there are no known conflicts of interest, this should be stated explicitly, for example, by writing 'None known'.

## Differences between protocol and review

It is sometimes necessary to use different methods from those described in the original protocol. This could be because:

- methods for dealing with a particular issue had not been specified in the protocol;

- methods in the protocol could not be applied (for example, due to insufficient data or a lack of information required to implement the methods); and

- methods are changed because a preferable alternative is discovered.

Some changes of methods from protocol to review are acceptable, but must be fully described in this section. The section provides a summary of the main changes in methods for the review over time.

- Point out any methods that were determined subsequent to the original published protocol (e.g. adding or changing outcomes; adding 'Risk of bias' or 'Summary of findings' tables).

- Summarize methods from the protocol that could not be implemented in the current review (e.g. because the review identified no eligible studies, or because no studies fell in a particular pre-defined subgroup).

- Explain any changes in methods from the protocol to the review, state when they were made and provide the rationale for the changes. Such changes should not be driven by findings on the effects of interventions. Consider the potential effect on the review's conclusions of any changes in methods, and consider sensitivity analyses to assess this.

## Published notes

Published notes will appear in the review in the *CDSR*. They may include editorial notes and comments from the CRG, for example where issues highlighted by editors or referees are believed worthy of publication alongside the review. The author or source of these comments should be specified (e.g. from an editor or a referee).

Published notes must be completed for all withdrawn protocols and reviews, giving the reason for withdrawal. Only basic citation information, sources of support and published notes are published for withdrawn protocols and reviews.

## 4.6   Tables

### 4.6.1   Characteristics of included studies

The 'Characteristics of included studies' table has five entries for each study: Methods, Participants, Interventions, Outcomes and Notes. Up to three further entries may be specified for items not conveniently covered by these categories, for example, to provide information on length of follow-up, funding source, or indications of study quality that are unlikely to lead directly to a risk of bias (see Section 4.6.2 for including information on the risk of bias). Codes or abbreviations may be used in the table to enable clear and succinct presentation of multiple pieces of information within an entry; for example, authors could include country, setting, age and sex under the Participants entry. Footnotes should be used to explain any codes or abbreviations used (these will be published in the *CDSR*). Detailed guidance on 'Characteristics of included studies' tables is provided in Chapter 11 (Section 11.2).

## 4.6.2 Risk of bias

A 'Risk of bias' table is an optional, although strongly recommended, extension of the 'Characteristics of included studies' table. The standard 'Risk of bias' table includes assessments for sequence generation, allocation sequence concealment, blinding, incomplete outcome data, selective outcome reporting and 'other issues'. For each item, the table provides a description of what was reported to have happened in the study and a subjective judgement regarding protection from bias ('Yes' for a low risk of bias, 'No' for a high risk of bias; 'Unclear' otherwise). 'Risk of bias' tables are discussed in Chapter 8 (Section 8.6).

## 4.6.3 Characteristics of excluded studies

Certain studies that may appear to meet the eligibility criteria, but which were excluded, should be listed and the reason for exclusion should be given (for example, inappropriate comparator intervention). This should be kept brief, and a single reason for exclusion is usually sufficient. Selection of which studies to list as excluded is discussed in Chapter 7 (Section 7.2.5).

## 4.6.4 Characteristics of studies awaiting classification

The 'Characteristics of studies awaiting classification' table (formerly 'Studies awaiting assessment') has the same structure as the 'Characteristics of included studies' table. It should be used for two categories of study:

- Studies about which an inclusion or exclusion decision cannot be made because sufficient information is not currently available. All reasonable attempts to obtain information must be made before studies are left here on publication of the review, but the review should not be delayed excessively waiting for this information, especially if the inclusion or exclusion of the study is unlikely to have an impact on the review's conclusions. When information is not available for a table entry, the text 'Not known' should be inserted.

- Studies that have been identified but are awaiting an update to the review. In particular, it is appropriate to mention studies that have the potential to impact on the review's conclusions, or studies that receive wide publicity, in the review in the period between updates. An amended review may therefore be produced with such studies summarized in this table. The full update, with such studies fully incorporated, should be completed as soon as possible. When information is not available for a table entry, the text 'Not yet assessed' or 'Not known' should be inserted, as appropriate.

### 4.6.5 Characteristics of ongoing studies

The 'Characteristics of ongoing studies' table has eight entries for each study: Study name, Methods, Participants, Interventions, Outcomes, Starting date, Contact information and Notes. The contents of these entries should be comparable to those in the table of 'Characteristics of included studies'. Footnotes should be used to explain any abbreviations used in the table (these will be published in the *CDSR*).

### 4.6.6 Summary of findings

A 'Summary of findings' table is an optional, although strongly recommended, means of presenting findings for the most important outcomes, whether or not evidence is available for them. A 'Summary of findings' table includes, where appropriate, a summary of the amount of evidence; typical absolute risks for people receiving experimental and control interventions; estimates of relative effect (e.g. risk ratio or odds ratio); a depiction of the quality of the body of evidence; comments; and footnotes. The assessment of the quality of the body of evidence should follow the GRADE framework, which combines considerations of risk of bias, directness, heterogeneity, precision and publication bias.

A full specification and discussion of 'Summary of findings' tables is provided in Chapter 11 (Section 11.5). The GRADE system is overviewed in Chapter 12 (Section 12.2).

### 4.6.7 Additional tables

Additional tables may be used for information that cannot be conveniently placed in the text or in fixed tables. Examples include:

- information to support the background; and

- summaries of study characteristics (such as detailed descriptions of interventions or outcomes); additional tables are discussed in Chapter 11 (Section 11.6).

## 4.7 Studies and references

### 4.7.1 References to studies

Studies are organized under four fixed headings.

Each of these headings can include multiple studies (or no studies). A study is identified by a 'Study ID' (usually comprising the last name of first author and the year of the primary reference for the study). A year can be explicitly associated with each study (usually the year of completion, or the publication year of the primary reference), as can identifiers such as an International Standard Randomised Controlled Trial Number (ISRCTN). In addition, each study should be assigned a category of 'Data source' from among the following:

- published data only;

- published and unpublished data;

- unpublished data only; and

- published data only (unpublished sought but not used).

Each study can have multiple references. Each reference may be given identifiers such as a MEDLINE ID or a DOI. One reference for each study should be awarded the status of 'Primary reference'.

Authors should check all references for accuracy.

### 4.7.1.1 Included studies

Studies that meet the eligibility criteria and are included in the review.

### 4.7.1.2 Excluded studies

Studies that do not meet the eligibility criteria and are excluded from the review.

### 4.7.1.3 Studies awaiting classification

Relevant studies that have been identified, but cannot be assessed for inclusion until additional data or information are obtained.

### 4.7.1.4 Ongoing studies

Studies that are ongoing and meet (or appear to meet) the eligibility criteria.

## 4.7.2 Other references

References other than those to studies are divided among the following two categories. Note that RevMan also includes a 'Classification pending' category to facilitate organization of references while preparing a review. All references should be moved out of this category before a review is marked for submission to the *CDSR*, since any references remaining in this category will not be published.

### *4.7.2.1   Additional references*

Other references cited in the text should be listed here, including those cited in the Background and Methods sections. If a report of a study is cited in the text for some reason other than referring to the study (for example, because of some background or methodological information in the reference), it should be listed here as well as under the relevant study.

### *4.7.2.2   Other published versions of this review*

References to other published versions of the review in a journal, textbook or the *CDSR* or elsewhere should be listed here.

## 4.8   Data and analyses

Results of studies included in a review are organized in a hierarchy: studies are nested within (optional) subgroups, which are nested within outcomes, which are nested within comparisons (see Figure 4.8.a). A study can be included several times among the analyses.

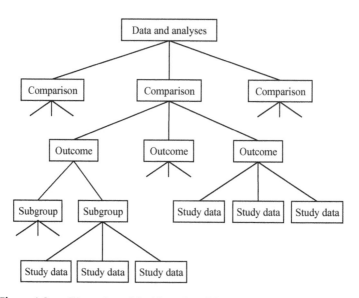

**Figure 4.8.a**   Illustration of the hierarchy of the 'Data and analyses' section.

RevMan automatically generates forest plots illustrating data, effect estimates and results of meta-analyses (where selected) from the data entered into the 'Data and analyses' structure. The author is able to control whether, and how, meta-analyses are performed.

Note: The 'Data and analyses' should be considered as supplementary information because they may not appear in some formats of the published review. Key forest plots (containing data for each study) may be selected to be *always* included with the full text of the review by selecting them as figures (see Section 4.9). The full published Cochrane review in the *CDSR* will, however, contain all of the 'Data and analyses' section as a series of forest plots or tables.

Authors should avoid listing comparisons or outcomes for which there are no data (i.e. have forest plots with no studies). Instead, authors should note in the text of the review that no data are available for the comparisons. However, if the review has a 'Summary of findings' table, the main outcomes should be included in this irrespective of whether data are available from the included studies.

Analyses are addressed in Chapter 9; including discussion of comparisons (Section 9.1.6), types of outcome data (Section 9.2) and subgroups (Section 9.6). Useful conversions from reported data to the required format are provided in Chapter 7 (Section 7.7).

### 4.8.1 Comparison

The comparisons should correspond to the questions or hypotheses under 'Objectives'.

### 4.8.2 Outcome

Five types of outcome data are possible: dichotomous data, continuous data, 'O – E' and 'V' statistics, generic inverse variance (estimate and standard error) and other data (text only).

### 4.8.3 Subgroup

Subgroups may relate to subsets of studies (for example, trials using different durations of physiotherapy) or to a subdivision of the outcome (for example, short-term, medium-term, long-term).

### 4.8.4 Study data

Data for each study must be entered in a particular format specific to the type of outcome data (e.g. a sample size, mean and standard deviation for each group for continuous data).

## 4.9    Figures

Five types of figures may be included within the text of the review (see Table 4.9.a). These figures will always be presented with the full-text publication of the review. Each figure must have a caption, providing a brief description (or explanation) of the figure, and must be referred to (with a link) in the review text. Issues in the selection of figures are discussed in Chapter 11 (Section 11.4.2).

### 4.9.1    RevMan plots and graphs

Forest plots and funnel plots from among those in the 'Data and analyses' may be selected as figures. Graphical representations of judgements on risk of bias can also be

**Table 4.9.a**    Types of figures that can be included in a Cochrane review

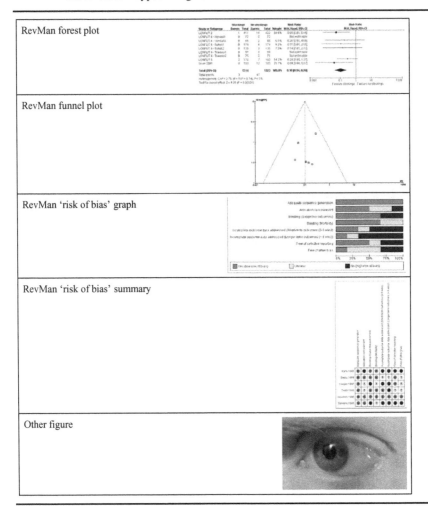

| RevMan forest plot |
| RevMan funnel plot |
| RevMan 'risk of bias' graph |
| RevMan 'risk of bias' summary |
| Other figure |

generated within RevMan and included as figures. Forest plots are discussed in Chapter 11 (Section 11.3.2). Funnel plots are discussed in Chapter 10 (Section 10.4). 'Risk of bias' graphs and 'Risk of bias' summaries are discussed in Chapter 8 (Section 8.6).

### 4.9.2 Other figures

Graphs and other images that are not generated by RevMan can be included as figures. These should never be used for content that can be generated in other ways within RevMan, for example as forest plots or as additional tables.

Authors are responsible for obtaining permission for images included in the review and for following guidance to ensure the images are fit for publication. If permission to publish a copyrighted figure is granted, the final phrase of the figure caption must be: "Copyright © [Year] [Name of copyright holder, or other required wording]: reproduced with permission.".

Figures showing statistical analyses should follow the relevant guidance prepared by the Statistical Methods Group (see Supplementary material on the *Handbook* web site: www.cochrane.org/resources/handbook).

## 4.10 Sources of support to the review

Authors should acknowledge grants that supported the review, and other forms of support, such as support from their university or institution in the form of a salary. Sources of support are divided into 'internal' (provided by the institutions at which the review was produced) and 'external' (provided by other institutions or funding agencies). Each source, its country of origin and what it supported should be provided.

## 4.11 Feedback

Each piece of Feedback incorporated into a review is identified by a short title and the date. **Summary, Reply** and **Contributors** are subheadings in this section. The summary should be prepared by the Feedback editor for the CRG in consultation, if necessary, with the person submitting the comment. The author(s) of the review should prepare a reply. The names of the people who contributed to the process of responding to the feedback should be given under 'Contributors'. Further information on Feedback is given in Chapter 3 (Section 3.6).

*See also*

• Further information on Feedback is given in Chapter 3 (Section 3.6).

## 4.12   Appendices

Appendices provide a place for supplementary information such as:

- detailed search strategies (appendices are the recommended place to put these);
- lengthy details of non-standard statistical methods;
- data collection forms; and
- details of outcomes (e.g. measurement scales).

Appendices may not appear in some formats of the published review.

## 4.13   Chapter information

**Editors:** Julian PT Higgins and Sally Green.

**This chapter should be cited as**: Higgins JPT, Green S (editors). Chapter 4: Guide to the contents of a Cochrane protocol and review. In: Higgins JPT, Green S (editors). *Cochrane Handbook for Systematic Reviews of Interventions*. Chichester (UK): John Wiley & Sons, 2008.

**Acknowledgements:** This chapter builds on earlier versions of the *Handbook*. For details of previous authors and editors of the *Handbook*, please refer to Chapter 1 (Section 1.4). The list of recommended headings was developed by Julian Higgins in discussion with Mike Clarke, Sally Hopewell, Jacqueline Birks, numerous Review Group Co-ordinators, a working group on assessing risk of bias, and members of the Handbook Advisory Group. Contributing authors in recent updates have included Ginny Brunton, Mike Clarke, Mark Davies, Frances Fairman, Sally Green, Julian Higgins, Nicki Jackson, Harriet MacLehose, Sandy Oliver, Peter Tugwell and Janet Wale. We thank Lisa Askie, Sonja Henderson, Monica Kjeldstrøm, Carol Lefebvre, Philippa Middleton, Rasmus Moustgaard and Rebecca Smyth for helpful comments.

## 4.14   References

**Docherty 1999**
   Docherty M, Smith R. The case for structuring the discussion of scientific papers. *BMJ* 1999; 318: 1224–1225.
**Flanagin 1998**
   Flanagin A, Carey LA, Fontanarosa PB, Phillips SG, Pace BP, Lundberg GD, Rennie D. Prevalence of articles with honorary authors and ghost authors in peer-reviewed medical journals. *JAMA* 1998; 280: 222–224.

**International Committee of Medical Journal Editors 2006**

International Committee of Medical Journal Editors. Uniform requirements for manuscripts submitted to biomedical journals: Writing and editing for biomedical publication [Updated February 2006]. Available from: http://www.icmje.org (accessed 1 January 2008).

**Rennie 1997**

Rennie D, Yank V, Emanuel L. When authorship fails. A proposal to make contributors accountable. *JAMA* 1997; 278: 579–585.

**Rennie 1998**

Rennie D, Yank V. If authors became contributors, everyone would gain, especially the reader. *American Journal of Public Health* 1998; 88: 828–830.

**Yank 1999**

Yank V, Rennie D. Disclosure of researcher contributions: a study of original research articles in The Lancet. *Annals of Internal Medicine* 1999; 130: 661–670.

# PART 2: General methods for Cochrane reviews

# 5 Defining the review question and developing criteria for including studies

**Edited by Denise O'Connor, Sally Green and Julian PT Higgins**

## Key Points

- A clearly defined, focused review begins with a well framed question. In Cochrane reviews, questions are stated broadly as review 'Objectives', and specified in detail as 'Criteria for considering studies for this review'.

- The review question should specify the types of population (participants), types of interventions (and comparisons), and the types of outcomes that are of interest. The acronym PICO (Participants, Interventions, Comparisons and Outcomes) helps to serve as a reminder of these. These components of the question, with the additional specification of types of study that will be included, form the basis of the pre-specified eligibility criteria for the review.

- Cochrane reviews should include all outcomes that are likely to be meaningful, and not include trivial outcomes. Primary outcomes should be limited to a very small number and include adverse as well as beneficial outcomes.

- Cochrane reviews can focus on broad questions, or be more narrowly defined. There are advantages and disadvantages of each.

## 5.1   Questions and eligibility criteria

### 5.1.1   Rationale for well-formulated questions

As with any research, the first and most important decision in preparing a systematic review is to determine its focus. This is best done by clearly framing the questions the review seeks to answer. Well-formulated questions will guide many aspects of the review process, including determining eligibility criteria, searching for studies, collecting data from included studies, and presenting findings (Jackson 1980, Cooper 1984, Hedges 1994). In Cochrane reviews, questions are stated broadly as review 'Objectives', and specified in detail as 'Criteria for considering studies for this review'. As well as focussing review conduct, the contents of these sections are used by readers in their initial assessments of whether the review is likely to be directly relevant to the issues they face.

A statement of the review's objectives should begin with a precise statement of the primary objective, ideally in a single sentence. Where possible the style should be of the form 'To assess the effects of [*intervention or comparison*] for [*health problem*] in [*types of people, disease or problem and setting if specified*]'. This might be followed by one or more secondary objectives, for example relating to different participant groups, different comparisons of interventions or different outcome measures.

The detailed specification of the review question requires consideration of several key components (Richardson 1995, Counsell 1997). The 'clinical question' should specify the types of population (participants), types of interventions (and comparisons), and the types of outcomes that are of interest. The acronym PICO (**P**articipants, **I**nterventions, **C**omparisons and **O**utcomes) helps to serve as a reminder of these. Equal emphasis in addressing each PICO component is not necessary. For example, a review might concentrate on competing interventions for a particular stage of breast cancer, with stage and severity of the disease being defined very precisely; or alternately focus on a particular drug for any stage of breast cancer, with the treatment formulation being defined very precisely.

### 5.1.2   Eligibility criteria

One of the features that distinguish a systematic review from a narrative review is the pre-specification of criteria for including and excluding studies in the review (eligibility criteria). Eligibility criteria are a combination of aspects of the clinical question plus specification of the types of studies that have addressed these questions. The participants, interventions and comparisons in the clinical question usually translate directly into eligibility criteria for the review. Outcomes usually are not part of the criteria for including studies: a Cochrane review would typically seek all rigorous studies (e.g. randomized trials) of a particular comparison of interventions in a particular population of participants, irrespective of the outcomes measured or reported. However, some reviews do legitimately restrict eligibility to specific outcomes. For example, the same intervention may be studied in the same population for different purposes (e.g. hormone replacement therapy, or aspirin); or a review may address specifically the adverse effects of an intervention used for several conditions (see Chapter 14, Section 14.2.3).

In Sections 5.2 to 5.5 we provide an overview of the key components of questions and study types with examples of useful issues to consider for each component and the subsequent development of eligibility criteria to guide inclusion of studies.

## 5.2 Defining types of participants: which people and populations?

The criteria for considering types of people included in studies in a review should be sufficiently broad to encompass the likely diversity of studies, but sufficiently narrow to ensure that a meaningful answer can be obtained when studies are considered in aggregate. It is often helpful to consider the types of people that are of interest in two steps. First, the diseases or conditions of interest should be defined using explicit criteria for establishing their presence or not. Criteria that will force the unnecessary exclusion of studies should be avoided. For example, diagnostic criteria that were developed more recently – which may be viewed as the current gold standard for diagnosing the condition of interest – will not have been used in earlier studies. Expensive or recent diagnostic tests may not be available in many countries or settings.

Second, the broad population and setting of interest should be defined. This involves deciding whether a special population group is of interest, determined by factors such as age, sex, race, educational status or the presence of a particular condition such as angina or shortness of breath. Interest may focus on a particular setting such as a community, hospital, nursing home, chronic care institution, or outpatient setting. Box 5.2.a outlines some factors to consider when developing criteria for the 'Types of participants'.

---

**Box 5.2.a    Factors to consider when developing criteria for 'Types of participants'**

- How is the disease/condition defined?
- What are the most important characteristics that describe these people (participants)?
- Are there any relevant demographic factors (e.g. age, sex, ethnicity)?
- What is the setting (e.g. hospital, community etc)?
- Who should make the diagnosis?
- Are there other types of people who should be excluded from the review (because they are likely to react to the intervention in a different way)?
- How will studies involving only a subset of relevant participants be handled?

---

The types of participants of interest usually determine directly the participant-related eligibility criteria for including studies. However, pre-specification of rules for dealing with studies that only partially address the population of interest can be challenging. For example, if interest focuses on children, a cut-point such as 16 years old might be desirable, but does not determine a strategy for dealing with studies with participants aged from 12 to 18. Use of arbitrary rules (such as "more than 80% of the participants are under 16") will not be practical if detailed information is not available from the study. A phrase such as "the majority of participants are under 16" may be sufficient. Although there is a risk of review authors' biases affecting *post hoc* inclusion decisions, this may be outweighed by a common sense strategy in which eligibility decisions keep faith with the objectives of the review rather than with arbitrary rules. Difficult decisions should be documented in the review, and sensitivity analyses can assess the impact of these decisions on the review's findings (see Chapter 9, Section 9.7).

Any restrictions with respect to specific population characteristics or settings should be based on a sound rationale. It is important that Cochrane reviews are globally relevant, so justification for the exclusion of studies based on population characteristics should be explained in the review. For example, focusing a review of the effectiveness of mammographic screening on women between 40 and 50 years old may be justified on the basis of biological plausibility, previously published systematic reviews and existing controversy. On the other hand, focusing a review on a particular subgroup of people on the basis of their age, sex or ethnicity simply because of personal interests when there is no underlying biologic or sociological justification for doing so should be avoided. When it is uncertain whether there are important differences in effects among various subgroups of people, it may be best to include all of the relevant subgroups and then test for important and plausible differences in effect in the analysis (see Chapter 9, Section 9.6). This should be planned *a priori*, stated as a secondary objective and not driven by the availability of data.

## 5.3 Defining types of interventions: which comparisons to make?

The second key component of a well-formulated question is to specify the interventions of interest and the interventions against which these will be compared (comparisons). In particular, are the interventions to be compared with an inactive control intervention (e.g. placebo, no treatment, standard care, or a waiting list control), or with an active control intervention (e.g. a different variant of the same intervention, a different drug, a different kind of therapy)?

When specifying drug interventions, factors such as the drug preparation, route of administration, dose, duration, and frequency should be considered. For more complex interventions (such as educational or behavioural interventions), the common or core features of the interventions will need to be defined. In general, it is useful to consider exactly what is delivered, at what intensity, how often it is delivered, who delivers it, and whether people involved in delivery of the intervention need to be trained. Review authors should also consider whether variation in the intervention (i.e. based on dosage/intensity, mode of delivery, frequency, duration etc) is so great that it would have substantially different effects on the participants and outcomes of interest, and hence may be important to restrict.

Box 5.3.a outlines some factors to consider when developing criteria for the 'Types of interventions' (and comparisons).

---

**Box 5.3.a    Factors to consider when developing criteria for 'Types of interventions'**

- What are the experimental and control (comparator) interventions of interest?
- Does the intervention have variations (e.g. dosage/intensity, mode of delivery, personnel who deliver it, frequency of delivery, duration of delivery, timing of delivery)?
- Are all variations to be included (for example is there a critical dose below which the intervention may not be clinically appropriate)?
- How will trials including only part of the intervention be handled?
- How will trials including the intervention of interest combined with another intervention (co-intervention) be handled?

---

## 5.4    Defining types of outcomes: which outcome measures are most important?

### 5.4.1    Listing relevant outcomes

Although reporting of outcomes should rarely determine eligibility of studies for a review, the third key component of a well-formulated question is the delineation of particular outcomes that are of interest. In general, Cochrane reviews should include all outcomes that are likely to be meaningful to clinicians, patients (consumers), the general public, administrators and policy makers, but should not include outcomes reported in included studies if they are trivial or meaningless to decision makers. Outcomes considered to be meaningful and therefore addressed in a review will not necessarily have been reported in individual studies. For example, quality of life is an important outcome, perhaps the most important outcome, for people considering whether or not to use chemotherapy for advanced cancer, even if the available studies are found to report only survival (see Chapter 17). Including all important outcomes in a review will highlight gaps in the primary research and encourage researchers to address these gaps in future studies.

Outcomes may include survival (mortality), clinical events (e.g. strokes or myocardial infarction), patient-reported outcomes (e.g. symptoms, quality of life), adverse events, burdens (e.g. demands on caregivers, frequency of tests, restrictions on lifestyle) and economic outcomes (e.g. cost and resource use). It is critical that outcomes used to assess adverse effects as well as outcomes used to assess beneficial effects are among those addressed by a review (see Chapter 14). If combinations of outcomes will be considered, these need to be specified. For example, if a study fails to make a distinction between non-fatal and fatal strokes, will these data be included in a meta-analysis if the question specifically relates to stroke death?

Review authors should consider how outcomes may be measured, both in terms of the type of scale likely to be used and the timing of measurement. Outcomes may be measured objectively (e.g. blood pressure, number of strokes) or subjectively as rated by a clinician, patient, or carer (e.g. disability scales). It may be important to specify whether measurement scales have been published or validated. When defining the timing of outcome measurement, authors may consider whether all time frames or only selected time-points will be included in the review. One strategy is to group time-points into pre-specified intervals to represent 'short-term', 'medium-term' and 'long-term' outcomes and to take no more than one of each from each study for any particular outcome. It is important to give the timing of outcome measure considerable thought as it can influence the results of the review (Gøtzsche 2007).

As Cochrane reviews are increasingly included in Overviews of reviews (see Chapter 22), harmonization of outcomes across reviews addressing related questions will facilitate this process. It may be helpful for review authors to consider those measures used in related reviews when defining the type and timing of measurement within their own review. In addition, several clinical areas are developing agreed core sets of outcome measures for use in randomized trials, and consideration of these in defining the detail of measurement of outcomes selected for the review is likely to be helpful.

Various sources can be used to develop a list of relevant outcomes, including the clinical experiences of the review authors, input from consumers and advisory groups (see Chapter 2), and evidence from the literature (including qualitative research about outcomes important to those affected). Further information about the use of qualitative research to inform the formulation of review questions, including types of outcome measures, can be found in Chapter 20.

While all important outcomes should be included in Cochrane reviews, trivial outcomes should not be included. Authors need to avoid overwhelming and potentially misleading readers with data that are of little or no importance. In addition, indirect or surrogate outcome measures, such as laboratory results or radiologic results (e.g. loss of bone mineral content as a surrogate for fractures in hormone replacement therapy), are potentially misleading and should be avoided or interpreted with caution because they may not predict clinically important outcomes accurately. Surrogate outcomes may provide information on how a treatment might work but not whether it actually does work. Many interventions reduce the risk for a surrogate outcome but have no effect or have harmful effects on clinically relevant outcomes, and some interventions have no effect on surrogate measures but improve clinical outcomes.

## 5.4.2 Prioritizing outcomes: main, primary and secondary outcomes

### Main outcomes

Once a full list of relevant outcomes has been compiled for the review, authors should prioritize the outcomes and select the main outcomes of relevance to the review question. The main outcomes are the essential outcomes for decision-making, and are those that would form the basis of a 'Summary of findings' table. 'Summary of findings' tables provide key information about the amount of evidence for important comparisons and outcomes, the quality of the evidence and the magnitude of effect (see Chapter 11, Section 11.5). There should be no more than seven main outcomes, which should generally not include surrogate or interim outcomes. They should not be chosen on the basis of any anticipated or observed magnitude of effect, or because they are likely to have been addressed in the studies to be reviewed.

### *Primary outcomes*

Primary outcomes for the review should be identified from among the main outcomes. Primary outcomes are the outcomes that would be expected to be analysed should the review identify relevant studies, and conclusions about the effects of the interventions under review will be based largely on these outcomes. There should in general be no more than three primary outcomes and they should include at least one desirable and at least one undesirable outcome (to assess beneficial and adverse effects respectively).

### *Secondary outcomes*

Main outcomes not selected as primary outcomes would be expected to be listed as secondary outcomes. In addition, secondary outcomes may include a limited number of additional outcomes the review intends to address. These may be specific to only some comparisons in the review. For example, laboratory tests and other surrogate measures may not be considered as main outcomes as they are less important than clinical endpoints in informing decisions, but they may be helpful in explaining effect or determining intervention integrity (see Chapter 7, Section 7.3.4).

Box 5.4.a summarizes the principal factors to consider when developing criteria for the 'Types of outcomes'.

---

**Box 5.4.a    Factors to consider when developing criteria for 'Types of outcomes'**

- Main outcomes, for inclusion in the 'Summary of findings' table, are those that are essential for decision-making, and should usually have an emphasis on patient-important outcomes.
- Primary outcomes are the two or three outcomes from among the main outcomes that the review would be likely to be able to address if sufficient studies are identified, in order to reach a conclusion about the effects (beneficial and adverse) of the intervention(s).
- Secondary outcomes include the remaining main outcomes (other than primary outcomes) plus additional outcomes useful for explaining effects.
- Ensure that outcomes cover potential as well as actual adverse effects.
- Consider outcomes relevant to all potential decision makers, including economic data.
- Consider the type and timing of outcome measurements.

---

### 5.4.3    Adverse outcomes

It is important that Cochrane reviews include information about the undesirable as well as desirable outcomes of the interventions examined. Review authors should consider carefully how they will include data on undesirable outcomes in their review, and at least one undesirable outcome should be defined as a primary outcome measure. Assessment of adverse effects is discussed in detail in Chapter 14.

### 5.4.4    Economic data

Decision makers need to consider the economic aspects of an intervention, such as whether its adoption will lead to a more efficient use of resources. Economic data such as resource use, costs or cost-effectiveness (or a combination of these) may therefore be included as outcomes in a review. It is useful to break down measures of resource use and costs to the level of specific items or categories. It is helpful to consider an international perspective in the discussion of costs. Economics issues are discussed in detail in Chapter 15.

## 5.5    Defining types of study

Certain study designs are more appropriate than others for answering particular questions. Authors should consider *a priori* what study designs are likely to provide reliable data with which to address the objectives of their review.

Because Cochrane reviews address questions about the effects of health care, they focus primarily on randomized trials. Randomization is the only way to prevent systematic differences between baseline characteristics of participants in different intervention groups in terms of both known and unknown (or unmeasured) confounders (see Chapter 8). For clinical interventions, deciding who receives an intervention and who does not is influenced by many factors, including prognostic factors. Empirical evidence suggests that, on average, non-randomized studies produce effect estimates that indicate more extreme benefits of the effects of health care than randomized trials. However, the extent, and even the direction, of the bias is difficult to predict. These issues are discussed at length in Chapter 13, which provides guidance on when it might be appropriate to include non-randomized studies in a Cochrane review.

A practical consideration also motivates the restriction of many Cochrane reviews to randomized trials. The efforts of The Cochrane Collaboration to identify randomized trials have not been matched for the identification of other types of studies. Consequently, including studies other than randomized trials in a review may require additional efforts to identify studies and to keep the review up to date, and might increase the risk that the result of the review will be influenced by publication bias. This issue and other bias-related issues important to consider when defining types of studies (e.g. whether to restrict study eligibility on the basis of language or publication status) are discussed in detail in Chapter 10.

Specific aspects of study design and conduct should also be considered when defining eligibility criteria, even if the review is restricted to randomized trials. For example, decisions over whether cluster-randomized trials (Chapter 16, Section 16.3) and cross-over trials (Chapter 16, Section 16.4) are eligible should be made, as should thresholds for eligibility based on aspects such as use of a placebo comparison group, evaluation of outcomes blinded to allocation, or a minimum period of follow-up. There will always be a trade-off between restrictive study design criteria (which might result in the inclusion of studies with low risk of bias, but which are very small in number) and more liberal design criteria (which might result in the inclusion of more studies, but which are at a higher risk of bias). Furthermore, excessively broad criteria might result in the inclusion of misleading evidence. If, for example, interest focuses on whether a therapy improves survival in patients with a chronic condition, it might be inappropriate to look at studies of very short duration, except to make explicit the point that they cannot address the question of interest.

## 5.6  Defining the scope of a review question (broad versus narrow)

The questions addressed by a review may be broad or narrow in scope. For example, a review might address a broad question regarding whether antiplatelet agents in general are effective in preventing all thrombotic events in humans. Alternatively, a review might address whether a particular antiplatelet agent, such as aspirin, is effective in decreasing the risks of a particular thrombotic event, stroke, in elderly persons with a previous history of stroke.

Determining the scope of a review question is a decision dependent upon multiple factors including perspectives regarding a question's relevance and potential impact; supporting theoretical, biologic and epidemiological information; the potential generalizability and validity of answers to the questions; and available resources.

There are advantages and disadvantages to both broad and narrow questions, some of which are summarized in Table 5.6.a. The validity of very broadly defined reviews may be criticized for 'mixing apples and oranges', particularly when good biologic or sociological evidence suggests that various formulations of an intervention behave very differently or that various definitions of the condition of interest are associated with markedly different effects of the intervention.

In practice, a Cochrane review may start (or have started) with a broad scope, and be divided up into narrower reviews as evidence accumulates and the original review becomes unwieldy. This may be done for practical and logistical reasons, for example to make updating easier as well as to make it easier for readers to keep up to date with the findings. Individual authors in consultation with their CRGs must decide if there are instances where splitting a broader focused review into a series of more narrowly focused reviews is appropriate and the methods that are implemented to achieve this (see Chapter 3, Section 3.4.4). If a major change is to be undertaken, such as splitting a broad review into a series of more narrowly focused reviews, a new protocol will need to be

**Table 5.6.a**   Some advantages and disadvantages of broad versus narrow review questions

|  | Broad scope | Narrow scope |
|---|---|---|
| **Choice of participants** e.g. corticosteroid injection for shoulder tendonitis (narrow) or corticosteroid injection for any tendonitis (broad) | *Advantages*: Comprehensive summary of the evidence. Ability to assess generalizability of findings across types of participants. | *Advantages*: Manageability for review team; ease of reading. |
|  | *Disadvantages*: May be more appropriate to prepare an Overview of reviews (see Chapter 22). Searching, data collection, analysis and writing may require more resources. Risk of 'mixing apples and oranges' (heterogeneity); interpretation may be difficult. | *Disadvantages*: Evidence may be sparse. Findings may not be generalizable to other settings or populations. Scope could be chosen by review authors to produce a desired result. |
| **Definition of an intervention** e.g. supervised running for depression (narrow) or any exercise for depression (broad) | *Advantages*: Comprehensive summary of the evidence. Ability to assess generalizability of findings across different implementations of the intervention. | *Advantages*: Manageability for review team; ease of reading. |
|  | *Disadvantages*: Searching, data collection, analysis and writing may require more resources. Risk of 'mixing apples and oranges' (heterogeneity); interpretation may be difficult. | *Disadvantages*: Evidence may be sparse. Findings may not be generalizable to other formulations of the intervention. Scope could be chosen by review authors to produce a desired result. |
| **Choice of interventions and comparisons** e.g. alarms for preventing bed-wetting (narrow) or interventions for preventing bed-wetting (broad) | *Advantages*: Comprehensive summary of the evidence. | *Advantages*: Manageability for review team. Clarity of objectives and ease of reading. |
|  | *Disadvantages*: May be unwieldy, and more appropriate to present as an Overview of reviews (see Chapter 22). Searching, data collection, analysis and writing may require more resources. | *Disadvantages*: May have limited value when not included in an Overview. |

published for each of the component reviews which clearly document the eligibility criteria for each one.

The advent of Cochrane Overviews of reviews (Chapter 22, Section 22.1.1), in which multiple Cochrane reviews are summarized, may affect scoping decisions for reviews. Overviews can summarize multiple Cochrane reviews of different interventions for the same condition, or multiple reviews of the same intervention for different types of participants. It may increasingly be considered desirable to plan a series of reviews with a relatively narrow scope, alongside an Overview to summarize their findings.

## 5.7 Changing review questions

While questions should be posed in the protocol before initiating the full review, these questions should not become a straitjacket that prevents exploration of unexpected issues (Khan 2001). Reviews are analyses of existing data that are constrained by previously chosen study populations, settings, intervention formulations, outcome measures and study designs. It is generally not possible to formulate an answerable question for a review without knowing some of the studies relevant to the question, and it may become clear that the questions a review addresses need to be modified in light of evidence accumulated in the process of conducting the review.

Although a certain fluidity and refinement of questions is to be expected in reviews as a fuller understanding of the evidence is gained, it is important to guard against bias in modifying questions. Data-driven questions can generate false conclusions based on spurious results. Any changes to the protocol that result from revising the question for the review should be documented in the section 'Differences between the protocol and the review'. Sensitivity analyses may be used to assess the impact of changes on the review findings (see Chapter 9, Section 9.7). When refining questions it is useful to ask the following questions:

- What is the motivation for the refinement?

- Could the refinement have been influenced by results from any of the included studies?

- Are search strategies appropriate for the refined question (especially any that have already been undertaken)?

- Are data collection methods appropriate to the refined question?

## 5.8 Chapter information

**Editors**: Denise O'Connor, Sally Green and Julian PT Higgins.

**This chapter should be cited as:** O'Connor D, Green S, Higgins JPT (editors). Chapter 5: Defining the review question and developing criteria for including studies.

In: Higgins JPT, Green S (editors), *Cochrane Handbook of Systematic Reviews of Interventions*. Chichester (UK): John Wiley & Sons, 2008.

**Acknowledgements**: This section builds on earlier versions of the *Handbook*. For details of previous authors and editors of the *Handbook*, see Chapter 1 (Section 1.4).

## 5.9   References

**Cooper 1984**

Cooper HM. The problem formulation stage. In: Cooper HM (editors). *Integrating Research: a Guide for Literature Reviews*. Newbury Park (CA): Sage Publications, 1984.

**Counsell 1997**

Counsell C. Formulating questions and locating primary studies for inclusion in systematic reviews. *Annals of Internal Medicine* 1997; 127: 380–387.

**Gøtzsche 2007**

Gøtzsche PC, Hróbjartsson A, Maric K, Tendal B. Data extraction errors in meta-analyses that use standardized mean differences. *JAMA* 2007; 298: 430–437.

**Hedges 1994**

Hedges LV. Statistical considerations. In: Cooper H, Hedges LV (editors). *The Handbook of Research Synthesis*. New York (NY): Russell Sage Foundation, 1994.

**Jackson 1980**

Jackson GB. Methods for integrative reviews. *Review of Educational Research* 1980; 50: 438–460.

**Khan 2001**

Khan KS, ter Riet G, Glanville J, Sowden AJ, Kleijnen J (editors). *Undertaking Systematic Reviews of Research on Effectiveness: CRD's Guidance for those Carrying Out or Commissioning Reviews (CRD Report Number 4)* (2nd edition). York (UK): NHS Centre for Reviews and Dissemination, University of York, 2001.

**Richardson 1995**

Richardson WS, Wilson MS, Nishikawa J, Hayward RSA. The well-built clinical question: a key to evidence based decisions. *ACP Journal Club* 1995: A12–A13.

# 6 Searching for studies

**Carol Lefebvre, Eric Manheimer and Julie Glanville on behalf of the Cochrane Information Retrieval Methods Group**

## Key Points

- Review authors should work closely from the start with the Trials Search Co-ordinator (TSC) of their Cochrane Review Group (CRG).

- Studies (not reports of studies) are included in Cochrane reviews but identifying reports of studies is currently the most convenient approach to identifying the majority of studies and obtaining information about them and their results.

- Trials registers and trials results registers are an increasingly important source of information.

- The Cochrane Central Register of Controlled Trials (CENTRAL), MEDLINE and EMBASE (if access is available to either the review author or TSC) should be searched for all Cochrane reviews, either directly or via the CRG's Specialized Register.

- Searches should seek high sensitivity, which may result in relatively low precision.

- Too many *different* search concepts should be avoided, but a wide variety of search terms should be combined with OR within *each* concept.

- Both free-text and subject headings should be used (for example Medical Subject Headings (MeSH) and EMTREE).

- Existing highly sensitive search strategies (filters) to identify randomized trials should be used, such as the newly revised Cochrane Highly Sensitive Search Strategies for identifying randomized trials in MEDLINE (but do not apply these filters in CENTRAL).

# 6.1    Introduction

Cochrane Review Groups (CRGs) are responsible for providing review authors with references to studies that are possibly relevant to their review. The majority of CRGs employ a dedicated Trials Search Co-ordinator to provide this service (see Section 6.1.1.1). The information in this chapter is designed to assist authors wishing to undertake supplementary searches for studies and to provide background information so that they can better understand the search process. In all cases review authors should contact the Trials Search Co-ordinator of their CRG before starting to search, in order to find out the level of support they provide.

This chapter will also be useful to Trials Search Co-ordinators who are new to their post, as well those who are more experienced, who may wish to consult this chapter as a reference source.

This chapter outlines some general issues in searching for studies; describes the main sources of potential studies; and discusses how to plan the search process, design and carry out search strategies, manage references found during the search process and correctly document and report the search process.

This chapter concentrates on searching for randomized trials. Many of the search principles discussed, however, will also apply to other study designs discussed elsewhere above. For some review topics, for example complex interventions, it may be necessary to adopt other approaches and to include studies other than randomized trials. Review authors are recommended to seek specific guidance from their CRG and refer also to the relevant chapters of this *Handbook*, such as Chapter 13 for non-randomized studies, Chapter 14 for adverse effects, Chapter 15 for economics data, Chapter 17 for patient-reported outcomes, Chapter 20 for qualitative research and Chapter 21 for reviews in health promotion and public health. Review authors searching for studies for inclusion in Cochrane reviews of diagnostic test accuracy should refer to the *Cochrane Handbook for Systematic Reviews of Diagnostic Test Accuracy*.

The numerous web sites listed in this chapter were checked in June 2008.

## 6.1.1    General issues

### *6.1.1.1    Role of the Trials Search Co-ordinator*

The Trials Search Co-ordinator for each CRG is responsible for providing assistance to authors with searching for studies for inclusion in their reviews. The range of assistance varies according to the resources available to individual CRGs but may include some or all of the following: providing relevant studies from the CRG's Specialized Register (see Section 6.3.2.4 for more detail), designing search strategies for the main bibliographic databases, running these searches in databases available to the CRG, saving search results and sending them to authors, advising authors on how to run searches in other databases and how to download results into their reference management software (see Section 6.5). Contact your Trials Search Co-ordinator before you start searching to find out the level of assistance offered.

If a CRG is currently without a Trials Search Co-ordinator authors should seek the guidance of a local healthcare librarian or information specialist, where possible one with experience of conducting searches for systematic reviews.

### 6.1.1.2 Minimizing bias

Systematic reviews of interventions require a thorough, objective and reproducible search of a range of sources to identify as many relevant studies as possible (within resource limits). This is a major factor in distinguishing systematic reviews from traditional narrative reviews and helps to minimize bias and therefore assist in achieving reliable estimates of effects.

A search of MEDLINE alone is not considered adequate. A systematic review showed that only 30%–80% of all known published randomized trials were identifiable using MEDLINE (depending on the area or specific question) (Dickersin 1994). Even if relevant records are in MEDLINE, it can be difficult to retrieve them (Golder 2006, Whiting 2008). Going beyond MEDLINE is important not only for ensuring that as many relevant studies as possible are identified but also to minimize selection bias for those that are found. Relying exclusively on a MEDLINE search may retrieve a set of reports unrepresentative of all reports that would have been identified through a comprehensive search of several sources.

Time and budget restraints require the review author to balance the thoroughness of the search with efficiency in use of time and funds and the best way of achieving this balance is to be aware of, and try to minimize, the biases such as publication bias and language bias that can result from restricting searches in different ways (see Chapter 10, Section 10.2).

### 6.1.1.3 Studies versus reports of studies

Systematic reviews have studies as the primary units of interest and analysis. However, a single study may have more than one report about it and each of these reports may contribute useful information for the review (see Chapter 7, Section 7.2). For most of the sources listed in Section 6.2, the search process will retrieve individual reports of studies, however there are some study-based resources, such as trials registers and trials results databases (see Sections 6.2.3.1 to 6.2.3.4).

### 6.1.1.4 Copyright and licensing

It is Cochrane Collaboration policy that all review authors and others involved in the Collaboration should adhere to copyright legislation and the terms of database licensing agreements. With respect to searching for studies, this refers in particular to adhering to the terms and conditions of use when searching databases and downloading records and adhering to copyright legislation when obtaining copies of articles. Review authors should seek guidance on this from their Trials Search Co-ordinator or local healthcare librarian, as copyright legislation varies across jurisdictions and licensing agreements across institutions.

### 6.1.2  Summary points

- Cochrane review authors should seek advice from the Trials Search Co-ordinator of their Cochrane Review Group (CRG) *before* starting a search.

- If the CRG is currently without a Trials Search Co-ordinator, seek the guidance of a local healthcare librarian or information specialist, where possible one with experience of searching for systematic reviews.

- Use the Table of Contents to navigate to specific sections of this chapter.

- A search of MEDLINE alone is not considered adequate.

- It is Cochrane Collaboration policy that all review authors and others involved in the Collaboration should adhere to database licensing terms and conditions of use and copyright legislation.

## 6.2  Sources to search

### 6.2.1  Bibliographic databases

#### 6.2.1.1  *Bibliographic databases – general introduction*

Searches of health-related bibliographic databases are generally the easiest and least time-consuming way to identify an initial set of relevant reports of studies. Some bibliographic databases, such as MEDLINE and EMBASE, include abstracts for the majority of recent records. A key advantage of these databases is that they can be searched electronically both for words in the title or abstract and by using the standardized indexing terms, or controlled vocabulary, assigned to each record (see Section 6.4.5).

   The Cochrane Collaboration has been developing a database or register of reports of controlled trials called The Cochrane Central Register of Controlled Trials (CENTRAL). This is considered to be the best single source of reports of trials that might be eligible for inclusion in Cochrane reviews. The three bibliographic databases generally considered to be the most important sources to search for reports of trials – CENTRAL, MEDLINE and EMBASE – are described in more detail in subsequent sections.

Databases are available to individuals for a fee, on a subscription or on a 'pay-as-you-go' basis. They can also be available free at the point of use through national provisions, site-wide licences at institutions such as universities or hospitals, through professional organizations as part of their membership packages or free of charge on the internet.

There are also a number of international initiatives to provide free or low-cost online access to databases (and full-text journals) over the internet. The Health InterNetwork Access to Research Initiative (HINARI) provides access to a wide range of databases including *The Cochrane Library* and nearly 4000 major journals from a wide range of publishers in biomedical and related social sciences, for healthcare professionals in local, not-for-profit institutions in over 100 low-income countries.

- www.who.int/hinari/en/

The International Network for the Availability of Scientific Publications (INASP) also provides access to a wide range of databases including *The Cochrane Library* and journals. Journal titles available vary by country. For further details see:

- www.inasp.info/file/68/about-inasp.html

Electronic Information for Libraries (eIFL) is a similar initiative based on library consortia to support affordable licensing of journals in 50 low-income and transition countries in central, eastern and south-east Europe, the former Soviet Union, Africa, the Middle-East and south-east Asia.

- www.eifl.net/cps/sections/about

For more detailed information about how to search these and other databases refer to Sections 6.3.3 and 6.4.

### *6.2.1.2   The Cochrane Central Register of Controlled Trials (CENTRAL)*

The Cochrane Central Register of Controlled Trials (CENTRAL) serves as the most comprehensive source of reports of controlled trials. CENTRAL is published as part of *The Cochrane Library* and is updated quarterly. As of January 2008 (Issue 1, 2008), CENTRAL contains nearly 530,000 citations to reports of trials and other studies potentially eligible for inclusion in Cochrane reviews, of which 310,000 trial reports are from MEDLINE, 50,000 additional trial reports are from EMBASE and the remaining 170,000 are from other sources such as other databases and handsearching.

Many of the records in CENTRAL have been identified through systematic searches of MEDLINE and EMBASE, as described in Sections 6.3.2.1 and 6.3.2.2. CENTRAL, however, includes citations to reports of controlled trials that are not indexed in MEDLINE, EMBASE or other bibliographic databases; citations published in many languages; and citations that are available only in conference proceedings or other sources that are difficult to access (Dickersin 2002). It also includes records from trials registers and trials results registers (see Section 6.2.3).

CENTRAL is available free of charge to all CRGs through access to *The Cochrane Library*. The web address for *The Cochrane Library* is: http://www.thecochranelibrary. com. Many health and academic institutions and organizations provide access to their members, and in many countries there is free access for the whole population (for example through funded national licences or arrangements for low-income countries). Information about access to *The Cochrane Library* for specific countries can be found under 'Access to Cochrane' at the top of *The Cochrane Library* home page.

### 6.2.1.3   MEDLINE and EMBASE

MEDLINE currently contains over 16 million references to journal articles from the 1950s onwards. Currently 5,200 journals in 37 languages are indexed for MEDLINE:

- www.nlm.nih.gov/pubs/factsheets/medline.html

PubMed provides access to a free version of MEDLINE that also includes up-to-date citations not yet indexed for MEDLINE:

- www.nlm.nih.gov/pubs/factsheets/pubmed.html

Additionally, PubMed includes records from journals that are not indexed for MEDLINE and records considered 'out-of-scope' from journals that are partially indexed for MEDLINE. For further information about the differences between MEDLINE and PubMed see:

- www.nlm.nih.gov/pubs/factsheets/dif_med_pub.html

MEDLINE is also available on subscription from a number of online database vendors, such as Ovid. Access is usually free to members of the institutions paying the subscriptions (e.g. hospitals and universities).

The US National Library of Medicine (NLM) has developed the NLM Gateway, which allows users to search MEDLINE or PubMed together with other NLM resources simultaneously such as the Health Services Research Projects database (HSRProj), Meeting Abstracts and the TOXLINE Subset for toxicology citations.

- gateway.nlm.nih.gov/gw/Cmd

EMBASE currently contains over 12 million records from 1974 onwards. Currently 4,800 journals are indexed for EMBASE in 30 languages

- www.info.embase.com/embase_suite/about/brochures/embase_fs.pdf

EMBASE.com is Elsevier's own version of EMBASE that, in addition to the 12 million EMBASE records from 1974 onwards, also includes over 7 million unique records from MEDLINE from 1966 to date, thus allowing both databases to be searched simultaneously.

- www.info.embase.com/embase_com/about/index.shtml

In 2007, Elsevier launched EMBASE Classic which now provides access to records digitized from the Excerpta Medica print journals (the original print indexes from which EMBASE was created) from 1947 to 1973.

- www.info.embaseclassic.com/pdfs/factsheet.pdf

EMBASE is only available by subscription. Authors should check if their CRG has access and, if not, whether it is available through their local institution's library.

For guidance on how to search MEDLINE and EMBASE for reports of trials, see Sections 6.3.3.2, 6.4.11.1 and 6.4.11.2.

*Database overlap*    Of the 4,800 journals indexed in EMBASE, 1,800 are not indexed in MEDLINE. Similarly, of the 5,200 journals indexed in MEDLINE, 1,800 are not indexed in EMBASE.

- www.info.embase.com/embase_suite/about/brochures/embase_fs.pdf

The actual degree of reference overlap varies widely according to the topic but studies comparing searches of the two databases have generally concluded that a comprehensive search requires that both databases be searched (Suarez-Almazor 2000). Although MEDLINE and EMBASE searches tend not to identify the same sets of references, they have been found to return similar numbers of relevant references.

### 6.2.1.4    *National and regional databases*

In addition to MEDLINE and EMBASE, which are generally considered to be the key international general healthcare databases, many countries and regions produce electronic bibliographic databases that concentrate on the literature produced in those regions, and which often include journals and other literature not indexed elsewhere. Access to many of these databases is available free of charge on the internet. Others are only available by subscription or on a 'pay-as-you-go' basis. Indexing complexity and consistency varies, as does the sophistication of the search interface, but they can be an important source of additional studies from journals not indexed in other international databases such as MEDLINE or EMBASE. Some examples are included in Box 6.2.a.

---

**Box 6.2.a    Examples of regional electronic bibliographic databases**

*Africa*: African Index Medicus
  ○ indexmedicus.afro.who.int/
*Australia*: Australasian Medical Index (fee-based)
  ○ www.nla.gov.au/ami/
*China*: Chinese Biomedical Literature Database (CBM) (in Chinese)
  ○ www.imicams.ac.cn/cbm/index.asp
*Eastern Mediterranean*: Index Medicus for the Eastern Mediterranean Region
  ○ www.emro.who.int/his/vhsl/
*Europe*: PASCAL (fee-based)
  ○ international.inist.fr/article21.html
*India*: IndMED
  ○ indmed.nic.in/
*Korea*: KoreaMed
  ○ www.koreamed.org/SearchBasic.php
*Latin America and the Caribbean*: LILACS
  ○ bases.bireme.br/cgi-bin/wxislind.exe/iah/online/?IsisScript=iah/
    iah.xis&base=LILACS&lang=i&Form=F
*South-East Asia*: Index Medicus for the South-East Asia Region (IMSEAR)
  ○ library.searo.who.int/modules.php?op=modload&name=websis&file=
    imsear
*Ukraine and the Russian Federation*: Panteleimon
  ○ www.panteleimon.org/maine.php3
*Western Pacific*: Western Pacific Region Index Medicus (WPRIM)
  ○ wprim.wpro.who.int/SearchBasic.php

---

### 6.2.1.5   Subject-specific databases

Which subject-specific databases to search in addition to CENTRAL, MEDLINE and EMBASE will be influenced by the topic of the review, access to specific databases and budget considerations. Most of the main subject-specific databases are available only on a subscription or 'pay-as-you-go' basis. Access to databases is therefore likely to be limited to those databases that are available to the Trials Search Co-ordinator at the CRG editorial base and those that are available at the institutions of the review authors. A selection of the main subject-specific databases that are more likely to be available through institutional subscriptions (and therefore 'free at the point of use') or are available free of charge on the internet are listed in Box 6.2.b, together with

---

**Box 6.2.b    Examples of subject-specific electronic bibliographic databases**

Biology and pharmacology

- Biological Abstracts/BIOSIS Previews:
  - biosis.org/
- Derwent Drug File:
  - scientific.thomson.com/support/products/drugfile/
- International Pharmaceutical Abstracts:
  - scientific.thomson.com/products/ipa/

Health promotion

- BiblioMap – EPPI-Centre database of health promotion research (free on the internet):
  - eppi.ioe.ac.uk/webdatabases/Intro.aspx?ID=7
- Database of Promoting Health Effectiveness Reviews (DoPHER) (free on the internet):
  - eppi.ioe.ac.uk/webdatabases/Intro.aspx?ID=2

International health

- Global Health:
  - www.cabi.org/datapage.asp?iDocID=169
- POPLINE (reproductive health) (free on the internet):
  - db.jhuccp.org/ics-wpd/popweb/

Nursing and allied health

- Allied and Complementary Medicine (AMED):
  - www.bl.uk/collections/health/amed.html
- British Nursing Index (BNI):
  - www.bniplus.co.uk/
- Cumulative Index to Nursing and Allied Health (CINAHL):
  - www.cinahl.com/
- EMCare:
  - www.elsevier.com/wps/find/bibliographicdatabasedescription.cws_home/708272/description#description
- MANTIS (osteopathy and chiropractic):
  - www.healthindex.com/
- OTseeker (systematic reviews and appraised randomized trials in occupational therapy) (free on the internet):
  - www.otseeker.com/

- Physiotherapy Evidence Database (PEDro) (systematic reviews and appraised randomized trials in physiotherapy) (free on the internet):
  - www.pedro.fhs.usyd.edu.au/

### Social and community health and welfare

- AgeLine (free on the internet):
  - www.aarp.org/research/ageline/
- Childdata:
  - www.childdata.org.uk/
- CommunityWISE:
  - www.oxmill.com/communitywise/
- Social Care Online (free on the internet):
  - www.scie-socialcareonline.org.uk/
- Social Services Abstracts:
  - www.csa.com/factsheets/ssa-set-c.php

### Social science, education, psychology and psychiatry

- Applied Social Sciences Index and Abstracts (ASSIA):
  - www.csa.com/factsheets/assia-set-c.php
- Campbell Collaboration's Social, Psychological, Educational and Criminological Trials Register (C2-SPECTR) (free on the internet):
  - geb9101.gse.upenn.edu/
- Education Resources Information Center (ERIC) (free on the internet)
  - www.eric.ed.gov/
- PsycINFO:
  - www.apa.org/psycinfo/
- Social Policy and Practice (evidence-based social science research):
  - www.ovid.com/site/catalog/DataBase/1859.pdf
- Sociological Abstracts:
  - www.csa.com/factsheets/socioabs-set-c.php

web addresses for further information. Access details vary according to institution. Review authors should seek advice from their local healthcare librarian for access at their institution.

In addition to subject-specific databases, general search engines include:

- Google Scholar (free on the internet):

  - scholar.google.com/advanced_scholar_search?hl=en&lr=

- Intute (free on the internet):

  ○ www.intute.ac.uk/

- Turning Research into Practice (TRIP) database (evidence-based healthcare resource) (free on the internet):

  ○ www.tripdatabase.com/

### 6.2.1.6    *Citation indexes*

Science Citation Index/Science Citation Index Expanded is a database that lists published articles from approximately 6,000 major scientific, technical and medical journals and links them to the articles in which they have been cited (a feature known as cited reference searching). It is available online as SciSearch and on the internet as Web of Science. Web of Science is also incorporated in Web of Knowledge. It can be searched as a source database like MEDLINE. It can also be used to identify studies for a review by identifying a known relevant source article, and checking each of the articles citing the source article, to see if they are also relevant to the review. It is a way of searching forward in time from the publication of an important relevant article to identify additional relevant articles published since then. Records also include the listed references from the original record, which in turn are another possible source of relevant trial reports. Citation searching is an important adjunct to database searching and handsearching (Greenhalgh 2005). Information about these products is available at:

- scientific.thomson.com/products/sci/
- scientific.thomson.com/products/wos/
- isiwebofknowledge.com/

A similar database exists for the social sciences known as Social Sciences Citation Index:

- scientific.thomson.com/products/ssci/

In 2004, Elsevier launched an abstract and citation database – Scopus. Scopus covers 15,000 journals (of which over 1,200 are open access journals) and 500 conference proceedings. It contains over 33 million abstracts, and results from nearly 400 million scientific web pages:

- info.scopus.com/overview/what/

### 6.2.1.7   Dissertations and theses databases

Dissertations and theses are not normally indexed in general bibliographic databases such as MEDLINE or EMBASE but there are exceptions, such as CINAHL, which indexes nursing dissertations. To identify relevant studies published in dissertations or theses it is advisable to search specific dissertation sources: see Box 6.2.c.

---

**Box 6.2.c   Examples of dissertations and theses databases**

- ProQuest Dissertations & Theses Database: indexes more than 2 million doctoral dissertations and masters' theses:
  - www.proquest.co.uk/products_pq/descriptions/pqdt.shtml
- Index to Theses in Great Britain and Ireland: lists over 500,000 theses:
  - www.theses.com/
- DissOnline: indexes 50,000 German dissertations:
  - www.dissonline.de/

---

### 6.2.1.8   Grey literature databases

There are many definitions of grey literature, but it is usually understood to mean literature that is not formally published in sources such as books or journal articles. Conference abstracts and other grey literature have been shown to be sources of approximately 10% of the studies referenced in Cochrane reviews (Mallett 2002). In a recently updated Cochrane methodology review, all five studies reviewed showed that published trials showed an overall greater treatment effect than grey literature trials (Hopewell 2007b). Thus, failure to identify trials reported in conference proceedings and other grey literature might affect the results of a systematic review.

Conference abstracts are a particularly important source of grey literature and are covered in Section 6.2.2.4.

EAGLE (the European Association for Grey Literature Exploitation), has closed the SIGLE (System for Information on Grey Literature) database, which was one of the most widely-used databases of grey literature. INIST in France (Institute for Scientific and Technical Information) has launched OpenSIGLE, which provides access to all the former SIGLE records, new data added by EAGLE members and information from Greynet.

- opensigle.inist.fr

The Healthcare Management Information Consortium (HMIC)   The HMIC database contains records from the Library & Information Services department of the Department of Health (DH) in England and the King's Fund Information & Library Service. It includes all DH publications including circulars and press releases.

The King's Fund is an independent health charity that works to develop and improve management of health and social care services. The database is considered to be a good source of grey literature on topics such as health and community care management, organizational development, inequalities in health, user involvement, and race and health.

- www.ovid.com/site/catalog/DataBase/99.jsp?top=2&mid=3&bottom= 7&subsection=10

The National Technical Information Service (NTIS) provides access to the results of both US and non-US government-sponsored research and can provide the full text of the technical report for most of the results retrieved. NTIS from 1964 is free on the internet.

- www.ntis.gov/

PsycEXTRA is a companion database to PsycINFO in psychology, behavioural science and health. It includes references from newsletters, magazines, newspapers, technical and annual reports, government reports and consumer brochures. PsycEXTRA is different from PsycINFO in its format, because it includes abstracts and citations plus full text for a major portion of the records. There is no coverage overlap with PsycINFO.

- www.apa.org/psycextra/

## 6.2.2 Journals and other non-bibliographic database sources

### 6.2.2.1 Handsearching

Handsearching involves a manual page-by-page examination of the entire contents of a journal issue or conference proceedings to identify all eligible reports of trials. In journals, reports of trials may appear in articles, abstracts, news columns, editorials, letters or other text. Handsearching healthcare journals and conference proceedings can be a useful adjunct to searching electronic databases for at least two reasons: 1) not all trial reports are included in electronic bibliographic databases, and 2) even when they are included, they may not contain relevant search terms in the titles or abstracts or be indexed with terms that allow them to be easily identified as trials (Dickersin 1994). Each journal year or conference proceeding should be handsearched thoroughly and competently by a well-trained handsearcher for all reports of trials, irrespective of topic, so that once it has been handsearched it will not need to be searched again. A Cochrane Methodology Review has found that a combination of handsearching and electronic searching is necessary for full identification of relevant reports published in journals, even for those that are indexed in MEDLINE (Hopewell 2007a). This was especially the case for articles published before 1991 when there was no indexing term for randomized trials in MEDLINE and for those articles that are in parts of journals (such as supplements and conference abstracts) which are not routinely indexed in databases such as MEDLINE.

To facilitate the identification of all published trials The Cochrane Collaboration has organized extensive handsearching efforts, predominantly through CRGs, Fields and Cochrane Centres. The US Cochrane Center oversees prospective registration of all potential handsearching and maintains files of handsearching activity in the Master List (Journals) and the Master List (Conference Proceedings) (see apps1.jhsph.edu/cochrane/masterlist.asp). Over 3,000 journals have been, or are being, searched within the Collaboration. The Master Lists enable search progress to be recorded and monitored for each title and also prevent duplication of effort which might occur if the same journal or conference proceeding were to be searched by more than one group or individual.

Cochrane entities and authors can prioritize handsearching based on where they expect to identify the most trial reports. This prioritization can be informed by searching CENTRAL, MEDLINE and EMBASE in a topic area and identifying which journals appear to be associated with the most retrieved citations. Preliminary evidence suggests that most of the journals with a high yield of trial reports are indexed in MEDLINE (Dickersin 2002) but this may reflect the fact that Cochrane contributors have concentrated early efforts on searching these journals. Therefore, journals not indexed in MEDLINE or EMBASE should also be considered for handsearching.

Authors are not routinely expected to handsearch journals for their reviews but they should discuss with their Trials Search Co-ordinator whether in their particular case handsearching of any journals or conference proceedings might be beneficial. Authors who wish to handsearch journals or conference proceedings should consult their Trials Search Co-ordinator who can determine whether the journal or conference proceedings has already been searched, and, if it has not, they can register the search on the relevant Master List and provide training in handsearching. Training material is available on the US Cochrane Center web site (apps1.jhsph.edu/cochrane/handsearcher_res.htm).

All correspondence regarding the initiation, progress and status of a journal or conference proceeding search should be between the CRG Trials Search Co-ordinator and staff at the US Cochrane Center.

### 6.2.2.2   Full text journals available electronically

The full text of an increasing number of journals is available electronically on a subscription basis or free of charge on the internet. In addition to providing a convenient method for retrieving the full article of already identified records, full-text journals can also be searched electronically, depending on the search interface, in a similar way to the way database records can be searched in a bibliographic database.

It is important to specify if the full text of a journal has been searched electronically. Some journals omit sections of the print version, for example letters, from the electronic version and some include extra articles in electronic format only.

Most academic institutions subscribe to a wide range of electronic journals and these are therefore available free of charge at the point of use to members of those institutions. Review authors should seek advice about electronic journal access from the library service at their local institution. Some professional organizations provide access to a range of journals as part of their membership package. In some countries similar arrangements exist for health service employees through national licences. There are also a number of international initiatives to provide free or low-cost online access to full-text journals (and databases) over the internet, including the Health InterNetwork Access to Research Initiative (HINARI), the International Network for the Availability of Scientific Publications (INASP) and Electronic Information for Libraries (eIFL). For further information on these initiatives see Section 6.2.1.1.

Examples of some full-text journal sources that are available worldwide free of charge without subscription are given in Box 6.2.d.

It is recommended that a local electronic copy or print copy be taken and filed of any possibly relevant article found electronically for subscription journals, as the subscription to that journal may not be in perpetuity. The journal may cease publication or change publishers and access to previously available articles may cease. The same applies to journals available free of charge on the internet, as the circumstances around availability of specific journals might change.

---

**Box 6.2.d   Examples of full-text journal sources available world-wide without charge**

- BioMed Central:
  - www.biomedcentral.com/browse/journals/
- Public Library of Science (PLoS):
  - www.plos.org/journals/
- PubMed Central (PMC):
  - www.pubmedcentral.nih.gov/

Web sites listing journals offering free full-text access include:
- Free Medical Journals:
  - freemedicaljournals.com/
- HighWire Press:
  - highwire.stanford.edu/lists/freeart.dtl

---

### 6.2.2.3   Tables of contents

Many journals, even those that are available by subscription only, offer Table of Contents (TOC) services free of charge, normally through e-mail alerts or RSS feeds. In addition a number of organizations offer TOC services: see Box 6.2.e.

---

**Box 6.2.e   Examples of organizations offering Table of Contents (TOC) services**

- British Library Direct (free):
  - direct.bl.uk/bld/Home.do
- British Library Direct Plus (subscription):
  - www.bl.uk/reshelp/atyourdesk/docsupply/productsservices/bldplus/
- British Library Inside (to be replaced by British Library Direct Plus) (subscription):
  - www.bl.uk/inside
- Current Contents Connect (subscription):
  - scientific.thomson.com/products/ccc/
- Scientific Electronic Library Online (SciELO) – Brazil (free):
  - www.scielo.br/
- Zetoc (Z39.50 Table Of Contents) (free as specified below);
  Zetoc provides access to the British Library's Electronic Table of Contents. It is free of charge for members of the Joint Information Systems Committee (JISC)-sponsored higher and further education institutions in the UK and all of NHS Scotland and Northern Ireland:
  - zetoc.mimas.ac.uk/

---

### 6.2.2.4   Conference abstracts or proceedings

Although conference proceedings are not indexed in MEDLINE and a number of other major databases, they are indexed in the BIOSIS databases (http://www.biosis.org/). Over one-half of trials reported in conference abstracts never reach full publication, and those that are eventually published in full have been shown to be systematically different from those that are never published in full (Scherer 2007). It is, therefore, important to try to identify possibly relevant studies reported in conference abstracts through specialist database sources and by handsearching or electronically searching those abstracts that are made available in print form, on CD-ROM or on the internet. Many conference proceedings are published as journal supplements. Specialist conference abstract sources are listed in Box 6.2.f.

Many conference abstracts are published free of charge on the internet, such as those of the American Society of Clinical Oncology (ASCO):

- www.asco.org/ASCO/Meetings

### 6.2.2.5   Other reviews, guidelines and reference lists as sources of studies

Some of the most convenient and obvious sources of references to potentially relevant studies are existing reviews. Copies of previously published reviews on, or relevant

---

**Box 6.2.f   Examples of specialist conference abstract sources**

- Biological Abstracts/RRM (Reports, Reviews, Meetings):
  - ○ scientific.thomson.com/products/barrm/
- British Library Inside (to be replaced by British Library Direct Plus):
  - ○ www.bl.uk/inside
- British Library Direct Plus:
  - ○ www.bl.uk/reshelp/atyourdesk/docsupply/productsservices/bldplus
- ISI Proceedings:
  - ○ scientific.thomson.com/products/proceedings/

---

to, the topic of interest should be obtained and checked for references to the included (and excluded) studies. As well as the *Cochrane Database of Systematic Reviews (CDSR)*, *The Cochrane Library* includes *The Database of Abstracts of Reviews of Effects* (DARE) and the *Health Technology Assessment Database* (HTA Database), both produced by the Centre for Reviews and Dissemination (CRD) at the University of York in the UK. Both databases provide information on published reviews of the effects of health care. As well as being published and updated quarterly in *The Cochrane Library,* more up-to-date versions of these databases are available free of charge on the CRD web site, where they are updated more frequently. For example, for the issue of *The Cochrane Library* published in January 2007, the DARE and HTA records were supplied by CRD staff in November 2006. The January 2007 publication of *The Cochrane Library* was the current issue until April 2007, so the DARE and HTA records in *The Cochrane Library* range between being two months to five months out of date.

- www.crd.york.ac.uk/crdweb

CRD used to produce the CRD Ongoing Reviews Database which was searchable through the UK National Research Register (NRR) but since that was archived in September 2007, records of ongoing reviews have been transferred to the HTA Database.

Reviews and guidelines may also provide useful information about the search strategies used in their development: see Box 6.2.g. Specific evidence-based search services such as Turning Research into Practice (TRIP) can be used to identify reviews and guidelines. For the range of systematic review sources searched by TRIP see:

- www.tripdatabase.com/Aboutus/Publications/index.html?catid=11

A key source for identifying guidelines in the National Guideline Clearinghouse.

- www.guideline.gov

MEDLINE, EMBASE and other bibliographic databases can also be used to identify review articles and guidelines. In MEDLINE, the most appropriate review articles should be indexed under the Publication Type term 'Meta-analysis', which was introduced in 1993, or 'Review', which was introduced in 1966. Guidelines should be indexed under the Publication Type term 'Practice Guideline', which was introduced in 1991. EM-BASE also has a thesaurus term 'Systematic Review', which was introduced in 2003, and 'Practice Guideline', which was introduced in 1994.

There is a so-called 'Systematic Review' search strategy or filter on PubMed under the Clinical Queries link:

- www.ncbi.nlm.nih.gov/entrez/query/static/clinical.shtml

It is very broad in its scope and retrieves many references that are not systematic reviews. The strategy is described as follows: "This strategy is intended to retrieve citations identified as systematic reviews, meta-analyses, reviews of clinical trials, evidence-based medicine, consensus development conferences, guidelines, and citations to articles from journals specializing in review studies of value to clinicians."

- www.nlm.nih.gov/bsd/pubmed_subsets/sysreviews_strategy.html

Search strategies or filters have been developed to identify systematic reviews in MEDLINE (White 2001, Montori 2005) and EMBASE (Wilczynski 2007). Search strategies for identifying systematic reviews in other databases and for identifying guidelines are listed on the InterTASC Information Specialists' Subgroup Search Filter Resource web site.

- www.york.ac.uk/inst/crd/intertasc/sr.htm

---

**Box 6.2.g Examples of evidence-based guidelines**

- Australian National Health and Medical Research Council: Clinical Practice Guidelines:
  - nhmrc.gov.au/publications/subjects/clinical.htm
- Canadian Medical Association – Infobase: Clinical Practice Guidelines:
  - mdm.ca/cpgsnew/cpgs/index.asp
- National Guideline Clearinghouse (US):
  - www.guideline.gov/
- National Library of Guidelines (UK):
  - www.library.nhs.uk/guidelinesFinder/
- New Zealand Guidelines Group:
  - www.nzgg.org.nz
- NICE Clinical Guidelines (UK):
  - www.nice.org.uk/aboutnice/whatwedo/aboutclinicalguidelines/ about_clinical_ guidelines.jsp

As well as searching the references cited in existing systematic reviews and meta-analyses, reference lists of identified studies may also be searched for additional studies (Greenhalgh 2005). Since investigators may selectively cite studies with positive results, reference lists should be used with caution as an adjunct to other search methods (see Chapter 10, Section 10.2.2.3).

#### 6.2.2.6   Web searching

There is little empirical evidence as to the value of using general internet search engines such as Google to identify potential studies (Eysenbach 2001). Searching research funders' and device manufacturers' web sites might be fruitful. Searching pharmaceutical industry web sites may be useful, in particular their trials registers, covered in Section 6.2.3.3. If internet searches are conducted, it is recommended that review authors should file a print copy or save locally an electronic copy of details of information about any possibly relevant study found on the internet, rather than simply 'book-marking' the site, in case the record of the trial is removed or altered at a later stage. It is important to keep a record of the date the web site was accessed for citation purposes.

### 6.2.3   Unpublished and ongoing studies

Some completed studies are never published. An association between 'significant' results and publication has been documented across a number of studies, as summarized in Chapter 10 (Section 10.2). Finding out about unpublished studies, and including them in a systematic review when eligible and appropriate, is important for minimizing bias. There is no easy and reliable way to obtain information about studies that have been completed but never published. This situation is improving as a result of a number of initiatives:

- The International Standard Randomised Controlled Trial Number Register scheme launched as the first online service that provided unique numbers to randomized controlled trials in all areas of health care and from all countries around the world and subsequently ClinicalTrials.gov (see Section 6.2.3.1);

- The increasing acceptance on behalf of investigators of the importance of registering trials at inception;

- The support of registration at inception by the leading medical journal publishers and their refusal to subsequently publish reports of trials not properly registered (De Angelis 2004, De Angelis 2005);

- The US National Institutes for Health (NIH) Public Access Policy (see publicaccess. nih.gov/), which until December 2007 was voluntary but now requires that "all in-vestigators funded by the NIH submit or have submitted for them to the National

Library of Medicine's PubMed Central an electronic version of their final, peer-reviewed manuscripts upon acceptance for publication to be made publicly available no later than 12 months after the official date of publication".

○ publicaccess.nih.gov/policy.htm

Colleagues can be an important source of information about unpublished studies, and informal channels of communication can sometimes be the only means of identifying unpublished data. Formal letters of request for information can also be used to identify completed but unpublished studies. One way of doing this is to send a comprehensive list of relevant articles along with the inclusion criteria for the review to the first author of reports of included studies, asking if they know of any additional studies (published or unpublished) that might be relevant. It may also be desirable to send the same letter to other experts and pharmaceutical companies or others with an interest in the area. It should be borne in mind that asking researchers for information about completed but never published studies has not always been found to be fruitful (Hetherington 1989, Horton 1997) though some researchers have reported that this is an important method for retrieving studies for systematic reviews (Royle 2003, Greenhalgh 2005). Some organizations set up web sites for systematic review projects listing the studies identified to date and inviting submission of information on studies not already listed. It has also been suggested that legislation such as the Freedom of Information Acts in countries such as the UK and the US might be used to gain access to information about unpublished trials (Bennett 2003, MacLean 2003).

It is also important to identify ongoing studies, so that when a review is later updated these can be assessed for possible inclusion. Information about possibly relevant ongoing studies should be included in the review in the 'Characteristics of ongoing studies' table (see Chapter 4, Section 4.6.5). Awareness of the existence of a possibly relevant ongoing study might also affect decisions with respect to when to update a specific review. Unfortunately, no single, comprehensive, centralized register of ongoing trials exists (Manheimer 2002). Efforts have, however, been made by a number of organizations, including organizations representing the pharmaceutical industry and pharmaceutical companies themselves, to begin to provide central access to ongoing trials and in some cases trial results on completion, either on a national or international basis. In an effort to improve this situation, the World Health Organization (WHO) launched the International Clinical Trials Registry Platform Search Portal in May 2007 to search across a range of trials registers, similar to the initiative launched some years earlier by Current Controlled Trials with their so-called *meta*Register. Currently (as at June 2008) the WHO portal only searches across three primary registers (the Australian and New Zealand Clinical Trials Registry, ClinicalTrials.gov and the Current Controlled Trials International Standard Randomised Controlled Trial Number Register) but it is anticipated that other registers will be included as the project progresses.

### 6.2.3.1 *National and international trials registers*

Box 6.2.h lists national and international trials registers.

## Box 6.2.h Examples of national and international trials registers

- The Association of the British Pharmaceutical Industry (ABPI) – Pharmaceutical Industry Clinical Trials database:
  ○ www.cmrinteract.com/clintrial/
- The Australian New Zealand Clinical Trials Registry:
  ○ www.anzctr.org.au/
- CenterWatch Clinical Trials Listing Service:
  ○ www.centerwatch.com/
- Chinese Clinical Trial Register:
  ○ www.chictr.org/Default.aspx
- ClinicalTrials.gov register:
  ○ clinicaltrials.gov/
- Community Research & Development Information Service (of the European Union) (trials and other research):
  ○ cordis.europa.eu/en/home.html
- Current Controlled Trials *meta*Register of Controlled Trials (*m*RCT) – active registers:
  ○ www.controlled-trials.com/mrct/
- Current Controlled Trials *meta*Register of Controlled Trials (*m*RCT) – archived registers:
  ○ www.controlled-trials.com/mrct/archived
- European Medicines Agency (EMEA):
  ○ www.emea.europa.eu/index/indexh1.htm
- German trials register – not yet launched. Final agreement reached 30 August 2007 – will be included under the WHO International Clinical Trials Registry Platform Search Portal – for further details as and when available see:
  ○ www.who.int/trialsearch
- Hong Kong clinical trials register - HKClinicalTrials.com:
  ○ www.hkclinicaltrials.com/
- Indian clinical trials registry - Clinical Trials Registry – India (CTRI):
  ○ www.ctri.in
- International Clinical Trials Registry Platform Search Portal:
  ○ www.who.int/trialsearch
- International Federation of Pharmaceutical Manufacturers and Associations (IFPMA) Clinical Trials Portal:
  ○ www.ifpma.org/clinicaltrials.html
- International Standard Randomised Controlled Trial Number Register:
  ○ www.controlled-trials.com/isrctn/
- Netherlands trial register (Nederlands Trialregister – in Dutch):
  ○ www.trialregister.nl/trialreg/index.asp
- South African National Clinical Trial Register:
  ○ www.sanctr.gov.za/

- UK Clinical Research Network Portfolio Database:
  - portal.nihr.ac.uk/Pages/Portfolio.aspx
- UK Clinical Trials Gateway:
  - www.controlled-trials.com/ukctr/
- UK National Research Register (NRR) (trials and other research – archived September 2007 – see UK Clinical Trials Gateway):
  - portal.nihr.ac.uk/Pages/NRRArchive.aspx
- University hospital Medical Information Network (UMIN) Clinical Trials Registry (for Japan) – UMIN CTR:
  - www.umin.ac.jp/ctr/

In addition, Drugs@FDA provides information about most of the drugs approved in the US since 1939. For those approved more recently (from 1998), there is often a 'review', which contains the scientific analyses that provided the basis for approval of the new drug.

- www.accessdata.fda.gov/scripts/cder/drugsatfda/index.cfm

Other national and regional drug approval agencies may also be useful sources of trial information.

### 6.2.3.2  Subject-specific trials registers

There are many condition-specific trials registers, especially in the field of cancer – which are too numerous to list. They can be identified by searching the internet and by searching within some of the resources listed above such as the Current Controlled Trials *meta*Register of Controlled Trials (*m*RCT).

### 6.2.3.3  Pharmaceutical industry trials registers

Some pharmaceutical companies make available information about their clinical trials though their own web sites, either instead of or in addition to the information they make available through national or international web sites such as those listed above. Some examples are included in Box 6.2.i.

### 6.2.3.4  Trials results registers and other sources

Registers of the results of completed trials are a more recent phenomenon, following on from ongoing trials registers that simply list details of the trial. They are of particular value because trial results are not always published, and even if published are not

---

**Box 6.2.i   Examples of pharmaceutical industry trials registers**

- AstraZeneca Clinical Trials web site:
  ○ www.astrazenecaclinicaltrials.com/
- Bristol-Myers Squibb Clinical Trial Registry:
  ○ ctr.bms.com/ctd/registry.do
- Eli Lilly and Company Clinical Trial Registry (also includes trial results)
  ○ www.lillytrials.com/
- GlaxoSmithKline clinical trial register:
  ○ ctr.gsk.co.uk/medicinelist.asp
- NovartisClinicalTrials.com:
  ○ www.novartisclinicaltrials.com/webapp/etrials/home.do
- Roche Clinical Trial Protocol Registry:
  ○ www.roche-trials.com/registry.html
- Wyeth Clinical Trial Listings:
  ○ www.wyeth.com/ClinicalTrialListings

---

always published in full. Recent legislation in the US known as Section 801 of the Food and Drug Administration Amendments Act of 2007 (FDAAA 801), enacted in September 2007, called for expanding ClinicalTrials.gov and adding a clinical trial results database.

Examples of trials results registers are provided in Box 6.2.j.

In addition, Clinical Trial Results is a web site that hosts slide presentations from clinical trialists reporting the results of clinical trials:

- www.clinicaltrialresults.org/

---

**Box 6.2.j   Examples of trials results registers**

- International Federation of Pharmaceutical Manufacturers and Associations (IFPMA) Clinical Trials Portal:
  ○ www.ifpma.org/clinicaltrials.html
- PhRMA Clinical Study Results Database:
  ○ www.clinicalstudyresults.org/about
- Bristol-Myers Squibb Clinical Trial Results:
  ○ ctr.bms.com/ctd/results.do
- Eli Lilly and Company Clinical Trial Registry:
  ○ www.lillytrials.com/
- Roche Clinical Trials Results Database:
  ○ www.roche-trials.com/results.html
- Wyeth Clinical Trial Results:
  ○ www.wyeth.com/ClinicalTrialResults

### 6.2.4  Summary points

- Cochrane review authors should seek advice from their Trials Search Co-ordinator on sources to search.

- CENTRAL is considered to be the best single source of reports of trials for inclusion in Cochrane reviews.

- The three bibliographic databases generally considered to be the most important sources to search for studies for inclusion in Cochrane reviews are CENTRAL, MEDLINE and EMBASE.

- National, regional and subject-specific databases should be selected for searching according to the topic of the review.

- Conference abstracts and other grey literature can be an important source of studies for inclusion in reviews.

- Reference lists in other reviews, guidelines, included (and excluded) studies and other related articles should be searched for additional studies.

- Efforts should be made to identify unpublished studies.

- Ongoing trials should be identified and tracked for possible inclusion in reviews on completion.

- Trials registers and trials results registers are an important source of ongoing and unpublished trials.

## 6.3  Planning the search process

### 6.3.1  Involving Trials Search Co-ordinators and healthcare librarians in the search process

It is the responsibility of each CRG to support review authors in identifying reports of studies for inclusion in their reviews, and most CRGs employ a Trials Search Co-ordinator to fulfil this role (see Section 6.1.1.1). Most CRGs offer support to authors in study identification from the early planning stage to the final write-up of the review for publication in the *CDSR*. This support might include designing search strategies or advising on their design, running searches, in particular in databases not available to the review author at their institution, and providing review authors with lists of references to studies from the CRG's Specialized Register and possibly from other databases. The range of services offered varies across CRGs according to the resources available.

Review authors are, therefore, encouraged to contact the Trials Search Co-ordinator of their CRG at the earliest stage for advice and support.

If authors are conducting their own searches, they should seek advice from their Trials Search Co-ordinator with respect to which database(s) to search and the exact strategies to be run. It should also be borne in mind that the search process needs to be documented in enough detail throughout to ensure that it can be reported correctly in the review, to the extent that all the searches of all the databases are reproducible. The full search strategies for each database should be included in the review in an Appendix. It is, therefore, important that review authors should save all search strategies and take notes at the time to enable the completion of that section at the appropriate time. For further guidance on this, authors should contact their Trials Search Co-ordinator, and see Section 6.6.

If the CRG is currently without a Trials Search Co-ordinator it is recommended that review authors seek guidance from a healthcare librarian or information specialist, where possible with experience of supporting systematic reviews.

## 6.3.2 Collaboration-wide search initiatives

In planning the search process it is necessary to take into account what other searching has already been undertaken to avoid unnecessary duplication of effort. For example, considerable efforts over the years have gone into searching MEDLINE and EMBASE and incorporating reports of trials from these two major international databases into the Cochrane Central Register of Controlled Trials (CENTRAL). It is necessary, therefore, that any additional searching for a specific review should take into account what has gone before. Figure 6.3.a illustrates the contents of CENTRAL.

### 6.3.2.1   *What is in The Cochrane Central Register of Controlled Trials (CENTRAL) from MEDLINE?*

CENTRAL contains all records from MEDLINE indexed with the Publication Type term 'Randomized Controlled Trial' or 'Controlled Clinical Trial' that are indexed as human studies. These records are downloaded quarterly from MEDLINE by Wiley-Blackwell as part of the build of CENTRAL for publication in *The Cochrane Library*. For further details see:

- www3.interscience.wiley.com/cgi-bin/mrwhome/106568753/CENTRALHelpFile.html

A substantial proportion of the MEDLINE records coded 'Randomized Controlled Trial' or 'Controlled Clinical Trial' in the Publication Type field have been coded as a result of the work of The Cochrane Collaboration (Dickersin 2002). Handsearch results from Cochrane entities, for journals indexed in MEDLINE, have been sent to the US National Library of Medicine (NLM), where the MEDLINE records have been re-tagged with the publication types 'Randomized Controlled Trial' or 'Controlled Clinical

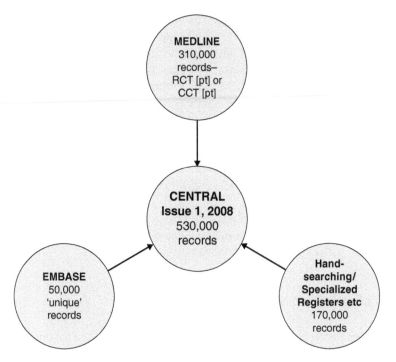

**Figure 6.3.a**   Illustration of the contents of CENTRAL

Trial' as appropriate. In addition, the US Cochrane Center (formerly the New England Cochrane Center, Providence Office and the Baltimore Cochrane Center) and the UK Cochrane Centre have conducted an electronic search of MEDLINE from 1966–2004 to identify reports of randomized controlled trials, identifiable from the MEDLINE titles and/or abstracts, not already indexed as such, using the first two phases of the Cochrane Highly Sensitive Search Strategy first published in 1994 (Dickersin 1994) and subsequently updated and included in the *Handbook*. The free text terms used were: clinical trial; (singl\$ OR doubl\$ OR trebl\$ OR tripl\$) AND (mask\$ OR blind\$); placebo\$; random\$. The \$ sign indicates the use of a truncation symbol. The following subject index terms (MeSH) used were exploded: randomized controlled trials; random allocation; double-blind method; single-blind method; clinical trials; placebos. The following subject heading (MeSH) was used unexploded: research design. The Publication Type terms used were: randomized controlled trial; controlled clinical trial; clinical trial.

A test was carried out using the terms in phase three of the 1994 Cochrane Highly Sensitive Search Strategy but the precision of those terms, having already searched on all the terms in phases one and two as listed above, was considered to be too low to warrant using these terms for the above project (Lefebvre 2001). It was, however, recognized that some of these terms might be useful when combined with subject terms to identify studies for some specific reviews (Eisinga 2007).

The above search was limited to humans. The following years were completed by the US Cochrane Center (1966–1984; 1998–2004) and by the UK Cochrane Centre (1985–1997). The results have been forwarded to the NLM and re-tagged in MEDLINE and are thus included in CENTRAL. This project is currently on hold. If the US Cochrane Center can attract funding for this project they will continue the electronic search of records entered into MEDLINE in 2005 and beyond. Any updates to this situation will be described in the CENTRAL Creation Details file in *The Cochrane Library*:

- www3.interscience.wiley.com/cgi-bin/mrwhome/106568753/ CENTRALHelpFile.html

CENTRAL includes from MEDLINE not only reports of trials that meet the more restrictive Cochrane definition for a controlled clinical trial (Box 6.3.a) but also trial reports that meet the less restrictive original NLM definition (Box 6.3.b), which used to include historical comparisons. There is currently no method of distinguishing, either in CENTRAL or in MEDLINE, which of these records meet the more restrictive Cochrane definition, as they are all indexed with the Publication Type term 'Controlled Clinical Trial'.

### 6.3.2.2    What is in The Cochrane Central Register of Controlled Trials (CENTRAL) from EMBASE?

In a study similar to that described above for MEDLINE, a search of EMBASE has been carried out by the UK Cochrane Centre for reports of trials not indexed as trials in MEDLINE (Lefebvre 2008). (Trials indexed as such in MEDLINE are already included in CENTRAL as described in Section 6.3.2.1, and are therefore de-duplicated against the EMBASE records as part of the search process.) The following terms are those currently used for the project and have been searched for the years 1980 to 2006: free-text terms: random$; factorial$; crossover$; cross over$; cross-over$; placebo$; doubl$ adj blind$; singl$ adj blind$; assign$; allocat$; volunteer$; and index terms, known as EMTREE terms: crossover-procedure; double-blind procedure; randomized controlled trial; single-blind procedure. A search for the years 1974 to 1979 inclusive has also been completed for the free-text terms: random$; factorial$; crossover$ and placebo$. The $ sign indicates the use of a truncation symbol.

These searches have yielded a total of 80,000 reports of trials not, at the time of the search, indexed as reports of trials in MEDLINE. All of these records are now published in CENTRAL, under contract between Elsevier, the publishers of EMBASE, and The Cochrane Collaboration. Of these 80,000 records, 50,000 are 'unique' to CENTRAL, that is they are not already included in CENTRAL with the records sourced from MEDLINE. This search is updated annually. Updates are described in the CENTRAL Creation Details file in *The Cochrane Library*:

- www3.interscience.wiley.com/cgi-bin/mrwhome/106568753/ CENTRALHelpFile.html

and the What's New section on *The Cochrane Library* home page:

- www3.interscience.wiley.com/cgi-bin/mrwhome/106568753/HOME

**Box 6.3.a   Cochrane definitions and criteria for randomized controlled trials (RCTs) and controlled clinical trials (CCTs)**

Records identified for inclusion should meet the eligibility criteria devised and agreed in November 1992, which were first published, in 1994, in the first version of the *Handbook* (see Chapter 1, Section 1.4). According to these eligibility criteria: A trial is eligible if, on the basis of the best available information (usually from one or more published reports), it is judged that:

- the individuals (or other units) followed in the trial were definitely or possibly assigned prospectively to one of two (or more) alternative forms of health care using
  - random allocation or
  - some quasi-random method of allocation (such as alternation, date of birth, or case record number).

Trials eligible for inclusion are classified according to the reader's degree of certainty that random allocation was used to form the comparison groups in the trial. If the author(s) state explicitly (usually by some variant of the term 'random' to describe the allocation procedure used) that the groups compared in the trial were established by random allocation, then the trial is classified as a RCT (randomized controlled trial). If the author(s) do not state explicitly that the trial was randomized, but randomization cannot be ruled out, the report is classified as a CCT (controlled clinical trial). The classification CCT is also applied to quasi-randomized studies, where the method of allocation is known but is not considered strictly random, and possibly quasi-randomized trials. Examples of quasi-random methods of assignment include alternation, date of birth, and medical record number.

The classification as RCT or CCT is based solely on what the author has written, not on the reader's interpretation; thus, it is not meant to reflect an assessment of the true nature or quality of the allocation procedure. For example, although 'double-blind' trials are nearly always randomized, many trial reports fail to mention random allocation explicitly and should therefore be classified as CCT.

Relevant reports are reports published in any year, of studies comparing at least two forms of health care (healthcare treatment, healthcare education, diagnostic tests or techniques, a preventive intervention, etc.) where the study is on either living humans or parts of their body or human parts that will be replaced in living humans (e.g., donor kidneys). Studies on cadavers, extracted teeth, cell lines, etc. are not relevant. *Searchers should identify all controlled trials meeting these criteria regardless of relevance to the entity with which they are affiliated.*

The highest possible proportion of all reports of controlled trials of health care should be included in CENTRAL. Thus, those searching the literature to identify trials should give reports the benefit of any doubts. Review authors will decide whether to include a particular report in a review.

---

**Box 6.3.b   US National Library of Medicine 2008 definitions for the Publication Type terms 'Randomized Controlled Trial' and 'Controlled Clinical Trial'**

### Randomized Controlled Trial

Work consisting of a clinical trial that involves at least one test treatment and one control treatment, concurrent enrolment and follow-up of the test- and control-treated groups, and in which the treatments to be administered are selected by a random process, such as the use of a random-numbers table.

### Controlled Clinical Trial

Work consisting of a clinical trial involving one or more test treatments, at least one control treatment, specified outcome measures for evaluating the studied intervention, and a bias-free method for assigning patients to the test treatment. The treatment may be drugs, devices, or procedures studied for diagnostic, therapeutic, or prophylactic effectiveness. Control measures include placebos, active medicine, no-treatment, dosage forms and regimens, historical comparisons, etc. When randomization using mathematical techniques, such as the use of a random-numbers table, is employed to assign patients to test or control treatments, the trial is characterized as a 'Randomized Controlled Trial'.

---

#### 6.3.2.3   *What is in The Cochrane Central Register of Controlled Trials (CENTRAL) from other databases and handsearching?*

Other general healthcare databases such as those published in Australia and China have undergone similar systematic searches to identify reports of trials for CENTRAL. The Australasian Cochrane Centre co-ordinated a search of the National Library of Australia's Australasian Medical Index from 1966 (McDonald 2002). This search has recently been updated to include records added up to 2007. The Chinese Cochrane Center, with support from the Australasian Cochrane Centre, co-ordinated a search of the Chinese Biomedical Literature Database from 1999 to 2001. In an ongoing project, the Chinese Cochrane Center, with support from the UK Cochrane Centre, is searching a number of Chinese sources with a view to including these records in CENTRAL. Similarly, the Brazilian Cochrane Centre in collaboration with the Regional Library of Medicine in Brazil (BIblioteca REgional de MEdicina – BIREME) is planning to co-ordinate a search of the Pan American Health Organization's database LILACS (Latin American Caribbean Health Sciences Literature).

Each of the Cochrane Centres has the responsibility for searching the general healthcare literature of its country or region. The CRGs and Fields are responsible for co-ordinating searching of the specialist healthcare literature in their areas of interest. More than 3000 journals have been, or are being, handsearched. Identified trial reports that are not relevant to a CRG's scope and thus are not appropriate for their Specialized Register (see below) are forwarded to Wiley-Blackwell as handsearch results. Handsearch records can be identified in CENTRAL as they are assigned the tag HS-HANDSRCH or HS-PRECENTRL.

- www3.interscience.wiley.com/cgi-bin/mrwhome/106568753/ CENTRALHelpFile.html

### 6.3.2.4 What is in The Cochrane Central Register of Controlled Trials (CENTRAL) from Specialized Registers of Cochrane Review Groups and Fields?

It is an 'essential core function' of CRGs that their "editorial bases develop and maintain a Specialized Register, containing all relevant studies in their area of interest, and submit this to CENTRAL on a quarterly basis", as outlined in Section 3.2.1.5 'Core functions of Cochrane Review Groups' in The Cochrane Manual (www.cochrane.org/admin/manual.htm).

The Specialized Register serves to ensure that individual review authors within the CRG have easy and reliable access to trials relevant to their review topic, normally through their Trials Search Co-ordinator. CRGs use the methods described in this chapter of the *Handbook* to identify trials for their Specialized Registers. Most CRGs also have systems in place to ensure that any additional eligible reports identified by authors for their review(s) are contributed to the CRG's Specialized Register. The registers are, in turn, submitted for inclusion in CENTRAL on a quarterly basis. Thus, records included in the Specialized Register of one CRG become accessible to all other CRGs through CENTRAL. Many Fields also develop subject-specific Specialized Registers and submit them for inclusion in CENTRAL as described above. To identify records in CENTRAL from within a specific Specialized Register it is possible to search on the Specialized Register tag, such as SR-STROKE. A list of all the Specialized Register tags can be found in the 'Appendix: Review Group or Field/Network Specialized Register Codes' in the 'CENTRAL Creation Details' Help File in *The Cochrane Library*:

- www3.interscience.wiley.com/cgi-bin/mrwhome/106568753/ CENTRALHelpFile.html

Records in a CRG's Specialized Register will often contain coding and other information not included in CENTRAL, so the Trials Search Co-ordinator will often be able to identify additional records in their Specialized Register, which could not be identified by searching in CENTRAL, by searching for these codes in the Specialized Register. Conversely, the search functionality of the bibliographic or other software used to manage Specialized Registers is usually less sophisticated than the search functionality available in *The Cochrane Library* so a search of CENTRAL will retrieve records from the Specialized Register that may not be easily retrievable from within the Specialized Register itself. It is therefore recommended that both CENTRAL and the Specialized Register itself are searched separately to maximize retrieval.

## 6.3.3   Searching CENTRAL, MEDLINE and EMBASE: specific issues

It is recommended that for all Cochrane reviews, CENTRAL and MEDLINE should be searched, as a minimum, together with EMBASE if it is available to either the CRG or the review author.

### *6.3.3.1   Searching The Cochrane Central Register of Controlled Trials (CENTRAL): specific issues*

CENTRAL is comprised of records from a wide range of sources (see Sections 6.2.1.2 and 6.3.2 and sub-sections), so there is no consistency in the format or content of the records.

The 310,000 records sourced from MEDLINE are best retrieved by a combination of Medical Subject Heading (MeSH) and free-text terms. The other records, including the 50,000 records sourced from EMBASE, are best retrieved using free-text searches across all fields.

Most of the records that do not come from MEDLINE or EMBASE (about 170,000 in *The Cochrane Library* Issue 1, 2008) do not have abstracts or any indexing terms. To retrieve these records, which consist predominantly of titles only, it is necessary to carry out a very broad search consisting of a wide range of free-text terms, which may be considered too broad to run across the whole of CENTRAL.

It is possible to identify the records that have been sourced from MEDLINE and EMBASE by searching in CENTRAL for those records that have PubMed or EMBASE accession numbers. It is possible then to exclude these records from a broad search of CENTRAL, as illustrated in the example in Box 6.3.c.

For general information about searching, which is relevant to searching CENTRAL, see Section 6.4.

### *6.3.3.2   Searching MEDLINE and EMBASE: specific issues*

Despite the fact that both MEDLINE and EMBASE have been searched systematically for reports of trials and that these reports of trials have been included in CENTRAL, as described in Sections 6.3.2.1 and 6.3.2.2, supplementary searches of both MEDLINE and EMBASE are recommended. Any such searches, however, should be undertaken in the knowledge of what searching has already been conducted to avoid duplication of effort.

*Searching MEDLINE*   There is a delay of some months between records being indexed in MEDLINE and appearing indexed as reports of trials in CENTRAL, since

---

**Box 6.3.c   Example of exclusion of MEDLINE and EMBASE records when searching CENTRAL**

Note: the example is for illustrative purposes only. A search of CENTRAL for a systematic review on this topic would require a wide range of alternative terms for both tamoxifen and breast cancer.

```
#1   "accession number" near pubmed
#2   "accession number" near2 embase
#3   #1 or #2
#4   tamoxifen
#5   (breast near cancer)
#6   #4 and #5
#7   #6 not #3
```

---

CENTRAL is only updated quarterly. For example, for the issue of *The Cochrane Library* published in January 2007, the MEDLINE records were downloaded by Wiley-Blackwell staff in November 2006. The January 2007 publication of *The Cochrane Library* was the current issue until April 2007, so the MEDLINE records range between being two to five months out of date. The most recent months of MEDLINE should, therefore, be searched, at least for records indexed as either 'Randomized Controlled Trial' or 'Controlled Clinical Trial' in the Publication Type, to identify those records recently indexed as RCTs or CCTs in MEDLINE.

Additionally, the most recent year to be searched under the project to identify reports of trials in MEDLINE and send them back to the US National Library of Medicine for re-tagging was 2004, so records added to MEDLINE during and since 2005 should be searched using one of the search strategies described in Section 6.4.11.1.

Finally, for extra sensitivity, or where the use of a randomized trial 'filter' is not appropriate, review authors should search MEDLINE for all years using subject terms only.

It should be remembered that the MEDLINE re-tagging project described in Section 6.3.2.1 assessed whether the records identified were reports of trials on the basis of the title and abstract only, so any supplementary search of MEDLINE that is followed up by accessing the full text of the articles will identify additional reports of trials, most likely through the methods sections, that were not identified through the titles or abstracts alone.

For guidance on running separate search strategies in the MEDLINE-indexed versions of MEDLINE and the versions of MEDLINE containing 'in process' and other non-indexed records please refer to Section 6.4.11.1.

Any reports of trials identified by the review author can be submitted to the Trials Search Co-ordinator who can ensure that they are added to CENTRAL. Any errors, in respect of records indexed as trials in MEDLINE that on the basis of the full article are definitely not reports of trials according to the definitions used by the National Library of Medicine (NLM) (see Section 6.3.2.1), should also be reported to the Trials Search Co-ordinator, so they can be referred to the NLM and corrected.

For general information about searching, which is relevant to searching MEDLINE, see Section 6.4.

***Searching EMBASE*** The project to identify reports of trials in EMBASE for inclusion in CENTRAL, described in Section 6.3.2.2, is carried out on an annual basis, so there is a time lag of approximately one to two years with respect to EMBASE records appearing in CENTRAL. The last two years of EMBASE should, therefore, be searched to cover work still in progress. Some suggested search terms are listed in Section 6.3.2.2. A search filter designed by the McMaster Hedges Team is also available (Wong 2006).

Finally, for extra sensitivity, or where the use of a randomized trial 'filter' is not appropriate, review authors should search EMBASE for all years using subject terms only, as described under similar circumstances for MEDLINE above. It should be remembered that the EMBASE project described above assessed whether the records identified were reports of trials on the basis of the title and abstract only, in the same way as the MEDLINE project described above. Therefore, any supplementary search of EMBASE that is followed up by accessing the full text of the articles will identify additional reports of trials, most likely through the methods sections, that were not identified through the titles or abstracts alone.

For general information about searching, which is relevant to searching EMBASE, see Section 6.4.

## 6.3.4  Summary points

- Cochrane review authors should seek advice from their Trials Search Co-ordinator throughout the search process.

- It is recommended that for all Cochrane reviews CENTRAL and MEDLINE should be searched, as a minimum, together with EMBASE if it is available to either the CRG or the review author.

- The full search strategies for each database searched will need to be included in an Appendix of the review, so all search strategies should be saved, and notes taken of the number of records retrieved for each database searched.

- CENTRAL contains over 350,000 records from MEDLINE and EMBASE, so care should be taken when searching MEDLINE and EMBASE to avoid unnecessary duplication of effort.

- MEDLINE should be searched from 2005 onwards inclusive using one of the revised and updated Cochrane Highly Sensitive Search Strategies for identifying randomized trials in MEDLINE as outlined in Section 6.4.11.1.

- EMBASE should be searched for the most recent two years as outlined in Section 6.4.11.2.

- Additional studies can be identified in MEDLINE and EMBASE by searching across the years already searched for CENTRAL, by obtaining the full article and by reading, in particular, the methods section.

## 6.4 Designing search strategies

### 6.4.1 Designing search strategies – an introduction

This section highlights some of the issues to consider when designing search strategies, but does not adequately address the many complexities in this area. It is in particular in this aspect of searching for studies that the skills of a Trials Search Co-ordinator or healthcare librarian are highly recommended. Many of the issues highlighted below relate to both the methodological aspect of the search (such as identifying reports of randomized trials) and the subject of the search. For a search to be robust both aspects require equal attention to be sure that relevant records are not missed.

The eligibility criteria for studies to be included in the review will inform how the search is conducted (see Chapter 5). The eligibility criteria will specify the types of designs, types of participants, types of intervention (experimental and comparator) and, in some cases, the types of outcomes to be addressed. Issues to consider in planning a search include the following:

- whether the review is limited to randomized trials or whether other study designs will be included (see also Chapter 13);

- the requirement to identify adverse effects data (see also Chapter 14);

- the nature of the intervention(s) being assessed;

- any geographic considerations such as the need to search the Chinese literature for studies in Chinese herbal medicine;

- the time period when any evaluations of these interventions may have taken place; and

- whether data from unpublished studies are to be included.

## 6.4.2 Structure of a search strategy

The structure of a search strategy should be based on the main concepts being examined in a review. For a Cochrane review, the review title should provide these concepts and the eligibility criteria for studies to be included will further assist in the selection of appropriate subject headings and text words for the search strategy.

It is usually unnecessary, and even undesirable, to search on every aspect of the review's clinical question (often referred to as PICO – that is Patient (or Participant or Population), Intervention, Comparison and Outcome). Although a research question may address particular populations, settings or outcomes, these concepts may not be well described in the title or abstract of an article and are often not well indexed with controlled vocabulary terms. They generally, therefore, do not lend themselves well to searching. In general databases, such as MEDLINE, a search strategy to identify studies for a Cochrane review will typically have three sets of terms: 1) terms to search for the health condition of interest, i.e. the population; 2) terms to search for the intervention(s) evaluated; and 3) terms to search for the types of study design to be included (typically a 'filter' for randomized trials). CENTRAL, however, aims to contain only reports with study designs possibly relevant for inclusion in Cochrane reviews, so searches of CENTRAL should not use a trials 'filter'. Filters to identify randomized trials and controlled trials have been developed specifically for MEDLINE and guidance is also given for searching EMBASE: see Section 6.4.11 and sub-sections. For reviews of complex interventions, it may be necessary to adopt a different approach, for example by searching only for the population or the intervention (Khan 2001).

## 6.4.3 Service providers and search interfaces

Both MEDLINE and EMBASE are offered by a number of service providers, via a range of search interfaces; for example Dialog offers both Dialog and DataStar. In addition the US National Library of Medicine and Elsevier both offer access to their own versions of MEDLINE and EMBASE respectively: MEDLINE through PubMed, which is available free of charge on the internet, and EMBASE through EMBASE.com which is available on subscription only. Search syntax varies across interfaces. For example, to search for the Publication Type term 'Randomized Controlled Trial' in the various search interfaces it is necessary to enter the term as:

randomized controlled trial.pt. (in Ovid)

randomized controlled trial [pt] (in PubMed)

randomized controlled trial in pt (in SilverPlatter)

Many service providers offer links to full-text versions of articles on other publishers' web sites, such as the PubMed 'Links/LinkOut' feature.

## 6.4.4　Sensitivity versus precision

Searches for systematic reviews aim to be as extensive as possible in order to ensure that as many as possible of the necessary and relevant studies are included in the review. It is, however, necessary to strike a balance between striving for comprehensiveness and maintaining relevance when developing a search strategy. Increasing the comprehensiveness (or sensitivity) of a search will reduce its precision and will retrieve more non-relevant articles.

Sensitivity is defined as the number of relevant reports identified divided by the total number of relevant reports in existence. Precision is defined as the number of relevant reports identified divided by the total number of reports identified.

Developing a search strategy is an iterative process in which the terms that are used are modified, based on what has already been retrieved. There are diminishing returns for search efforts; after a certain stage, each additional unit of time invested in searching returns fewer references that are relevant to the review. Consequently there comes a point where the rewards of further searching may not be worth the effort required to identify the additional references. The decision as to how much to invest in the search process depends on the question a review addresses, the extent to which the CRG's Specialized Register is developed, and the resources that are available. It should be noted, however, that article abstracts identified through a literature search can be 'scan-read' very quickly to ascertain potential relevance. At a conservatively-estimated reading rate of two abstracts per minute, the results of a database search can be 'scan-read' at the rate of 120 per hour (or approximately 1000 over an 8-hour period), so the high yield and low precision associated with systematic review searching is not as daunting as it might at first appear in comparison with the total time to be invested in the review.

## 6.4.5　Controlled vocabulary and text words

MEDLINE and EMBASE (and many other databases) can be searched using standardized subject terms assigned by indexers. Standardized subject terms (as part of a controlled vocabulary or thesaurus) are useful because they provide a way of retrieving articles that may use different words to describe the same concept and because they can provide information beyond that which is simply contained in the words of the title and abstract. When searching for studies for a systematic review, however, the extent to which subject terms are applied to references should be viewed with caution. Authors may not describe their methods or objectives well and indexers are not always experts in the subject areas or methodological aspects of the articles that they are indexing. In addition, the available indexing terms might not correspond to the terms the searcher wishes to use.

The controlled vocabulary search terms for MEDLINE (MeSH) and EMBASE (EMTREE) are not identical, and neither is the approach to indexing. For example, the pharmaceutical or pharmacological aspects of an EMBASE record are generally indexed in greater depth than the equivalent MEDLINE record, and in recent years

Elsevier has increased the number of index terms assigned to each EMBASE record. Searches of EMBASE may, therefore, retrieve additional articles that were not retrieved by a MEDLINE search, even if the records were present in both databases. Search strategies need to be customized for each database.

One way to begin to identify controlled vocabulary terms for a particular database is to retrieve articles from that database that meet the inclusion criteria for the review, and to note common text words and the subject terms the indexers have applied to the articles, which can then be used for a full search. Having identified a key article, additional relevant articles can be located, for example by using the 'Find Similar' option in Ovid or the 'Related Articles' option in PubMed. Additional controlled vocabulary terms should be identified using the search tools provided with the database, such as the Permuted Index under Search Tools in Ovid and the MeSH Database option in PubMed.

Many database thesauri offer the facility to 'explode' subject terms to include more specific terms automatically in the search. For example, a MEDLINE search using the MeSH term BRAIN INJURIES, if exploded, will automatically search not only for the term BRAIN INJURIES but also for the more specific term SHAKEN BABY SYNDROME. As articles in MEDLINE on the subject of shaken baby syndrome should only be indexed with the more specific term SHAKEN BABY SYNDROME and not also with the more general term BRAIN INJURIES it is important that MeSH terms are 'exploded' wherever appropriate, in order not to miss relevant articles. The same principle applies to EMTREE when searching EMBASE and also to a number of other databases. For further guidance on this topic, review authors should consult their Trials Search Co-ordinator or healthcare librarian.

It is particularly important in MEDLINE to distinguish between Publication Type terms and other related MeSH terms. For example, a report of a randomized trial would be indexed in MEDLINE with the Publication Type term 'Randomized Controlled Trial' whereas an article about randomized controlled trials would be indexed with the MeSH term RANDOMIZED CONTROLLED TRIALS AS TOPIC (note the latter is plural). The same applies to other indexing terms for trials, reviews and meta-analyses.

Review authors should assume that earlier articles are even harder to identify than recent articles. For example, abstracts are not included in MEDLINE for most articles published before 1976 and, therefore, text word searches will only apply to titles. In addition, few MEDLINE indexing terms relating to study design were available before the 1990s, so text word searches are necessary to retrieve older records.

In order to identify as many relevant records as possible searches should comprise a combination of subject terms selected from the controlled vocabulary or thesaurus ('exploded' where appropriate) with a wide range of free-text terms.

### 6.4.6  Synonyms, related terms, variant spellings, truncation and wildcards

When designing a search strategy, in order to be as comprehensive as possible, it is necessary to include a wide range of free-text terms for each of the concepts selected.

For example:

- synonyms: 'pressure sore' OR 'decubitus ulcer', etc;

- related terms: 'brain' OR 'head', etc; and

- variant spellings: 'tumour' OR 'tumor'.

Service providers offer facilities to capture these variations through truncation and wildcards:

- truncation: random* (for random or randomised or randomized or randomly, etc); and

- wildcard: wom?n (for woman or women).

These features vary across service providers. For further details refer to the service provider help files for the database in question.

### 6.4.7   Boolean operators (AND, OR and NOT)

A search strategy should build up the controlled vocabulary terms, text words, synonyms and related terms for each concept at a time, joining together each of the terms within each concept with the Boolean 'OR' operator: see demonstration search strategy (Figure 6.4.f). This means articles will be retrieved that contain at least one of these search terms. Sets of terms should usually be developed for the healthcare condition, intervention(s) and study design. These three sets of terms can then be joined together with the 'AND' operator. This final step of joining the three sets with the 'AND' operator limits the retrieved set to articles of the appropriate study design that address both the health condition of interest and the intervention(s) to be evaluated. A note of caution about this approach is warranted however: if an article does not contain at least one term from each of the three sets, it will not be identified. For example, if an index term has not been added to the record for the intervention and the intervention is not mentioned in the title and abstract, the article would be missed. A possible remedy is to omit one of the three sets of terms and decide which records to check on the basis of the number retrieved and the time available to check them. The 'NOT' operator should be avoided where possible to avoid the danger of inadvertently removing from the search set records that are relevant. For example, when searching for records indexed as female, 'NOT male' would remove any record that was about both males and females.

   Searches for Cochrane reviews can be extremely long, often including over 100 search statements. It can be tedious to type in the combinations of these search sets, for example as '#1 OR #2 OR #3 OR #4 .... OR #100'. Some service providers offer alternatives to this. For example, in Ovid it is possible to combine sets using the syntax 'or/1-100'. For those service providers where this is not possible, including *The*

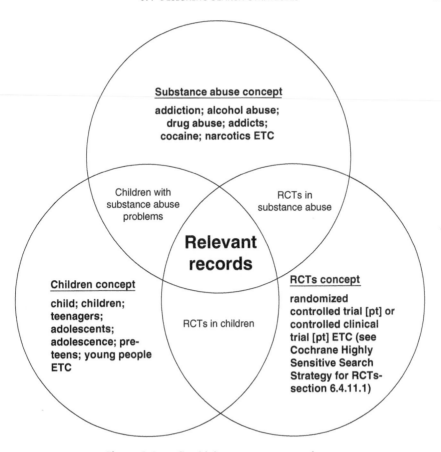

**Figure 6.4.a**   Combining concepts as search sets

*Cochrane Library* for searches of CENTRAL, it has been recommended that the search string above could be typed in full and saved, for example, as a Word document and the requisite number of combinations copied and pasted into the search as required. Having typed the string with the # symbols as above, a second string can be generated by globally replacing the # symbol with nothing to create the string '1 OR 2 OR 3 OR 4 .... OR 100' to be used for those service providers where the search interface does not use the # symbol.

## 6.4.8   Proximity operators (NEAR, NEXT and ADJ)

In some search interfaces it is necessary to specify, for example by using the 'NEXT' or 'ADJ' operator, that two search terms should be adjacent to each other, as the search might simply default to finding both words in the document as if the 'AND' operator had been used. It should be noted that the 'NEXT' operator in *The Cochrane Library* is more sensitive (i.e. retrieves more hits) than the alternative method of phrase searching using quotation marks, since quotation marks specify that exact phrase whereas the 'NEXT' operator incorporates auto-pluralization and auto-singularization as well as other variant word endings.

In addition, it is possible in many search interfaces to specify that the words should be within a specific number of words of each other. For example, the 'NEAR' operator in *The Cochrane Library* will find the search terms within six words of each other. This results in higher sensitivity than simple phrase searching or use of the 'NEXT' operator but greater precision than use of the 'AND' operator. It is, therefore, desirable to use this operator where available and relevant.

## 6.4.9    Language, date and document format restrictions

Research related to identifying trials has recently focused on the effect of excluding versus including from meta-analyses trials reported in languages other than English. This question is particularly important because the identification and translation of, or at least data extraction from, trials reported in languages other than English can substantially add to the costs of a review and the time taken to complete it. For further discussion of these issues, see Chapter 10 (Section 10.2.2.4). Whenever possible review authors should attempt to identify and assess for eligibility all possibly relevant reports of trials irrespective of language of publication. No language restrictions should be included in the search strategy. Date restrictions should be applied only if it is known that relevant studies could only have been reported during a specific time period, for example if the intervention was only available after a certain time point. Format restrictions such as excluding letters are not recommended because letters may contain important additional information relating to an earlier trial report or new information about a trial not reported elsewhere.

## 6.4.10    Identifying fraudulent studies, other retracted publications, errata and comments

When considering the eligibility of studies for inclusion in a Cochrane review, it is important to be aware that some studies may have been found to be fraudulent or may for other reasons have been retracted since publication. Reports of studies indexed in MEDLINE that have been retracted (as fraudulent or for other reasons) will have the Publication Type term 'Retracted Publication' added to the record. The article giving notice of the retraction will have the Publication Type term 'Retraction of Publication' assigned. Prior to any decision being taken to retract an article, articles may be published that refer to an original article and raise concerns of this sort. Such articles would be classified as a Comment. The US National Library of Medicine's (NLM's) policy on this is that "Among the types of articles that will be considered comments are: . . . . .

announcements or notices that report questionable science or investigations of scientific misconduct (sometimes published as 'Expression of concern')".

- www.nlm.nih.gov/pubs/factsheets/errata.html

In addition, articles may have been partially retracted, corrected through a published erratum or may have been corrected and re-published in full. When updating a review, it is important to search MEDLINE for the latest version of the citations to the records for the included studies. In some display formats of some versions of MEDLINE the retracted publication, erratum and comment statements are included in the citation data immediately after the title and are, therefore, highly visible. This is not, however, always the case so care should be taken to ensure that this information is always retrieved in all searches by downloading the appropriate fields together with the citation data (see Section 6.5.2). For further details of NLM's policy and practice in this area see:

- www.nlm.nih.gov/pubs/factsheets/errata.html

### 6.4.11   Search filters

Search filters are search strategies that are designed to retrieve specific types of records, such as those of a particular methodological design. They may be subjectively derived strategies such as the original Cochrane Highly Sensitive Search Strategy for identifying reports of randomized trials in MEDLINE (Dickersin 1994) or they may be objectively derived by word frequency analysis and tested on data sets of relevant records to assess their sensitivity and precision, such as the search strategies below for identifying randomized trials in MEDLINE (Glanville 2006). Recently a search filters web site has been developed by the UK InterTASC Information Specialists Subgroup (ISSG), which is the group of information professionals supporting research groups within England and Scotland providing technology assessments to the National Institute for Health and Clinical Excellence (NICE) (Glanville 2008). The purpose of the web site is to list methodological search filters and to provide critical appraisals of the various filters. The site includes, amongst others, filters for identifying systematic reviews, randomized and non-randomized studies and qualitative research in a range of databases and across a range of service providers.

- www.york.ac.uk/inst/crd/intertasc/

Search filters should be used with caution. They should be assessed not only for the reliability of their development and reported performance but also for their current accuracy, relevance and effectiveness given the frequent interface and indexing changes affecting databases. The ISSG offer a search filter appraisal tool to assist with assessing search filters and examples can be seen on the website.

- www.york.ac.uk/inst/crd/intertasc/qualitat.htm

### 6.4.11.1  The Cochrane Highly Sensitive Search Strategies for identifying randomized trials in MEDLINE

The first Cochrane Highly Sensitive Search Strategy for identifying randomized trials in MEDLINE was designed by Carol Lefebvre and published in 1994 (Dickersin 1994). This strategy was subsequently published in the *Handbook* and has been adapted and updated as necessary over time. The Cochrane Highly Sensitive Search Strategies for MEDLINE in subsequent sections are adapted from strategies first published in 2006 as a result of a frequency analysis of MeSH terms and free-text terms occurring in the titles and abstracts of MEDLINE-indexed records of reports of randomized controlled trials (Glanville 2006), using methods of search strategy design first developed by the authors to identify systematic reviews in MEDLINE (White 2001).

Two strategies are offered: a sensitivity-maximizing version and a sensitivity- and precision-maximizing version. It is recommended that searches for trials for inclusion in Cochrane reviews begin with the sensitivity-maximizing version in combination with a highly sensitive subject search. If this retrieves an unmanageable number of references the sensitivity- and precision-maximizing version should be used instead. It should be borne in mind that MEDLINE abstracts can be read quite quickly as they are relatively short and, at a conservative estimate of 30 seconds per abstract, 1000 abstracts can be read in approximately 8 hours.

The strategies have been updated, after re-analysis of the data used to derive those strategies, to reflect changes in indexing policy introduced by the US National Library of Medicine since the original analysis and changes in search syntax. These changes include:

- no longer assigning 'Clinical Trial' as a Publication Type to all records indexed with 'Randomized Controlled Trial' or 'Controlled Clinical Trial' as a Publication Type; and

- the change of the MeSH term CLINICAL TRIALS to CLINICAL TRIALS AS TOPIC.

The strategies are given in Box 6.4.a and Box 6.4.b for PubMed, and in Box 6.4.c and Box 6.4.d for Ovid.

It must be borne in mind that the strategies below are based on data derived from MEDLINE-indexed records and were designed to be run in MEDLINE. These strategies are not designed to retrieve 'in process' and other records not indexed with MeSH terms. It is, therefore, recommended that these strategies are run in the MEDLINE-indexed versions of MEDLINE and separate searches for non-indexed records are run in the database containing the 'in process' and non-indexed records. For example, in Ovid the strategies below should be run and updated in databases such as 'Ovid MEDLINE(R) 1950 to Month Week X 200X' and non-indexed records should be searched for in 'Ovid MEDLINE(R) In-Process & Other Non-Indexed Citations Month X, 200X'. For identifying non-indexed records a range of truncated free-text terms would be required,

---

**Box 6.4.a    Cochrane Highly Sensitive Search Strategy for identifying randomized trials in MEDLINE: sensitivity-maximizing version (2008 revision); PubMed format**

#1    randomized controlled trial [pt]
#2    controlled clinical trial [pt]
#3    randomized [tiab]
#4    placebo [tiab]
#5    drug therapy [sh]
#6    randomly [tiab]
#7    trial [tiab]
#8    groups [tiab]
#9    #1 OR #2 OR #3 OR #4 OR #5 OR #6 OR #7 OR #8
#10    animals [mh] NOT humans [mh]
#11    #9 NOT #10

---

*PubMed search syntax*
[pt] denotes a Publication Type term;
[tiab] denotes a word in the title or abstract;
[sh] denotes a subheading;
[mh] denotes a Medical Subject Heading (MeSH) term ('exploded');
[mesh: noexp] denotes a Medical Subject Heading (MeSH) term (not 'exploded');
[ti] denotes a word in the title.

---

**Box 6.4.b    Cochrane Highly Sensitive Search Strategy for identifying randomized trials in MEDLINE: sensitivity- and precision-maximizing version (2008 revision); PubMed format**

#1    randomized controlled trial [pt]
#2    controlled clinical trial [pt]
#3    randomized [tiab]
#4    placebo [tiab]
#5    clinical trials as topic [mesh: noexp]
#6    randomly [tiab]
#7    trial [ti]
#8    #1 OR #2 OR #3 OR #4 OR #5 OR #6 OR #7
#9    animals [mh] NOT humans [mh]
#10    #8 NOT #9

---

The search syntax is explained in Box 6.4.a.

---

**Box 6.4.c   Cochrane Highly Sensitive Search Strategy for identifying randomized trials in MEDLINE: sensitivity-maximizing version (2008 revision); Ovid format**

1   randomized controlled trial.pt.
2   controlled clinical trial.pt.
3   randomized.ab.
4   placebo.ab.
5   drug therapy.fs.
6   randomly.ab.
7   trial.ab.
8   groups.ab.
9   1 or 2 or 3 or 4 or 5 or 6 or 7 or 8
10   exp animals/ not humans.sh.
11   9 not 10

---

*Ovid search syntax*
.pt. denotes a Publication Type term;
.ab. denotes a word in the abstract;
.fs. denotes a 'floating' subheading;
.sh. denotes a Medical Subject Heading (MeSH) term;
.ti. denotes a word in the title.

---

**Box 6.4.d   Cochrane Highly Sensitive Search Strategy for identifying randomized trials in MEDLINE: sensitivity- and precision-maximizing version (2008 revision); Ovid format**

1   randomized controlled trial.pt.
2   controlled clinical trial.pt.
3   randomized.ab.
4   placebo.ab.
5   clinical trials as topic.sh.
6   randomly.ab.
7   trial.ti.
8   1 or 2 or 3 or 4 or 5 or 6 or 7
9   exp animals/ not humans.sh.
10   8 not 9

---

The search syntax is explained in Box 6.4.c.

such as random, placebo, trial, etc, and the search must not be limited to humans (as the records are not yet indexed as humans).

As discussed in Section 6.3.2.1, MEDLINE has been searched from 1966 to 2004 inclusive, using previous versions of the Cochrane Highly Sensitive Search Strategy for identifying randomized trials, and records of reports of trials (on the basis of the titles and abstracts only) have been re-indexed in MEDLINE and included in CENTRAL. Refer to Sections 6.3.2.1 and 6.3.3.2 for further guidance as to the appropriate use of these Highly Sensitive Search Strategies.

### 6.4.11.2  *Search filters for identifying randomized trials in EMBASE*

The UK Cochrane Centre is working on designing an objectively derived highly sensitive search strategy for identifying reports of randomized trials in EMBASE, using word frequency analysis methods similar to those used to design the highly sensitive search strategies for identifying randomized trials in MEDLINE described in Section 6.4.11.1 (Glanville 2006). Review authors wishing to conduct their own searches of EMBASE in the meanwhile might wish to consider using the search terms listed in Section 6.3.2.2 that are currently used by the UK Cochrane Centre to identify EMBASE reports of randomized trials for inclusion in CENTRAL (Lefebvre 2008). Alternatively, the search filter designed by Wong and colleagues for identifying what they define as "clinically sound treatment studies" in EMBASE may be used (Wong 2006).

As discussed in Section 6.3.2.2, EMBASE has been searched from 1980 to 2006 inclusive, using the terms listed in that section, and records of reports of trials (on the basis of the titles and abstracts only) have been included in CENTRAL.

## 6.4.12  Updating searches

When a Cochrane review is updated, the search process (i.e. deciding which databases and other sources to search for which years) will have to be reviewed. Those databases that were previously searched and are considered relevant for the update will need to be searched again. The previous search strategies will need to be updated to reflect issues such as: changes in indexing such as the addition or removal of controlled vocabulary terms (MeSH, EMTREE etc); changes in search syntax; comments or criticisms of the previous search strategies. If any of the databases originally searched are not to be searched for the update this should be explained and justified. New databases or other sources may have been produced or become available to the review author or Trials Search Co-ordinator and these should also be considered.

Caution should be exercised with the use of update limits when searching across MEDLINE-indexed and un-indexed records simultaneously such as in PubMed or in the Ovid MEDLINE 'In-Process & Other Non-Indexed Citations and Ovid MEDLINE 1950 to Present' file. Where possible, separate files should be selected and searched separately, such as the Ovid MEDLINE '1950 to Month Week X 200X', and the non-indexed records should be searched for in the Ovid MEDLINE 'In-Process & Other

**Box 6.4.e Demonstration search strategy for CENTRAL, for the topic 'Tamoxifen for breast cancer'**

#1  MeSH descriptor Breast Neoplasms explode all trees
#2  breast near cancer*
#3  breast near neoplasm*
#4  breast near carcinoma*
#5  breast near tumour*
#6  breast near tumor*
#7  #1 OR #2 OR #3 OR #4 OR #5 OR #6
#8  MeSH descriptor Tamoxifen explode all trees
#9  tamoxifen
#10  #8 OR #9
#11  #7 AND #10

The 'near' operator defaults to within six words;
'*' indicates truncation.

**Box 6.4.f Demonstration search strategy for MEDLINE (Ovid format), for the topic 'Tamoxifen for breast cancer'**

1   randomized controlled trial.pt.
2   controlled clinical trial.pt.
3   randomized.ab.
4   placebo.ab.
5   drug therapy.fs.
6   randomly.ab.
7   trial.ab.
8   groups.ab.
9   1 or 2 or 3 or 4 or 5 or 6 or 7 or 8
10  animals.sh. not (humans.sh. and animals.sh.)
11.  9 not 10
12.  exp Breast Neoplasms/
13.  (breast adj6 cancer$).mp.
14.  (breast adj6 neoplasm$).mp.
15.  (breast adj6 carcinoma$).mp.
16.  (breast adj6 tumour$).mp.
17.  (breast adj6 tumor$).mp.
18.  12 or 13 or 14 or 15 or 16 or 17
19.  exp Tamoxifen/
20.  tamoxifen.mp.
21.  19 or 20
22.  11 and 18 and 21

The 'adj6' operator indicates within six words;
'$' indicates truncation;
.mp. indicates a search of title, original title, abstract, name of substance word and subject heading word.

Non-Indexed Citations Month X, 200X' file. For further guidance on this issue, contact a Trials Search Co-ordinator.

## 6.4.13    Demonstration search strategies

Box 6.4.e provides a demonstration search strategy for CENTRAL for the topic 'Tamoxifen for breast cancer'. Note that it includes topic terms only (a randomized trial filter is not appropriate for CENTRAL). There is no limiting to humans only. The strategy is provided for illustrative purposes only: searches of CENTRAL for studies to include in a systematic review would have many more search terms for each of the concepts.

Box 6.4.f provides a demonstration search strategy for MEDLINE (Ovid format) for the topic 'Tamoxifen for breast cancer'. Note that both topic terms and a randomized trial filter are used for MEDLINE. The search is limited to humans. The strategy is provided for illustrative purposes only: searches of MEDLINE for systematic reviews would have many more search terms for each of the concepts.

## 6.4.14    Summary points

- Cochrane review authors should contact their Trials Search Co-ordinator *before* starting a search.

- For most Cochrane reviews, the search structure in most databases will be comprised of a subject search for population or condition and intervention together with a methodological filter for the study design, such as randomized trials.

- For searches of CENTRAL, do not apply a randomized trial filter and do not limit to human.

- Avoid too many *different* search concepts but use a wide variety of synonyms and related terms (both free text and controlled vocabulary terms) combined with 'OR' within *each* concept.

- Combine different concepts with 'AND'.

- Avoid use of the 'NOT' operator in combining search sets.

- Aim for high sensitivity and be prepared to accept low precision.

- Do not apply language restrictions to the search strategy.

- Searches designed for a specific database and service provider will need to be 'translated' for use in another database or service provider.

- Ensure awareness of any retracted publications (e.g. fraudulent publications), errata and comments.

- For identifying randomized trials in MEDLINE, begin with the sensitivity-maximizing version of the Cochrane Highly Sensitive Search Strategy. If this retrieves an unmanageable number of references, use the sensitivity- and precision-maximizing version instead.

- For update searches, where possible, separate database files should be selected and searched separately for the MEDLINE-indexed records and the non-indexed in-process records.

## 6.5 Managing references

### 6.5.1 Bibliographic software

Specially designed bibliographic or reference management software such as EndNote, ProCite, Reference Manager and RefWorks is useful and relatively easy to use to keep track of references to and reports of studies. The choice of which software to use is likely to be influenced by what is available and thus supported at the review author's institution. For a comparison of the above products and links to reviews of other bibliographic software packages see:

- www.burioni.it/forum/dellorso/bms-dasp/text/

Of the packages listed above, ProCite is generally considered to be very efficient for identifying duplicate references but is no longer updated by the suppliers. It does not support the wider range of character sets allowing references to be entered correctly in languages other than English, whereas EndNote does. Bibliographic software also facilitates storage of information about the methods and process of a search. For example, separate unused fields can be used to store information such as 1) the name of the database or other source details from which a trial report was identified, 2) when and from where an article was ordered and the date of article receipt and 3) whether the study associated with an article was included in or excluded from a review and, if excluded, the reasons for exclusion.

Files for importing references from CENTRAL into bibliographic software are available from the Cochrane Information Retrieval Methods Group web site at:

- www.cochrane.org/docs/import.htm

### 6.5.2 Which fields to download

In addition to the full record citation a number of key fields should be considered for downloading from databases where they are available.

Further detailed guidance on which fields to download has been compiled by the Trials Search Co-ordinators' Working Group and is available in a document entitled 'TSC User Guide to Managing Specialized Registers and Handsearch Records' at:

- www.cochrane.org/resources/hsearch.htm

**Abstract:** abstracts can be used to eliminate clearly irrelevant reports, obviating the need to obtain the full text of those reports or to return to the bibliographic database at a later time.

**Accession number/unique identifier:** it is advisable to set aside an unused field for storing the unique identifier/accession number of records downloaded, such as the PubMed ID number (PMID). This allows subsequent linkage to the full database record and also facilitates information management such as duplicate detection and removal.

**Affiliation/address:** may include the institutional affiliation and/or e-mail address of the author(s).

**Article identifier/digital object identifier (DOI):** can be used to cite and link to the full record.

**Clinical trial number:** if the record contains a clinical trial number such as those assigned by the ClinicalTrials.gov or ISRCTN schemes or a number allocated by the sponsor of the trial, these should be downloaded to aid linking of trial reports to the original studies. An example of this is the Clinical Trial Number (CN) field recently introduced in EMBASE.

**Index terms/thesaurus terms/keywords:** see Section 6.4.5. These help indicate why records were retrieved if the title and abstract lack detail.

**Language:** language of publication of the original article.

**Comments, corrections, errata, retractions and updates:** it is important to ensure that any fields that relate to subsequently published comments, corrections, errata, retractions and updates are selected for inclusion in the download, so that any impact of these subsequent publications can be taken into account. The most important fields to consider, together with their field labels in PubMed, are provided in Box 6.5.a.

- http://www.nlm.nih.gov/bsd/mms/medlineelements.html#cc

## 6.5.3  Summary points

- Use bibliographic software to manage references.

- Ensure that all the necessary fields are downloaded.

---

**Box 6.5.a   Important field labels in PubMed**

CIN: 'Comment in'
CON: 'Comment on'
CRI: 'Corrected and Republished in'
CRF: "Corrected and Republished from'
EIN: 'Erratum in'
EFR: 'Erratum for'
PRIN: 'Partial retraction in'
PROF: 'Partial retraction of'
RIN: 'Retraction in'
ROF: 'Retraction of'
RPI: 'Republished in'
RPF: ''Republished from'
UIN: 'Update in'
UOF: 'Update of'

---

# 6.6   Documenting and reporting the search process

## 6.6.1   Documenting the search process

The search process needs to be documented in enough detail throughout the process to ensure that it can be reported correctly in the review, to the extent that all the searches of all the databases are reproducible. It should be borne in mind at the outset that the full search strategies for each database will need to be included in an Appendix of the review. The search strategies will need to be copied and pasted exactly as run and included in full, together with the search set numbers and the number of records retrieved. The number of records retrieved will need to be recorded in the Results section of the review, under the heading 'Results of the search' (see Chapter 4, Section 4.5). The search strategies should not be re-typed as this can introduce errors. A recent study has shown lack of compliance with guidance in the *Handbook* with respect to search strategy description in Cochrane reviews (Sampson 2006). In the majority of CRGs, the Trials Search Co-ordinators are now asked to comment on the search strategy sections of a review as part of the sign-off process prior to a review being considered ready for publication in the *CDSR*. It is, therefore, recommended that review authors should seek guidance from their Trials Search Co-ordinator at the earliest opportunity with respect to documenting the process to facilitate writing up this section of the review. As mentioned elsewhere in this chapter, it is particularly important to save locally or file print copies of any information found on the internet, such as information about ongoing trials, as this information may no longer be accessible at the time the review is written up.

## 6.6.2 Reporting the search process

### 6.6.2.1 *Reporting the search process in the protocol*

The inclusion of any search strategies in the protocol for a Cochrane review is optional. Where searches have already been undertaken at the protocol stage it is considered useful to include them in the protocol so that they can be commented upon in the same way as other aspects of the protocol. Some CRGs are of the view that no searches should be undertaken until the protocol is finalized for publication as knowledge of the available studies might influence aspects of the protocol such as inclusion criteria.

### 6.6.2.2 *Reporting the search process in the review*

**Reporting the search process in the review abstract**

- List all databases searched.

- Note the dates of the last search for each database or the period searched.

- Note any language or publication status restrictions (but refer to Section 6.4.9).

- List individuals or organizations contacted.

For further guidance on how this information should be listed see Chapter 11 (Section 11.8).

**Reporting the search process in the Methods section**    In the 'Search methods for identification of studies' section(s):

- List all databases searched.

- Note the dates of the last search for each database AND the period searched.

- Note any language or publication status restrictions (but refer to Section 6.4.9).

- List grey literature sources.

- List individuals or organizations contacted.

- List any journals and conference proceedings specifically handsearched for the review.

- List any other sources searched (e.g. reference lists, the internet).

The full search strategies for each database should be included in an Appendix of the review to avoid interrupting the flow of the text of the review. The search strategies should be copied and pasted exactly as run and included in full together with the line numbers for each search set. They should not be re-typed as this can introduce errors. For further detailed guidance on this contact the Trials Search Co-ordinator.

***Reporting the search process in the Results section***    The number of hits retrieved by the electronic searches should be included in the Results section.

***Reporting the date of the search***    A single date should be specified in the 'date of search' field, to indicate when the most recent comprehensive search was started. For more information on specifying this date, see Chapter 3 (Section 3.3.3).

### 6.6.3  Summary points

- Seek guidance on documenting the search process from a Trials Search Co-ordinator before starting searching.

- The full strategy for each search of each database should be copied and pasted into an Appendix of the review.

- The total number of hits retrieved by each search strategy should be included in the Results section.

- Save locally or file print copies of any information found on the internet, such as information about ongoing trials.

- Refer to Chapter 4 (Section 4.5) and Chapter 11 (Section 11.8) for more information on what to report in the review and the abstract, respectively.

## 6.7  Chapter information

**Authors**: Carol Lefebvre, Eric Manheimer and Julie Glanville on behalf of the Cochrane Information Retrieval Methods Group.

**This chapter should be cited as**: Lefebvre C, Manheimer E, Glanville J. Chapter 6: Searching for studies. In: Higgins JPT, Green S (editors). *Cochrane Handbook for Systematic Reviews of Interventions*. Wiley, 2008.

**Acknowledgements**: This chapter has been developed from sections of previous editions of the *Handbook* co-authored since 1995 by Kay Dickersin, Kristen Larson, Carol Lefebvre and Eric Manheimer. Many of the sources listed in this chapter have been brought to our attention by a variety of people over the years and we should like to acknowledge this. We should like to thank the information specialists who shared with us information and documentation about their search processes. We should also like to thank Cochrane Trials Search Co-ordinators, members of the Cochrane Information

Retrieval Methods Group (see Box 6.7.a), the Health Technology Assessment International Special Interest Group on Information Resources and the InterTASC Information Specialists' Subgroup for comments on earlier drafts of this chapter, Anne Eisinga for proof-reading the search strategies, and the two peer reviewers, Steve McDonald and Ruth Mitchell, for their detailed and constructive comments.

---

### Box 6.7.a   The Cochrane Information Retrieval Methods Group

The Information Retrieval Methods Group (IRMG) aims to provide advice and support, to conduct research and to facilitate information exchange regarding methods to support the information retrieval activities of The Cochrane Collaboration. The group was officially registered with the Collaboration in November 2004. Members concentrate on providing practical support for the development of information retrieval techniques and facilities for information searchers. The group's aims are realized by the following activities:

- Offering advice on information retrieval policy and practice;
- Providing training and support;
- Conducting empirical research (including systematic reviews) into information retrieval methods;
- Helping to monitor the quality of searching techniques employed in systematic reviews;
- Liaising with members of the Campbell Collaboration to avoid duplication of effort in areas of information retrieval of interest to both the Cochrane and Campbell Collaborations;
- Serving as a forum for discussion.

*Web site*: www.cochrane.org/docs/irmg.htm

---

## 6.8   References

**Bennett 2003**
 Bennett DA, Jull A. FDA: untapped source of unpublished trials. *The Lancet* 2003; 361: 1402–1403.
**De Angelis 2004**
 De Angelis CD, Drazen JM, Frizelle FA, Haug C, Hoey J, Horton R, Kotzin S, Laine C, Marusic A, Overbeke AJ, Schroeder TV, Sox HC, Van der Weyden MB, International Committee of Medical Journal Editors. Clinical trial registration: a statement from the International Committee of Medical Journal Editors. *JAMA* 2004; 292: 1363–1364.
**De Angelis 2005**
 De Angelis CD, Drazen JM, Frizelle FA, Haug C, Hoey J, Horton R, Kotzin S, Laine C, Marusic A, Overbeke AJ, Schroeder TV, Sox HC, Van der Weyden MB, International Committee of Medical Journal Editors. Is this clinical trial fully registered? A statement from the International Committee of Medical Journal Editors. *JAMA* 2004; 293: 2927–2929.

**Dickersin 1994**

Dickersin K, Scherer R, Lefebvre C. Identifying relevant studies for systematic reviews. *BMJ* 1994; 309: 1286–1291.

**Dickersin 2002**

Dickersin K, Manheimer E, Wieland S, Robinson KA, Lefebvre C, McDonald S, CENTRAL Development Group. Development of the Cochrane Collaboration's CENTRAL Register of controlled clinical trials. *Evaluation and the Health Professions* 2002; 25: 38–64.

**Eisinga 2007**

Eisinga A, Siegfried N, Clarke M. The sensitivity and precision of search terms in Phases I, II and III of the Cochrane Highly Sensitive Search Strategy for identifying reports of randomized trials in MEDLINE in a specific area of health care – HIV/AIDS prevention and treatment interventions. *Health Information and Libraries Journal* 2007; 24: 103–109.

**Eysenbach 2001**

Eysenbach G, Tuische J, Diepgen TL. Evaluation of the usefulness of Internet searches to identify unpublished clinical trials for systematic reviews. *Medical Informatics and the Internet in Medicine* 2001; 26: 203–218.

**Glanville 2006**

Glanville JM, Lefebvre C, Miles JN, Camosso-Stefinovic J. How to identify randomized controlled trials in MEDLINE: ten years on. *Journal of the Medical Library Association* 2006; 94: 130–136.

**Glanville 2008**

Glanville J, Bayliss S, Booth A, Dundar Y, Fleeman ND, Foster L, Fraser C, Fernandes H, Fry-Smith A, Golder S, Lefebvre C, Miller C, Paisley S, Payne L, Price AM, Welch K, InterTASC Information Specialists' Subgroup. So many filters, so little time: the development of a Search Filter Appraised Checklist. *Journal of the Medical Library Association* (in press, 2008).

**Golder 2006**

Golder S, McIntosh HM, Duffy S, Glanville J, Centre for Reviews and Dissemination and UK Cochrane Centre Search Filters Design Group. Developing efficient search strategies to identify reports of adverse effects in MEDLINE and EMBASE. *Health Information and Libraries Journal* 2006; 23: 3–12.

**Greenhalgh 2005**

Greenhalgh T, Peacock R. Effectiveness and efficiency of search methods in systematic reviews of complex evidence: audit of primary sources. *BMJ* 2005; 331: 1064–1065.

**Hetherington 1989**

Hetherington J, Dickersin K, Chalmers I, Meinert CL. Retrospective and prospective identification of unpublished controlled trials: lessons from a survey of obstetricians and pediatricians. *Pediatrics* 1989; 84: 374–380.

**Hopewell 2007a**

Hopewell S, Clarke M, Lefebvre C, Scherer R. Handsearching versus electronic searching to identify reports of randomized trials. *Cochrane Database of Systematic Reviews* 2007, Issue 2. Art No: MR000001.

**Hopewell 2007b**

Hopewell S, McDonald S, Clarke M, Egger M. Grey literature in meta-analyses of randomized trials of health care interventions. *Cochrane Database of Systematic Reviews* 2007, Issue 2. Art No: MR000010.

**Horton 1997**

Horton R. Medical editors trial amnesty. *The Lancet* 1997; 350: 756.

**Khan 2001**

Khan KS, ter Riet G, Glanville J, Sowden AJ, Kleijnen J (editors). *Undertaking Systematic Reviews of Research on Effectiveness: CRD's Guidance for those Carrying Out or Commissioning Reviews (CRD Report Number 4)* (2nd edition). York (UK): NHS Centre for Reviews and Dissemination, University of York, 2001.

**Lefebvre 2001**

Lefebvre C, Clarke M. Identifying randomised trials. In: Egger M, Davey Smith G, Altman DG (editors). *Systematic Reviews in Health Care: Meta-analysis in Context* (2nd edition). London (UK): BMJ Publication Group, 2001.

**Lefebvre 2008**

Lefebvre C, Eisinga A, McDonald S, Paul N. Enhancing access to reports of clinical trials published world-wide – the contribution of EMBASE records to the Cochrane Central Register of Controlled Trials (CENTRAL) in The Cochrane Library. *Emerging Themes in Epidemiology* (in press, 2008).

**MacLean 2003**

MacLean CH, Morton SC, Ofman JJ, Roth EA, Shekelle PG. How useful are unpublished data from the Food and Drug Administration in meta-analysis? *Journal of Clinical Epidemiology* 2003; 56: 44–51.

**Mallett 2002**

Mallett S, Hopewell S, Clarke M. Grey literature in systematic reviews: The first 1000 Cochrane systematic reviews. *Fourth Symposium on Systematic Reviews: Pushing the Boundaries*, Oxford (UK), 2002.

**Manheimer 2002**

Manheimer E, Anderson D. Survey of public information about ongoing clinical trials funded by industry: evaluation of completeness and accessibility. *BMJ* 2002; 325: 528–531.

**McDonald 2002**

McDonald S. Improving access to the international coverage of reports of controlled trials in electronic databases: a search of the Australasian Medical Index. *Health Information and Libraries Journal* 2002; 19: 14–20.

**Montori 2005**

Montori VM, Wilczynski NL, Morgan D, Haynes RB. Optimal search strategies for retrieving systematic reviews from Medline: analytical survey. *BMJ* 2005; 330: 68.

**Royle 2003**

Royle P, Milne R. Literature searching for randomized controlled trials used in Cochrane reviews: rapid versus exhaustive searches. *International Journal of Technology Assessment in Health Care* 2003; 19: 591–603.

**Sampson 2006**

Sampson M, McGowan J. Errors in search strategies were identified by type and frequency. *Journal of Clinical Epidemiology* 2006; 59: 1057–1063.

**Scherer 2007**

Scherer RW, Langenberg P, von Elm E. Full publication of results initially presented in abstracts. *Cochrane Database of Systematic Reviews* 2007, Issue 2. Art No: MR000005.

**Suarez-Almazor 2000**

Suarez-Almazor ME, Belseck E, Homik J, Dorgan M, Ramos-Remus C. Identifying clinical trials in the medical literature with electronic databases: MEDLINE alone is not enough. *Controlled Clinical Trials* 2000; 21: 476–487.

**White 2001**

White VJ, Glanville JM, Lefebvre C, Sheldon TA. A statistical approach to designing search filters to find systematic reviews: objectivity enhances accuracy. *Journal of Information Science* 2001; 27: 357–370.

**Whiting 2008**

Whiting P, Westwood M, Burke M, Sterne J, Glanville J. Systematic reviews of test accuracy should search a range of databases to identify primary studies. *Journal of Clinical Epidemiology* 2008; 61: 357.e1–357.e10.

**Wilczynski 2007**

Wilczynski NL, Haynes RB, Hedges Team. EMBASE search strategies achieved high sensitivity and specificity for retrieving methodologically sound systematic reviews. *Journal of Clinical Epidemiology* 2007; 60: 29–33.

**Wong 2006**

Wong SS, Wilczynski NL, Haynes RB. Developing optimal search strategies for detecting clinically sound treatment studies in EMBASE. *Journal of the Medical Library Association* 2006; 94: 41–47.

# 7 Selecting studies and collecting data

**Edited by Julian PT Higgins and Jonathan J Deeks**

## Key Points

- Assessment of eligibility of studies, and extraction of data from study reports, should be done by at least two people, independently.

- Cochrane Intervention reviews have studies, rather than reports, as the unit of interest, and so multiple reports of the same study need to be linked together.

- Data collection forms are invaluable. They should be designed carefully to target the objectives of the review, and should be piloted for each new review (or review team).

- Tips are available for helping with the design and use of data collection forms.

- Data may be reported in diverse formats, but can often be converted into a format suitable for meta-analysis.

## 7.1  Introduction

The findings of a systematic review depend critically on decisions relating to which studies are included, and on decisions relating to which data from these studies are presented and analysed. Methods used for these decisions must be transparent, and they should be chosen to minimize biases and human error. Here we describe approaches that should be used in Cochrane reviews for selecting studies and deciding which of their data to present.

## 7.2   Selecting studies

### 7.2.1   Studies (not reports) as the unit of interest

A Cochrane review is a review of *studies* that meet pre-specified criteria for inclusion in the review. Since each study may have been reported in several articles, abstracts or other reports, a comprehensive search for studies for the review may identify many *reports* from potentially relevant studies. Two distinct processes are therefore required to determine which studies can be included in the review. One is to link together multiple reports of the same study; and the other is to use the information available in the various reports to determine which studies are eligible for inclusion. Although sometimes there is a single report for each study, it should never be assumed that this is the case.

### 7.2.2   Identifying multiple reports from the same study

Duplicate publication can introduce substantial biases if studies are inadvertently included more than once in a meta-analysis (Tramèr 1997). Duplicate publication can take various forms, ranging from identical manuscripts to reports describing different numbers of participants and different outcomes (von Elm 2004). It can be difficult to detect duplicate publication, and some 'detective work' by the review authors may be required.
   Some of the most useful criteria for comparing reports are:

- author names (most duplicate reports have authors in common, although it is not always the case);

- location and setting (particularly if institutions, such as hospitals, are named);

- specific details of the interventions (e.g. dose, frequency);

- numbers of participants and baseline data; and

- date and duration of the study (which can also clarify whether different sample sizes are due to different periods of recruitment).

Where uncertainties remain after considering these and other factors, it may be necessary to correspond with the authors of the reports.

### 7.2.3   A typical process for selecting studies

A typical process for selecting studies for inclusion in a review is as follows (the process should be detailed in the protocol for the review).

1. Merge search results using reference management software, and remove duplicate records of the same report (see Chapter 6, Section 6.5).

2. **Examine titles and abstracts** to remove obviously irrelevant reports (authors should generally be over-inclusive at this stage).

3. Retrieve full text of the potentially relevant reports.

4. Link together multiple reports of the same study (see Section 7.2.2).

5. **Examine full-text reports** for compliance of studies with eligibility criteria.

6. Correspond with investigators, where appropriate, to clarify study eligibility (it may be appropriate to request further information, such as missing results, at the same time).

7. Make final decisions on study inclusion and proceed to data collection.

## 7.2.4  Implementation of the selection process

Decisions about which studies to include in a review are among the most influential decisions that are made in the review process. However, they involve judgement. To help ensure that these judgements are reproducible, it is desirable for more than one author to repeat parts of the process. In practice, the exact approach may vary from review to review, depending in part on the experience and expertise of the review authors.

Authors must first decide if more than one of them will assess the titles and abstracts of records retrieved from the search (step 2 in Section 7.2.3). Using at least two authors may reduce the possibility that relevant reports will be discarded (Edwards 2002). It is most important that the final selection of studies into the review is undertaken by more than one author (step 5 in Section 7.2.3).

Experts in a particular area frequently have pre-formed opinions that can bias their assessments of both the relevance and validity of articles (Cooper 1989, Oxman 1993). Thus, while it is important that at least one author is knowledgeable in the area under review, it may be an advantage to have a second author who is not a content expert. Some authors may decide that assessments of relevance should be made by people who are blind or masked to information about the article, such as the journal that published it, the authors, the institution, and the magnitude and direction of the results. They could attempt to do this by editing copies of the articles. However, this takes much time, and may not be warranted given the resources required and the uncertain benefit in terms of protecting against bias (Berlin 1997).

Disagreements about whether a study should be included can generally be resolved by discussion. Often the cause of disagreement is a simple oversight on the part of one of the review authors. When the disagreement is due to a difference in interpretation, this may require arbitration by another person. Occasionally, it will not be possible to resolve disagreements about whether to include a study without additional information. In these cases, authors may choose to categorize the study in their review as one that is awaiting assessment until the additional information is obtained from the study authors.

In summary, the methods section of both the protocol and the review should detail:

- whether more than one author examines each title and abstract to exclude obviously irrelevant reports;

- whether those who examine each full-text report to determine eligibility will do so independently (this should be done by at least two people);

- whether the decisions on the above are made by content area experts, methodologists, or both;

- whether the people assessing the relevance of studies know the names of the authors, institutions, journal of publication and results when they apply the eligibility criteria; and

- how disagreements are handled.

A single failed eligibility criterion is sufficient for a study to be excluded from a review. In practice, therefore, eligibility criteria for each study should be assessed in order of importance, so that the first 'no' response can be used as the primary reason for exclusion of the study, and the remaining criteria need not be assessed.

For most reviews it will be worthwhile to pilot test the eligibility criteria on a sample of reports (say ten to twelve papers, including ones that are thought to be definitely eligible, definitely not eligible and doubtful). The pilot test can be used to refine and clarify the eligibility criteria, train the people who will be applying them and ensure that the criteria can be applied consistently by more than one person.

## 7.2.5   Selecting 'excluded studies'

A Cochrane review includes a list of excluded studies, detailing any studies that a reader might plausibly expect to see among the included studies. This covers all studies that may on the surface appear to meet the eligibility criteria but on further inspection do not, and also those that do not meet all of the criteria but are well known and likely to be thought relevant by some readers. By listing such studies as excluded and giving the primary reason for exclusion, the review authors can show that consideration has been given to these studies. The list of excluded studies should be as brief as possible. It should not list all of the reports that were identified by a comprehensive search. It should not list studies that obviously do not fulfil the entry criteria for the review as listed under 'Types of studies', 'Types of participants', and 'Types of interventions', and in particular should not list studies that are obviously not randomized if the review includes only randomized trials.

## 7.2.6   Measuring agreement

Formal measures of agreement are available to describe the extent to which assessments by multiple authors were the same (Orwin 1994). We describe in Section 7.2.6.1 how a kappa statistic may be calculated for measuring agreement between two authors making simple inclusion/exclusion decisions. Values of kappa between 0.40 and 0.59 have been considered to reflect fair agreement, between 0.60 and 0.74 to reflect good agreement and 0.75 or more to reflect excellent agreement (Orwin 1994).

It is not recommended that kappa statistics are calculated as standard in Cochrane reviews, although they can reveal problems, especially in the early stages of piloting. Comparison of a value of kappa with arbitrary cut-points is unlikely to convey the real impact of any disagreements on the review. For example, disagreement about the eligibility of a large, well conducted, study will have more substantial implications for the review than disagreement about a small study with risks of bias. The reasons for any disagreement should be explored. They may reveal the need to revisit eligibility criteria or coding schemes for data collection, and any resulting changes should be reported.

### 7.2.6.1   Calculations for a simple kappa statistic

Suppose the K studies are distributed according to numbers $a$ to $i$ as in Table 7.2.a. Then

$$kappa = \frac{P_O - P_E}{1 - P_E},$$

where

$$P_O = \frac{a + e + i}{K}$$

**Table 7.2.a**   Data for calculation of a simple kappa statistic

|  |  | Review author 2 | | | |
|  |  | Include | Exclude | Unsure | Total |
|---|---|---|---|---|---|
| Review author 1 | Include | $a$ | $b$ | $c$ | $I_1$ |
|  | Exclude | $d$ | $e$ | $f$ | $E_1$ |
|  | Unsure | $g$ | $h$ | $i$ | $U_1$ |
|  | Total | $I_2$ | $E_2$ | $U_2$ | K |

**Table 7.2.b**  Example data for calculation of a simple kappa statistic

|  |  | Review author 2 | | | |
|  |  | Include | Exclude | Unsure | Total |
|---|---|---|---|---|---|
| Review author 1 | Include | 5 | 3 | 4 | 12 |
|  | Exclude | 0 | 7 | 3 | 10 |
|  | Unsure | 0 | 0 | 3 | 3 |
|  | Total | 5 | 10 | 10 | 25 |

is the proportion of studies for which there was agreement, and

$$P_E = \frac{I_1 \times I_2 + E_1 \times E_2 + U_1 \times U_2}{K^2}$$

is the proportion of studies in which one would expect there to be agreement by chance alone. As an example, from the data in Table 7.2.b,

$$P_O = \frac{5 + 7 + 3}{25} = 0.6,$$

$$P_E = \frac{12 \times 5 + 10 \times 10 + 3 \times 10}{25^2} = 0.304,$$

and so

$$kappa = \frac{0.6 - 0.304}{1 - 0.304} = 0.43.$$

# 7.3   What data to collect

## 7.3.1   What are data?

For the purposes of this chapter, we define 'data' to be any information about (or deriving from) a study, including details of methods, participants, setting, context, interventions, outcomes, results, publications and investigators. Review authors should plan in advance what data will be required for their systematic review, and develop a strategy for obtaining them. The following sections review the types of information that should be sought, and these are summarized in Table 7.3.a. Section 7.4 reviews the main sources of the data.

**Table 7.3.a** Checklist of items to consider in data collection or data extraction

Items not in square brackets should normally be collected in all reviews; items in square brackets may be relevant to some reviews and not others.

---

**Source**
- Study ID (created by review author);
- Report ID (created by review author);
- Review author ID (created by review author);
- Citation and contact details;

**Eligibility**
- Confirm eligibility for review;
- Reason for exclusion;

**Methods**
- Study design;
- Total study duration;
- Sequence generation*;
- Allocation sequence concealment*;
- Blinding*;
- Other concerns about bias*;

**Participants**
- Total number;
- Setting;
- Diagnostic criteria;
- Age;
- Sex;
- Country;
- [Co-morbidity];
- [Socio-demographics];
- [Ethnicity];
- [Date of study];

**Interventions**
- Total number of intervention groups;

*For each intervention and comparison group of interest*:
- Specific intervention;
- Intervention details (sufficient for replication, if feasible);
- [Integrity of intervention];

**Outcomes**
- Outcomes and time points (i) collected; (ii) reported*;

*For each outcome of interest*:
- Outcome definition (with diagnostic criteria if relevant);
- Unit of measurement (if relevant);
- For scales: upper and lower limits, and whether high or low score is good;

**Results**
- Number of participants allocated to each intervention group;

*For each outcome of interest*:
- Sample size;
- Missing participants*;
- Summary data for each intervention group (e.g. $2 \times 2$ table for dichotomous data; means and SDs for continuous data);
- [Estimate of effect with confidence interval; P value];
- [Subgroup analyses];

**Miscellaneous**
- Funding source;
- Key conclusions of the study authors;
- Miscellaneous comments from the study authors;
- References to other relevant studies;
- Correspondence required;
- Miscellaneous comments by the review authors.

---

*Full description required for standard items in the 'Risk of bias' tool (see Chapter 8, Section 8.5).

## 7.3.2   Methods and potential sources of bias

Different research methods can influence study outcomes by introducing different biases into results. Basic study design characteristics should be collected for presentation in the table of 'Characteristics of included studies', including whether the study is randomized, whether the study has a cluster or cross-over design, and the duration of the study. If the review includes non-randomized studies, appropriate features of the studies should be described (see Chapter 13, Section 13.4).

Information should also be collected to facilitate assessments of the risk of bias in each included study using the tool described in Chapter 8 (Section 8.5). The tool covers issues such as sequence generation, allocation sequence concealment, blinding, incomplete outcome data and selective outcome reporting. For each item in the tool, a description of what happened in the study is required, which may include verbatim quotes from study reports. Information for assessment of incomplete outcome data and selective outcome reporting may be most conveniently collected alongside information on outcomes and results. Chapter 8 (Section 8.3.4) discusses some issues in the collection of information for assessments of risk of bias.

## 7.3.3   Participants and setting

Details of participants and setting are collected primarily for presentation in the table of 'Characteristics of included studies'. Some Cochrane Review Groups have developed standards regarding which characteristics should be collected. Typically, aspects that should be collected are those that could (or are believed to) affect presence or magnitude of an intervention effect, and those that could help users assess applicability. For example, if the review authors suspect important differences in intervention effect between different socio-economic groups (examples of this are rare), this information should be collected. If intervention effects are thought constant over such groups, and if such information would not be useful to help apply results, it should not be collected.

Participant characteristics that are often useful for assessing applicability include age and sex, and summary information about these should always be collected if they are not obvious from the context. These are likely to be presented in different formats (e.g. ages as means or medians, with SDs or ranges; sex as percentages or counts; and either of these for the whole study or for each intervention group separately). Review authors should seek consistent quantities where possible, and decide whether it is more relevant to summarize characteristics for the study as a whole or broken down, for example, by intervention group. Other characteristics that are sometimes important include ethnicity, socio-demographic details (e.g. education level) and the presence of co-morbid conditions.

If the settings of studies may influence intervention effects or applicability, then information on these should be collected. Typical settings of healthcare intervention studies include acute care hospitals, emergency facilities, general practice, extended care facilities such as nursing homes, offices, schools and communities. Sometimes studies are conducted in different geographical regions with important differences in cultural characteristics that could affect delivery of an intervention and its outcomes. Timing of the study may be associated with important technology differences or trends over time. If such information is important for the interpretation of the review, it should be collected.

Diagnostic criteria that were used to define the condition of interest can be a particularly important source of diversity across studies and should be collected. For example, in a review of drug therapy for congestive heart failure, it is important to know how the definition and severity of heart failure was determined in each study (e.g. systolic or diastolic dysfunction, severe systolic dysfunction with ejection fractions below 20%). Similarly, in a review of antihypertensive therapy, it is important to describe baseline levels of blood pressure of participants.

## 7.3.4 Interventions

Details of all experimental and comparison interventions of relevance to the review should be collected, primarily for presentation in the 'Characteristics of included studies' table. Again, details are required for aspects that could affect presence or magnitude of effect, or that could help users assess applicability. Where feasible, information should be sought (and presented in the review) that is sufficient for replication of the interventions under study, including any co-interventions administered as part of the study.

For many clinical trials of many non-complex interventions such as drugs or physical interventions, routes of delivery (e.g., oral or intravenous delivery, surgical technique used), doses (e.g. amount or intensity of each treatment, frequency of delivery), timing (e.g. within 24 hours of diagnosis) and length of treatment may be relevant. For complex interventions, such as those that evaluate psychotherapy, behavioural and educational approaches or healthcare delivery strategies, it is important to collect information about the contents of the intervention, who delivered it, and the format and timing of delivery.

### 7.3.4.1 Integrity of interventions

The degree to which specified procedures or components of the intervention are implemented as planned can have important consequences for the findings from a study. We will describe this as intervention integrity; related terms include compliance and fidelity. The verification of intervention integrity may be particularly important in reviews of preventive interventions and complex interventions, which are often implemented in conditions that present numerous obstacles to idealized delivery (Dane 1998). Information about integrity can help determine whether unpromising results are due to a poorly conceptualized intervention or to an incomplete delivery of the prescribed components. Assessment of the implementation of the intervention also reveals important information about the feasibility of an intervention in real life settings, and in particular how likely it is that the intervention can and will be implemented as planned. If it is difficult to achieve full implementation in practice, the program will have low feasibility (Dusenbury 2003).

The following five aspects of integrity of preventive programs are described by Dane and Schneider (Dane 1998):

1. The extent to which specified intervention components were delivered as prescribed (*adherence*);

2. Number, length and frequency of implementation of intervention components (*exposure*);

3. Qualitative aspects of intervention delivery that are not directly related to the implementation of prescribed content, such as implementer enthusiasm, training of implementers, global estimates of session effectiveness, and leader attitude towards the intervention (*quality of delivery*);

4. Measures of participant response to the intervention, which may include indicators such as levels of participation and enthusiasm (*participant responsiveness*);

5. Safeguard checks against the diffusion of treatments, that is, to ensure that the subjects in each experimental group received only the planned interventions (*program differentiation*).

The integrity of an intervention may be monitored during a study using process measures, and feedback from such an evaluation may lead to evolution of the intervention itself. Process evaluation studies are characterized by a flexible approach to data collection and the use of numerous methods generating a range of different types of data. They may encompass both quantitative and qualitative methods. Process evaluations may be published separately from the outcome evaluation of the intervention. When it is considered important, review authors should aim to address whether the trial accounted for, or measured, key process factors and whether the trials that thoroughly addressed integrity showed a greater impact. Process evaluations can be a useful source of factors that potentially influence the effectiveness of an intervention. Note, however, that measures of the success of blinding (e.g. in a placebo-controlled drug trial) may not be valuable (see Chapter 8, Section 8.11.1).

An example of a Cochrane review evaluating intervention integrity is provided by a review of smoking cessation in pregnancy (Lumley 2004). The authors found that process evaluation of the intervention occurred in only some trials, and in others the implementation was less than ideal (including some of the largest trials). The review highlighted how the transfer of an intervention from one setting to another may reduce its effectiveness if elements are changed or aspects of the materials are culturally inappropriate.

## 7.3.5    Outcome measures

Review authors should decide in advance whether they will collect information about all outcomes measured in a study, or about only those outcomes of (pre-specified) interest in the review. Because we recommend in Section 7.3.6 that results should only be collected for pre-specified outcomes, we also suggest that only the outcomes listed in the protocol be described in detail. However, a complete list of the names of all outcomes measured allows a more detailed assessment of the risk of bias due to selective outcome reporting (see Chapter 8, Section 8.13).

Information about outcomes that is likely to be important includes:

- definition (diagnostic method, name of scale, definition of threshold, type of behaviour);

- timing;

- unit of measurement (if relevant); and

- for scales: upper and lower limits, and whether a high or low score is favourable.

It may be useful to collect details of cited reports associated with scales, since these may contain further information about upper and lower limits, direction of benefit, typical averages and standard deviations, minimally important effect magnitudes, and information about validation.

Further considerations for economics outcomes are discussed in Chapter 15 (Section 15.4.2), and for patient-reported outcomes in Chapter 17.

### 7.3.5.1    Adverse outcomes

Collection of adverse effect outcomes can pose particular difficulties, discussed in detail in Chapter 14. Information falling under any of the terms 'adverse effect', 'adverse drug reaction', 'side effect', 'toxic effect', 'adverse event' and 'complication' may be considered as being potentially suitable for data extraction when evaluating the harmful effects of an intervention. Furthermore, it may be unclear whether an outcome should be classified as an adverse outcome (and the same outcome may be considered to be an adverse effect in some studies and not in others). No mention of adverse effects does not necessarily mean that no adverse effects occurred. It is usually safest to assume that they were not ascertained or not recorded. Quality of life measures are usually general measures that do not look specifically at particular adverse effects of the intervention. While quality of life scales can be used to gauge the overall well-being, they should not be regarded as substitutes for a detailed evaluation of safety and tolerability.

Precise definitions of adverse effect outcomes and their intensity should be recorded, since they may vary between studies. For example, in a review of aspirin and gastrointestinal haemorrhage, some trials simply reported gastrointestinal bleeds, while others reported specific categories of bleeding, such as haematemesis, melaena, and proctorrhagia (Derry 2000). The definition and reporting of severity of the haemorrhages (for example, major, severe, requiring hospital admission) also varied considerably among the trials (Zanchetti 1999). Moreover, a particular adverse effect may be described or measured in different ways among the studies. For example, the terms 'tiredness', 'fatigue' or 'lethargy' might all be used in reporting of adverse effects. Study authors may also use different thresholds for 'abnormal' results (for example, hypokalaemia diagnosed at a serum potassium concentration of 3.0 mmol/l or 3.5 mmol/l).

## 7.3.6  Results

Results should be collected only for the outcomes specified to be of interest in the protocol. Results for other outcomes should not be extracted unless the protocol is modified to add them, and this modification should be reported in the review. However, review authors should be alert to the possibility of important, unexpected findings, particularly serious adverse effects.

Reports of studies often include several results for the same outcome. For example, different measurement scales might be used, results may be presented separately for different subgroups, and outcomes may have been measured at different points in time. Variation in the results can be very large, depending on which data are selected (Gøtzsche 2007), and protocols should be as specific as possible about which outcome measures, time-points and summary statistics (e.g. final values versus change from baseline) are to be collected. Refinements to the protocol may be needed to facilitate decisions on which results should be extracted.

Section 7.7 describes the numbers that will be required in order to perform meta-analysis. The unit of analysis (e.g. participant, cluster, body part, treatment period) should be recorded for each result if it is not obvious (see Chapter 9, Section 9.3). The type of outcome data determines the nature of the numbers that will be sought for each outcome. For example, for a dichotomous ('yes' or 'no') outcome, the number of participants and the number who experienced the outcome will be sought for each group. It is important to collect the sample size relevant to each result, although this is not always obvious. Drawing a flow diagram as recommended in the CONSORT Statement (Moher 2001) can help to determine the flow of participants through a study if one is not available in a published report (available from www.consort-statement.org).

The numbers required for meta-analysis are not always available, and sometimes other statistics can be collected and converted into the required format. For example, for a continuous outcome, it is usually most convenient to seek the number of participants, the mean and the standard deviation for each intervention group. These are often not available directly, especially the standard deviation, and alternative statistics enable calculation or estimation of the missing standard deviation (such as a standard error, a confidence interval, a test statistic (e.g. from a t-test or F-test) or a P value). Details are provided in Section 7.7. Further considerations for dealing with missing data are discussed in Chapter 16 (Section 16.1).

### 7.3.7   Other information to collect

Other information will be required from each report of a study, including the citation, contact details for the authors of the study and any other details of sources of additional information about it (for example an identifier for the study that would allow it to be found in a register of trials). Of particular importance in many areas is the funding source of the study, or potential conflicts of interest of the study authors. Some review authors will wish to collect information on study characteristics that bear on the quality of the study's conduct but that are unlikely to lead directly to a risk of bias, such as whether ethical approval was obtained and whether a sample size calculation was performed.

We recommend that review authors collect the key conclusions of the included study as reported by its authors. It is not necessary to report these conclusions in the review, but they should be used to verify results of analyses undertaken by the review authors, particularly in relation to the direction of effect. Further comments by the study authors, for example any explanations they provide for unexpected findings, might be noted. References to other studies that are cited in the study report may be useful, although review authors should be aware of the possibility of citation bias (see Chapter 10, Section 10.2.2.3).

## 7.4   Sources of data

### 7.4.1   Reports

Most Cochrane reviews obtain the majority of their data from study reports. Study reports include journal articles, books, dissertations, conference abstracts and web sites. Note, however, that these are highly variable in their reliability as well as their level of detail. For example, conference abstracts may present preliminary findings and confirmation of final results may be required. It is strongly recommended that a data collection form is used for extracting data from study reports (see Section 7.6).

### 7.4.2   Correspondence with investigators

Review authors will often find that they are unable to extract all of the information they seek from available reports, with regard to both the details of the study and the numerical results. In such circumstances, authors are recommended to contact the original investigators. Review authors will need to consider whether they will contact study authors with a request that is open-ended, seeks specific pieces of information, includes a data collection form (either uncompleted or partially completed), or seeks data at the level of individual participants. Contact details of study authors, if not available from the study reports, can often be obtained from an alternative recent publication, from university staff listings, or by a general search of the world wide web.

### 7.4.3   Individual patient data

Rather than extracting data from study publications, the original research data may be sought directly from the researchers responsible for each study. Individual patient data (IPD) reviews, in which data are provided on each of the participants in each of the studies, are the gold standard in terms of availability of data. IPD can be re-analysed centrally and, if appropriate, combined in meta-analyses. IPD reviews are addressed in detail in Chapter 18.

## 7.5   Data collection forms

### 7.5.1   Rationale for data collection forms

The data collection form is a bridge between what is reported by the original investigators (e.g in journal articles, abstracts, personal correspondence) and what is ultimately reported by the review authors. The data collection form serves several important functions (Meade 1997). First, the form is linked directly to the review question and criteria for assessing eligibility of studies, and provides a clear summary of these that can be applied to identified study reports. Second, the data collection form is the historical record of the multitude of decisions (and changes to decisions) that occur throughout the review process. Third, the form is the source of data for inclusion in an analysis.

   Given the important functions of data collection forms, ample time and thought should be invested in their design. Because each review is different, data collection forms will vary across reviews. However, there are many similarities in the types of information that are important, and forms can be adapted from one review to the next. Although we use the term 'data collection form' in the singular, in practice it may be a series of forms used for different purposes: for example, a separate form for assessing eligibility of studies for inclusion in the review to facilitate the quick determination of studies that should be excluded.

### 7.5.2   Electronic versus paper data collection forms

The decision between data collection using paper forms and data collection using electronic forms is largely down to review authors' preferences. Potential advantages of paper forms include:

- convenience or preference;

- data extraction can be undertaken almost anywhere;

- easier to create and implement (no need for computer programming or specialist software);

- provides a permanent record of all manipulations and modifications (providing these manipulations and modifications are not erased); and

- simple comparison of forms completed by different review authors.

Potential advantages of electronic forms include:

- convenience or preference;

- combines data extraction and data entry into one step;

- forms may be programmed (e.g. using Microsoft Access) to 'lead' the author through the data collection process, for example, by posing questions that depend on answers to previous questions;

- data from reviews involving large numbers of studies are more easily stored, sorted and retrieved;

- allows simple conversions at the time of data extraction (e.g. standard deviations from standard errors; pounds to kilograms);

- rapid comparison of forms completed by different review authors; and

- environmental considerations.

Electronic systems have been developed that offer most of the advantages of both approaches (including the commercial SRS software: see www.trialstat.com). If review authors plan to develop their own electronic forms using spreadsheet or database programs, we recommend that (i) a paper form is designed first, and piloted using more than one author and several study reports; (ii) the data entry is structured in a logical manner with coding of responses as consistent and straightforward as possible; (iii) compatibility of output with RevMan is checked; and (iv) mechanisms are considered for recording, assessing and correcting data entry errors.

## 7.5.3 Design of a data collection form

When adapting or designing a data collection form, review authors should first consider how much information should be collected. Collecting too much information can lead to forms that are longer than original study reports, and can be very wasteful of time. Collection of too little information, or omission of key data, can lead to the need to return to study reports later in the review process.

Here are some tips for designing a data collection form, based on the informal collation of experiences from numerous review authors. The checklist in Table 7.3.a should also be consulted.

- Include the title of the review or a unique identifier. Data collection forms are adaptable across reviews and some authors participate in multiple reviews.

- Include a revision date or version number for the data collection form. Forms occasionally have to be revised, and this reduces the chances of using an outdated form by mistake.

- Record the name (or ID) of the person who is completing the form.

- Leave space for notes near the beginning of the form. This avoids placing notes, questions or reminders on the last page of the form where they are least likely to be noticed. Important notes may be entered into RevMan in the 'Notes' column of the 'Characteristics of included studies' table, or in the text of the review.

- Include a unique study ID as well as a unique report ID. This provides a link between multiple reports of the same study. Each included study must be given a study identifier that is used in RevMan (usually comprising the last name of first author and the year of the primary reference for the study).

- Include assessment (or verification) of eligibility of the study for the review near the beginning of the form. Then the early sections of the form can be used for the process of assessing eligibility. Reasons for exclusion of a study can readily be deduced from such assessments. For example, if only truly randomized trials are eligible, a query on the data collection form might be: 'Randomized? Yes, No, Unclear'. If a study used alternate allocation, the answer to the query is 'No', and this information may be entered into the 'Characteristics of excluded studies' table as the reason for exclusion.

- Record the source of each key piece of information collected, including where it was found in a report (this can be done by highlighting the data in hard copy, for example) or if information was obtained from unpublished sources or personal communications. Any unpublished information that is used should be coded in the same way as published information.

- Use tick boxes or coded responses to save time.

- Include 'not reported' or 'unclear' options alongside any 'yes' or 'no' responses.

- Consider formatting sections for collecting results to match RevMan data tables. However, data collection forms should incorporate sufficient flexibility to allow for variation in how data are reported. It is strongly recommended that outcome data be collected in the format in which they were reported (and then transformed in a subsequent step).

- Always collect sample sizes when collecting outcome data, in addition to collecting initial (e.g. randomized) numbers. There may be different sample sizes for different outcomes because of attrition or exclusions.

- Leave plenty of space for notes.

### 7.5.4   Coding and explanations

It is important to provide detailed instructions to all authors who will use the data collection form (Stock 1994). These might be inserted adjacent or near to the data field on the form, directly in the cell that contains the data (e.g. as a comment in Microsoft Excel) or, if they are lengthy, might be provided on a separate page. Use of coding schemes is efficient and facilitates a systematic presentation of study characteristics in the review. Accurate coding is important, and the coding should not be so complicated that the data collector is easily confused or likely to make poor classifications. Checks should be made that coding schemes are being used consistently by different review authors.

## 7.6   Extracting data from reports

### 7.6.1   Introduction

In most Cochrane reviews, the primary source of information about each study is published reports of studies, usually in the form of journal articles. One of the most important and time-consuming parts of a systematic review is extracting data from such reports. The data collection form will usually be designed with data extraction in mind.

Electronic searches for text can provide a useful aid to locating information within a report, for example using search facilities in PDF viewers, internet browsers and word processing software. Text searching should not be considered a replacement for reading the report, however, since information may be presented using variable terminology.

### 7.6.2   Who should extract data?

It is strongly recommended that more than one person extract data from every report to minimize errors and reduce potential biases being introduced by review authors. As a minimum, information that involves subjective interpretation and information that is critical to the interpretation of results (e.g. outcome data) should be extracted independently by at least two people. In common with implementation of the selection process (Section 7.2.4), it is preferable that data extractors are from complementary disciplines, for example a methodologist and a topic area specialist. It is important that everyone involved in data extraction has practice using the form and, if the form was designed by someone else, receives appropriate training.

Evidence in support of duplicate data extraction comes from several indirect sources. One study observed that independent data extraction by two authors resulted in fewer errors than a data extraction by a single author followed by verification by a second (Buscemi 2006). A high prevalence of data extraction errors (errors in 20 out of 34 reviews) has been observed (Jones 2005). A further study of data extraction to compute standardized mean differences found that a minimum of seven out of 27 reviews had substantial errors (Gøtzsche 2007).

### 7.6.3   Preparing for data extraction

All forms should be pilot tested using a representative sample of the studies to be reviewed. This testing may identify data that are missing from the form, or likely to be superfluous. It is wise to draft entries for the 'Characteristics of included studies' table (Chapter 11, Section 11.2) and the 'Risk of bias' table (Chapter 8, Section 8.5) using these pilot reports. Users of the form may provide feedback that certain coding instructions are confusing or incomplete (e.g. a list of options may not cover all situations). A consensus between review authors may be required before the form is modified to avoid any misunderstandings or later disagreements. It might be necessary to repeat the pilot testing on a new set of reports if major changes are needed after the first testing.

Problems with the data collection form will occasionally surface after pilot testing has been completed and the form may need to be revised after data extraction has started. In fact, it is common for a data collection form to require modifications after it has been piloted. When changes are made to the form or coding instructions, it may be necessary to return to reports that have already undergone data extraction. In some situations, it may only be necessary to clarify coding instructions without modifying the actual data collection form.

Some have proposed that some information in a report, such as its authors, be blinded to the review author prior to data extraction and assessment of risk of bias (Jadad 1996); see also Chapter 9 (Section 8.3.4). However, blinding of review authors to aspects of study reports is not generally recommended for Cochrane reviews (Berlin 1997).

### 7.6.4   Extracting data from multiple reports of the same study

Studies are frequently reported in more than one publication (Tramèr 1997, von Elm 2004). However, the unit of interest in a Cochrane Intervention review is the study and not the report. Thus, information from multiple reports needs to be collated. It is not appropriate to discard any report of an included study, since it may contain valuable information not included in the primary report. Review authors will need to decide between two strategies:

- Extract data from each report separately, then combine information across multiple data collection forms.

- Extract data from all reports directly into a single data collection form.

The choice of which strategy to use will depend on the nature of the reports and may vary across studies and across reports. For example, if a full journal article and multiple conference abstracts are available, it is likely that the majority of information will be obtained from the journal article, and completing a new data collection form for each conference abstract may be a waste of time. Conversely, if there are two or more detailed journal articles, perhaps relating to different periods of follow-up, then it is likely to be easier to perform data extraction separately for these articles and collate information from the data collection forms afterwards.

Drawing flow diagrams for participants in a study, such as those recommended in the CONSORT Statement (Moher 2001), can be particularly helpful when collating information from multiple reports.

## 7.6.5 Reliability and reaching consensus

When more than one author extracts data from the same reports, there is potential for disagreement. An explicit procedure or decision rule should be identified in the protocol for identifying and resolving disagreements. Most often, the source of the disagreement is an error by one of the extractors and is easily resolved. Thus, discussion among the authors is a sensible first step. More rarely, a disagreement may require arbitration by another person. Any disagreements that cannot be resolved should be addressed by contacting the study authors; if this is unsuccessful, the disagreement should be reported in the review.

The presence and resolution of disagreements should be carefully recorded. Maintaining a copy of the data 'as extracted' (in addition to the consensus data) allows assessment of reliability of coding. Examples of ways in which this can be achieved include:

- Use one author's (paper) data collection form and record changes after consensus in a different ink colour.

- Use a separate (paper) form for consensus data.

- Enter consensus data onto an electronic form.

Agreement of coded items can be quantified, for example using kappa statistics (Orwin 1994), although this is not routinely done in Cochrane reviews. A simple calculation for agreement between two authors is described in Section 7.2.6. If agreement is assessed, this should be done only for the most important data (e.g. key risk of bias assessments, or availability of key outcomes).

Informal consideration of the reliability of data extraction should be borne in mind throughout the review process, however. For example, if after reaching consensus on the first few studies, the authors note a frequent disagreement for specific data, then coding instructions may need modification. Furthermore, an author's coding strategy may change over time, as the coding rules are forgotten, indicating a need for re-training and, possibly, some re-coding.

### 7.6.6   Summary

In summary, the methods section of both the protocol and the review should detail:

- the data categories that are to be collected;

- how verification of extracted data from each report will be verified (e.g. extraction by two review authors, independently);

- whether data extraction is undertaken by content area experts, methodologists, or both;

- piloting, training and existence of coding instructions for the data collection form;

- how data are extracted from multiple reports of the same study; and

- how disagreements are handled if more than one author extracts data from each report.

## 7.7   Extracting study results and converting to the desired format

### 7.7.1   Introduction

We now outline the data that need to be collected from each study for analyses of dichotomous outcomes, continuous outcomes and other types of outcome data. These types of data are discussed in Chapter 9 (Section 9.2). It is usually desirable to collect summary data separately for each intervention group and to enter these into RevMan, where effect estimates can be calculated. Sometimes the required data may be obtained only indirectly, and the relevant results may not be obvious. This section provides some useful tips and techniques to deal with some of these situations. If summary data cannot be obtained from each intervention group, effect estimates may be presented directly. In Section 7.7.7 we describe how standard errors of such effect estimates can be obtained from confidence intervals and P values.

### 7.7.2   Data extraction for dichotomous outcomes

Dichotomous data are described in Chapter 9, Section 9.2.2, and their meta-analysis is described in Chapter 9, Section 9.4.4. The only data required for a dichotomous outcome are the numbers in each of the two outcome categories in each of the intervention groups (the numbers needed to fill in the four boxes $S_E$, $F_E$, $S_C$, $F_C$ in Chapter 9, Box 9.2.a). These are entered into RevMan as the numbers with the outcomes and the total sample sizes for the two groups. It is most reliable to collect dichotomous outcome data as the numbers who specifically did, and specifically did not, experience the outcome in each group. Although in theory this is equivalent to collecting the total numbers and the numbers experiencing the outcome, it is not always clear whether the reported total numbers are those on whom the outcome was measured. Occasionally the numbers incurring the event need to be derived from percentages (although it is not always clear which denominator to use, and rounded percentages may be compatible with more than one numerator).

Sometimes the numbers of participants and numbers of events are not available, but an effect estimate such as an odds ratio or risk ratio may be reported, for example in a conference abstract. Such data may be included in meta-analyses using the generic inverse variance method only if they are accompanied by measures of uncertainty such as a standard error, 95% confidence interval or an exact P value: see Section 7.7.7.

### 7.7.3    Data extraction for continuous outcomes

Continuous data are described in Chapter 9, Section 9.2.3, and their meta-analysis is discussed in Chapter 9, Section 9.4.5. To perform a meta-analysis of continuous data using either mean differences or standardized mean differences review authors should seek:

- mean value of the outcome measurements in each intervention group ($M_E$ and $M_C$);

- standard deviation of the outcome measurements in each intervention group ($SD_E$ and $SD_C$); and

- number of participants on whom the outcome was measured in each intervention group ($N_E$ and $N_C$).

Due to poor and variable reporting it may be difficult or impossible to obtain the necessary information from the data summaries presented. Studies vary in the statistics they use to summarize the average (sometimes using medians rather than means) and variation (sometimes using standard errors, confidence intervals, interquartile ranges and ranges rather than standard deviations). They also vary in the scale chosen to analyse the data (e.g. post-intervention measurements versus change from baseline; raw scale versus logarithmic scale).

A particularly misleading error is to misinterpret a standard error as a standard deviation. Unfortunately it is not always clear what is being reported and some intelligent reasoning, and comparison with other studies, may be required. Standard deviations and standard errors are occasionally confused in the reports of studies, and the terminology is used inconsistently.

When needed, missing information and clarification about the statistics presented should always be sought from the authors. However, for several of the measures of variation there is an approximate or direct algebraic relationship with the standard deviation, so it may be possible to obtain the required statistic even if it is not published in the paper, as explained in Sections 7.7.3.2 to 7.7.3.7. More details and examples are available elsewhere (Deeks 1997a, Deeks 1997b). Chapter 16 (Section 16.1.3) discusses options if standard deviations remain missing after attempts to obtain them.

Sometimes the numbers of participants, means and standard deviations are not available, but an effect estimate such as a mean difference or standardized mean difference may be reported, for example in a conference abstract. Such data may be included in meta-analyses using the generic inverse variance method only if they are accompanied by measures of uncertainty such as a standard error, 95% confidence interval or an exact P value. A suitable standard error from a confidence interval for a mean difference should be obtained using the early steps of the process described in Section 7.7.3.3. For standardized mean differences, see Section 7.7.7.

### 7.7.3.1  Post-intervention versus change from baseline

A common feature of continuous data is that a measurement used to assess the outcome of each participant is also measured at baseline, that is before interventions are administered. This gives rise to the possibility of using differences in **changes from baseline** (also called a **change score**) as the primary outcome. Review authors are advised not to focus on change from baseline unless this method of analysis was used in some of the study reports.

When addressing change from baseline, a single measurement is created for each participant, obtained either by subtracting the final measurement from the baseline measurement or by subtracting the baseline measurement from the final measurement. Analyses then proceed as for any other type of continuous outcome variable using the changes rather than the final measurements.

Commonly, studies in a review will have used a mixture of changes from baseline and final values. Some studies will report both; others will report only change scores or only final values. As explained in Chapter 9 (Section 9.4.5.2), both final values and change scores can sometimes be combined in the same analysis so this is not necessarily a problem. Authors may wish to extract data on both change from baseline and final value outcomes if the required means and standard deviations are available. A key problem associated with the choice of which analysis to use is the possibility of selective reporting of the one with the more exaggerated results, and review authors should seek evidence of whether this may be the case (see Chapter 8, Section 8.13).

A final problem with extracting information on change from baseline measures is that often baseline and final measurements will be reported for different numbers of participants due to missed visits and study withdrawals. It may be difficult to identify the subset of participants who report both baseline and final value measurements for whom change scores can be computed.

### 7.7.3.2 Obtaining standard deviations from standard errors and confidence intervals for group means

A standard deviation can be obtained from the standard error of a mean by multiplying by the square root of the sample size:

$$SD = SE \times \sqrt{N}$$

When making this transformation, standard errors must be of means calculated from within an intervention group and not standard errors of the difference in means computed between intervention groups.

Confidence intervals for means can also be used to calculate standard deviations. Again, the following applies to confidence intervals for mean values calculated within an intervention group and not for estimates of differences between interventions (for these, see Section 7.7.3.3). Most confidence intervals are 95% confidence intervals. If the sample size is large (say bigger than 100 in each group), the 95% confidence interval is 3.92 standard errors wide (3.92 = 2 × 1.96). The standard deviation for each group is obtained by dividing the length of the confidence interval by 3.92, and then multiplying by the square root of the sample size:

$$SD = \sqrt{N} \times (\text{upper limit} - \text{lower limit})/3.92$$

For 90% confidence intervals 3.92 should be replaced by 3.29, and for 99% confidence intervals it should be replaced by 5.15.

If the sample size is small (say less than 60 in each group) then confidence intervals should have been calculated using a value from a t distribution. The numbers 3.92, 3.29 and 5.15 need to be replaced with slightly larger numbers specific to the t distribution, which can be obtained from tables of the t distribution with degrees of freedom equal to the group sample size minus 1. Relevant details of the t distribution are available as appendices of many statistical textbooks, or using standard computer spreadsheet packages. For example the t value for a 95% confidence interval from a sample size of 25 can be obtained by typing **=tinv(1-0.95,25-1)** in a cell in a Microsoft Excel spreadsheet (the result is 2.0639). The divisor, 3.92, in the formula above would be replaced by 2 × 2.0639 = 4.128.

For moderate sample sizes (say between 60 and 100 in each group), either a t distribution or a standard normal distribution may have been used. Review authors should look for evidence of which one, and might use a t distribution if in doubt.

As an example, consider data presented as follows:

| Group | Sample size | Mean | 95% CI |
|---|---|---|---|
| Experimental intervention | 25 | 32.1 | (30.0, 34.2) |
| Control intervention | 22 | 28.3 | (26.5, 30.1) |

The confidence intervals should have been based on t distributions with 24 and 21 degrees of freedom respectively. The divisor for the experimental intervention group is 4.128, from above. The standard deviation for this group is $\sqrt{25} \times (34.2 - 30.0)/4.128 = 5.09$. Calculations for the control group are performed in a similar way.

It is important to check that the confidence interval is symmetrical about the mean (the distance between the lower limit and the mean is the same as the distance between the mean and the upper limit). If this is not the case, the confidence interval may have been calculated on transformed values (see Section 7.7.3.4).

### 7.7.3.3    *Obtaining standard deviations from standard errors, confidence intervals, t values and P values for differences in means*

Standard deviations can be obtained from standard errors, confidence intervals, t values or P values that relate to the differences between means in two groups. The difference in means itself (MD) is required in the calculations from the t value or the P value. An assumption that the standard deviations of outcome measurements are the same in both groups is required in all cases, and the standard deviation would then be used for both intervention groups. We describe first how a t value can be obtained from a P value, then how a standard error can be obtained from a t value or a confidence interval, and finally how a standard deviation is obtained from the standard error. Review authors may select the appropriate steps in this process according to what results are available to them. Related methods can be used to derive standard deviations from certain F statistics, since taking the square root of an F value may produce the same t value. Care is often required to ensure that an appropriate F value is used, and advice of a knowledgeable statistician is recommended.

***From P value to t value***    Where actual P values obtained from t tests are quoted, the corresponding t value may be obtained from a table of the t distribution. The degrees of freedom are given by $N_E + N_C - 2$, where $N_E$ and $N_C$ are the sample sizes in the experimental and control groups. We will illustrate with an example. Consider a trial of an experimental intervention ($N_E = 25$) versus a control intervention ($N_C = 22$), where the difference in means was MD = 3.8. It is noted that the P value for the comparison was P = 0.008, obtained using a two-sample t-test.

The t value that corresponds with a P value of 0.008 and $25 + 22 - 2 = 45$ degrees of freedom is t = 2.78. This can be obtained from a table of the t distribution with 45 degrees of freedom or a computer (for example, by entering = **tinv(0.008, 45)** into any cell in a Microsoft Excel spreadsheet).

Difficulties are encountered when levels of significance are reported (such as P < 0.05 or even P = NS which usually implies P > 0.05) rather than exact P values. A conservative approach would be to take the P value at the upper limit (e.g. for P < 0.05 take P = 0.05, for P < 0.01 take P = 0.01 and for P < 0.001 take P = 0.001). However, this is not a solution for results which are reported as P = NS: see Section 7.7.3.7.

***From t value to standard error***    The t value is the ratio of the difference in means to the standard error of the difference in means. The standard error of the difference in means can therefore be obtained by dividing the difference in means (MD) by the t value:

$$SE = \frac{MD}{t}.$$

In the example, the standard error of the difference in means is obtained by dividing 3.8 by 2.78, which gives 1.37.

***From confidence interval to standard error*** If a 95% confidence interval is available for the difference in means, then the same standard error can be calculated as:

$$SE = (\text{upper limit} - \text{lower limit})/3.92$$

as long as the trial is large. For 90% confidence intervals 3.92 should be replaced by 3.29, and for 99% confidence intervals it should be replaced by 5.15. If the sample size is small then confidence intervals should have been calculated using a t distribution. The numbers 3.92, 3.29 and 5.15 need to be replaced with larger numbers specific to both the t distribution and the sample size, and can be obtained from tables of the t distribution with degrees of freedom equal to $N_E + N_C - 2$, where $N_E$ and $N_C$ are the sample sizes in the two groups. Relevant details of the t distribution are available as appendices of many statistical textbooks, or using standard computer spreadsheet packages. For example, the t value for a 95% confidence interval from a comparison of a sample size of 25 with a sample size of 22 can be obtained by typing **=tinv(1-0.95,25+22-2)** in a cell in a Microsoft Excel spreadsheet.

***From standard error to standard deviation*** The within-group standard deviation can be obtained from the standard error of the difference in means using the following formula:

$$SD = \frac{SE}{\sqrt{\frac{1}{N_E} + \frac{1}{N_C}}}$$

In the example,

$$SD = \frac{1.37}{\sqrt{\frac{1}{25} + \frac{1}{22}}} = 4.69.$$

Note that this standard deviation is the average of the standard deviations of the experimental and control arms, and should be entered into RevMan twice (once for each intervention group).

### 7.7.3.4 Transformations and skewed data

Summary statistics may be presented after a transformation has been applied to the raw data. For example, means and standard deviations of logarithmic values may be available (or, equivalently, a geometric mean and its confidence interval). Such results should be collected, as they may be included in meta-analyses, or – with certain assumptions – may be transformed back to the raw scale.

For example, a trial reported meningococcal antibody responses 12 months after vaccination with meningitis C vaccine and a control vaccine (MacLennan 2000) as geometric mean titres of 24 and 4.2 with 95% confidence intervals of 17 to 34 and 3.9 to 4.6 respectively. These summaries were obtained by finding the means and confidence intervals of the natural logs of the antibody responses (for vaccine 3.18: 95%CI (2.83 to 3.53), and control 1.44 (1.36 to 1.53)), and taking their exponentials (anti-logs). A meta-analysis may be performed on the scale of these natural log antibody responses. Standard deviations of the log-transformed data may be derived from the latter pair of confidence intervals using methods described in Section 7.7.3.2. For further discussion of meta-analysis with skewed data, see Chapter 9 (Section 9.4.5.3).

### 7.7.3.5 Medians and interquartile ranges

The median is very similar to the mean when the distribution of the data is symmetrical, and so occasionally can be used directly in meta-analyses. However, means and medians can be very different from each other if the data are skewed, and medians are often reported *because* the data are skewed (see Chapter 9, Section 9.4.5.3).

Interquartile ranges describe where the central 50% of participants' outcomes lie. When sample sizes are large and the distribution of the outcome is similar to the normal distribution, the width of the interquartile range will be approximately 1.35 standard deviations. In other situations, and especially when the outcomes distribution is skewed, it is not possible to estimate a standard deviation from an interquartile range. Note that the use of interquartile ranges rather than standard deviations can often be taken as an indicator that the outcomes distribution is skewed.

### 7.7.3.6 Ranges

Ranges are very unstable and, unlike other measures of variation, increase when the sample size increases. They describe the extremes of observed outcomes rather than the average variation. Ranges should not be used to estimate standard deviations. One common approach has been to make use of the fact that, with normally distributed data, 95% of values will lie within $2 \times SD$ either side of the mean. The SD may therefore be estimated to be approximately one quarter of the typical range of data values. This method is not robust and we recommend that it should not be used.

### 7.7.3.7  No information on variability

If none of the above methods allow calculation of the standard deviations from the trial report (and the information is not available from the trialists) then, in order to perform a meta-analysis, an author may be forced to impute ('fill in') the missing data or to exclude the study from the meta-analysis: see Chapter 16 (Section 16.1.3). A narrative approach to synthesis may also be used. It is valuable to tabulate available results for all studies included in the systematic review, even if they cannot be included in a formal meta-analysis.

### 7.7.3.8  Combining groups

Sometimes it is desirable to combine two reported subgroups into a single group. This might be the case, for example, if a study presents sample sizes, means and standard deviations separately for males and females in each of the intervention groups. The formulae in Table 7.7.a can be used to combine numbers into a single sample size, mean and standard deviation for each intervention group (i.e. combining across males and females in this example). Note that the rather complex-looking formula for the SD produces the SD of outcome measurements *as if the combined group had never been divided into two*. An approximation to this standard deviation is obtained by using the usual pooled standard deviation, which provides a slight underestimate of the desired standard deviation.

These formulae are also appropriate for use in studies that compare more than two interventions, to combine two intervention groups into a single intervention group (see Chapter 16, Section 16.5). For example, 'Group 1' and 'Group 2' might refer to two alternative variants of an intervention to which participants were randomized.

If there are more than two groups to combine, the simplest strategy is to apply the above formula sequentially (i.e. combine group 1 and group 2 to create group '1 + 2', then combine group '1 + 2' and group 3 to create group '1 + 2 + 3', and so on).

**Table 7.7.a**  Formulae for combining groups

| | Group 1 (e.g. males) | Group 2 (e.g. females) | Combined groups |
|---|---|---|---|
| **Sample size** | $N_1$ | $N_2$ | $N_1 + N_2$ |
| **Mean** | $M_1$ | $M_2$ | $\dfrac{N_1 M_1 + N_2 M_2}{N_1 + N_2}$ |
| **SD** | $SD_1$ | $SD_2$ | $\sqrt{\dfrac{(N_1 - 1)\,SD_1^2 + (N_2 - 1)\,SD_2^2 + \dfrac{N_1 N_2}{N_1 + N_2}\left(M_1^2 + M_2^2 - 2M_1 M_2\right)}{N_1 + N_2 - 1}}$ |

## 7.7.4    Data extraction for ordinal outcomes

Ordinal data, when outcomes are categorized into several, ordered, categories, are described in Chapter 9, Section 9.2.4, and their meta-analysis is discussed in Chapter 9, Section 9.4.7. The data that need to be extracted for ordinal outcomes depend on whether the ordinal scale will be dichotomized for analysis (see Section 7.7.2), treated as a continuous outcome (see Section 7.7.3) or analysed directly as ordinal data. This decision, in turn, will be influenced by the way in which authors of the studies analysed their data. Thus it may be impossible to pre-specify whether data extraction will involve calculation of numbers of participants above and below a defined threshold, or mean values and standard deviations. In practice, it is wise to extract data in all forms in which they are given as it will not be clear which is the most common until all studies have been reviewed, and in some circumstances more than one form of analysis may justifiably be included in a review.

Where ordinal data are being dichotomized and there are several options for selecting a cut-point (or the choice of cut-point is arbitrary) it is sensible to plan from the outset to investigate the impact of choice of cut-point in a sensitivity analysis (see Chapter 9, Section 9.7). To do this it is necessary to collect the data that would be used for each alternative dichotomization. Hence it is preferable to record the numbers in each category of short ordinal scales to avoid having to extract data from a paper more than once. This approach of recording all categorizations is also sensible when studies use slightly different short ordinal scales, and it is not clear whether there will be a cut-point that is common across all the studies which can be used for dichotomization.

It is also necessary to record the numbers in each category of the ordinal scale for each intervention group if the proportional odds ratio method will be used (see Chapter 9, Section 9.2.4).

## 7.7.5    Data extraction for counts

Counts are described in Chapter 9, Section 9.2.5, and their meta-analysis is discussed in Chapter 9, Section 9.4.8. Data that are inherently counts may be analysed in several ways. The essential decision is whether to make the outcome of interest dichotomous, continuous, time-to-event or a rate. A common error is to treat counts directly as dichotomous data, using as sample sizes either the total number of participants or the total number of, say, person-years of follow-up. Neither of these approaches is appropriate for an event that may occur more than once for each participant. This becomes obvious when the total number of events exceeds the sample size, leading to nonsensical results. Although it is preferable to decide how count data will be analysed in advance, the choice is often determined by the format of the available data, and thus cannot be decided until the majority of studies have been reviewed. Review authors should generally, therefore, extract count data in the form in which they are reported.

Sometimes detailed data on events and person-years at risk are not available, but results calculated from them are. For example, an estimate of a rate ratio or rate difference may be presented in a conference abstract. Such data may be included in meta-analyses only if they are accompanied by measures of uncertainty such as a 95% confidence interval: see Section 7.7.7. From this a standard error can be obtained and the generic inverse variance method used for meta-analysis.

### 7.7.5.1   *Extracting counts as dichotomous data*

To consider the outcome as a dichotomous outcome, the author must determine the number of participants in each intervention group, and the number of participants in each intervention group who experience *at least one event* (or some other appropriate criterion which classified all participants into one of two possible groups). Any time element in the data is lost through this approach, though it may be possible to create a series of dichotomous outcomes, for example at least one stroke during the first year of follow-up, at least one stroke during the first two years of follow-up, and so on. It may be difficult to derive such data from published reports.

### 7.7.5.2   *Extracting counts as continuous data*

To extract counts as continuous data (i.e. average number of events per patient), guidance in Section 7.7.3 should be followed, although particular attention should be paid to the likelihood that the data will be highly skewed.

### 7.7.5.3   *Extracting counts as time-to-event data*

For rare events that can happen more than once, an author may be faced with studies that treat the data as time-to-*first*-event. To extract counts as time-to-event data, guidance in Section 7.7.6 should be followed.

### 7.7.5.4   *Extracting counts as rate data*

If it is possible to extract the total number of events in each group, and the total amount of person-time at risk in each group, then count data can be analysed as rates (see Chapter 9, Section 9.4.8). Note that the total number of participants is not required for an analysis of rate data but should be recorded as part of the description of the study.

## 7.7.6   Data extraction for time-to-event outcomes

Time-to-event outcomes are described in Chapter 9, Section 9.2.6, and their meta-analysis is discussed in Chapter 9, Section 9.4.9. Meta-analysis of time-to-event data commonly involves obtaining individual patient data from the original investigators, re-analysing the data to obtain estimates of the log hazard ratio and its standard error, and then performing a meta-analysis (see Chapter 18). Conducting a meta-analysis using summary information from published papers or trial reports is often problematic as the most appropriate summary statistics are typically not presented. Two approaches can be used to obtain estimates of log hazard ratios and their standard errors, for inclusion in a meta-analysis using the generic inverse variance methods, regardless of whether individual patient data or aggregate data are being used. For practical guidance, review authors should consult Tierney et al. (Tierney 2007).

In the first approach an estimate of the log hazard ratio can be obtained from statistics computed during a log-rank analysis. Collaboration with a knowledgeable statistician is advised if this approach is followed. The log hazard ratio (experimental relative to control) is estimated by $(O - E)/V$, which has standard error $1/\sqrt{V}$, where O is the observed number of events on the experimental intervention, E is the log-rank expected number of events on the experimental intervention, $O - E$ is the log rank statistic and V is the variance of the log-rank statistic. It is therefore necessary to obtain values of $O - E$ and V for each study.

These statistics are easily computed if individual patient data are available, and can sometimes be extracted from quoted statistics and survival curves (Parmar 1998, Williamson 2002). Alternatively, use can sometimes be made of aggregated data for each intervention group in each trial. For example, suppose that the data comprise the number of participants who have the event during the first year, second year, etc., and the number of participants who are event free and still being followed up at the end of each year. A log-rank analysis can be performed on these data, to provide the $O - E$ and V values, although careful thought needs to be given to the handling of censored times. Because of the coarse grouping the log hazard ratio is estimated only approximately, and in some reviews it has been referred to as a log odds ratio (Early Breast Cancer Trialists' Collaborative Group 1990). If the time intervals are large, a more appropriate approach is one based on interval-censored survival (Collett 1994).

The second approach can be used if trialists have analysed the data using a Cox proportional hazards model, or if a Cox model is fitted to individual patient data. Cox models produce direct estimates of the log hazard ratio and its standard error (so that a generic inverse variance meta-analysis can be performed). If the hazard ratio is quoted in a report together with a confidence interval or P value, estimates of standard error can be obtained as described in Section 7.7.7.

## 7.7.7  Data extraction for estimates of effects

### 7.7.7.1  *Effect estimates and generic inverse variance meta-analysis*

In some reviews, an overall estimate of effect will be sought from each study rather than summary data for each intervention group. This may be the case, for example, for non-randomized studies, cross-over trials, cluster-randomized trials, or studies with time-to-event outcomes. Meta-analysis can be applied to such effect estimates if their standard errors are available, using the generic inverse variance outcome type in RevMan (see Chapter 9, Section 9.4.3). When extracting data from non-randomized studies, and from some randomized studies, adjusted effect estimates may be available (e.g. adjusted odds ratios from logistic regression analyses, or adjusted rate ratios from Poisson regression analyses). The process of data extraction, and analysis using the generic inverse variance method, is the same as for unadjusted estimates, although the variables that have been adjusted for should be recorded (see Chapter 13, Section 13.6.2).

On occasion, summary data for each intervention group (for example, numbers of events and participants, or means and standard deviations) may be sought, but cannot be extracted. In such situations it may still be possible to include the study in a meta-analysis using the generic inverse variance method. A limitation of this approach is that estimates and standard errors of the same effect measure must be calculated for all the other studies in the same meta-analysis, even if they provide the summary data by intervention group. For example, if numbers in each outcome category by intervention group are known for some studies, but only odds ratios (ORs) are available for other studies, then ORs would need to be calculated for the first set of studies and entered into RevMan under the generic inverse variance outcome type to enable meta-analysis with the second set of studies. RevMan may be used to calculate these ORs (entering them as dichotomous data), and the confidence intervals that RevMan presents may be transformed to standard errors using the methods that follow.

Estimates of an effect measure of interest may be presented along with a confidence interval or a P value. It is usually desirable to obtain a standard error from these numbers, so that the generic inverse variance outcome type in RevMan can be used to perform a meta-analysis. The procedure for obtaining a standard error depends on whether the effect measure is an absolute measure (e.g. mean difference, standardized mean difference, risk difference) or a ratio measure (e.g. odds ratio, risk ratio, hazard ratio, rate ratio). We describe these procedures in Section 7.7.7.2 and Section 7.7.7.3, respectively. However, for continuous outcome measures, the special cases of extracting results for a mean from one intervention arm, and extracting results for the difference between two means, are addressed in Section 7.7.3.

### 7.7.7.2    Obtaining standard errors from confidence intervals and P values: absolute (difference) measures

If a 95% confidence interval is available for an absolute measure of intervention effect (e.g. SMD, risk difference, rate difference), then the standard error can be calculated as

$$SE = (\text{upper limit} - \text{lower limit})/3.92.$$

For 90% confidence intervals divide by 3.29 rather than 3.92; for 99% confidence intervals divide by 5.15.

Where exact P values are quoted alongside estimates of intervention effect, it is possible to estimate standard errors. While all tests of statistical significance produce P values, different tests use different mathematical approaches to obtain a P value. The method here assumes P values have been obtained through a particularly simple approach of dividing the effect estimate by its standard error and comparing the result (denoted Z) with a standard normal distribution (statisticians often refer to this as a Wald test). Where significance tests have used other mathematical approaches the estimated standard errors may not coincide exactly with the true standard errors.

The first step is to obtain the Z value corresponding to the reported P value from a table of the standard normal distribution. A standard error may then be calculated as

$$SE = \text{intervention effect estimate}/Z.$$

As an example, suppose a conference abstract presents an estimate of a risk difference of 0.03 (P = 0.008). The Z value that corresponds to a P value of 0.008 is Z = 2.652. This can be obtained from a table of the standard normal distribution or a computer (for example, by entering **=abs(normsinv(0.008/2)** into any cell in a Microsoft Excel spreadsheet). The standard error of the risk difference is obtained by dividing the risk difference (0.03) by the Z value (2.652), which gives 0.011.

### 7.7.7.3    Obtaining standard errors from confidence intervals and P values: ratio measures

The process of obtaining standard errors for ratio measures is similar to that for absolute measures, but with an additional first step. Analyses of ratio measures are performed on the natural log scale (see Chapter 9, Section 9.2.7). For a ratio measure, such as a risk ratio, odds ratio or hazard ratio (which we will denote generically as RR here), first calculate

$$\text{lower limit} = \ln(\text{lower confidence limit given for RR})$$

$$\text{upper limit} = \ln(\text{upper confidence limit given for RR})$$

$$\text{intervention effect estimate} = \ln RR$$

Then the formulae in Section 7.7.7.2 can be used. Note that the standard error refers to the log of the ratio measure. When using the generic inverse variance method in RevMan, the data should be entered on the natural log scale, that is as lnRR and the standard error of lnRR, as calculated here (see Chapter 9, Section 9.4.3).

## 7.8   Managing data

It is possible to collect data on paper data collection forms and to enter them directly into RevMan. Often, however, there will be a need or desire to manage data in intermediate computer software before entry into RevMan. A variety of software and data management programs may be helpful for this, including spreadsheet software (e.g. Microsoft Excel) and database programs (e.g. Microsoft Access). For example, tabulation of extracted information about studies in a spreadsheet can facilitate the classifying of studies into comparisons and subgroups. Furthermore, statistical conversions, for example from standard errors to standard deviations, should ideally be undertaken with a computer rather than using a hand calculator, since it allows a permanent record to be kept of the original and calculated numbers as well as the actual calculations used.

## 7.9 Chapter information

**Editors**: Julian PT Higgins and Jonathan J Deeks.

**This chapter should be cited as**: Higgins JPT, Deeks JJ (editors). Chapter 7: Selecting studies and collecting data. In: Higgins JPT, Green S (editors), *Cochrane Handbook for Systematic Reviews of Interventions*. Chichester (UK): John Wiley & Sons, 2008.

**Acknowledgements**: This section builds on earlier versions of the *Handbook*. For details of previous authors and editors of the *Handbook*, see Chapter 1 (Section 1.4). Andrew Herxheimer, Nicki Jackson, Yoon Loke, Deirdre Price and Helen Thomas contributed text. Stephanie Taylor and Sonja Hood contributed suggestions for designing data collection forms. We are grateful to Judith Anzures, Mike Clarke, Miranda Cumpston and Peter Gøtzsche for helpful comments.

## 7.10 References

**Berlin 1997**
Berlin JA. Does blinding of readers affect the results of meta-analyses? University of Pennsylvania Meta-analysis Blinding Study Group. *The Lancet* 1997; 350: 185–186.

**Buscemi 2006**
Buscemi N, Hartling L, Vandermeer B, Tjosvold L, Klassen TP. Single data extraction generated more errors than double data extraction in systematic reviews. *Journal of Clinical Epidemiology* 2006; 59: 697–703.

**Collett 1994**
Collett D. *Modelling Survival Data in Medical Research*. London: Chapman and Hall, 1994.

**Cooper 1989**
Cooper H, Ribble RG. Influences on the outcome of literature searches for integrative research reviews. *Knowledge* 1989; 10: 179–201.

**Dane 1998**
Dane AV, Schneider BH. Program integrity in primary and early secondary prevention: are implementation effects out of control? *Clinical Psychology Review* 1998; 18: 23–45.

**Deeks 1997a**
Deeks J. Are you sure that's a standard deviation? (part 1). *Cochrane News* 1997; Issue No. 10: 11–12. (Available from www.cochrane.org/newslett/ccnewsbi.htm).

**Deeks 1997b**

Deeks J. Are you sure that's a standard deviation? (part 2). *Cochrane News* 1997; Issue No. 11: 11–12. (Available from www.cochrane.org/newslett/ccnewsbi.htm).

**Derry 2000**

Derry S, Loke YK. Risk of gastrointestinal haemorrhage with long term use of aspirin: meta-analysis. *BMJ* 2000; 321: 1183–1187.

**Dusenbury 2003**

Dusenbury L, Brannigan R, Falco M, Hansen WB. A review of research on fidelity of implementation: implications for drug abuse prevention in school settings. *Health Education Research* 2003; 18: 237–256.

**Early Breast Cancer Trialists' Collaborative Group 1990**

Early Breast Cancer Trialists' Collaborative Group. *Treatment of Early Breast Cancer. Volume 1: Worldwide Evidence 1985–1990*. Oxford (UK): Oxford University Press, 1990. (Available from www.ctsu.ox.ac.uk).

**Edwards 2002**

Edwards P, Clarke M, DiGuiseppi C, Pratap S, Roberts I, Wentz R. Identification of randomized controlled trials in systematic reviews: accuracy and reliability of screening records. *Statistics in Medicine* 2002; 21: 1635–1640.

**Gøtzsche 2007**

Gøtzsche PC, Hróbjartsson A, Maric K, Tendal B. Data extraction errors in meta-analyses that use standardized mean differences. *JAMA* 2007; 298: 430–437.

**Jadad 1996**

Jadad AR, Moore RA, Carroll D, Jenkinson C, Reynolds DJM, Gavaghan DJ, McQuay H. Assessing the quality of reports of randomized clinical trials: Is blinding necessary? *Controlled Clinical Trials* 1996; 17: 1–12.

**Jones 2005**

Jones AP, Remington T, Williamson PR, Ashby D, Smyth RL. High prevalence but low impact of data extraction and reporting errors were found in Cochrane systematic reviews. *Journal of Clinical Epidemiology* 2005; 58: 741–742.

**Lumley 2004**

Lumley J, Oliver SS, Chamberlain C, Oakley L. Interventions for promoting smoking cessation during pregnancy. *Cochrane Database of Systematic Reviews* 2004, Issue 4. Art No: CD001055.

**MacLennan 2000**

MacLennan JM, Shackley F, Heath PT, Deeks JJ, Flamank C, Herbert M, Griffiths H, Hatzmann E, Goilav C, Moxon ER. Safety, immunogenicity, and induction of immunologic memory by a serogroup C meningococcal conjugate vaccine in infants: A randomized controlled trial. *JAMA* 2000; 283: 2795–2801.

**Meade 1997**

Meade MO, Richardson WS. Selecting and appraising studies for a systematic review. *Annals of Internal Medicine* 1997; 127: 531–537.

**Moher 2001**

Moher D, Schulz KF, Altman DG. The CONSORT Statement: revised recommendations for improving the quality of reports of parallel-group randomised trials. *The Lancet* 2001; 357: 1191–1194. (Available from www.consort-statement.org).

**Orwin 1994**

Orwin RG. Evaluating coding decisions. In: Cooper H, Hedges LV (editors). *The Handbook of Research Synthesis*. New York (NY): Russell Sage Foundation, 1994.

**Oxman 1993**

Oxman AD, Guyatt GH. The science of reviewing research. *Annals of the New York Academy of Sciences* 1993; 703: 125–133.

**Parmar 1998**

Parmar MKB, Torri V, Stewart L. Extracting summary statistics to perform meta-analyses of the published literature for survival endpoints. *Statistics in Medicine* 1998; 17: 2815–2834.

**Stock 1994**

Stock WA. Systematic coding for research synthesis. In: Cooper H, Hedges LV (editors). *The Handbook of Research Synthesis*. New York (NY): Russell Sage Foundation, 1994.

**Tierney 2007**

Tierney JF, Stewart LA, Ghersi D, Burdett S, Sydes MR. Practical methods for incorporating summary time-to-event data into meta-analysis. *Trials* 2007; 8: 16.

**Tramèr 1997**

Tramèr MR, Reynolds DJ, Moore RA, McQuay HJ. Impact of covert duplicate publication on meta-analysis: a case study. *BMJ* 1997; 315: 635–640.

**von Elm 2004**

von Elm E, Poglia G, Walder B, Tramèr MR. Different patterns of duplicate publication: an analysis of articles used in systematic reviews. *JAMA* 2004; 291: 974–980.

**Williamson 2002**

Williamson PR, Smith CT, Hutton JL, Marson AG. Aggregate data meta-analysis with time-to-event outcomes. *Statistics in Medicine* 2002; 21: 3337–3351.

**Zanchetti 1999**

Zanchetti A, Hansson L. Risk of major gastrointestinal bleeding with aspirin (Authors' reply). *The Lancet* 1999; 353: 149–150.

# 8 Assessing risk of bias in included studies

**Edited by Julian PT Higgins and Douglas G Altman on behalf of the Cochrane Statistical Methods Group and the Cochrane Bias Methods Group**

## Key Points

- Problems with the design and execution of individual studies of healthcare interventions raise questions about the validity of their findings; empirical evidence provides support for this concern.

- An assessment of the validity of studies included in a Cochrane review should emphasize the risk of bias in their results, i.e. the risk that they will overestimate or underestimate the true intervention effect.

- Numerous tools are available for assessing methodological quality of clinical trials. We recommend against the use of scales yielding a summary score.

- The Cochrane Collaboration recommends a specific tool for assessing risk of bias in each included study. This comprises a description and a judgement for each entry in a 'Risk of bias' table, where each entry addresses a specific feature of the study. The judgement for each entry involves answering a question, with answers 'Yes' indicating low risk of bias, 'No' indicating high risk of bias, and 'Unclear' indicating either lack of information or uncertainty over the potential for bias.

- Plots of 'Risk of bias' assessments can be created in RevMan.

- For parallel group trials, the features of interest in a standard 'Risk of bias' table of a Cochrane review are sequence generation, allocation sequence concealment, blinding, incomplete outcome data, selective outcome reporting and other potential sources of bias.

- Detailed considerations for the assessment of these features are provided in this chapter.

## 8.1    Introduction

The extent to which a Cochrane review can draw conclusions about the effects of an intervention depends on whether the data and results from the included studies are valid. In particular, a meta-analysis of invalid studies may produce a misleading result, yielding a narrow confidence interval around the wrong intervention effect estimate. The evaluation of the validity of the included studies is therefore an essential component of a Cochrane review, and should influence the analysis, interpretation and conclusions of the review.

The validity of a study may be considered to have two dimensions. The first dimension is whether the study is asking an appropriate research question. This is often described as 'external validity', and its assessment depends on the purpose for which the study is to be used. External validity is closely connected with the generalizability or applicability of a study's findings, and is addressed in Chapter 12.

The second dimension of a study's validity relates to whether it answers its research question 'correctly', that is, in a manner free from bias. This is often described as 'internal validity', and it is this aspect of validity that we address in this chapter. As most Cochrane reviews focus on randomized trials, we concentrate on how to appraise the validity of this type of study. Chapter 13 addresses further issues in the assessment of non-randomized studies, and Chapter 14 includes further considerations for adverse effects. Assessments of internal validity are frequently referred to as 'assessments of methodological quality' or 'quality assessment'. However, we will avoid the term quality, for reasons explained below. In the next section we define 'bias' and distinguish it from the related concepts of random error and quality.

## 8.2    What is bias?

### 8.2.1    'Bias' and 'risk of bias'

A **bias** is a systematic error, or deviation from the truth, in results or inferences. Biases can operate in either direction: different biases can lead to underestimation or overestimation of the true intervention effect. Biases can vary in magnitude: some are small (and trivial compared with the observed effect) and some are substantial (so that an apparent finding may be entirely due to bias). Even a particular source of bias may vary in direction: bias due to a particular design flaw (e.g. lack of allocation concealment) may lead to underestimation of an effect in one study but overestimation in another study. It is usually impossible to know to what extent biases have affected the results of a particular study, although there is good empirical evidence that particular flaws in the design, conduct and analysis of randomized clinical trials lead to bias (see Section 8.2.3). Because the results of a study may in fact be unbiased despite a methodological flaw, it is more appropriate to consider **risk of bias**.

Differences in risks of bias can help explain variation in the results of the studies included in a systematic review (i.e. can explain heterogeneity of results). More rigorous studies are more likely to yield results that are closer to the truth. Meta-analysis of results from studies of variable validity can result in false positive conclusions (erroneously concluding an intervention is effective) if the less rigorous studies are biased toward overestimating an intervention's effect. They might also come to false negative conclusions (erroneously concluding no effect) if the less rigorous studies are biased towards underestimating an intervention's effect (Detsky 1992).

It is important to assess risk of bias in all studies in a review irrespective of the anticipated variability in either the results or the validity of the included studies. For instance, the results may be consistent among studies but all the studies may be flawed. In this case, the review's conclusions should not be as strong as if a series of rigorous studies yielded consistent results about an intervention's effect. In a Cochrane review, this appraisal process is described as the *assessment of risk of bias in included studies*. A tool that has been developed and implemented in RevMan for this purpose is described in Section 8.5. The rest of this chapter provides the rationale for this tool as well as explaining how bias assessments should be summarized and incorporated in analyses (Sections 8.6 to 8.8). Sections 8.9 to 8.14 provide background considerations to assist review authors in using the tool.

Bias should not be confused with **imprecision**. Bias refers to *systematic error*, meaning that multiple replications of the same study would reach the wrong answer on average. Imprecision refers to *random error*, meaning that multiple replications of the same study will produce different effect estimates because of sampling variation even if they would give the right answer on average. The results of smaller studies are subject to greater sampling variation and hence are less precise. Imprecision is reflected in the confidence interval around the intervention effect estimate from each study and in the weight given to the results of each study in a meta-analysis. More precise results are given more weight.

## 8.2.2 'Risk of bias' and 'quality'

Bias may be distinguished from **quality**. The phrase 'assessment of methodological quality' has been used extensively in the context of systematic review methods to refer to the critical appraisal of included studies. The term suggests an investigation of the extent to which study authors conducted their research to the highest possible standards. This *Handbook* draws a distinction between assessment of methodological quality and assessment of risk of bias, and recommends a focus on the latter. The reasons for this distinction include:

1. The key consideration in a Cochrane review is the extent to which results of included studies should be *believed*. Assessing risk of bias targets this question squarely.

2. A study may be performed to the highest possible standards yet still have an important risk of bias. For example, in many situations it is impractical or impossible to blind participants or study personnel to intervention group. It is inappropriately judgemental to describe all such studies as of 'low quality', but that does not mean they are free of bias resulting from knowledge of intervention status.

3. Some markers of quality in medical research, such as obtaining ethical approval, performing a sample size calculation and reporting a study in line with the CONSORT Statement (Moher 2001d), are unlikely to have direct implications for risk of bias.

4. An emphasis on risk of bias overcomes ambiguity between the quality of reporting and the quality of the underlying research (although does not overcome the problem of having to rely on reports to assess the underlying research).

Notwithstanding these concerns about the term 'quality', the term 'quality of evidence' is used in 'Summary of findings' tables in Cochrane reviews to describe the extent to which one can be confident that an estimate of effect is near the true value for an outcome, across studies, as described in Chapter 11 (Section 11.5) and Chapter 12 (Section 12.2). The risk of bias in the results of each study contributing to an estimate of effect is one of several factors that must be considered when judging the quality of a body of evidence, as defined in this context.

### 8.2.3   Establishing empirical evidence of biases

Biases associated with particular characteristics of studies may be examined using a technique often known as **meta-epidemiology** (Naylor 1997, Sterne 2002). A meta-epidemiological study analyses a collection of meta-analyses, in each of which the component studies have been classified according to some study-level characteristic. An early example was the study of clinical trials with dichotomous outcomes included in meta-analyses from the *Cochrane Pregnancy and Childbirth Database* (Schulz 1995b). This study demonstrated that trials in which randomization was inadequately concealed or inadequately reported yielded exaggerated estimates of intervention effect compared with trials reporting adequate concealment, and found a similar (but smaller) association for trials that were not described as double-blind.

A simple analysis of a meta-epidemiological study is to calculate the 'ratio of odds ratios' within each meta-analysis (for example, the intervention odds ratio in trials with inadequate/unclear allocation concealment divided by the odds ratio in trials with adequate allocation concealment). These ratios of odds ratios are then combined across meta-analyses, in a meta-analysis. Thus, such analyses are also known as 'meta-meta-analyses'. In subsequent sections of this chapter, empirical evidence of bias from meta-epidemiological studies is cited where available as part of the rationale for assessing each domain of potential bias.

## 8.3   Tools for assessing quality and risk of bias

### 8.3.1   Types of tools

Many tools have been proposed for assessing the quality of studies for use in the context of a systematic review and elsewhere. Most tools are **scales**, in which various components of quality are scored and combined to give a summary score; or **checklists**, in which specific questions are asked (Jüni 2001).

In 1995, Moher and colleagues identified 25 scales and 9 checklists that had been used to assess the validity or 'quality' of randomized trials (Moher 1995, Moher 1996). These scales and checklists included between 3 and 57 items and were found to take from 10 to 45 minutes to complete for each study. Almost all of the items in the instruments were based on suggested or 'generally accepted' criteria that are mentioned in clinical trial textbooks. Many instruments also contained items that were not directly related to internal validity, such as whether a power calculation was done (an item that relates more to the precision of the results) or whether the inclusion and exclusion criteria were clearly described (an item that relates more to applicability than validity). Scales were more likely than checklists to include criteria that do not directly relate to internal validity.

The Collaboration's recommended tool for assessing risk of bias is neither a scale nor a checklist. It is a **domain-based evaluation**, in which critical assessments are made separately for different domains, described in Section 8.5. It was developed between 2005 and 2007 by a working group of methodologists, editors and review authors. Because it is impossible to know the extent of bias (or even the true risk of bias) in a given study, the possibility of validating any proposed tool is limited. The most realistic assessment of the validity of a study may involve subjectivity: for example an assessment of whether lack of blinding of patients might plausibly have affected recurrence of a serious condition such as cancer.

## 8.3.2 Reporting versus conduct

A key difficulty in the assessment of risk of bias or quality is the obstacle provided by incomplete reporting. While the emphasis should be on the risk of bias in the actual design and conduct of a study, it can be tempting to resort to assessing the adequacy of reporting. Many of the tools reviewed by Moher et al. were liable to confuse these separate issues (Moher 1995). Moreover, scoring in scales was often based on whether something was reported (such as stating how participants were allocated) rather than whether it was done appropriately in the study.

## 8.3.3 Quality scales and Cochrane reviews

The use of scales for assessing quality or risk of bias is explicitly discouraged in Cochrane reviews. While the approach offers appealing simplicity, it is not supported by empirical evidence (Emerson 1990, Schulz 1995b). Calculating a summary score inevitably involves assigning 'weights' to different items in the scale, and it is difficult to justify the weights assigned. Furthermore, scales have been shown to be unreliable assessments of validity (Jüni 1999) and they are less likely to be transparent to users of the review. It is preferable to use simple approaches for assessing validity that can be fully reported (i.e. how each trial was rated on each criterion).

One commonly-used scale was developed by Jadad and colleagues for randomized trials in pain research (Jadad 1996). The use of this scale is explicitly discouraged. As well as suffering from the generic problems of scales, it has a strong emphasis on reporting rather than conduct, and does not cover one of the most important potential biases in randomized trials, namely allocation concealment (see Section 8.10.1).

## 8.3.4 Collecting information for assessments of risk of bias

Despite the limitations of reports, information about the design and conduct of studies will often be obtained from published reports, including journal papers, book chapters, dissertations, conference abstracts and web sites (including trials registries). Published protocols are a particularly valuable source of information when they are available. The extraction of information from such reports is discussed in Chapter 7. Data collection forms should include space to extract sufficient details to allow implementation of the Collaboration's 'Risk of bias' tool (Section 8.5). When extracting this information, it is particularly desirable to record the source of each piece of information (including the precise location within a document). It is helpful to test data collection forms and assessments of risk of bias within a review team on a pilot sample of articles to ensure that criteria are applied consistently, and that consensus can be reached. Three to six papers that, if possible, span a range from low to high risk of bias might provide a suitable sample for this.

Authors must also decide whether those assessing risk of bias will be blinded to the names of the authors, institutions, journal and results of a study when they assess its methods. One study suggested that blind assessment of reports might produce lower and more consistent ratings than open assessments (Jadad 1996), whereas other studies suggested little benefit from blind assessments (Berlin 1997, Kjaergard 2001). Blinded assessments are very time consuming, they may not be possible when the studies are well known to the review authors, and not all domains of bias can be assessed independently of the outcome data. Furthermore, knowledge of who undertook a study can sometimes allow reasonable assumptions to be made about how the study was conducted (although such assumptions must be reported by the review author). Authors must weigh the potential benefits against the costs involved when deciding whether or not to blind assessment of certain information in study reports.

Review authors with different levels of methodological training and experience may identify different sources of evidence and reach different judgements about risk of bias. Although experts in content areas may have pre-formed opinions that can influence their assessments (Oxman 1993), they may nonetheless give more consistent assessments of the validity of studies than people without content expertise (Jadad 1996). Content experts may have valuable insights into the magnitudes of biases, and experienced methodologists may have valuable insights into potential biases that are not at first apparent. It is desirable that review authors should include both content experts and methodologists and ensure that all have an adequate understanding of the relevant methodological issues.

Attempts to assess risk of bias are often hampered by incomplete reporting of what happened during the conduct of the study. One option for collecting missing information is to contact the study investigators. Unfortunately, contacting authors of trial reports may lead to overly positive answers. In a survey of 104 trialists, using direct questions about blinding with named categories of trial personnel, 43% responded that the data analysts in their double-blind trials were blinded, and 19% responded that the manuscript writers were blinded (Haahr 2006). This is unlikely to be true, given that such procedures were reported in only 3% and 0% of the corresponding published articles, and that they are very rarely described in other trial reports.

To reduce the risk of overly positive answers, review authors should use open-ended questions when asking trial authors for information about study design and conduct. For example, to obtain information about blinding, a request of the following form might be appropriate: "Please describe all measures used, if any, to ensure blinding of trial participants and key trial personnel from knowledge of which intervention a participant had received." To obtain information about the randomization process, a request of the following form might be appropriate: "How did you decide which treatment the next patient should get?" More focused questions can then be asked to clarify remaining uncertainties.

# 8.4  Introduction to sources of bias in clinical trials

The reliability of the results of a randomized trial depends on the extent to which potential sources of bias have been avoided. A key part of a review is to consider the risk of bias in the results of each of the eligible studies. We introduce six issues to consider briefly here, then describe a tool for assessing them in Section 8.5. We provide more detailed consideration of each issue in Sections 8.9 to 8.14.

The unique strength of randomization is that, if successfully accomplished, it prevents selection bias in allocating interventions to participants. Its success in this respect depends on fulfilling several interrelated processes. A rule for allocating interventions to participants must be specified, based on some chance (random) process. We call this **sequence generation**. Furthermore, steps must be taken to secure strict implementation of that schedule of random assignments by preventing foreknowledge of the forthcoming allocations. This process if often termed **allocation concealment**, although could more accurately be described as allocation sequence concealment. Thus, one suitable method for assigning interventions would be to use a simple random (and therefore unpredictable) sequence, and to conceal the upcoming allocations from those involved in enrolment into the trial.

After enrolment into the study, **blinding** (or masking) of study participants and personnel may reduce the risk that knowledge of which intervention was received, rather than the intervention itself, affects outcomes and outcome measurements. Blinding can be especially important for assessment of subjective outcomes, such as degree of postoperative pain. Effective blinding can also ensure that the compared groups receive a similar amount of attention, ancillary treatment and diagnostic investigations. Blinding may also be important for objective outcomes in trials where enthusiasm for participation or follow-up may be influenced by group allocation. Blinding is not always possible, however. For example, it is usually impossible to blind people to whether or not major surgery has been undertaken.

**Incomplete outcome data** raise the possibility that effect estimates are biased. There are two reasons for incomplete (or missing) outcome data in clinical trials. *Exclusions* refer to situations in which some participants are omitted from reports of analyses, despite outcome data being available to the trialists. *Attrition* refers to situations in which outcome data are not available.

Within a published report those analyses with statistically significant differences between intervention groups are more likely to be reported than non-significant differences. This sort of 'within-study publication bias' is usually known as outcome reporting bias or **selective reporting** bias, and may be one of the most substantial biases affecting results from individual studies (Chan 2005).

In addition there are **other sources of bias** that are relevant only in certain circumstances. Some can be found only in particular trial designs (e.g. carry-over in cross-over trials and recruitment bias in cluster-randomized trials); some can be found across a broad spectrum of trials, but only for specific circumstances (e.g. bias due to early stopping); and there may be sources of bias that are only found in a particular clinical setting. There are also some complex interrelationships between elements of allocation and elements of blinding in terms of whether bias may be introduced. For example, one approach to sequence generation is through 'blocking', whereby a set number of experimental group allocations and a set number of control group allocations are randomly ordered within a 'block' of sequentially recruited participants. If there is a lack of blinding after enrolment, such that allocations are revealed to the clinician recruiting to the trial, then it may be possible for some future allocations to be predicted, thus compromising the assignment process.

For all potential sources of bias, it is important to consider the likely magnitude and the likely direction of the bias. For example, if all methodological limitations of studies were expected to bias the results towards a lack of effect, and the evidence indicates that the intervention is effective, then it may be concluded that the intervention is effective even in the presence of these potential biases.

A useful classification of biases is into selection bias, performance bias, attrition bias, detection bias and reporting bias. Table 8.4a describes each of these and shows how the domains of assessment in the Collaboration's 'Risk of bias' tool fit with these categories.

# 8.5 The Cochrane Collaboration's tool for assessing risk of bias

## 8.5.1 Overview

This section describes the recommended approach for assessing risk of bias in studies included in Cochrane reviews. It is a two-part tool, addressing the six specific domains discussed in Sections 8.9 to 8.14 (namely sequence generation, allocation concealment,

**Table 8.4.a**   A common classification scheme for bias

| Type of bias | Description | Relevant domains in the Collaboration's 'Risk of bias' tool |
|---|---|---|
| Selection bias. | Systematic differences between baseline characteristics of the groups that are compared. | • Sequence generation.<br>• Allocation concealment. |
| Performance bias. | Systematic differences between groups in the care that is provided, or in exposure to factors other than the interventions of interest. | • Blinding of participants, personnel and outcome assessors.<br>• Other potential threats to validity. |
| Attrition bias. | Systematic differences between groups in withdrawals from a study. | • Incomplete outcome data.<br>• Blinding of participants, personnel and outcome assessors. |
| Detection bias. | Systematic differences between groups in how outcomes are determined. | • Blinding of participants, personnel and outcome assessors.<br>• Other potential threats to validity. |
| Reporting bias. | Systematic differences between reported and unreported findings. | • Selective outcome reporting (see also Chapter 10). |

blinding, incomplete outcome data, selective outcome reporting and 'other issues'). The tool is summarized in Table 8.5.a. Each domain includes one or more specific entries in a 'Risk of bias' table. Within each entry, the first part of the tool involves describing what was reported to have happened in the study. The second part of the tool involves assigning a judgement relating to the risk of bias for that entry. This is achieved by answering a pre-specified question about the adequacy of the study in relation to the entry, such that a judgement of 'Yes' indicates low risk of bias, 'No' indicates high risk of bias, and 'Unclear' indicates unclear or unknown risk of bias.

The domains of sequence generation, allocation concealment and selective outcome reporting should each be addressed in the tool by a single entry for each study. For blinding and for incomplete outcome data, two or more entries may be used because assessments generally need to be made separately for different outcomes (or for the same outcome at different time points). Review authors should try to limit the number of entries used by grouping outcomes, for example, as 'subjective' or 'objective' outcomes for the purposes of assessing blinding; or as 'patient-reported at 6 months' or 'patient-reported at 12 months' for incomplete outcome data. The same groupings of outcomes will be applied to every study in the review. The final domain ('other sources of bias') can be assessed as a single entry for studies as a whole (the default in RevMan). It is recommended, however, that multiple, pre-specified, entries be used to address specific other risks of bias. Such author-specified entries may be for studies as a whole or for individual (or grouped) outcomes within every study. Adding new entries involves specifying a question that should be answerable as 'Yes' to indicate a low risk of bias.

**Table 8.5.a**   The Cochrane Collaboration's tool for assessing risk of bias

| Domain | Description | Review authors' judgement |
|---|---|---|
| **Sequence generation.** | Describe the method used to generate the allocation sequence in sufficient detail to allow an assessment of whether it should produce comparable groups. | Was the allocation sequence adequately generated? |
| **Allocation concealment.** | Describe the method used to conceal the allocation sequence in sufficient detail to determine whether intervention allocations could have been foreseen in advance of, or during, enrolment. | Was allocation adequately concealed? |
| **Blinding of participants, personnel and outcome assessors** *Assessments should be made for each main outcome (or class of outcomes).* | Describe all measures used, if any, to blind study participants and personnel from knowledge of which intervention a participant received. Provide any information relating to whether the intended blinding was effective. | Was knowledge of the allocated intervention adequately prevented during the study? |
| **Incomplete outcome data** *Assessments should be made for each main outcome (or class of outcomes).* | Describe the completeness of outcome data for each main outcome, including attrition and exclusions from the analysis. State whether attrition and exclusions were reported, the numbers in each intervention group (compared with total randomized participants), reasons for attrition/exclusions where reported, and any re-inclusions in analyses performed by the review authors. | Were incomplete outcome data adequately addressed? |
| **Selective outcome reporting.** | State how the possibility of selective outcome reporting was examined by the review authors, and what was found. | Are reports of the study free of suggestion of selective outcome reporting? |
| **Other sources of bias.** | State any important concerns about bias not addressed in the other domains in the tool. | Was the study apparently free of other problems that could put it at a high risk of bias? |
|  | If particular questions/entries were pre-specified in the review's protocol, responses should be provided for each question/entry. |  |

**Table 8.5.b**   Examples of summary descriptions for sequence generation entry

| | |
|---|---|
| Sequence generation. | Comment: No information provided. |
| Sequence generation. | Quote: "patients were randomly allocated". |
| Sequence generation. | Quote: "patients were randomly allocated". |
| | Comment: Probably done, since earlier reports from the same investigators clearly describe use of random sequences (Cartwright 1980). |
| Sequence generation. | Quote: "patients were randomly allocated". |
| | Comment: Probably not done, as a similar trial by these investigators included the same phrase yet used alternate allocation (Winrow 1983). |
| Sequence generation. | Quote (from report): "patients were randomly allocated". |
| | Quote (from correspondence): "randomization was performed according to day of treatment". |
| | Comment: Not randomized. |

## 8.5.2   The description

The description provides a succinct summary from which judgements of risk of bias can be made, and aims to ensure transparency in how these judgements are reached. For a specific study, information for the description will often come from a single published study report, but may be obtained from a mixture of study reports, protocols, published comments on the study and contacts with the investigators. Where appropriate, the description should include verbatim quotes from reports or correspondence. Alternatively, or in addition, it may include a summary of known facts, or a comment from the review authors. In particular, it should include other information that influences any judgements made (such as knowledge of other studies performed by the same investigators). A helpful construction to supplement an ambiguous quote is to state 'Probably done' or 'Probably not done', providing the rationale for such assertions. When no information is available from which to make a judgement, this should be stated explicitly. Examples of proposed formatting for the description are provided in Table 8.5.b.

## 8.5.3   The judgement

Review authors' judgements involve answering a specific question for each entry. In all cases, **an answer 'Yes' indicates a low risk of bias**, and **an answer 'No' indicates high risk of bias**.

Table 8.5.c provides criteria for making judgements about risk of bias from each of the six domains in the tool. If insufficient detail is reported of what happened in the study, the judgement will usually be 'Unclear' risk of bias. An 'Unclear' judgement should also be made if what happened in the study is known, but the risk of bias is

**Table 8.5.c**   Criteria for judging risk of bias in the 'Risk of bias' assessment tool

---

**SEQUENCE GENERATION**
**Was the allocation sequence adequately generated? [Short form: *Adequate sequence generation?*]**

---

| | |
|---|---|
| Criteria for a judgement of 'YES' (i.e. low risk of bias). | The investigators describe a random component in the sequence generation process such as:<br>• Referring to a random number table;<br>• Using a computer random number generator;<br>• Coin tossing;<br>• Shuffling cards or envelopes;<br>• Throwing dice;<br>• Drawing of lots;<br>• Minimization*.<br><br>*Minimization may be implemented without a random element, and this is considered to be equivalent to being random. |
| Criteria for the judgement of 'NO' (i.e. high risk of bias). | The investigators describe a non-random component in the sequence generation process. Usually, the description would involve some systematic, non-random approach, for example:<br>• Sequence generated by odd or even date of birth;<br>• Sequence generated by some rule based on date (or day) of admission;<br>• Sequence generated by some rule based on hospital or clinic record number.<br><br>Other non-random approaches happen much less frequently than the systematic approaches mentioned above and tend to be obvious. They usually involve judgement or some method of non-random categorization of participants, for example:<br>• Allocation by judgement of the clinician;<br>• Allocation by preference of the participant;<br>• Allocation based on the results of a laboratory test or a series of tests;<br>• Allocation by availability of the intervention. |
| Criteria for the judgement of 'UNCLEAR' (uncertain risk of bias). | Insufficient information about the sequence generation process to permit judgement of 'Yes' or 'No'. |

---

**ALLOCATION CONCEALMENT**
**Was allocation adequately concealed? [Short form: *Allocation concealment?*]**

---

| | |
|---|---|
| Criteria for a judgement of 'YES' (i.e. low risk of bias). | Participants and investigators enrolling participants could not foresee assignment because one of the following, or an equivalent method, was used to conceal allocation:<br>• Central allocation (including telephone, web-based and pharmacy-controlled randomization);<br>• Sequentially numbered drug containers of identical appearance;<br>• Sequentially numbered, opaque, sealed envelopes. |

**Table 8.5.c**  (*continued*)

| | |
|---|---|
| Criteria for the judgement of 'NO' (i.e. high risk of bias). | Participants or investigators enrolling participants could possibly foresee assignments and thus introduce selection bias, such as allocation based on:<br>• Using an open random allocation schedule (e.g. a list of random numbers);<br>• Assignment envelopes were used without appropriate safeguards (e.g. if envelopes were unsealed or non-opaque or not sequentially numbered);<br>• Alternation or rotation;<br>• Date of birth;<br>• Case record number;<br>• Any other explicitly unconcealed procedure. |
| Criteria for the judgement of 'UNCLEAR' (uncertain risk of bias). | Insufficient information to permit judgement of 'Yes' or 'No'. This is usually the case if the method of concealment is not described or not described in sufficient detail to allow a definite judgement – for example if the use of assignment envelopes is described, but it remains unclear whether envelopes were sequentially numbered, opaque and sealed. |

---

**BLINDING OF PARTICIPANTS, PERSONNEL AND OUTCOME ASSESSORS**
**Was knowledge of the allocated interventions adequately prevented during the study?**
**[Short form: *Blinding*?]**

| | |
|---|---|
| Criteria for a judgement of 'YES' (i.e. low risk of bias). | Any one of the following:<br>• No blinding, but the review authors judge that the outcome and the outcome measurement are not likely to be influenced by lack of blinding;<br>• Blinding of participants and key study personnel ensured, and unlikely that the blinding could have been broken;<br>• Either participants or some key study personnel were not blinded, but outcome assessment was blinded and the non-blinding of others unlikely to introduce bias. |
| Criteria for the judgement of 'NO' (i.e. high risk of bias). | Any one of the following:<br>• No blinding or incomplete blinding, and the outcome or outcome measurement is likely to be influenced by lack of blinding;<br>• Blinding of key study participants and personnel attempted, but likely that the blinding could have been broken;<br>• Either participants or some key study personnel were not blinded, and the non-blinding of others likely to introduce bias. |
| Criteria for the judgement of 'UNCLEAR' (uncertain risk of bias). | Any one of the following:<br>• Insufficient information to permit judgement of 'Yes' or 'No';<br>• The study did not address this outcome. |

**Table 8.5.c** *(continued)*

---

**INCOMPLETE OUTCOME DATA**
**Were incomplete outcome data adequately addressed? [Short form:** *Incomplete outcome data addressed***?]**

---

| | |
|---|---|
| Criteria for a judgement of 'YES' (i.e. low risk of bias). | Any one of the following:<br>• No missing outcome data;<br>• Reasons for missing outcome data unlikely to be related to true outcome (for survival data, censoring unlikely to be introducing bias);<br>• Missing outcome data balanced in numbers across intervention groups, with similar reasons for missing data across groups;<br>• For dichotomous outcome data, the proportion of missing outcomes compared with observed event risk not enough to have a clinically relevant impact on the intervention effect estimate;<br>• For continuous outcome data, plausible effect size (difference in means or standardized difference in means) among missing outcomes not enough to have a clinically relevant impact on observed effect size;<br>• Missing data have been imputed using appropriate methods. |
| Criteria for the judgement of 'NO' (i.e. high risk of bias). | Any one of the following:<br>• Reason for missing outcome data likely to be related to true outcome, with either imbalance in numbers or reasons for missing data across intervention groups;<br>• For dichotomous outcome data, the proportion of missing outcomes compared with observed event risk enough to induce clinically relevant bias in intervention effect estimate;<br>• For continuous outcome data, plausible effect size (difference in means or standardized difference in means) among missing outcomes enough to induce clinically relevant bias in observed effect size;<br>• 'As-treated' analysis done with substantial departure of the intervention received from that assigned at randomization;<br>• Potentially inappropriate application of simple imputation. |
| Criteria for the judgement of 'UNCLEAR' (uncertain risk of bias). | Any one of the following:<br>• Insufficient reporting of attrition/exclusions to permit judgement of 'Yes' or 'No' (e.g. number randomized not stated, no reasons for missing data provided);<br>• The study did not address this outcome. |

**Table 8.5.c**  *(continued)*

---

**SELECTIVE OUTCOME REPORTING**
**Are reports of the study free of suggestion of selective outcome reporting? [Short form:**
*Free of selective reporting?***]**

---

| | |
|---|---|
| Criteria for a judgement of 'YES' (i.e. low risk of bias). | Any of the following:<br>● The study protocol is available and all of the study's pre-specified (primary and secondary) outcomes that are of interest in the review have been reported in the pre-specified way;<br>● The study protocol is not available but it is clear that the published reports include all expected outcomes, including those that were pre-specified (convincing text of this nature may be uncommon). |
| Criteria for the judgement of 'NO' (i.e. high risk of bias). | Any one of the following:<br>● Not all of the study's pre-specified primary outcomes have been reported;<br>● One or more primary outcomes is reported using measurements, analysis methods or subsets of the data (e.g. subscales) that were not pre-specified;<br>● One or more reported primary outcomes were not pre-specified (unless clear justification for their reporting is provided, such as an unexpected adverse effect);<br>● One or more outcomes of interest in the review are reported incompletely so that they cannot be entered in a meta-analysis;<br>● The study report fails to include results for a key outcome that would be expected to have been reported for such a study. |
| Criteria for the judgement of 'UNCLEAR' (uncertain risk of bias). | Insufficient information to permit judgement of 'Yes' or 'No'. It is likely that the majority of studies will fall into this category. |

---

**OTHER POTENTIAL THREATS TO VALIDITY**
**Was the study apparently free of other problems that could put it at a risk of bias?**
**[Short form:** *Free of other bias?***]**

---

| | |
|---|---|
| Criteria for a judgement of 'YES' (i.e. low risk of bias). | The study appears to be free of other sources of bias. |
| Criteria for the judgement of 'NO' (i.e. high risk of bias). | There is at least one important risk of bias. For example, the study:<br>● Had a potential source of bias related to the specific study design used; or<br>● Stopped early due to some data-dependent process (including a formal-stopping rule); or<br>● Had extreme baseline imbalance; or |

---

**Table 8.5.c** (*continued*)

|  | • Has been claimed to have been fraudulent; or |
|  | • Had some other problem. |
| Criteria for the judgement of 'UNCLEAR' (uncertain risk of bias). | There may be a risk of bias, but there is either: |
|  | • Insufficient information to assess whether an important risk of bias exists; or |
|  | • Insufficient rationale or evidence that an identified problem will introduce bias. |

unknown; or if an entry is not relevant to the study at hand (particularly for assessing blinding and incomplete outcome data, when the outcome being assessed by the entry has not been measured in the study).

# 8.6 Presentation of assessments of risk of bias

A 'Risk of bias' table is available in RevMan for inclusion in a Cochrane review as part of the 'Table of characteristics of included studies'. For each question-based entry, the judgement ('Yes' for low risk of bias; 'No' for high risk of bias, or 'Unclear') is followed by a text box providing a description of the design, conduct or observations that underlie the judgement. Figure 8.6.a provides an example of how it might look. If the text box is left empty, and the judgement is left as 'Unclear', then the entry will be omitted from the 'Risk of bias' table for the study on publication in the CDSR.

Considerations for presentation of 'Risk of bias' assessments in the review text are discussed in Chapter 4 (Section 4.5) (under the Results sub-heading 'Risk of bias in included studies' and the Discussion subheading 'Quality of the evidence').

Two figures may be generated using RevMan for inclusion in a published review. A 'Risk of bias graph' figure illustrates the proportion of studies with each of the judgements ('Yes', 'No', 'Unclear') for each entry in the tool (see Figure 8.6.b). A 'Risk of bias summary' figure presents all of the judgements in a cross-tabulation of study by entry (see Figure 8.6.c).

# 8.7 Summary assessments of risk of bias

The Collaboration's recommended tool for assessing risk of bias in included studies involves the assessment and presentation of individual domains, such as allocation concealment and blinding. To draw conclusions about the overall risk of bias for an outcome it is necessary to summarize these. The use of scales (in which scores for multiple items are added up to produce a total) is discouraged for reasons outlined in Section 8.3.1.

Nonetheless, any assessment of the overall risk of bias involves consideration of the relative importance of different domains. A review author will have to make judgements about which domains are most important in the current review. For example, for highly subjective outcomes such as pain, authors may decide that blinding of participants is

| Entry | Judgement | Description |
|---|---|---|
| Adequate sequence generation? | Yes. | Quote: "patients were randomly allocated." Comment: Probably done, since earlier reports from the same investigators clearly describe use of random sequences (Cartwright 1980). |
| Allocation concealment? | No. | Quote: "...using a table of random numbers." Comment: Probably not done. |
| Blinding? (Patient-reported outcomes) | Yes. | Quote: "double blind, double dummy"; "High and low dose tablets or capsules were indistinguishable in all aspects of their outward appearance. For each drug an identically matched placebo was available (the success of blinding was evaluated by examining the drugs before distribution)." Comment: Probably done. |
| Blinding? (Mortality) | Yes. | Obtained from medical records; review authors do not believe this will introduce bias. |
| Incomplete outcome data addressed?(Short-term outcomes (2-6 wks)) | No. | 4 weeks: 17/110 missing from intervention group (9 due to 'lack of efficacy'); 7/113 missing from control group (2 due to 'lack of efficacy'). |
| Incomplete outcome data addressed? (Longer-term outcomes (>6 wks)) | No. | 12 weeks: 31/110 missing from intervention group; 18/113 missing from control group. Reasons differ across groups. |
| Free of selective reporting? | No. | Three rating scales for cognition listed in Methods, but only one reported. |
| Free of other bias? | No. | Trial stopped early due to apparent benefit. |

**Figure 8.6.a**   Example of a 'Risk of bias' table for a single study (fictional)

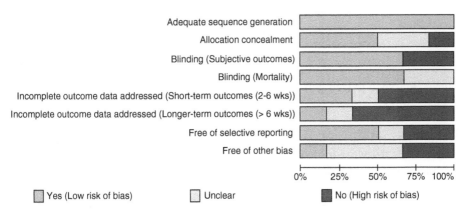

**Figure 8.6.b**   Example of a 'Risk of bias graph' figure

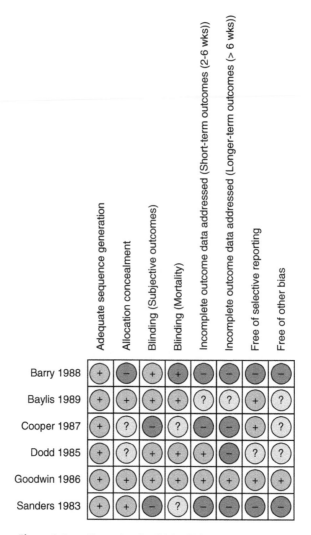

**Figure 8.6.c**    Example of a 'Risk of bias summary' figure

critical. How such judgements are reached should be made explicit and they should be informed by:

• **Empirical evidence of bias**: Sections 8.5 to 8.14 summarize empirical evidence of the association between domains such as allocation concealment and blinding and estimated magnitudes of effect. However, the evidence base remains incomplete.

• **Likely direction of bias**: The available empirical evidence suggests that failure to meet most criteria, such as adequate allocation concealment, is associated with over-estimates of effect. If the likely direction of bias for a domain is such that effects will be underestimated (biased towards the null), then, providing the review demonstrates an important effect of the intervention, such a domain may be of less concern.

- **Likely magnitude of bias**: The likely magnitude of bias associated with any domain may vary. For example, the magnitude of bias associated with inadequate blinding of participants is likely to be greater for more subjective outcomes. Some indication of the likely magnitude of bias may be provided by the empirical evidence base (see above), but this does not yet provide clear information on the particular scenarios in which biases may be large or small. It may, however, be possible to consider the likely magnitude of bias relative to the estimated magnitude of effect. For example, inadequate allocation sequence concealment and a small estimate of effect might substantially reduce one's confidence in the estimate, whereas minor inadequacies in how incomplete outcome data were addressed might not substantially reduce one's confidence in a large estimate of effect.

Summary assessment of risk of bias might be considered at four levels:

- **Summarizing risk of bias for a study across outcomes**: Some domains affect the risk of bias across outcomes in a study: e.g. sequence generation and allocation sequence concealment. Other domains, such as blinding and incomplete outcome data, may have different risks of bias for different outcomes within a study. Thus, review authors should not assume that the risk of bias is the same for all outcomes in a study. Moreover, a summary assessment of the risk of bias across all outcomes for a study is generally of little interest.

- **Summarizing risk of bias for an outcome within a study (across domains)**: This is the recommended level at which to summarize the risk of bias in a study, because some risks of bias may be different for different outcomes. A summary assessment of the risk of bias for an outcome should include all of the entries relevant to that outcome: i.e. both study-level entries, such as allocation sequence concealment, and outcome specific entries, such as blinding.

- **Summarizing risk of bias for an outcome across studies (e.g. for a meta-analysis)**: These are the main summary assessments that will be made by review authors and incorporated into judgements about the 'quality of evidence' in 'Summary of findings' tables, as described in Chapter 11 (Section 11.5).

- **Summarizing risk of bias for a review as a whole (across studies and outcomes)**: It may be tempting to summarize the overall risk of bias in a review, but this should be avoided for two reasons. First, this requires value judgements about which outcomes are critical to a decision and, therefore, should be included in this assessment. Frequently no data are available from the studies included in a review for some outcomes that may be critical, such as adverse effects, and the risk of bias is rarely the same across all of the outcomes that are critical to such an assessment. Second, judgements about which outcomes are critical to a decision may vary from setting to setting, both due to differences in values and due to differences in other factors, such as baseline risk. Thus, judgements about the overall risk of bias of evidence across studies and outcomes should be made in a specific context, for example in the context of clinical practice guidelines, and not in the context of systematic reviews that are intended to inform decisions across a variety of settings.

Review authors should make explicit judgements about the risk of bias for important outcomes both within and across studies. This requires identifying the most important domains ('key domains') that feed into these summary assessments. Table 8.7.a provides a possible approach to making summary assessments of the risk of bias for important outcomes within and across studies.

**Table 8.7.a**  Possible approach for summary assessments of the risk of bias for each important outcome (across domains) within and across studies

| Risk of bias | Interpretation | Within a study | Across studies |
|---|---|---|---|
| Low risk of bias. | Plausible bias unlikely to seriously alter the results. | Low risk of bias for all key domains. | Most information is from studies at low risk of bias. |
| Unclear risk of bias. | Plausible bias that raises some doubt about the results. | Unclear risk of bias for one or more key domains. | Most information is from studies at low or unclear risk of bias. |
| High risk of bias. | Plausible bias that seriously weakens confidence in the results. | High risk of bias for one or more key domains. | The proportion of information from studies at high risk of bias is sufficient to affect the interpretation of results. |

# 8.8    Incorporating assessments into analyses

## 8.8.1    Introduction

Statistical considerations often involve a trade-off between bias and precision. A meta-analysis that includes all eligible studies may produce a result with high precision (narrow confidence interval), but be seriously biased because of flaws in the conduct of some of the studies. On the other hand, including only the studies at low risk of bias in all domains assessed may produce a result that is unbiased but imprecise (if there are only a few high-quality studies).

When performing and presenting meta-analyses, review authors must address risk of bias in the results of included studies. It is not appropriate to present analyses and interpretations based on all studies, ignoring flaws identified during the assessment of risk of bias. The higher the proportion of studies assessed to be at high risk of bias, the more cautious should be the analysis and interpretation of their results.

## 8.8.2 Exploring the impact of risk of bias

### 8.8.2.1 Graphing results according to risk of bias

In the discussion that follows, we refer to comparisons of results according to individual bias domains. However, such comparisons can also be made according to risk of bias summarized at the study level (see Section 8.7).

Plots of intervention effect estimates (e.g. forest plots) stratified according to risk of bias are likely to be a useful way to begin examining the potential for bias to affect the results of a meta-analysis. Forest plots ordered by judgements on each 'Risk of bias' entry are available in RevMan 5. Such plots give a visual impression both of the relative contributions of the studies at low, unclear and high risk of bias, and also of the extent of differences in intervention effect estimates between studies at low, unclear and high risk of bias. It will usually be sensible to restrict such plots to key bias domains (see Section 8.7).

### 8.8.2.2 Studies assessed as at unclear risk of bias

Studies are assessed as at unclear risk of bias when too few details are available to make a judgement of 'high' or 'low' risk; when the risk of bias is genuinely unknown despite sufficient information about the conduct; or when an entry is not relevant to a study (for example because the study did not address any of the outcomes in the group of outcomes to which the entry applies). When the first reason dominates, it is reasonable to assume that the average bias in results from such studies will be less than in studies at high risk of bias, because the conduct of some studies assessed as unclear will in fact have avoided bias. Limited evidence from empirical studies that examined the 'high' and 'unclear' categories separately confirms this: for example, the study of Schulz et al. found that intervention odds ratios were exaggerated by 41% for trials with inadequate concealment (high risk of bias) and by 30% for trials with unclear concealment (unclear risk of bias) (Schulz 1995b). However, most empirical studies have combined the 'high' and 'unclear' categories, which were then compared with the 'low' category.

It is recommended that review authors do not combine studies at 'low' and 'unclear' risk of bias in analyses, unless they provide specific reasons for believing that these studies are likely to have been conducted in a manner that avoided bias. In the rest of this section, we will assume that studies assessed as at low risk of bias will be treated as a separate category.

### 8.8.2.3    *Meta-regression and comparisons of subgroups*

Formal comparisons of intervention effects according to risk of bias can be done using meta-regression (see Chapter 9, Section 9.6.4). For studies with dichotomous outcomes, results of meta-regression analyses are most usefully expressed as ratios of odds ratios (or risk ratios) comparing results of studies at high or unclear risk of bias with those of studies at low risk of bias.

$$\text{Ratio of odds ratios} = \frac{\text{Intervention odds ratio in studies at high or unclear risk of bias}}{\text{Intervention odds ratio in studies at low risk of bias}}$$

Alternatively, separate comparisons of high versus low and unclear versus low can be made. For studies with continuous outcomes (e.g. blood pressure), intervention effects are expressed as mean differences between intervention groups, and results of meta-regression analyses correspond to differences of mean differences.

If the estimated effect of the intervention is the same in studies at high and unclear risk of bias as in studies at low risk of bias then the ratio of odds ratios (or risk ratios) equals 1, while the difference between mean differences will equal zero. As explained in Section 8.2.3, empirical evidence from collections of meta-analyses assembled in meta-epidemiological studies suggests that, on average, intervention effect estimates tend to be more exaggerated in studies at high or unclear risk of bias than in studies at low risk of bias.

When a meta-analysis includes many studies, meta-regression analyses can include more than one domain (e.g. both allocation concealment and blinding).

Results of meta-regression analyses include a confidence interval for the ratio of odds ratios, and a P value for the null hypothesis that there is no difference between the results of studies at high or unclear and low risk of bias. Because meta-analyses usually contain a small number of studies, the ratio of odds ratios is usually imprecisely estimated. It is therefore important not to conclude, on the basis of a non-significant P value, that there is no difference between the results of studies at high or unclear and low risk of bias, and therefore no impact of bias on the results. Examining the confidence interval will often show that the difference between studies at high or unclear and low risk of bias is consistent with both no bias and a substantial effect of bias.

A test for differences across subgroups provides an alternative to meta-regression for examination of a single entry (e.g. comparing studies with adequate versus inadequate allocation concealment). Within a fixed-effect meta-analysis framework, such tests are available in RevMan 5. However, such P values are of limited use without corresponding confidence intervals, and they will in any case be too small in the presence of heterogeneity, either within or between subgroups.

## 8.8.3    Including 'risk of bias' assessments in analyses

Broadly speaking, studies at high or unclear risk of bias should be given reduced weight in meta-analyses, compared with studies at low risk of bias (Spiegelhalter 2003).

However, formal statistical methods to combine the results of studies at high and low risk of bias are not sufficiently well developed that they can currently be recommended for use in Cochrane reviews (see Section 8.8.4.2). Therefore, the major approach to incorporating risk of bias assessments in Cochrane reviews is to **restrict** meta-analyses to studies at low (or lower) risk of bias.

### 8.8.3.1 Possible analysis strategies

When risks of bias vary across studies in a meta-analysis, three broad strategies are available for choosing which result to present as the main finding for a particular outcome (for instance, in deciding which result to present in the Abstract). The intended strategy should be described in the protocol for the review.

***Present all studies and provide a narrative discussion of risk of bias***    The simplest approach to incorporating bias assessments in results is to present an estimated intervention effect based on all available studies, together with a description of the risk of bias in individual domains, or a description of the summary risk of bias, across studies. This is the only feasible option when all studies are at high risk, all are at unclear risk or all are at low risk of bias. However, when studies have different risks of bias, we discourage such an approach for two reasons. First, detailed descriptions of risk of bias in the results section, together with a cautious interpretation in the discussion section, will often be lost in the conclusions, abstract and summary of findings, so that the final interpretation ignores the risk of bias. Second, such an analysis fails to down-weight studies at high risk of bias and hence will lead to an overall intervention that is too precise as well as being potentially biased.

***Primary analysis restricted to studies at low (or low and unclear) risk of bias***    The second approach involves defining a threshold, based on key bias domains (see Section 8.7), such that only studies meeting specific criteria are included in the primary analysis. The threshold may be determined using the original review eligibility criteria, or using reasoned argument (which may draw on empirical evidence of bias from meta-epidemiological studies). If the primary analysis includes studies at unclear risk of bias, review authors must provide justification for this choice. Ideally the threshold, or the method for determining it, should be specified in the review protocol. Authors should keep in mind that all thresholds are arbitrary, and that studies may in theory lie anywhere on the spectrum from 'free of bias' to 'undoubtedly biased'. The higher the threshold, the more similar the studies will be in their risks of bias, but they may end up being few in number.

Having presented a restricted primary analysis, review authors are encouraged to perform **sensitivity analyses** showing how conclusions might be affected if studies at high risk of bias were included in analyses. When analyses are presented that include studies judged to be at high risk of bias, review authors must present these judgements alongside their presentation of results in the text.

***Present multiple analyses***     Two or more analyses incorporating different inclusion criteria might be presented with equal prominence, for example, one including all studies and one including only those at low risk of bias. This avoids the need to make a difficult decision, but may be confusing for readers. In particular, people who need to make a decision usually require a single estimate of effect. Further, 'Summary of findings' tables will usually only present a single result for each outcome.

### 8.8.4   Other methods for addressing risk of bias

#### 8.8.4.1   Direct weighting

Methods have been described for weighting studies in the meta-analysis according to their validity or risk of bias (Detsky 1992). The usual statistical method for combining results of multiple studies is to weight studies by the amount of information they contribute (more specifically, by the inverse variances of their effect estimates). This gives studies with more precise results (narrower confidence intervals) more weight. It is also possible to weight studies additionally according to validity, so that more valid studies have more influence on the summary result. A combination of inverse variances and validity assessments can be used. The main objection to this approach is that it requires a numerical summary of validity for each study, and there is no empirical basis for determining how much weight to assign to different domains of bias. Furthermore, the resulting weighted average will be biased if some of the studies are biased. Direct weighting of effect estimates by validity or assessments of risk of bias should be avoided (Greenland 2001).

#### 8.8.4.2   Bayesian approaches

Bayesian analyses allow for the incorporation of external information or opinion on the nature of bias (see Chapter 16, Section 16.8) (Turner 2008). Prior distributions for specific biases in intervention effect estimates might be based on empirical evidence of bias, on elicited prior opinion of experts, or on reasoned argument. Bayesian methods for adjusting meta-analyses for biases are a subject of current research; they are not currently sufficiently well developed for widespread adoption.

## 8.9   Sequence generation

### 8.9.1   Rationale for concern about bias

Under the domain of sequence generation in the Collaboration's tool for assessing risk of bias, we address whether or not the study used a randomized sequence of assignments. This is the first of two domains in the Collaboration's tool that address the allocation process, the second being concealment of the allocation sequence (allocation concealment). We start by explaining the distinction between these domains.

The starting point for an unbiased intervention study is the use of a mechanism that ensures that the same sorts of participants receive each intervention. Several interrelated processes need to be considered. First, an allocation sequence must be used that, if perfectly implemented, would balance prognostic factors, on average, evenly across intervention groups. Randomization plays a fundamental role here. It can be argued that other assignment rules, such as alternation (alternating between two interventions) or rotation (cycling through more than two interventions), can achieve the same thing (Hill 1990). However, a theoretically unbiased rule is insufficient to prevent bias in practice. If future assignments can be anticipated, either by predicting them or by knowing them, then selection bias can arise due to the selective enrolment and non-enrolment of participants into a study in the light of the upcoming intervention assignment.

Future assignments may be anticipated for several reasons. These include (i) knowledge of a deterministic assignment rule, such as by alternation, date of birth or day of admission; (ii) knowledge of the sequence of assignments, whether randomized or not (e.g. if a sequence of random assignments is posted on the wall); (iii) ability to predict assignments successfully, based on previous assignments (which may sometimes be possible when randomization methods are used that attempt to ensure an exact ratio of allocations to different interventions). Complex interrelationships between theoretical and practical aspects of allocation in intervention studies make the assessment of selection bias challenging. Perhaps the most important among the practical aspects is concealment of the allocation sequence, that is the use of mechanisms to prevent foreknowledge of the next assignment. This has historically been assessed in Cochrane reviews, with empirical justification. We address allocation sequence concealment as a separate domain in the tool (see Section 8.10).

Randomization allows for the sequence to be unpredictable. An unpredictable sequence, combined with allocation sequence concealment, should be sufficient to prevent selection bias. However, selection bias may arise despite randomization if the random allocations are not concealed, and selection bias may (in theory at least) arise despite allocation sequence concealment if the underlying sequence is not random. We acknowledge that a randomized sequence is not always completely unpredictable, even if mechanisms for allocation concealment are in place. This may sometimes be the case, for example, if blocked randomization is used, and all allocations are known after enrolment. Nevertheless, we do not consider this special situation under either sequence generation or allocation concealment, and address it as a separate consideration in Section 8.14.1.4.

Methodological studies have assessed the importance of sequence generation. At least four of those studies have avoided confounding by disease or intervention, which is critical to the assessment (Schulz 1995b, Moher 1998, Kjaergard 2001, Siersma 2007). The inadequate generation of allocation sequences was observed to be associated with biased intervention effects across the studies (Als-Nielsen 2004). In one study that restricted the analysis to 79 trials that had reported an adequately concealed allocation sequence, trials with inadequate sequence generation yielded exaggerated estimates of intervention effects, on average, than trials with adequate sequence generation (relative odds ratio of 0.75; 95% CI of 0.55 to 1.02; P = 0.07). These results suggest that if assignments are non-random, some deciphering of the sequence can occur, even with apparently adequate concealment of the allocation sequence (Schulz 1995b).

## 8.9.2   Assessing risk of bias in relation to adequate or inadequate sequence generation

Sequence generation is often improperly addressed in the design and implementation phases of RCTs, and is often neglected in published reports, which causes major problems in assessing the risk of bias. The following considerations may help review authors assess whether sequence generation is suitable to protect against bias, when using the Collaboration's tool (Section 8.5).

### 8.9.2.1   Adequate methods of sequence generation

The use of a random component should be sufficient for adequate sequence generation.
   Randomization with no constraints to generate an allocation sequence is called **simple randomization** or **unrestricted randomization**. In principle, this could be achieved by allocating interventions using methods such as repeated coin-tossing, throwing dice or dealing previously shuffled cards (Schulz 2002c, Schulz 2006). More usually it is achieved by referring to a published list of random numbers, or to a list of random assignments generated by a computer. In trials using large samples (usually meaning at least 100 in each randomized group (Schulz 2002c, Schulz 2002d, Schulz 2006), simple randomization generates comparison groups of relatively similar sizes. In trials using small samples, simple randomization will sometimes result in an allocation sequence leading to groups that differ, by chance, quite substantially in size or in the occurrence of prognostic factors (i.e. 'case-mix' variation) (Altman 1999).

*Example (of low risk of bias): We generated the two comparison groups using simple randomization, with an equal allocation ratio, by referring to a table of random numbers.*

   Sometimes **restricted randomization** is used to generate a sequence to ensure particular allocation ratios to the intervention groups (e.g. 1:1). Blocked randomization (random permuted blocks) is a common form of restricted randomization (Schulz 2002c, Schulz 2006). Blocking ensures that the numbers of participants to be assigned to each of the comparison groups will be balanced within blocks of, for example, five in one group and five in the other for every 10 consecutively entered participants. The block size may be randomly varied to reduce the likelihood of foreknowledge of intervention assignment.

*Example (of low risk of bias): We used blocked randomization to form the allocation list for the two comparison groups. We used a computer random number generator to select random permuted blocks with a block size of eight and an equal allocation ratio.*

Also common is stratified randomization, in which restricted randomization is performed separately within strata. This generates separate randomization schedules for subsets of participants defined by potentially important prognostic factors, such as disease severity and study centres. If simple (rather than restricted) randomization was used in each stratum, then stratification would have no effect but the randomization would still be valid. Risk of bias may be judged in the same way whether or not a trial claims to have stratified.

Another approach that incorporates both the general concepts of stratification and restricted randomization is minimization, which can be used to make small groups closely similar with respect to several characteristics. The use of minimization should not automatically be considered to put a study at risk of bias. However, some methodologists remain cautious about the acceptability of minimization, particularly when it is used without any random component, while others consider it to be very attractive (Brown 2005).

Other adequate types of randomization that are sometimes used are biased coin or urn randomization, replacement randomization, mixed randomization, and maximal randomization (Schulz 2002c, Schulz 2002d, Berger 2003). If these or other approaches are encountered, consultation with a statistician may be necessary.

### 8.9.2.2   Inadequate methods of sequence generation

Systematic methods, such as alternation, assignment based on date of birth, case record number and date of presentation, are sometimes referred to as 'quasi-random'. Alternation (or rotation, for more than two intervention groups) might in principle result in similar groups, but many other systematic methods of sequence generation may not. For example, the day on which a patient is admitted to hospital is not solely a matter of chance.

An important weakness with all systematic methods is that concealing the allocation schedule is usually impossible, which allows foreknowledge of intervention assignment among those recruiting participants to the study, and biased allocations (see Section 8.10).

*Example (of high risk of bias): We allocated patients to the intervention group based on the week of the month.*

*Example (of high risk of bias): Patients born on even days were assigned to Treatment A and patients born on odd days were assigned to Treatment B.*

### 8.9.2.3   Methods of sequence generation with unclear risk of bias

A simple statement such as 'we randomly allocated' or 'using a randomized design' is often insufficient to be confident that the allocation sequence was genuinely randomized. It is not uncommon for authors to use the term 'randomized' even when it is not justified: many trials with declared systematic allocation are described by the authors as randomized. If there is doubt, then the adequacy of sequence generation should be considered to be unclear.

Sometimes trial authors provide some information, but they incompletely define their approach and do not confirm some random component in the process. For example, authors may state that blocked randomization was used, but the process of selecting the blocks, such as a random number table or a computer random number generator, was not specified. The adequacy of sequence generation should then be classified as unclear.

# 8.10  Allocation sequence concealment

## 8.10.1  Rationale for concern about bias

Randomized sequence generation is a necessary but not a sufficient safeguard against bias in intervention allocation. Efforts made to generate unpredictable and unbiased sequences are likely to be ineffective if those sequences are not protected by adequate concealment of the allocation sequence from those involved in the enrolment and assignment of participants.

Knowledge of the next assignment – for example, from a table of random numbers openly posted on a bulletin board – can cause selective enrolment of participants on the basis of prognostic factors. Participants who would have been assigned to an intervention deemed to be 'inappropriate' may be rejected. Other participants may be deliberately directed to the 'appropriate' intervention, which can often be accomplished by delaying a participant's entry into the trial until the next appropriate allocation appears. Deciphering of allocation schedules may occur even if concealment was attempted. For example, unsealed allocation envelopes may be opened, while translucent envelopes may be held against a bright light to reveal the contents (Schulz 1995a, Schulz 1995b, Jüni 2001). Personal accounts suggest that many allocation schemes have been deciphered by investigators because the methods of concealment were inadequate (Schulz 1995a).

Avoidance of such selection biases depends on preventing foreknowledge of intervention assignment. Decisions on participants' eligibility and their decision whether to give informed consent should be made in ignorance of the upcoming assignment. Adequate **concealment of allocation sequence** shields those who admit participants to a study from knowing the upcoming assignments.

Several methodological studies have looked at whether concealment of allocation sequence is associated with magnitude of effect estimates in controlled clinical trials while avoiding confounding by disease or intervention. A pooled analysis of seven methodological studies found that effect estimates from trials with inadequate concealment of allocation or unclear reporting of the technique used for concealment of allocation were on average 18% more 'beneficial' than effect estimates from trials with adequate concealment of allocation (95% confidence interval 5 to 29%) (Pildal 2007). A recent detailed analysis of three of these data sets combined (1346 trials from 146 meta-analyses) sheds some light on the heterogeneity of these studies. Intervention effect estimates were exaggerated when there was inadequate allocation concealment in trials where a subjective outcome was analysed, but there was little evidence of bias in trials with objective outcomes (Wood 2008).

## 8.10.2 Assessing risk of bias in relation to adequate or inadequate allocation sequence concealment

The following considerations may help review authors assess whether concealment of allocation was sufficient to protect against bias, when using the Collaboration's tool (Section 8.5).

Proper allocation sequence concealment secures strict implementation of an allocation sequence without foreknowledge of intervention assignments. Methods for allocation concealment refer to techniques used to implement the sequence, **not** to generate it (Schulz 1995b). However, most allocation *sequences* that are deemed inadequate, such as allocation based on day of admission or case record number, cannot be adequately concealed, and so fail on both counts. It is theoretically possible, yet unlikely, that an inadequate sequence is adequately concealed (the person responsible for recruitment and assigned interventions would have to be unaware that the sequence being implemented was inappropriate). However, it is not uncommon for an adequate (i.e. randomized) allocation sequence to be inadequately concealed, for example if the sequence is posted on the staff room wall.

Some review authors confuse allocation concealment with blinding of allocated interventions. Allocation concealment seeks to prevent selection bias in intervention assignment by protecting the allocation sequence *before and until* assignment, and can always be successfully implemented regardless of the study topic (Schulz 1995b, Jüni 2001). In contrast, blinding seeks to prevent performance and detection bias by protecting the sequence *after* assignment (Jüni 2001, Schulz 2002a), and cannot always be implemented – for example, in trials comparing surgical with medical treatments. Thus, allocation concealment up to the point of assignment of the intervention and blinding after that point address different sources of bias and differ in their feasibility.

The importance of allocation concealment may depend on the extent to which potential participants in the study have different prognoses, whether strong beliefs exist among investigators and participants regarding the benefits or harms of assigned interventions, and whether uncertainty about the interventions is accepted by all people involved (Schulz 1995a). Among the different methods used to conceal allocation, central randization by a third party is perhaps the most desirable. Methods using envelopes are more susceptible to manipulation than other approaches (Schulz 1995b). If investigators use envelopes, they should develop and monitor the allocation process to preserve concealment. In addition to use of sequentially numbered, opaque, sealed envelopes, they should ensure that the envelopes are opened sequentially, and only after the envelope has been irreversibly assigned to the participant.

**Table 8.10.a** Minimal and extended criteria for judging concealment of allocation sequence to be adequate (low risk of bias)

| Minimal criteria for a judgement of adequate concealment of the allocation sequence | Extended criteria providing additional assurance |
|---|---|
| Central randomization. | The central randomization office was remote from patient recruitment centres. Participant details were provided, for example, by phone, fax or email and the allocation sequence was concealed to individuals staffing the randomization office until a participant was irreversibly registered. |
| Sequentially numbered drug containers. | Drug containers prepared by an independent pharmacy were sequentially numbered and opened sequentially. Containers were of identical appearance, tamper-proof and equal in weight. |
| Sequentially numbered, opaque, sealed envelopes. | Envelopes were sequentially numbered and opened sequentially only after participant details were written on the envelope. Pressure sensitive or carbon paper inside the envelope transferred the participant's details to the assignment card. Cardboard or aluminium foil inside the envelope rendered the envelope impermeable to intense light. Envelopes were sealed using tamper-proof security tape. |

### 8.10.2.1   Adequate methods of allocation sequence concealment

Table 8.10.a provides minimal criteria for a judgement of adequate concealment of allocation sequence (left) and extended criteria which provide additional assurance that concealment of the allocation sequence was indeed adequate (right).

*Examples (of low risk of bias) [published descriptions of concealment procedures judged to be adequate, as compiled by Schulz and Grimes (Schulz 2002b)]:*

" *. . . that combined coded numbers with drug allocation. Each block of ten numbers was transmitted from the central office to a person who acted as the randomization authority in each centre. This individual (a pharmacist or a nurse not involved in care of the trial patients and independent of the site investigator) was responsible for allocation, preparation, and accounting of trial infusion. The trial infusion was prepared at a separate site, then taken to the bedside nurse every 24 h. The nurse infused it into the patient at the appropriate rate. The randomization schedule was thus concealed from all care providers, ward physicians, and other research personnel."* (Bellomo 2000).

" *. . . concealed in sequentially numbered, sealed, opaque envelopes, and kept by the hospital pharmacist of the two centres." (Smilde 2001).*

*"Treatments were centrally assigned on telephone verification of the correctness of inclusion criteria . . ." (de Gaetano 2001).*

*"Glenfield Hospital Pharmacy Department did the randomization, distributed the study agents, and held the trial codes, which were disclosed after the study." (Brightling 2000).*

# 8.11  Blinding of participants, personnel and outcome assessors

## 8.11.1  Rationale for concern about bias

Blinding (sometimes called masking) refers to the process by which study participants and personnel, including people assessing outcomes, are kept unaware of intervention allocations after inclusion of participants into the study. Blinding may reduce the risk that knowledge of which intervention was received, rather than the intervention itself, affects outcomes and assessments of outcomes.

Different types of participants and personnel can be blinded in a clinical trial (Gøtzsche 1996, Haahr 2006):

1. participants (e.g. patients or healthy people);

2. healthcare providers (e.g. the doctors or nurses responsible for care);

3. outcome assessors, including primary data collectors (e.g. interview staff responsible for measurement or collection of outcome data) and any secondary assessors (e.g. external outcome adjudication committees);

4. data analysts (e.g. statisticians); and

5. Manuscript writers.

Lack of blinding of participants or healthcare providers could bias the results by affecting the *actual* outcomes of the participants in the trial. This may be due to a lack of expectations in a control group, or due to differential behaviours across intervention groups (for example, differential drop-out, differential cross-over to an alternative intervention, or differential administration of co-interventions). If participants, providers or outcome assessors are aware of assignments, bias could be introduced into *assessments* of outcome, depending on who measures the outcomes. If data analysts and writers are unblinded, reporting biases may be introduced. In assessing blinding in Cochrane reviews, the emphasis should be placed on participants, providers and outcome assessors. Given the overlapping considerations when participants or healthcare providers are also those assessing outcomes, we consider all types of participants jointly in assessing risk of bias.

In empirical studies, lack of blinding in randomized trials has been shown to be associated with more exaggerated estimated intervention effects, by 9% on average, measured as odds ratio (Pildal 2007). These studies have dealt with a variety of outcomes, some of which are objective. The estimated effect has been observed to be more biased, on average, in trials with more subjective outcomes (Wood 2008). Lack of blinding might also lead to bias caused by additional investigations or co-interventions regardless of the type of outcomes, if these occur differentially across intervention groups.

All outcome assessments can be influenced by lack of blinding, although there are particular risks of bias with more subjective outcomes (e.g. pain or number of days with a common cold). It is therefore important to consider how subjective or objective an outcome is when considering blinding. The importance of blinding and whether blinding is possible may differ across outcomes within a study. Seemingly objective assessments, e.g. doctors assessing the degree of psychological or physical impairment, can also be somewhat subjective (Noseworthy 1994).

Blinding can be impossible for at least some people (e.g. most patients receiving surgery). However, such studies can take other measures to reduce the risk of bias, such as treating patients according to a strict protocol to reduce the risk of differential behaviours by patients and healthcare providers.

An attempt to blind participants and personnel does not ensure successful blinding in practice. Blinding can be compromised for most interventions. For many blinded drug trials, the side effects of the drugs allow the possible detection of which intervention is being received for some participants, unless the study compares two rather similar interventions, e.g. drugs with similar side effects, or uses an active placebo (Boutron 2006).

In blinded studies, especially placebo-controlled trials, there may be concern about whether the participants truly were blinded (and sometimes also whether those caring for the patients were). Several groups have suggested that it would be sensible to ask trial participants at the end of the trial to guess which treatment they had been receiving (Fergusson 2004, Rees 2005), and some reviews of such reports have been published (Fergusson 2004, Hróbjartsson 2007). Evidence of correct guesses exceeding 50% would seem to suggest that blinding may have been broken, but in fact can simply reflect the patients' experiences in the trial: a good outcome, or a marked side effect, will tend to be more often attributed to an active treatment, and a poor outcome to a placebo (Sackett 2007). It follows that we would expect to see some successful 'guessing' when there is a difference in either efficacy or adverse effects, but none when the interventions have very similar effects, even when the blinding has been preserved. As a consequence, review authors should consider carefully whether to take any notice of the findings of such an exercise.

## 8.11.2  Assessing risk of bias in relation to adequate or inadequate blinding

Study reports often describe blinding in broad terms, such as 'double blind'. This term makes it impossible to know who was blinded (Schulz 2002a). Such terms are also used very inconsistently (Devereaux 2001, Boutron 2005, Haahr 2006), and the frequency of explicit reporting of the blinding status of study participants and personnel remains low even in trials published in top journals (Montori 2002), despite recommendations to be explicit in the CONSORT Statement (Moher 2001c). A review of methods used for blinding highlights the variety of methods used in practice (Boutron 2006). The following considerations may help review authors assess whether any blinding used in a study was likely to be sufficient to protect against bias, when using the Collaboration's tool (Section 8.5).

When considering the risk of bias from lack of blinding it is important to consider specifically:

1. who was and was not blinded;

2. risk of bias in actual outcomes due to lack of blinding during the study (e.g. due to co-intervention or differential behaviour); and

3. risk of bias in outcome assessments (considering how subjective or objective an outcome is).

Assessors of some outcomes may be blinded while assessors of other outcomes are not. For example, in a surgical trial in which patients are aware of their own intervention, patient-reported outcomes (e.g. quality of life) would obviously be collected in knowledge of the intervention received, whereas other outcomes, measured by an independent clinician (e.g. physical ability), might be blinded. Furthermore, risk of bias may be high for some outcomes and low for others, even if the same people were unblinded in the study. For example, knowledge of the assigned intervention may impact on behavioural outcomes (such as number of clinic visits), while not impacting on physiological outcomes or mortality. In many circumstances assessment of total mortality might be considered to be unbiased, even if outcome assessors were aware of intervention assignments. Thus, assessments of risk of bias resulting from lack of blinding may need to be made separately for different outcomes.

Rather than assessing risk of bias for each outcome separately, it is often convenient to group outcomes with similar risks of bias (see Section 8.5). For example, there may be a common assessment of risk of bias for all subjective outcomes that is different from a common assessment of blinding for all objective outcomes.

## 8.12 Incomplete outcome data

### 8.12.1 Rationale for concern about bias

Missing outcome data, due to attrition (drop-out) during the study or exclusions from the analysis, raise the possibility that the observed effect estimate is biased. We shall use the term **incomplete outcome data** to refer to both attrition and exclusions. When an individual participant's outcome is not available we shall refer to it as **missing**.

Attrition may occur for the following reasons.

- Participants withdraw, or are withdrawn, from the study.

- Participants do not attend an appointment at which outcomes should have been measured.

- Participants attend an appointment but do not provide relevant data.

- Participants fail to complete diaries or questionnaires.

- Participants cannot be located (lost to follow-up).

- The study investigators decide, usually inappropriately, to cease follow-up.

- Data or records are lost, or are unavailable for other reasons.

In addition, some participants may be excluded from analysis for the following reasons.

- Some enrolled participants were later found to be ineligible.

- An 'as-treated' (or per-protocol) analysis is performed (in which participants are included only if they received the intended intervention in accordance with the protocol; see Section 8.12.2).

- The study analysis excluded some participants for other reasons.

Some exclusions of participants may be justifiable, in which case they need not be considered as leading to missing outcome data (Fergusson 2002). For example, participants who are randomized but are subsequently found not to have been eligible for the trial may be excluded, as long as the discovery of ineligibility could not have been affected by the randomized intervention, and preferably on the basis of decisions made blinded to assignment. The intention to exclude such participants should be specified before the outcome data are seen.

An intention-to-treat (ITT) analysis is often recommended as the least biased way to estimate intervention effects in randomized trials (Newell 1992): see Chapter 16 (Section 16.2). The principles of ITT analyses are

1. keep participants in the intervention groups to which they were randomized, regardless of the intervention they actually received;

2. measure outcome data on all participants; and

3. include all randomized participants in the analysis.

The first principle can always be applied. However, the second is often impossible due to attrition beyond the control of the trialists. Consequently, the third principle of conducting an analysis that includes all participants can only be followed by making assumptions about the missing values (see below). Thus very few trials can perform a true ITT analysis without making imputations, especially when there is extended follow-up. In practice, study authors may describe an analysis as ITT even when some outcome data are missing. The term 'ITT' does not have a clear and consistent definition, and it is used inconsistently in study reports (Hollis 1999). Review authors should use the term only to imply all three of the principles above, and should interpret with care any studies that use the term without clarification.

Review authors may also encounter analyses described as "modified intention-to-treat", which usually means that participants were excluded if they did not receive a specified minimum amount of the intended intervention. This term is also used in a variety of ways so review authors should always seek information about precisely who was included.

Note that it might be possible to conduct analyses that include participants who were excluded by the study authors (**re-inclusions**), if the reasons for exclusions are considered inappropriate and the data are available to the review author. Review authors are encouraged to do this when possible and appropriate.

Concerns over bias resulting from incomplete outcome data are driven mainly by theoretical considerations. Several empirical studies have looked at whether various aspects of missing data are associated with the magnitude of effect estimates. Most found no clear evidence of bias (Schulz 1995b, Kjaergard 2001, Balk 2002, Siersma 2007). Tierney et al. observed a tendency for analyses conducted after trial authors excluded participants to favour the experimental intervention compared with analyses including all participants (Tierney 2005). There are notable examples of biased 'per-protocol' analyses, however (Melander 2003) and a review has found more exaggerated effect estimates from 'per-protocol' analyses compared with 'ITT' analyses of the same trials (Porta 2007). Interpretation of empirical studies is difficult because exclusions are poorly reported, particularly before 1996 in the pre-CONSORT era (Moher 2001b). For example, Schulz observed that the *apparent* lack of exclusions was associated with more 'beneficial' effect sizes as well as with less likelihood of adequate allocation concealment (Schulz 1996). Hence, failure to report exclusions in trials in Schulz's study may have been a marker of poor trial conduct rather than true absence of any exclusions.

Empirical research has also investigated the adequacy with which incomplete outcome data are addressed in reports of trials. One study, of 71 trial reports from four general medical journals, concluded that missing data are common and often inadequately handled in the statistical analysis (Wood 2004).

## 8.12.2 Assessing risk of bias from incomplete outcome data

The risk of bias arising from incomplete outcome data depends on several factors, including the amount and distribution across intervention groups, the reasons for outcomes being missing, the likely difference in outcome between participants with and without data, what study authors have done to address the problem in their reported analyses, and the clinical context. Therefore it is not possible to formulate a simple rule for judging a study to be at low or high risk of bias. The following considerations may help review authors assess whether incomplete outcome data could be addressed in a way that protects against bias, when using the Collaboration's tool (Section 8.5).

It is often assumed that a high proportion of missing outcomes, or a large difference in proportions between intervention groups, is the main cause for concern over bias. However, these characteristics on their own are insufficient to introduce bias. Here we elaborate on situations in which an analysis can be judged to be at low or high risk of bias. It is essential to consider the reasons for outcomes being missing as well as the numbers missing.

### 8.12.2.1   Low risk of bias due to incomplete outcome data

To conclude that there are no missing outcome data, review authors should be confident that the participants included in the analysis are exactly those who were randomized into the trial. If the numbers randomized into each intervention group are not clearly reported, the risk of bias is unclear. As noted above, participants randomized but subsequently found not to be eligible need not always be considered as having missing outcome data.

**Example (of low risk of bias): "All patients completed the study and there were no losses to follow up, no treatment withdrawals, no trial group changes and no major adverse events".**

**Acceptable reasons for missing data**   A healthy person's decision to move house away from the geographical location of a clinical trial is unlikely to be connected with their subsequent outcome. For studies with a long duration of follow-up, some withdrawals for such reasons are inevitable.

For studies reporting time-to-event data, all participants who did not experience the event of interest are considered to be 'censored' on the date of their last follow-up (we do not know whether the outcome event occurred after follow-up ended). The important consideration for this type of analysis is whether such censoring can be assumed to be unbiased, i.e. that the intervention effect (e.g. assessed by a hazard ratio) in individuals who were censored before the *scheduled* end of follow-up is the same as the hazard ratio in other individuals. In other words, there is no bias if censoring is unrelated to prognosis.

If outcome data are missing in both intervention groups, but reasons for these are both reported and balanced across groups, then important bias would not be expected unless the reasons have different implications in the compared groups. For example, 'refusal to participate' may mean unwillingness to exercise in an exercise group, whereas refusal might imply dissatisfaction with the advice not to exercise in the other group. In practice, incomplete reporting of reasons for missing outcomes may prevent review authors from making this assessment.

*Potential impact of missing data on effect estimates*   The potential impact of missing **dichotomous outcomes** depends on the frequency (or risk) of the outcome. For example, if 10% of participants have missing outcomes, then their potential impact on the results is much greater if the risk of the event is 10% than if it is 50%. The following table illustrates the potential impact of observed risks. A and B represent two hypothetical trials of 1000 participants in which 90% of the individuals are observed, and the risk ratio among these 900 observed participants is 1. Furthermore, in both trials we suppose that missing participants in the intervention group have a high risk of event (80%) and those in the control group have a much lower risk (20%). The only difference between trials A and B is the risk among the observed participants. In trial A the risk is 50%, and the impact of the missing data, had they been observed, is low. In trial B the risk is 10%, and the impact of the same missing data, had they been observed, is large. Generally, the higher the ratio of participants with missing data to participants with events, the greater potential there is for bias. In trial A this ratio was 100/450 (0.2), whereas in Trial B it was 100/90 (1.1).

| | Number randomized | Risk among observed | Observed data | Hypothetical extreme risks among missing participants | Missing data | Complete data | Risk ratio based on all participants |
|---|---|---|---|---|---|---|---|
| Trial A | | | | | | | |
| Intervention | 500 | **50%** | 225/450 | 80% | 40/50 | 265/500 | |
| | | | | | | | **1.13** |
| Control | 500 | **50%** | 225/450 | 20% | 10/50 | 235/500 | |
| Trial B | | | | | | | |
| Intervention | 500 | **10%** | 45/450 | 80% | 40/50 | 85/500 | |
| | | | | | | | **1.55** |
| Control | 500 | **10%** | 45/450 | 20% | 10/50 | 55/500 | |

The potential impact of missing **continuous outcomes** increases with the proportion of participants with missing data. It is also necessary to consider the plausible intervention effect among participants with missing outcomes. The following table illustrates the impact of different proportions of missing outcomes. A and B represent two hypothetical trials of 1000 participants in which the difference in mean response between intervention and control among the observed participants is 0. Furthermore, in both trials we suppose that missing participants in the intervention arm have a higher mean and those in the control arm have a lower mean. The only difference between trials A and B is the number of missing participants. In trial A, 90% of participants are observed and 10% missing, and the impact of the missing data on the observed mean difference is low. In trial B, half of the participants are missing, and the impact of the same missing data on the observed mean difference is large.

|  | Number randomized | Number observed | Observed mean | Number missing | Hypothetical extreme mean among missing participants | Overall mean (weighted average) | Mean difference based on all participants |
|---|---|---|---|---|---|---|---|
| **Trial A** | | | | | | | |
| Intervention | 500 | **450** | 10 | **50** | 15 | 10.5 | |
| Control | 500 | **450** | 10 | **50** | 5 | 9.5 | **1** |
| **Trial B** | | | | | | | |
| Intervention | 500 | **250** | 10 | **250** | 15 | 12.5 | |
| Control | 500 | **250** | 10 | **250** | 5 | 7.5 | **5** |

### 8.12.2.2   High risk of bias due to incomplete outcome data

***Unacceptable reasons for missing data***   A difference in the proportion of incomplete outcome data across groups is of concern if the availability of outcome data is determined by the participants' true outcomes. For example, if participants with poorer clinical outcomes are more likely to drop out due to adverse effects, and this happens mainly in the experimental group, then the effect estimate will be biased in favour of the experimental intervention. Exclusion of participants due to 'inefficacy' or 'failure to improve' will introduce bias if the numbers excluded are not balanced across intervention groups. Note that a non-significant result of a statistical test for differential missingness does not confirm the absence of bias, especially in small studies.

***Example (of high risk of bias): "In a trial of sibutramine versus placebo to treat obesity, 13/35 were withdrawn from the sibutramine group, 7 of these due to lack of efficacy. 25/34 were withdrawn from the placebo group, 17 due to lack of efficacy. An 'intention-to-treat' analysis included only those remaining" (Cuellar 2000) (i.e. only 9 of 34 in the placebo group).***

Even if incomplete outcome data are balanced in numbers across groups, bias can be introduced if the reasons for missing outcomes differ. For example, in a trial of an experimental intervention aimed at smoking cessation it is feasible that a proportion of the control intervention participants could leave the study due to a lack of enthusiasm at receiving nothing novel (and continue to smoke), and that a similar proportion of the experimental intervention group could leave the study due to successful cessation of smoking.

The common approach to dealing with missing outcome data in smoking cessation studies (to assume that everyone who leaves the study continues to smoke) may therefore not always be free from bias. The example highlights the importance of considering *reasons* for incomplete outcome data when assessing risk of bias. In practice, knowledge of why most participants drop out is often unavailable, although an empirical study has observed that 38 out of 63 trials with missing data provided information on reasons (Wood 2004), and this is likely to improve through the use of the CONSORT Statement (Moher 2001a).

*'As-treated' (per-protocol) analyses*   Eligible participants should be analysed in the groups to which they were randomized, regardless of the intervention that they actually received. Thus, in a study comparing surgery with radiotherapy for treatment of localized prostate cancer, patients who refused surgery and chose radiotherapy subsequent to randomization should be included in the surgery group for analysis. This is because participants' propensity to change groups may be related to prognosis, in which case switching intervention groups introduces selection bias. Although this is strictly speaking an issue of inappropriate analysis rather than incomplete outcome data, studies in which 'as treated' analyses are reported should be rated as at high risk of bias due to incomplete outcome data, unless the number of switches is too small to make any important difference to the estimated intervention effect.

A similarly inappropriate approach to analysis of a study is to focus only on participants who complied with the protocol. A striking example is provided by a trial of the lipid lowering drug, clofibrate (Coronary Drug Project Research Group 1980). The five-year mortality in 1103 men assigned to clofibrate was 20.0%, and in 2789 men assigned to placebo was 20.9% (P = 0.55). Those who adhered well to the protocol in the clofibrate group had lower five-year mortality (15.0%) than those who did not (24.6%). However, a similar difference between 'good adherers' and 'poor adherers' was observed in the placebo group (15.1% vs 28.3%). Thus, adherence was a marker of prognosis rather than modifying the effect of clofibrate. These findings show the serious difficulty of evaluating intervention efficacy in subgroups determined by patient responses to the interventions. Because non-receipt of intervention can be more informative than non-availability of outcome data, there is a high risk of bias in analyses restricted to compliers, even with low rates of incomplete data.

### 8.12.2.3   *Attempts to address missing data in reports: imputation*

A common, but potentially dangerous, approach to dealing with missing outcome data is to **impute** outcomes and treat them as if they were real measurements (see also Chapter 16, Section 16). For example, individuals with missing outcome data might be assigned the mean outcome for their intervention group, or be assigned a treatment success or failure. Such procedures can lead both to serious bias and to confidence intervals that are too narrow. A variant of this, the validity of which is more difficult to assess, is the use of 'last observation carried forward' (LOCF). Here, the most recently observed outcome measure is assumed to hold for all subsequent outcome assessment times (Lachin 2000, Unnebrink 2001). LOCF procedures can also lead to serious bias. For example, in a trial of a drug for a degenerative condition, such as Alzheimer's disease, attrition may be related to side effects of the drug. Because outcomes tend to deteriorate with time, using LOCF will bias the effect estimate in favour of the drug. On the other hand, use of LOCF might be appropriate if most people for whom outcomes are carried forward had a genuine measurement relatively recently.

There is a substantial literature on statistical methods that deal with missing data in a valid manner: see Chapter 16 (Section 16.1). There are relatively few practical applications of these methods in clinical trial reports (Wood 2004). Statistical advice is recommended if review authors encounter their use. A good starting point for learning about them is www.missingdata.org.uk.

# 8.13    Selective outcome reporting

## 8.13.1    Rationale for concern about bias

Selective outcome reporting has been defined as the selection of a subset of the original variables recorded, on the basis of the results, for inclusion in publication of trials (Hutton 2000); see also Chapter 10 (Section 10.2.2.5). The particular concern is that statistically non-significant results might be selectively withheld from publication. Until recently, published evidence of selective outcome reporting was limited. There were initially a few case studies. Then a small study of a complete cohort of applications approved by a single Local Research Ethics Committee found that the primary outcome was stated in only six of the protocols for the 15 publications obtained. Eight protocols made some reference to an intended analysis, but seven of the publications did not follow this analysis plan (Hahn 2002). Within-study selective reporting was evident or suspected in several trials included in a review of a cohort of five meta-analyses in the *Cochrane Database of Systematic Reviews* (Williamson 2005a).

Convincing direct empirical evidence for the existence of within-study selective reporting bias comes from three recent studies. In the first study (Chan 2004a), 102 trials with 122 publications and 3736 outcomes were identified. Overall, (a median of) 38% of efficacy and 50% of safety outcomes per parallel group trial were incompletely reported, i.e. with insufficient information to be included in a meta-analysis. Statistically significant outcomes had a higher odds ratio of being fully reported when compared with non-significant outcomes, both for efficacy (pooled odds ratio 2.4; 95% confidence interval 1.4 to 4.0) and for harms (4.7, 1.8 to 12) data. Further, when comparing publications with protocols, 62% of trials had at least one primary outcome that was changed, introduced or omitted. A second study of 48 trials funded by the Canadian Institutes of Health Research found closely similar results (Chan 2004b). A third study, involving a retrospective review of 519 trial publications and a follow-up survey of authors, compared the presented results with the outcomes mentioned in the methods section of the same article (Chan 2005). On average, over 20% of the outcomes measured in parallel group trials were incompletely reported. Within trials, such outcomes had a higher odds of being statistically non-significant compared with fully reported outcomes (odds ratio 2.0 (1.6 to 2.7) for efficacy outcomes; 1.9 (1.1 to 3.5) for harm outcomes). These three studies suggest an odds ratio of about 2.4 associated with selective outcome reporting which corresponds, for example, to about 50% of non-significant outcomes being published compared to 72% of significant ones.

In all three studies, authors were asked whether there were unpublished outcomes, whether those showed significant differences and why those outcomes had not been published. The most common reasons for non-publication of results were 'lack of clinical importance' or lack of statistical significance. Therefore, meta-analyses excluding unpublished outcomes are likely to overestimate intervention effects. Further, authors commonly failed to mention the existence of unpublished outcomes even when those outcomes had been mentioned in the protocol or publication.

Recent studies have found similar results (Ghersi 2006, von Elm 2006). In a different type of study, the effect in meta-analyses was larger when fewer of the available trials contributed data to that meta-analysis (Furukawa 2007). This finding also suggests that results may have been selectively withheld by trialists on the basis of the magnitude of effect.

Bias associated with selective reporting of different measures of the same characteristic seems likely. In trials of treatments for schizophrenia, an intervention effect has been observed to be more likely when unpublished, rather than published, rating scales were used (Marshall 2000). The authors hypothesized that data from unpublished scales may be less likely to be published when they are not statistically significant or that, following analysis, unfavourable items may have been dropped to create an apparent beneficial effect.

In many systematic reviews, only a few eligible studies can be included in a meta-analysis for a specific outcome because the necessary information was not reported by the other studies. While that outcome may not have been assessed in some studies, there is almost always a risk of biased reporting for some studies. Review authors need to consider whether an outcome was collected but not reported or simply not collected.

Selective reporting of outcomes may arise in several ways, some affecting the study as a whole (point 1 below) and others relating to specific outcomes (points 2–6 below):

1. Selective omission of outcomes from reports: Only some of the analysed outcomes may be included in the published report. If that choice is made based on the results, in particular the statistical significance, the corresponding meta-analytic estimates are likely to be biased.

2. Selective choice of data for an outcome: For a specific outcome there may be different time points at which the outcome has been measured, or there may have been different instruments used to measure the outcome at the same time point (e.g. different scales, or different assessors). For example, in a report of a trial in osteoporosis, there were 12 different data sets to choose from for estimating bone mineral content. The standardized mean difference for these 12 possibilities varied between $-0.02$ and $1.42$ (Gøtzsche 2007). If study authors make choices in relation to such results, then the meta-analytic estimate will be biased.

3. Selective reporting of analyses using the same data: There are often several different ways in which an outcome can be analysed. For example, continuous outcomes such as blood pressure reduction might be analysed as a continuous or dichotomous variable, with the further possibility of selecting from multiple cut-points. Another

common analysis choice is between endpoint scores versus changes from baseline (Williamson 2005b). Switching from an intended comparison of final values to a comparison of changes from baseline because of an observed baseline imbalance actually introduces bias rather than removes it (as the study authors may suppose) (Senn 1991, Vickers 2001).

4. Selective reporting of subsets of the data: Selective reporting may occur if outcome data can be subdivided, for example selecting sub-scales of a full measurement scale or a subset of events. For example, fungal infections may be identified at baseline or within a couple of days after randomization or may be so-called 'break-through' fungal infections that are detected some days after randomization, and selection of a subset of these infections may lead to reporting bias (Jørgensen 2006, Jørgensen 2007).

5. Selective under-reporting of data: Some outcomes may be reported but with inadequate detail for the data to be included in a meta-analysis. Sometimes this is explicitly related to the result, for example reported only as "not significant" or "P > 0.05".

Yet other forms of selective reporting are not addressed here; they include selected reporting of subgroup analyses or adjusted analyses, and presentation of the first period results in cross-over trials (Williamson 2005a). Also, descriptions of outcomes as 'primary', 'secondary' etc may sometimes be altered retrospectively in the light of the findings (Chan 2004a, Chan 2004b). This issue alone should not generally be of concern to review authors (who do not take note of which outcomes are so labelled in each study), provided it does not influence which results are published.

## 8.13.2   Assessing risk of bias from selective reporting of outcomes

Although the possibility of *between-study* publication bias can be examined only by considering a complete set of studies (see Chapter 10), the possibility of *within-study* selective outcome reporting can be examined for each study included in a systematic review. The following considerations may help review authors assess whether outcome reporting is sufficiently complete and transparent to protect against bias using the Collaboration's tool (Section 8.5).

Statistical methods to detect within-study selective reporting are, as yet, not well developed. There are, however, other ways of detecting such bias although a thorough assessment is likely to be labour intensive. If the protocol is available, then outcomes in the protocol and published report can be compared. If not, then outcomes listed in the methods section of an article can be compared with those whose results are reported. If non-significant results are mentioned but not reported adequately, bias in a meta-analysis is likely to occur. Further information can also be sought from authors of the study reports, although it should be realized that such information may be unreliable (Chan 2004a).

Some differences between protocol and publication may be explained by legitimate changes to the protocol. Although such changes should be reported in publications, none of the 150 studies in the two samples of Chan et al. did so (Chan 2004a, Chan 2004b).

Review authors should look hard for evidence of collection by study investigators of a small number of key outcomes that are routinely measured in the area in question, and report which studies report data on these and which do not. Review authors should consider the *reasons* why data might be missing from a meta-analysis (Williamson 2005b). Methods for seeking such evidence are not well-established, but we describe some possible strategies.

A useful first step is to construct a matrix indicating which outcomes were recorded in which studies, for example with rows as studies and columns as outcomes. Complete and incomplete reporting can also be indicated. This matrix will show to the review authors which studies did not report outcomes reported by most other studies.

PubMed, other major reference databases and the internet should be searched for a study protocol; in rare cases the web address will be given in the study report. Alternatively, and more often in the future as mandatory registration of trials becomes more common, a detailed description of the study may be available in a trial registry. Abstracts of presentations relating to the study may contain information about outcomes not subsequently mentioned in publications. In addition, review authors should examine carefully the methods section of published articles for details of outcomes that were assessed.

Of particular interest is missing information that seems sure to have been recorded. For example, some measurements are expected to appear together, such as systolic and diastolic blood pressure, so we should wonder why if only one is reported. An alternative example is a study reporting the proportion of participants whose change in a continuous variable exceeded some threshold; the investigators must have had access to the raw data and so could have shown the results as mean and SD of the changes. Williamson et al. give several examples, including a Cochrane review in which nine trials reported the outcome treatment failure but only five reported mortality. Yet mortality was part of the definition of treatment failure so those data must have been collected in the four trials missing from the analysis of mortality. Bias was suggested by the marked difference in results for treatment failure for trials with or without separate reporting of mortality (Williamson 2005a).

When there is suspicion of or direct evidence for selective outcome reporting it is desirable to ask the study authors for additional information. For example, authors could be asked to supply the study protocol and full information for outcomes reported inadequately. In addition, for outcomes mentioned in article or protocol but not reported, they could be asked to clarify whether those outcome measures were in fact analysed, and if so to supply the data.

It is not generally recommended to try to 'adjust for' reporting bias in the main meta-analysis. Sensitivity analysis is a better approach to investigate the possible impact of selective outcome reporting (Hutton 2000, Williamson 2005a).

The assessment of risk of bias due to selective reporting of outcomes should be made for the study as a whole, rather than for each outcome. Although it may be clear for a particular study that some specific outcomes are subject to selective reporting while others are not, we recommend the study-level approach because it is not practical to list all fully reported outcomes in the 'Risk of bias' table. The Description part of the tool (see Section 8.5.2) should be used to describe the outcomes for which there is particular evidence of selective (or incomplete) reporting. The study-level judgement provides an assessment of the overall susceptibility of the study to selective reporting bias.

# 8.14   Other potential threats to validity

## 8.14.1   Rationale for concern about bias

The preceding domains (sequence generation, allocation concealment, blinding, incomplete outcome data and selective outcome reporting) relate to important potential sources of bias in clinical trials across all healthcare areas. Beyond these specific domains, however, review authors should be alert for further issues that may raise concerns about the possibility of bias. This sixth domain in the 'Risk of bias' assessment tool is a 'catch-all' for other such sources of bias. For reviews in some topic areas, there may be additional questions that should be asked of all studies. In particular, some study designs warrant special consideration when they are encountered. If particular study designs are anticipated (e.g. cross-over trials, or types of non-randomized study), additional questions relating to the risk of bias in these types of studies may be posed. Assessing risk of bias in non-randomized studies is addressed in Chapter 13, and risk of bias for cluster-randomized trials, cross-over trials and trials with multiple intervention groups is addressed in Chapter 16. Furthermore, some major, unanticipated, problems with specific studies may be identified during the course of the systematic review or meta-analysis. For example, a trial may stop early, or may have substantial imbalance of participant characteristics at baseline. Several examples are discussed in the sections that follow.

### 8.14.1.1   Design-specific risks of bias

The principal concern over risk of bias in non-randomized studies is selection bias in the form of differences in types of participants between experimental and control intervention groups. Review authors should refer to the full discussion in Chapter 13 (Section 13.5). The main concerns over risk of bias in cluster-randomized trials are: (i) recruitment bias (differential participant recruitment in clusters for different interventions); (ii) baseline imbalance; (iii) loss of clusters; (iv) incorrect analysis; and (v) comparability with individually randomized trials. The main concerns over risk of bias in cross-over trials are: (i) whether the cross-over design is suitable; (ii) whether there is a carry-over effect; (iii) whether only first period data are available; (iv) incorrect analysis; and (v) comparability of results with those from parallel-group trials. These are discussed in detail in Chapter 16 (Sections 16.3 and 16.4). Risk of bias in studies with more than two intervention groups is also discussed in Chapter 16 (Section 16.5).

### 8.14.1.2 Early stopping

Studies that were stopped early (whether or not as a result of a formal stopping rule) are more likely to show extreme intervention effects than those that continue to the end, particularly if they have very few events (Montori 2005). This is especially the case when a study stops because early results show a large, statistically significant, intervention effect, although it may also be the case if a study stops early because of harm. If a study does not describe having a pre-specified sample size, or any formal stopping rules, or the attained sample size is much less than the intended size but no explanation is given, then the study may have stopped at a point chosen because of the observed results, and so the available results may be biased. Early stopping may be more common than is reported. For example, in a study of 44 industry-initiated trials, the trial protocols showed that the sponsor had access to accumulating data in 16 (e.g. through interim analyses and participation in data and safety monitoring committees), but such access was disclosed in only one corresponding trial report. An additional 16 protocols noted that the sponsor had the right to stop the trial at any time, for any reason; this was not noted in any of the trial publications (Gøtzsche 2006). Even when trials are known to have stopped early, systematic reviews frequently fail to note this (Bassler 2007).

 Bias-adjusted analyses are available for studies that stop early due to a formal stopping rule, but such analyses are seldom implemented, and there is not consensus on an appropriate method (Montori 2005).

 Studies that fail to attain a pre-specified sample size for reasons unrelated to the observed intervention effect (e.g. a lower than expected recruitment rate, insufficient funds, no supply of drug) are not more likely to show extreme results, and should not generally be considered to be prone to bias due to early stopping.

*Example (of high risk of bias): The data and safety monitoring board recommended stopping the trial because the test statistic for the primary outcome measure exceeded the stopping boundary for benefit.*

### 8.14.1.3 Baseline imbalance

Baseline imbalance in factors that are strongly related to outcome measures can cause bias in the intervention effect estimate. This can happen through chance alone, but imbalance may also arise through non-randomized (unconcealed) allocation of interventions. Sometimes trial authors may exclude some randomized individuals, causing imbalance in participant characteristics in the different intervention groups. Sequence generation, lack of allocation concealment or exclusion of participants should each be addressed using the specific entries for these in the tool. If further inexplicable baseline imbalance is observed that is sufficient to lead to important exaggeration of effect estimates, then it should be noted. Tests of baseline imbalance have no value in truly randomized trials, but very small P values could suggest bias in the intervention allocation.

*Example (of high risk of bias): A trial of captopril vs conventional anti-hypertensive had small but highly significant imbalances in height, weight, systolic and diastolic BP: P = 10⁻⁴ to 10⁻¹⁸ (Hansson 1999). Such an imbalance suggests failure of randomization (which was by sealed envelopes) at some centres (Peto 1999).*

### 8.14.1.4   Blocked randomization in unblinded trials

Some combinations of methods for sequence generation, allocation concealment and blinding act together to create a risk of selection bias in the allocation of interventions. One particular combination is the use of blocked randomization in an unblinded trial, or in a blinded trial where the blinding is broken, for example because of characteristic side effects. When blocked randomization is used, and when the assignments are revealed subsequent to the person recruiting into the trial, then it is sometimes possible to predict future assignments. This is particularly the case when blocks are of a fixed size and are not divided across multiple recruitment centres. This ability to predict future assignments can happen even when allocation concealment is adequate according to the criteria suggested in Table 8.5.c (Berger 2005).

### 8.14.1.5   Differential diagnostic activity

Outcome assessments can be biased despite effective blinding. In particular, increased diagnostic activity could lead to increased diagnosis of true but harmless cases of disease. For example, many stomach ulcers give no symptoms and have no clinical relevance, but such cases could be detected more frequently on gastroscopy in patients who receive a drug that causes unspecific stomach discomfort and therefore leads to more gastroscopies. Similarly, if a drug causes diarrhoea, this could lead to more digital rectal examinations, and, therefore, also to the detection of more harmless cases of prostatic cancer. Obviously, assessment of beneficial effects can also become biased through such a mechanism. Interventions may also lead to different diagnostic activity, for example if the experimental intervention is a nurse visiting a patient at home, and the control intervention is no visit.

### 8.14.1.6   Further examples of potential biases

The following list of other potential sources of bias in a clinical study may aid detection of further problems.

- The conduct of the study is affected by interim results (e.g. recruiting additional participants from a subgroup showing more benefit).

- There is deviation from the study protocol in a way that does not reflect clinical practice (e.g. *post-hoc* stepping-up of doses to exaggerated levels).

- There is pre-randomization administration of an intervention that could enhance or diminish the effect of a subsequent, randomized, intervention.

- Inappropriate administration of an intervention (or co-intervention).

- Contamination (e.g. participants pooling drugs).

- Occurrence of 'null bias' due to interventions being insufficiently well delivered or overly wide inclusion criteria for participants (Woods 1995).

- An insensitive instrument is used to measure outcomes (which can lead to under-estimation of both beneficial and harmful effects).

- Selective reporting of subgroups.

- Fraud.

- Inappropriate influence of funders (e.g. in one empirical study, more than half of the protocols for industry-initiated trials stated that the sponsor either owns the data or needs to approve the manuscript, or both; none of these constraints were stated in any of the trial publications (Gøtzsche 2006)).

## 8.14.2  Assessing risk of bias from other sources

Some general guidelines for determining suitable topics for assessment as 'other sources of bias' are provided below. In particular, suitable topics should constitute potential sources of bias and not sources of imprecision, sources of diversity (heterogeneity) or measures of research quality that are unrelated to bias. The topics covered in this domain of the tool include primarily the examples provided in Section 8.14.1. Beyond these specific issues, however, review authors should be alert for study-specific issues that may raise concerns about the possibility of bias, and should formulate judgements about them under this domain of the tool. The following considerations may help review authors assess whether a study is free of risk of bias from other sources using the Collaboration's tool (Section 8.5).

Wherever possible, a review protocol should pre-specify any questions to be addressed, which would lead to separate entries in the 'Risk of bias' table. For example, if cross-over trials are the usual study design for the question being addressed by the review, then specific questions related to bias in cross-over trials should be formulated in advance.

Issues covered by the risk of bias tool must be a potential source of bias, and not just a cause of *imprecision* (see Section 8.2), and this applies to aspects that are assessed under this 'other sources of bias' domain. A potential source of bias must be able to change the magnitude of the effect estimate, whereas sources of imprecision affect only the uncertainty in the estimate (i.e. its confidence interval). Potential factors affecting precision of an estimate include technological variability (e.g. measurement error) and observer variability.

Because the tool addresses only internal biases, any issue covered by this domain should be a potential source of internal bias, and not a source of *diversity*. Possible causes of diversity include differences in dose of drug, length of follow-up, and characteristics of participants (e.g. age, stage of disease). Studies may select doses that favour the experimental drug over the control drug. For example, old drugs are often overdosed (Safer 2002) or may be given under clearly suboptimal circumstances that do not reflect clinical practice (Johansen 2000, Jørgensen 2007). Alternatively, participants may be selectively chosen for inclusion in a study on the basis of previously demonstrated 'response' to the experimental intervention. It is important that such biased choices are addressed in Cochrane reviews. Although they may not be covered by the 'Risk of bias' tool described in the current chapter, they may sometimes be addressed in the analysis (e.g. by subgroup analysis and meta-regression) and should be considered in the grading and interpretation of evidence in a 'Summary of findings' table (see Chapters 11 and 12).

Many judgements can be made about the design and conduct of a clinical trial, but not all of them may be associated with bias. Measures of 'quality' alone are often strongly associated with aspects that could introduce bias. However, review authors should focus on the mechanisms that lead to bias rather than descriptors of studies that reflect only 'quality'. Some examples of 'quality' indicators that should not be assessed within this domain include criteria related to applicability, 'generalizability' or 'external validity, (including those noted above), criteria related to precision (e.g. sample size or use of a sample size (or power) calculation), reporting standards, and ethical criteria (e.g. whether the study had ethical approval or participants gave informed consent). Such factors may be important, and would be presented in the table of 'Characteristics of included studies' or in Additional tables (see Chapter 11).

Finally, to avoid double-counting, potential sources of bias should not be included as 'bias from other sources' if they are more appropriately covered by earlier domains in the tool. For example, in Alzheimer's disease, patients deteriorate significantly over time during the trial. Generally, the effects of treatments are small and treatments have appreciable toxicity. Dealing satisfactorily with participant losses is very difficult. Those on treatment are likely to drop out earlier due to adverse effects or death, and hence the measurements on these people, tending to be earlier in the study, will favour the intervention. It is often difficult to get continued monitoring of these participants in order to carry out an analysis of all randomized participants. This issue, although it might at first seem to be a topic-specific cause of bias, would be more appropriately covered under Incomplete Outcome Data.

## 8.15    Chapter information

**Editors**: Julian PT Higgins and Douglas G Altman on behalf of the Cochrane Statistical Methods Group and the Cochrane Bias Methods Group.

**This chapter should be cited as**: Higgins JPT, Altman DG (editors). Chapter 8: Assessing risk of bias in included studies. In: Higgins JPT, Green S (editors). *Cochrane*

*Handbook for Systematic Reviews of Interventions.* Chichester (UK): John Wiley & Sons, 2008.

**Contributing authors**: Doug Altman, Gerd Antes, Peter Gøtzsche, Julian Higgins, Peter Jüni, Steff Lewis, David Moher, Andy Oxman, Ken Schulz, Jonathan Sterne and Simon Thompson.

**Acknowledgements**: The material in this chapter was developed by a working group consisting of Doug Altman (co-lead), Gerd Antes, Chris Cates, Mike Clarke, Jon Deeks, Peter Gøtzsche, Julian Higgins (co-lead), Sally Hopewell, Peter Jüni (core group), Steff Lewis, Philippa Middleton, David Moher (core group), Andy Oxman, Ken Schulz (core group), Nandi Siegfried, Jonathan Sterne Simon Thompson. We thank Hilda Bastian, Rachelle Buchbinder, Iain Chalmers, Miranda Cumpston, Sally Green, Peter Herbison, Victor Montori, Hannah Rothstein, Georgia Salanti, Guido Schwarzer, Ian Shrier, Jayne Tierney, Ian White and Paula Williamson for helpful comments. For details of the Cochrane Statistical Methods Group, see Chapter 9 (Box 9.8.a) and for the Cochrane Bias Methods Group, see Chapter 10 (Box 10.5.a).

# 8.16 References

**Als-Nielsen 2004**
Als-Nielsen B, Gluud LL, Gluud C. Methodological quality and treatment effects in random-ized trials: a review of six empirical studies. *12th Cochrane Colloquium*, Ottawa (Canada), 2004.

**Altman 1999**
Altman DG, Bland JM. How to randomize. *BMJ* 1999; 319: 703–704.

**Balk 2002**
Balk EM, Bonis PAL, Moskowitz H, Schmid CH, Ioannidis JPA, Wang C, Lau J. Correlation of quality measures with estimates of treatment effect in meta-analyses of randomized controlled trials. *JAMA* 2002; 287: 2973–2982.

**Bassler 2007**
Bassler D, Ferreira-Gonzalez I, Briel M, Cook DJ, Devereaux PJ, Heels-Ansdell D, Kir-palani H, Meade MO, Montori VM, Rozenberg A, Schunemann HJ, Guyatt GH. Systematic reviewers neglect bias that results from trials stopped early for benefit. *Journal of Clinical Epidemiology* 2007; 60: 869–873.

**Bellomo 2000**
Bellomo R, Chapman M, Finfer S, Hickling K, Myburgh J. Low-dose dopamine in patients with early renal dysfunction: a placebo-controlled randomised trial. Australian and New Zealand Intensive Care Society (ANZICS) Clinical Trials Group. *The Lancet* 2000; 356: 2139–2143.

**Berger 2003**
Berger VW, Ivanova A, Knoll MD. Minimizing predictability while retaining balance through the use of less restrictive randomization procedures. *Statistics in Medicine* 2003; 22: 3017–3028.

**Berger 2005**
Berger VW. Quantifying the magnitude of baseline covariate imbalances resulting from selection bias in randomized clinical trials. *Biometrical Journal* 2005; 47: 119–127.

**Berlin 1997**

Berlin JA. Does blinding of readers affect the results of meta-analyses? University of Pennsylvania Meta-analysis Blinding Study Group. *The Lancet* 1997; 350: 185–186.

**Boutron 2005**

Boutron I, Estellat C, Ravaud P. A review of blinding in randomized controlled trials found results inconsistent and questionable. *Journal of Clinical Epidemiology* 2005; 58: 1220–1226.

**Boutron 2006**

Boutron I, Estellat C, Guittet L, Dechartres A, Sackett DL, Hróbjartsson A, Ravaud P. Methods of blinding in reports of randomized controlled trials assessing pharmacologic treatments: a systematic review. *PLOS Medicine* 2006; 3: 1931–1939.

**Brightling 2000**

Brightling CE, Monteiro W, Ward R, Parker D, Morgan MD, Wardlaw AJ, Pavord ID. Sputum eosinophilia and short-term response to prednisolone in chronic obstructive pulmonary disease: a randomised controlled trial. *The Lancet* 2000; 356: 1480–1485.

**Brown 2005**

Brown S, Thorpe H, Hawkins K, Brown J. Minimization: reducing predictability for multi-centre trials whilst retaining balance within centre. *Statistics in Medicine* 2005; 24: 3715–3727.

**Chan 2004a**

Chan AW, Hróbjartsson A, Haahr MT, Gøtzsche PC, Altman DG. Empirical evidence for selective reporting of outcomes in randomized trials: comparison of protocols to published articles. *JAMA* 2004; 291: 2457–2465.

**Chan 2004b**

Chan AW, Krleža-Jeric K, Schmid I, Altman DG. Outcome reporting bias in randomized trials funded by the Canadian Institutes of Health Research. *Canadian Medical Association Journal* 2004; 171: 735–740.

**Chan 2005**

Chan AW, Altman DG. Identifying outcome reporting bias in randomised trials on PubMed: review of publications and survey of authors. *BMJ* 2005; 330: 753.

**Coronary Drug Project Research Group 1980**

Coronary Drug Project Research Group. Influence of adherence to treatment and response of cholesterol on mortality in the coronary drug project. *New England Journal of Medicine* 1980; 303: 1038–1041.

**Cuellar 2000**

Cuellar GEM, Ruiz AM, Monsalve MCR, Berber A. Six-month treatment of obesity with sibutramine 15 mg; a double-blind, placebo-controlled monocenter clinical trial in a Hispanic population. *Obesity Research* 2000; 8: 71–82.

**de Gaetano 2001**

de Gaetano G. Low-dose aspirin and vitamin E in people at cardiovascular risk: a randomised trial in general practice. Collaborative Group of the Primary Prevention Project. *The Lancet* 2001; 357: 89–95.

**Detsky 1992**

Detsky AS, Naylor CD, O'Rourke K, McGeer AJ, L'Abbe KA. Incorporating variations in the quality of individual randomized trials into meta-analysis. *Journal of Clinical Epidemiology* 1992; 45: 255–265.

**Devereaux 2001**

Devereaux PJ, Manns BJ, Ghali WA, Quan H, Lacchetti C, Montori VM, Bhandari M, Guyatt GH. Physician interpretations and textbook definitions of blinding terminology in randomized controlled trials. *JAMA* 2001; 285: 2000–2003.

**Emerson 1990**

Emerson JD, Burdick E, Hoaglin DC, Mosteller F, Chalmers TC. An empirical study of the possible relation of treatment differences to quality scores in controlled randomized clinical trials. *Controlled Clinical Trials* 1990; 11: 339–352.

**Fergusson 2002**

Fergusson D, Aaron SD, Guyatt G, Hébert P. Post-randomisation exclusions: the intention to treat principle and excluding patients from analysis. *BMJ* 2002; 325: 652–654.

**Fergusson 2004**

Fergusson D, Glass KC, Waring D, Shapiro S. Turning a blind eye: the success of blinding reported in a random sample of randomised, placebo controlled trials. *BMJ* 2004; 328: 432.

**Furukawa 2007**

Furukawa TA, Watanabe N, Omori IM, Montori VM, Guyatt GH. Association between unreported outcomes and effect size estimates in Cochrane meta-analyses. *JAMA* 2007; 297: 468–470.

**Ghersi 2006**

Ghersi D, Clarke M, Simes J. Selective reporting of the primary outcomes of clinical trials: a follow-up study. *14th Cochrane Colloquium*, Dublin (Ireland), 2006.

**Gøtzsche 1996**

Gøtzsche PC. Blinding during data analysis and writing of manuscripts. *Controlled Clinical Trials* 1996; 17: 285–290.

**Gøtzsche 2006**

Gøtzsche PC, Hróbjartsson A, Johansen HK, Haahr MT, Altman DG, Chan AW. Constraints on publication rights in industry-initiated clinical trials. *JAMA* 2006; 295: 1645–1646.

**Gøtzsche 2007**

Gøtzsche PC, Hróbjartsson A, Maric K, Tendal B. Data extraction errors in meta-analyses that use standardized mean differences. *JAMA* 2007; 298: 430–437.

**Greenland 2001**

Greenland S, O'Rourke K. On the bias produced by quality scores in meta-analysis, and a hierarchical view of proposed solutions. *Biostatistics* 2001; 2: 463–471.

**Haahr 2006**

Haahr MT, Hróbjartsson A. Who is blinded in randomised clinical trials? A study of 200 trials and a survey of authors. *Clinical Trials* 2006; 3: 360–365.

**Hahn 2002**

Hahn S, Williamson PR, Hutton JL. Investigation of within-study selective reporting in clinical research: follow-up of applications submitted to a local research ethics committee. *Journal of Evaluation in Clinical Practice* 2002; 8: 353–359.

**Hansson 1999**

Hansson L, Lindholm LH, Niskanen L, Lanke J, Hedner T, Niklason A, Luomanmaki K, Dahlof B, de Faire U, Morlin C, Karlberg BE, Wester PO, Bjorck JE. Effect of angiotensin-converting-enzyme inhibition compared with conventional therapy on cardiovascular morbidity and mortality in hypertension: the Captopril Prevention Project (CAPPP) randomised trial. *The Lancet* 1999; 353: 611–616.

**Hill 1990**

Hill AB. Memories of the British streptomycin trial in tuberculosis: the first randomized clinical trial. *Controlled Clinical Trials* 1990; 11: 77–79.

**Hollis 1999**

Hollis S, Campbell F. What is meant by intention to treat analysis? Survey of published randomised controlled trials. *BMJ* 1999; 319: 670–674.

**Hróbjartsson 2007**

Hróbjartsson A, Forfang E, Haahr MT, ls-Nielsen B, Brorson S. Blinded trials taken to the test: an analysis of randomized clinical trials that report tests for the success of blinding. *International Journal of Epidemiology* 2007; 36: 654–663.

**Hutton 2000**

Hutton JL, Williamson PR. Bias in meta-analysis due to outcome variable selection within studies. *Journal of the Royal Statistical Society Series C* 2000; 49: 359–370.

**Jadad 1996**

Jadad AR, Moore RA, Carroll D, Jenkinson C, Reynolds DJM, Gavaghan DJ, McQuay H. Assessing the quality of reports of randomized clinical trials: Is blinding necessary? *Controlled Clinical Trials* 1996; 17: 1–12.

**Johansen 2000**

Johansen HK, Gøtzsche PC. Amphotericin B lipid soluble formulations versus amphotericin B in cancer patients with neutropenia. *Cochrane Database of Systematic Reviews* 2000, Issue 3. Art No: CD000969.

**Jørgensen 2006**

Jørgensen KJ, Johansen HK, Gøtzsche PC. Voriconazole versus amphotericin B in cancer patients with neutropenia. *Cochrane Database of Systematic Reviews* 2006, Issue 1. Art No: CD004707.

**Jørgensen 2007**

Jørgensen KJ, Johansen HK, Gøtzsche PC. Flaws in design, analysis and interpretation of Pfizer's antifungal trials of voriconazole and uncritical subsequent quotations. *Trials* 2007; 7: 3.

**Jüni 1999**

Jüni P, Witschi A, Bloch R, Egger M. The hazards of scoring the quality of clinical trials for meta-analysis. *JAMA* 1999; 282: 1054–1060.

**Jüni 2001**

Jüni P, Altman DG, Egger M. Systematic reviews in health care: Assessing the quality of controlled clinical trials. *BMJ* 2001; 323: 42–46.

**Kjaergard 2001**

Kjaergard LL, Villumsen J, Gluud C. Reported methodologic quality and discrepancies between large and small randomized trials in meta-analyses. *Annals of Internal Medicine* 2001; 135: 982–989.

**Lachin 2000**

Lachin JM. Statistical considerations in the intent-to-treat principle. *Controlled Clinical Trials* 2000; 21: 167–189.

**Marshall 2000**

Marshall M, Lockwood A, Bradley C, Adams C, Joy C, Fenton M. Unpublished rating scales: a major source of bias in randomised controlled trials of treatments for schizophrenia. *British Journal of Psychiatry* 2000; 176: 249–252.

**Melander 2003**

Melander H, Ahlqvist-Rastad J, Meijer G, Beermann B. Evidence b(i)ased medicine – selective reporting from studies sponsored by pharmaceutical industry: review of studies in new drug applications. *BMJ* 2003; 326: 1171–1173.

**Moher 1995**

Moher D, Jadad AR, Nichol G, Penman M, Tugwell P, Walsh S. Assessing the quality of randomized controlled trials: An annotated bibliography of scales and checklists. *Controlled Clinical Trials* 1995; 16: 62–73.

**Moher 1996**

Moher D, Jadad AR, Tugwell P. Assessing the quality of randomized controlled trials: Current issues and future directions. *International Journal of Technology Assessment in Health Care* 1996; 12: 195–208.

**Moher 1998**

Moher D, Pham B, Jones A, Cook DJ, Jadad AR, Moher M, Tugwell P, Klassen TP. Does quality of reports of randomised trials affect estimates of intervention efficacy reported in meta-analyses? *The Lancet* 1998; 352: 609–613.

**Moher 2001a**

Moher D, Schulz KF, Altman DG. The CONSORT statement: revised recommendations for improving the quality of reports of parallel-group randomised trials. *The Lancet* 2001; 357: 1191–1194.

**Moher 2001b**

Moher D, Schulz KF, Altman DG. The CONSORT statement: revised recommendations for improving the quality of reports of parallel-group randomised trials. *The Lancet* 2001; 357: 1191–1194.

**Moher 2001c**

Moher D, Schulz KF, Altman DG. The CONSORT statement: revised recommendations for improving the quality of reports of parallel-group randomised trials. *The Lancet* 2001; 357: 1191–1194.

**Moher 2001d**

Moher D, Schulz KF, Altman DG. The CONSORT statement: revised recommendations for improving the quality of reports of parallel-group randomised trials. *The Lancet* 2001; 357: 1191–1194.

**Montori 2002**

Montori VM, Bhandari M, Devereaux PJ, Manns BJ, Ghali WA, Guyatt GH. In the dark: the reporting of blinding status in randomized controlled trials. *Journal of Clinical Epidemiology* 2002; 55: 787–790.

**Montori 2005**

Montori VM, Devereaux PJ, Adhikari NK, Burns KE, Eggert CH, Briel M, Lacchetti C, Leung TW, Darling E, Bryant DM, Bucher HC, Schünemann HJ, Meade MO, Cook DJ, Erwin PJ, Sood A, Sood R, Lo B, Thompson CA, Zhou Q, Mills E, Guyatt GH. Randomized trials stopped early for benefit: a systematic review. *JAMA* 2005; 294: 2203–2209.

**Naylor 1997**

Naylor CD. Meta-analysis and the meta-epidemiology of clinical research. *BMJ* 1997; 315: 617–619.

**Newell 1992**

Newell DJ. Intention-to-treat analysis: implications for quantitative and qualitative research. *International Journal of Epidemiology* 1992; 21: 837–841.

**Noseworthy 1994**

Noseworthy JH, Ebers GC, Vandervoort MK, Farquhar RE, Yetisir E, Roberts R. The impact of blinding on the results of a randomized, placebo-controlled multiple sclerosis clinical trial. *Neurology* 1994; 44: 16–20.

**Oxman 1993**

Oxman AD, Guyatt GH. The science of reviewing research. *Annals of the New York Academy of Sciences* 1993; 703: 125–133.

**Peto 1999**

Peto R. Failure of randomisation by "sealed" envelope. *The Lancet* 1999; 354: 73.

**Pildal 2007**

Pildal J, Hróbjartsson A, Jørgensen KJ, Hilden J, Altman DG, Gøtzsche PC. Impact of allocation concealment on conclusions drawn from meta-analyses of randomized trials. *International Journal of Epidemiology* 2007; 36: 847–857.

**Porta 2007**

Porta N, Bonet C, Cobo E. Discordance between reported intention-to-treat and per protocol analyses. *Journal of Clinical Epidemiology* 2007; 60: 663–669.

**Rees 2005**

Rees JR, Wade TJ, Levy DA, Colford JM, Jr., Hilton JF. Changes in beliefs identify unblinding in randomized controlled trials: a method to meet CONSORT guidelines. *Contemporary Clinical Trials* 2005; 26: 25–37.

**Sackett 2007**

Sackett DL. Commentary: Measuring the success of blinding in RCTs: don't, must, can't or needn't? *International Journal of Epidemiology* 2007; 36: 664–665.

**Safer 2002**

Safer DJ. Design and reporting modifications in industry-sponsored comparative psychopharmacology trials. *Journal of Nervous and Mental Disease* 2002; 190: 583–592.

**Schulz 1995a**

Schulz KF. Subverting randomization in controlled trials. *JAMA* 1995; 274: 1456–1458.

**Schulz 1995b**

Schulz KF, Chalmers I, Hayes RJ, Altman DG. Empirical evidence of bias. Dimensions of methodological quality associated with estimates of treatment effects in controlled trials. *JAMA* 1995; 273: 408–412.

**Schulz 1996**

Schulz KF, Grimes DA, Altman DG, Hayes RJ. Blinding and exclusions after allocation in randomised controlled trials: survey of published parallel group trials in obstetrics and gynaecology. *BMJ* 1996; 312: 742–744.

**Schulz 2002a**

Schulz KF, Chalmers I, Altman DG. The landscape and lexicon of blinding in randomized trials. *Annals of Internal Medicine* 2002; 136: 254–259.

**Schulz 2002b**

Schulz KF, Grimes DA. Allocation concealment in randomised trials: defending against deciphering. *The Lancet* 2002; 359: 614–618.

**Schulz 2002c**

Schulz KF, Grimes DA. Generation of allocation sequences in randomised trials: chance, not choice. *The Lancet* 2002; 359: 515–519.

**Schulz 2002d**

Schulz KF, Grimes DA. Unequal group sizes in randomised trials: guarding against guessing. *The Lancet* 2002; 359: 966–970.

**Schulz 2006**

Schulz KF, Grimes DA. *The Lancet Handbook of Essential Concepts in Clinical Research.* Edinburgh (UK): Elsevier, 2006.

**Senn 1991**

Senn S. Baseline comparisons in randomized clinical trials. *Statistics in Medicine* 1991; 10: 1157–1159.

**Siersma 2007**

Siersma V, ls-Nielsen B, Chen W, Hilden J, Gluud LL, Gluud C. Multivariable modelling for meta-epidemiological assessment of the association between trial quality and treatment effects estimated in randomized clinical trials. *Statistics in Medicine* 2007; 26: 2745–2758.

**Smilde 2001**

Smilde TJ, van Wissen S, Wollersheim H, Trip MD, Kastelein JJ, Stalenhoef AF. Effect of aggressive versus conventional lipid lowering on atherosclerosis progression in familial hypercholesterolaemia (ASAP): a prospective, randomised, double-blind trial. *The Lancet* 2001; 357: 577–581.

**Spiegelhalter 2003**

Spiegelhalter DJ, Best NG. Bayesian approaches to multiple sources of evidence and uncertainty in complex cost-effectiveness modelling. *Statistics in Medicine* 2003; 22: 3687–3709.

**Sterne 2002**

Sterne JA, Jüni P, Schulz KF, Altman DG, Bartlett C, Egger M. Statistical methods for assessing the influence of study characteristics on treatment effects in 'meta-epidemiological' research. *Statistics in Medicine* 2002; 21: 1513–1524.

**Tierney 2005**

Tierney JF, Stewart LA. Investigating patient exclusion bias in meta-analysis. *International Journal of Epidemiology* 2005; 34: 79–87.

**Turner 2008**

Turner RM, Spiegelhalter DJ, Smith GCS, Thompson SG. Bias modelling in evidence synthesis. *Journal of the Royal Statistical Society Series* (in press, 2008).

**Unnebrink 2001**

Unnebrink K, Windeler J. Intention-to-treat: methods for dealing with missing values in clinical trials of progressively deteriorating diseases. *Statistics in Medicine* 2001; 20: 3931–3946.

**Vickers 2001**

Vickers AJ. The use of percentage change from baseline as an outcome in a controlled trial is statistically inefficient: a simulation study. *BMC Medical Research Methodology* 2001; 1:6.

**von Elm 2006**

von Elm E, Röllin A, Blümle A, Senessie C, Low N, Egger M. Selective reporting of outcomes of drug trials. Comparison of study protocols and pulbished articles. *14th Cochrane Colloquium*, Dublin (Ireland), 2006.

**Williamson 2005a**

Williamson PR, Gamble C. Identification and impact of outcome selection bias in meta-analysis. *Statistics in Medicine* 2005; 24: 1547–1561.

**Williamson 2005b**

Williamson PR, Gamble C, Altman DG, Hutton JL. Outcome selection bias in meta-analysis. *Statistical Methods in Medical Research* 2005; 14: 515–524.

**Wood 2004**

Wood AM, White IR, Thompson SG. Are missing outcome data adequately handled? A review of published randomized controlled trials in major medical journals. *Clinical Trials* 2004; 1: 368–376.

**Wood 2008**

Wood L, Egger M, Gluud LL, Schulz K, Jüni P, Altman DG, Gluud C, Martin RM, Wood AJG, Sterne JAC. Empirical evidence of bias in treatment effect estimates in controlled trials with different interventions and outcomes: meta-epidemiological study. *BMJ* 2008; 336: 601–605.

**Woods 1995**

Woods KL. Mega-trials and management of acute myocardial infarction. *The Lancet* 1995; 346: 611–614.

# 9 Analysing data and undertaking meta-analyses

**Edited by Jonathan J Deeks, Julian PT Higgins and Douglas G Altman on behalf of the Cochrane Statistical Methods Group**

## Key Points

- Meta-analysis is the statistical combination of results from two or more separate studies.

- Potential advantages of meta-analyses include an increase in power, an improvement in precision, the ability to answer questions not posed by individual studies, and the opportunity to settle controversies arising from conflicting claims. However, they also have the potential to mislead seriously, particularly if specific study designs, within-study biases, variation across studies, and reporting biases are not carefully considered.

- It is important to be familiar with the type of data (e.g. dichotomous, continuous) that result from measurement of an outcome in an individual study, and to choose suitable effect measures for comparing intervention groups.

- Most meta-analysis methods are variations on a weighted average of the effect estimates from the different studies.

- Variation across studies (heterogeneity) must be considered, although most Cochrane reviews do not have enough studies to allow the reliable investigation of the reasons for it. Random-effects meta-analyses allow for heterogeneity by assuming that underlying effects follow a normal distribution.

- Many judgements are required in the process of preparing a Cochrane review or meta-analysis. Sensitivity analyses should be used to examine whether overall findings are robust to potentially influential decisions.

# 9.1    Introduction

### 9.1.1    Do not start here!

It can be tempting to jump prematurely into a statistical analysis when undertaking a systematic review. The production of a diamond at the bottom of a plot is an exciting moment for many authors, but results of meta-analyses can be very misleading if suitable attention has not been given to formulating the review question; specifying eligibility criteria; identifying, selecting and critically appraising studies; collecting appropriate data; and deciding what would be meaningful to analyse. Review authors should consult the chapters that precede this one before a meta-analysis is undertaken.

### 9.1.2    Planning the analysis

While in primary studies the investigators select and collect data from individual patients, in systematic reviews the investigators select and collect data from primary studies. While primary studies include analyses of their participants, Cochrane reviews contain analyses of the primary studies. Analyses may be narrative, such as a structured summary and discussion of the studies' characteristics and findings, or quantitative, that is involving statistical analysis. **Meta-analysis** – the statistical combination of results from two or more separate studies – is the most commonly used statistical technique. Cochrane review writing software (RevMan) can perform a variety of meta-analyses, but it must be stressed that meta-analysis is not appropriate in all Cochrane reviews. Issues to consider when deciding whether a meta-analysis is appropriate in a review are discussed in this section and in Section 9.1.4.

Studies comparing healthcare interventions, notably randomized trials, use the outcomes of participants to compare the effects of different interventions. Meta-analyses focus on pair-wise comparisons of interventions, such as an experimental intervention versus a control intervention, or the comparison of two experimental interventions. The terminology used here (experimental versus control interventions) implies the former, although the methods apply equally to the latter.

The contrast between the outcomes of two groups treated differently is known as the 'effect', the 'treatment effect' or the 'intervention effect'. Whether analysis of included studies is narrative or quantitative, a general framework for synthesis may be provided by considering four questions:

1. What is the direction of effect?

2. What is the size of effect?

3. Is the effect consistent across studies?

4. What is the strength of evidence for the effect?

Meta-analysis provides a statistical method for questions 1 to 3. Assessment of question 4 relies additionally on judgements based on assessments of study design and risk of bias, as well as statistical measures of uncertainty.

Narrative synthesis uses subjective (rather than statistical) methods to follow through questions 1 to 4, for reviews where meta-analysis is either not feasible or not sensible. In a narrative synthesis the method used for each stage should be pre-specified, justified and followed systematically. Bias may be introduced if the results of one study are inappropriately stressed over those of another.

The analysis plan follows from the scientific aim of the review. Reviews have different types of aims, and may therefore contain different approaches to analysis.

1. The most straightforward Cochrane review assembles studies that make one particular comparison between two treatment options, for example, comparing kava extract versus placebo for treating anxiety (Pittler 2003). Meta-analysis and related techniques can be used if there is a consistent outcome measure to:

   ○ Establish whether there is evidence of an effect;

   ○ Estimate the size of the effect and the uncertainty surrounding that size; and

   ○ Investigate whether the effect is consistent across studies.

2. Some reviews may have a broader focus than a single comparison. The first is where the intention is to identify and collate studies of numerous interventions for the same disease or condition. An example of such a review is that of topical treatments for fungal infections of the skin and nails of the foot, which included studies of any topical treatment (Crawford 2007). The second, related aim is that of identifying a 'best' intervention. A review of interventions for emergency contraception sought that which was most effective (while also considering potential adverse effects). Such reviews may include multiple comparisons and meta-analyses between all possible pairs of treatments, and require care when it comes to planning analyses (see Section 9.1.6 and Chapter 16, Section 16.6).

3. Occasionally review comparisons have particularly wide scopes that make the use of meta-analysis problematic. For example, a review of workplace interventions for smoking cessation covered diverse types of interventions (Moher 2005). When reviews contain very diverse studies a meta-analysis might be useful to answer the overall question of whether there is evidence that, for example, work-based interventions can work (but see Section 9.1.4). But use of meta-analysis to describe the size of effect may not be meaningful if the implementations are so diverse that an effect estimate cannot be interpreted in any specific context.

4. An aim of some reviews is to investigate the relationship between the size of an effect and some characteristic(s) of the studies. This is uncommon as a primary

aim in Cochrane reviews, but may be a secondary aim. For example, in a review of beclomethasone versus placebo for chronic asthma, there was interest in whether the administered dose of beclomethasone affected its efficacy (Adams 2005). Such investigations of heterogeneity need to be undertaken with care (see Section 9.6).

## 9.1.3   Why perform a meta-analysis in a review?

The value a meta-analysis can add to a review depends on the context in which it is used, as described in Section 9.1.2. The following are reasons for considering including a meta-analysis in a review.

1. To increase power. Power is the chance of detecting a real effect as statistically significant if it exists. Many individual studies are too small to detect small effects, but when several are combined there is a higher chance of detecting an effect.

2. To improve precision. The estimation of an intervention effect can be improved when it is based on more information.

3. To answer questions not posed by the individual studies. Primary studies often involve a specific type of patient and explicitly defined interventions. A selection of studies in which these characteristics differ can allow investigation of the consistency of effect and, if relevant, allow reasons for differences in effect estimates to be investigated.

4. To settle controversies arising from apparently conflicting studies or to generate new hypotheses. Statistical analysis of findings allows the degree of conflict to be formally assessed, and reasons for different results to be explored and quantified.

Of course, the use of statistical methods does not guarantee that the results of a review are valid, any more than it does for a primary study. Moreover, like any tool, statistical methods can be misused.

## 9.1.4   When not to use meta-analysis in a review

If used appropriately, meta-analysis is a powerful tool for deriving meaningful conclusions from data and can help prevent errors in interpretation. However, there are situations in which a meta-analysis can be more of a hindrance than a help.

- A common criticism of meta-analyses is that they 'combine apples with oranges'. If studies are clinically diverse then a meta-analysis may be meaningless, and genuine differences in effects may be obscured. A particularly important type of diversity is in the comparisons being made by the primary studies. Often it is nonsensical to combine all included studies in a single meta-analysis: sometimes there is a mix of comparisons of different treatments with different comparators, each combination of which may need to be considered separately. Further, it is important not to combine outcomes that are too diverse. Decisions concerning what should and should not be combined are inevitably subjective, and are not amenable to statistical solutions but require discussion and clinical judgement. In some cases consensus may be hard to reach.

- Meta-analyses of studies that are at risk of bias may be seriously misleading. If bias is present in each (or some) of the individual studies, meta-analysis will simply compound the errors, and produce a 'wrong' result that may be interpreted as having more credibility.

- Finally, meta-analyses in the presence of serious publication and/or reporting biases are likely to produce an inappropriate summary.

## 9.1.5   What does a meta-analysis entail?

While the use of statistical methods in reviews can be extremely helpful, the most essential element of an analysis is a thoughtful approach, to both its narrative and quantitative elements. This entails consideration of the following questions:

1. Which comparisons should be made?

2. Which study results should be used in each comparison?

3. What is the best summary of effect for each comparison?

4. Are the results of studies similar within each comparison?

5. How reliable are those summaries?

The first step in addressing these questions is to decide which comparisons to make (see Section 9.1.6) and what sorts of data are appropriate for the outcomes of interest (see Section 9.2). The next step is to prepare tabular summaries of the characteristics and results of the studies that are included in each comparison (extraction of data and conversion to the desired format is discussed in Chapter 7, Section 7.7). It is then possible to derive estimates of effect across studies in a systematic way (Section 9.4), to measure and investigate differences among studies (Sections 9.5 and 9.6) and to interpret the findings and conclude how much confidence should be placed in them (see Chapter 12).

## 9.1.6    Which comparisons should be made?

The first and most important step in planning the analysis is to specify the pair-wise comparisons that will be made. The comparisons addressed in the review should relate clearly and directly to the questions or hypotheses that are posed when the review is formulated (see Chapter 5). It should be possible to specify in the protocol of a review the main comparisons that will be made. However, it will often be necessary to modify comparisons and add new ones in light of the data that are collected. For example, important variations in the intervention may only be discovered after data are collected.

Decisions about which studies are similar enough for their results to be grouped together require an understanding of the problem that the review addresses, and judgement by the author and the user. The formulation of the questions that a review addresses is discussed in Chapter 5. Essentially the same considerations apply to deciding which comparisons to make, which outcomes to combine and which key characteristics (of study design, participants, interventions and outcomes) to consider when investigating variation in effects (heterogeneity). These considerations must be addressed when setting up the 'Data and analyses' tables in RevMan and in deciding what information to put in the table of 'Characteristics of included studies'.

## 9.1.7    Writing the analysis section of the protocol

The analysis section of a Cochrane review protocol may be more susceptible to change than other protocol sections (such as criteria for including studies and how methodological quality will be assessed). It is rarely possible to anticipate all the statistical issues that may arise, for example, finding outcomes that are similar but not the same as each other; outcomes measured at multiple or varying time-points; and use of concomitant treatments.

However the protocol should provide a strong indication as to how the author will approach the statistical evaluation of studies' findings. At least one member of the review team should be familiar with the majority of the contents of this chapter when the protocol is written. As a guideline we recommend that the following be addressed:

1. Ensure that the analysis strategy firmly addresses the stated objectives of the review (see Section 9.1.2).

2. Consider which types of study design would be appropriate for the review. Parallel group trials are the norm, but other randomized designs may be appropriate to the topic (e.g. cross-over trials, cluster-randomized trials, factorial trials). Decide how such studies will be addressed in the analysis (see Section 9.3).

3. Decide whether a meta-analysis is intended and consider how the decision as to whether a meta-analysis is appropriate will be made (see Sections 9.1.3 and 9.1.4).

4. Determine the likely nature of outcome data (e.g. dichotomous, continuous etc) (see Section 9.2).

5. Consider whether it is possible to specify in advance what intervention effect measures will be used (e.g. risk ratio, odds ratio or risk difference for dichotomous outcomes; mean difference or standardized mean difference for continuous outcomes) (see Sections 9.4.4.4 and 9.4.5.1).

6. Decide how statistical heterogeneity will be identified or quantified (see Section 9.5.2).

7. Decide whether random-effects meta-analyses, fixed-effect meta-analyses or both methods will be used for each planned meta-analysis (see Section 9.5.4).

8. Consider how clinical and methodological diversity (heterogeneity) will be assessed and whether (and how) these will be incorporated into the analysis strategy (see Sections 9.5 and 9.6).

9. Decide how the risk of bias in included studies will be assessed and addressed in the analysis (see Chapter 8).

10. Pre-specify characteristics of the studies that may be examined as potential causes of heterogeneity (see Section 9.6.5).

11. Consider how missing data will be handled (e.g. imputing data for intention-to-treat analyses) (see Chapter 16, Sections 16.1 and 16.2).

12. Decide whether (and how) evidence of possible publication and/or reporting biases will be sought (see Chapter 10).

It may become apparent when writing the protocol that additional expertise is likely to be required; and if so, a statistician should be sought to join the review team.

## 9.2 Types of data and effect measures

### 9.2.1 Types of data

The starting point of all meta-analyses of studies of effectiveness involves the identification of the data type for the outcome measurements. Throughout this chapter we consider outcome data to be of five different types:

1. dichotomous (or binary) data, where each individual's outcome is one of only two possible categorical responses;

2. continuous data, where each individual's outcome is a measurement of a numerical quantity;

3. ordinal data (including measurement scales), where the outcome is one of several ordered categories, or generated by scoring and summing categorical responses;

4. counts and rates calculated from counting the number of events that each individual experiences; and

5. time-to-event (typically survival) data that analyse the time until an event occurs, but where not all individuals in the study experience the event (censored data).

The ways in which the effect of an intervention can be measured depend on the nature of the data being collected. In this section we briefly examine the types of outcome data that might be encountered in systematic reviews of clinical trials, and review definitions, properties and interpretation of standard measures of intervention effect. In Sections 9.4.4.4 and 9.4.5.1 we discuss issues in the selection of one of these measures for a particular meta-analysis.

## 9.2.2   Effect measures for dichotomous outcomes

Dichotomous (binary) outcome data arise when the outcome for every participant is one of two possibilities, for example, dead or alive, or clinical improvement or no clinical improvement. This section considers the possible summary statistics when the outcome of interest has such a binary form. The most commonly encountered effect measures used in clinical trials with dichotomous data are:

- the risk ratio (RR) (also called the relative risk);

- the odds ratio (OR);

- the risk difference (RD) (also called the absolute risk reduction); and

- the number needed to treat (NNT).

Details of the calculations of the first three of these measures are given in Box 9.2.a. Numbers needed to treat are discussed in detail in Chapter 12 (Section 12.5).

*Aside: As events may occasionally be desirable rather than undesirable, it would be preferable to use a more neutral term than risk (such as probability), but for the sake of convention we use the terms risk ratio and risk difference throughout. We also use the term 'risk ratio' in preference to 'relative risk' for consistency with other terminology. The two are interchangeable and both conveniently abbreviate to 'RR'. Note also that we have been careful with the use of the words 'risk' and 'rates'. These words are often treated synonymously. However, we have tried to reserve use of the word 'rate' for the data type 'counts and rates' where it describes the frequency of events in a measured period of time.*

---

**Box 9.2.a  Calculation of risk ratio (RR), odds ratio (OR) and risk difference (RD) from a 2 × 2 table**

The results of a clinical trial can be displayed as a 2 × 2 table:

|  | Event ('Success') | No event ('Fail') | Total |
|---|---|---|---|
| **Experimental intervention** | $S_E$ | $F_E$ | $N_E$ |
| **Control intervention** | $S_C$ | $F_C$ | $N_C$ |

where $S_E$, $S_C$, $F_E$ and $F_C$ are the numbers of participants with each outcome ('S' or 'F') in each group ('E' or 'C'). The following summary statistics can be calculated:

$$RR = \frac{\text{risk of event in experimental group}}{\text{risk of event in control group}} = \frac{S_E/N_E}{S_C/N_C}$$

$$OR = \frac{\text{odds of event in experimental group}}{\text{odds of event in control group}} = \frac{S_E/F_E}{S_C/F_C} = \frac{S_E F_C}{F_E S_C}$$

$$RD = \text{risk of event in experimental group} - \text{risk of event in control group}$$

$$= \frac{S_E}{N_E} - \frac{S_C}{N_C}$$

---

### 9.2.2.1  *Risk and odds*

In general conversation the terms 'risk' and 'odds' are used interchangeably (as are the terms 'chance', 'probability' and 'likelihood') as if they describe the same quantity. In statistics, however, risk and odds have particular meanings and are calculated in different ways. When the difference between them is ignored, the results of a systematic review may be misinterpreted.

**Risk** is the concept more familiar to patients and health professionals. Risk describes the probability with which a health outcome (usually an adverse event) will occur. In research, risk is commonly expressed as a decimal number between 0 and 1, although it is occasionally converted into a percentage. In 'Summary of findings' tables in Cochrane reviews, it is often expressed as a number of individuals per 1000 (see Chapter 11, Section 11.5). It is simple to grasp the relationship between a risk and the likely occurrence of events: in a sample of 100 people the number of events observed will on average be the risk multiplied by 100. For example, when the risk is 0.1, about 10 people out of every 100 will have the event; when the risk is 0.5, about 50 people out of every 100 will have the event. In a sample of 1000 people, these numbers are 100 and 500 respectively.

**Odds** is a concept that is more familiar to gamblers. The odds is the ratio of the probability that a particular event will occur to the probability that it will not occur, and can be any number between zero and infinity. In gambling, the odds describes the ratio of the size of the potential winnings to the gambling stake; in health care it is the ratio of the number of people with the event to the number without. It is commonly expressed as a ratio of two integers. For example, an odds of 0.01 is often written as 1:100, odds of 0.33 as 1:3, and odds of 3 as 3:1. Odds can be converted to risks, and risks to odds, using the formulae:

$$\text{risk} = \frac{\text{odds}}{1 + \text{odds}}; \quad \text{odds} = \frac{\text{risk}}{1 - \text{risk}}$$

The interpretation of an odds is more complicated than for a risk. The simplest way to ensure that the interpretation is correct is to first convert the odds into a risk. For example, when the odds are 1:10, or 0.1, one person will have the event for every 10 who do not, and, using the formula, the risk of the event is $0.1/(1 + 0.1) = 0.091$. In a sample of 100, about 9 individuals will have the event and 91 will not. When the odds is equal to 1, one person will have the event for every one who does not, so in a sample of 100, $100 \times 1/(1 + 1) = 50$ will have the event and 50 will not.

The difference between odds and risk is small when the event is rare (as illustrated in the first example above where a risk of 0.091 was seen to be similar to an odds of 0.1). When events are common, as is often the case in clinical trials, the differences between odds and risks are large. For example, a risk of 0.5 is equivalent to an odds of 1; and a risk of 0.95 is equivalent to odds of 19.

Measures of effect for clinical trials with dichotomous outcomes involve comparing either risks or odds from two intervention groups. To compare them we can look at their ratio (risk ratio or odds ratio) or their difference in risk (risk difference).

### 9.2.2.2  Measures of relative effect: the risk ratio and odds ratio

Measures of relative effect express the outcome in one group relative to that in the other. The **risk ratio** (or relative risk) is the ratio of the risk of an event in the two groups, whereas the **odds ratio** is the ratio of the odds of an event (see Box 9.2.a). For both measures a value of 1 indicates that the estimated effects are the same for both interventions.

Neither the risk ratio nor the odds ratio can be calculated for a study if there are no events in the control group. This is because, as can be seen from the formulae in Box 9.2.a, we would be trying to divide by zero. The odds ratio also cannot be calculated if everybody in the intervention group experiences an event. In these situations, and others where standard errors cannot be computed, it is customary to add $1/2$ to each cell of the 2 × 2 table (RevMan automatically makes this correction when necessary). In the case where no events (or all events) are observed in both groups the study provides no information about relative probability of the event and is automatically omitted from the meta-analysis. This is entirely appropriate. Zeros arise particularly when the event of interest is rare – such events are often unintended adverse outcomes. For further discussion of choice of effect measures for such sparse data (often with lots of zeros) see Chapter 16 (Section 16.9).

Risk ratios describe the multiplication of the risk that occurs with use of the experimental intervention. For example, a risk ratio of 3 for a treatment implies that events with treatment are three times more likely than events without treatment. Alternatively we can say that treatment increases the risk of events by $100 \times (RR - 1)\% = 200\%$. Similarly a risk ratio of 0.25 is interpreted as the probability of an event with treatment being one-quarter of that without treatment. This may be expressed alternatively by saying that treatment decreases the risk of events by $100 \times (1 - RR)\% = 75\%$. This is known as the relative risk reduction (see also Chapter 12, Section 12.5.1). The interpretation of the clinical importance of a given risk ratio cannot be made without knowledge of the typical risk of events without treatment: a risk ratio of 0.75 could correspond to a clinically important reduction in events from 80% to 60%, or a small, less clinically important reduction from 4% to 3%.

The numerical value of the observed risk ratio must always be between 0 and 1/ CGR, where CGR (abbreviation of 'control group risk', sometimes referred to as the control event rate) is the observed risk of the event in the control group (expressed as a number between 0 and 1). This means that for common events large values of risk ratio are impossible. For example, when the observed risk of events in the control group is 0.66 (or 66%) then the observed risk ratio cannot exceed 1.5. This problem applies only for increases in risk, and causes problems only when the results are extrapolated to risks above those observed in the study.

Odds ratios, like odds, are more difficult to interpret (Sinclair 1994, Sackett 1996). Odds ratios describe the multiplication of the odds of the outcome that occur with use of the intervention. To understand what an odds ratio means in terms of changes in numbers of events it is simplest to first convert it into a risk ratio, and then interpret the risk ratio in the context of a typical control group risk, as outlined above. The formula for converting an odds ratio to a risk ratio is provided in Chapter 12 (Section 12.5.4.4). Sometimes it may be sensible to calculate the RR for more than one assumed control group risk.

### 9.2.2.3 Warning: OR and RR are not the same

Because risk and odds are different when events are common, the risk ratio and the odds ratio also differ when events are common. The non-equivalence of the risk ratio and odds ratio does not indicate that either is wrong: both are entirely valid ways of describing an intervention effect. Problems may arise, however, if the odds ratio is misinterpreted as a risk ratio. For interventions that increase the chances of events, the odds ratio will be larger than the risk ratio, so the misinterpretation will tend to overestimate the intervention effect, especially when events are common (with, say, risks of events more than 20%). For interventions that reduce the chances of events, the odds ratio will be smaller than the risk ratio, so that again misinterpretation overestimates the effect of the intervention. This error in interpretation is unfortunately quite common in published reports of individual studies and systematic reviews.

### 9.2.2.4   Measure of absolute effect: the risk difference

The **risk difference** is the difference between the observed risks (proportions of individuals with the outcome of interest) in the two groups (see Box 9.2.a). The risk difference can be calculated for any study, even when there are no events in either group. The risk difference is straightforward to interpret: it describes the actual difference in the observed risk of events between experimental and control interventions; for an individual it describes the estimated difference in the probability of experiencing the event. However, the clinical importance of a risk difference may depend on the underlying risk of events. For example, a risk difference of 0.02 (or 2%) may represent a small, clinically insignificant change from a risk of 58% to 60% or a proportionally much larger and potentially important change from 1% to 3%. Although the risk difference provides more directly relevant information than relative measures (Laupacis 1988, Sackett 1997) it is still important to be aware of the underlying risk of events and consequences of the events when interpreting a risk difference. Absolute measures, such as the risk difference, are particularly useful when considering trade-offs between likely benefits and likely harms of an intervention.

The risk difference is naturally constrained (like the risk ratio), which may create difficulties when applying results to other patient groups and settings. For example, if a study or meta-analysis estimates a risk difference of $-0.1$ (or $-10\%$), then for a group with an initial risk of, say, 7% the outcome will have an impossible estimated negative probability of $-3\%$. Similar scenarios for increases in risk occur at the other end of the scale. Such problems can arise only when the results are applied to patients with different risks from those observed in the studies.

The number needed to treat is obtained from the risk difference. Although it is often used to summarize results of clinical trials, NNTs cannot be combined in a meta-analysis (see Section 9.4.4.4). However, odds ratios, risk ratios and risk differences may be usefully converted to NNTs and used when interpreting the results of a meta-analysis as discussed in Chapter 12 (Section 12.5).

### 9.2.2.5   What is the event?

In the context of dichotomous outcomes, healthcare interventions are intended either to reduce the risk of occurrence of an adverse outcome or increase the chance of a good outcome. All of the effect measures described in Section 9.2.2 apply equally to both scenarios.

In many situations it is natural to talk about one of the outcome states as being an event. For example, when participants have particular symptoms at the start of the study the event of interest is usually recovery or cure. If participants are well or alternatively at risk of some adverse outcome at the beginning of the study, then the event is the onset of disease or occurrence of the adverse outcome. Because the focus is usually on the experimental intervention group, a study in which the experimental intervention reduces the occurrence of an adverse outcome will have an odds ratio and risk ratio less than 1, and a negative risk difference. A study in which the experimental intervention increases the occurrence of a good outcome will have an odds ratio and risk ratio greater than 1, and a positive risk difference (see Box 9.2.a).

However, it is possible to switch events and non-events and consider instead the proportion of patients not recovering or not experiencing the event. For meta-analyses using risk differences or odds ratios the impact of this switch is of no great consequence: the switch simply changes the sign of a risk difference, whilst for odds ratios the new odds ratio is the reciprocal ($1/x$) of the original odds ratio.

By contrast, switching the outcome can make a substantial difference for risk ratios, affecting the effect estimate, its significance, and the consistency of intervention effects across studies. This is because the precision of a risk ratio estimate differs markedly between situations where risks are low and situations where risks are high. In a meta-analysis the effect of this reversal cannot easily be predicted. The identification, before data analysis, of which risk ratio is more likely to be the most relevant summary statistic is therefore important and discussed further in Section 9.4.4.4.

## 9.2.3   Effect measures for continuous outcomes

The term 'continuous' in statistics conventionally refers to data that can take any value in a specified range. When dealing with numerical data, this means that any number may be measured and reported to arbitrarily many decimal places. Examples of truly continuous data are weight, area and volume. In practice, in Cochrane reviews we can use the same statistical methods for other types of data, most commonly measurement scales and counts of large numbers of events (see Section 9.2.4).

Two summary statistics are commonly used for meta-analysis of continuous data: the mean difference and the standardized mean difference. These can be calculated whether the data from each individual are single assessments or change from baseline measures. It is also possible to measure effects by taking ratios of means, or by comparing statistics other than means (e.g. medians). However, methods for these are not addressed here.

### *9.2.3.1   The mean difference (or difference in means)*

The **mean difference** (more correctly, 'difference in means') is a standard statistic that measures the absolute difference between the mean value in two groups in a clinical trial. It estimates the amount by which the experimental intervention changes the outcome on average compared with the control. It can be used as a summary statistic in meta-analysis when outcome measurements in all studies are made on the same scale.

*Aside: Analyses based on this effect measure have historically been termed weighted mean difference (WMD) analyses in the* Cochrane Database of Systematic Reviews (CDSR). *This name is potentially confusing: although the meta-analysis computes a weighted average of these differences in means, no weighting is involved in calculation of a statistical summary of a single study. Furthermore, all meta-analyses involve a weighted combination of estimates, yet we do not use the word 'weighted' when referring to other methods.*

### 9.2.3.2 The standardized mean difference

The **standardized mean difference** is used as a summary statistic in meta-analysis when the studies all assess the same outcome but measure it in a variety of ways (for example, all studies measure depression but they use different psychometric scales). In this circumstance it is necessary to standardize the results of the studies to a uniform scale before they can be combined. The standardized mean difference expresses the size of the intervention effect in each study relative to the variability observed in that study. (Again in reality the intervention effect is a difference in means and not a mean of differences):

$$\text{SMD} = \frac{\text{difference in mean outcome between groups}}{\text{standard deviation of outcome among participants}}.$$

Thus studies for which the difference in means is the same proportion of the standard deviation will have the same SMD, regardless of the actual scales used to make the measurements.

However, the method assumes that the differences in standard deviations among studies reflect differences in measurement scales and not real differences in variability among study populations. This assumption may be problematic in some circumstances where we expect real differences in variability between the participants in different studies. For example, where pragmatic and explanatory trials are combined in the same review, pragmatic trials may include a wider range of participants and may consequently have higher standard deviations. The overall intervention effect can also be difficult to interpret as it is reported in units of standard deviation rather than in units of any of the measurement scales used in the review, but in some circumstances it is possible to transform the effect back to the units used in a specific study (see Chapter 12, Section 12.6).

The term 'effect size' is frequently used in the social sciences, particularly in the context of meta-analysis. Effect sizes typically, though not always, refer to versions of the standardized mean difference. It is recommended that the term 'standardized mean difference' be used in Cochrane reviews in preference to 'effect size' to avoid confusion with the more general medical use of the latter term as a synonym for 'intervention effect' or 'effect estimate'. The particular definition of standardized mean difference used in Cochrane reviews is the effect size known in social science as Hedges' (adjusted) $g$.

It should be noted that the SMD method does not correct for differences in the direction of the scale. If some scales increase with disease severity whilst others decrease it is essential to multiply the mean values from one set of studies by $-1$ (or alternatively to subtract the mean from the maximum possible value for the scale) to ensure that all the scales point in the same direction. Any such adjustment should be described in the statistical methods section of the review. The standard deviation does not need to be modified.

### 9.2.4   Effect measures for ordinal outcomes and measurement scales

**Ordinal outcome data** arise when each participant is classified in a category and when the categories have a natural order. For example, a 'trichotomous' outcome with an ordering to the categories, such as the classification of disease severity into 'mild', 'moderate' or 'severe', is of ordinal type. As the number of categories increases, ordinal outcomes acquire properties similar to continuous outcomes, and probably will have been analysed as such in a clinical trial.

**Measurement scales** are one particular type of ordinal outcome frequently used to measure conditions that are difficult to quantify, such as behaviour, depression, and cognitive abilities. Measurement scales typically involve a series of questions or tasks, each of which is scored and the scores then summed to yield a total 'score'. If the items are not considered of equal importance a weighted sum may be used.

It is important to know whether scales have been validated: that is, that they have been proven to measure the conditions that they claim to measure. When a scale is used to assess an outcome in a clinical trial, the cited reference to the scale should be studied in order to understand the objective, the target population and the assessment questionnaire. As investigators often adapt scales to suit their own purpose by adding, changing or dropping questions, review authors should check whether an original or adapted questionnaire is being used. This is particularly important when pooling outcomes for a meta-analysis. Clinical trials may appear to use the same rating scale, but closer examination may reveal differences that must be taken into account. It is possible that modifications to a scale were made in the light of the results of a study, in order to highlight components that appear to benefit from an experimental intervention.

Specialist methods are available for analysing ordinal outcome data that describe effects in terms of **proportional odds ratios**, but they are not available in RevMan, and become unwieldy (and unnecessary) when the number of categories is large. In practice longer ordinal scales are often analysed in meta-analyses as continuous data, whilst shorter ordinal scales are often made into dichotomous data by combining adjacent categories together. The latter is especially appropriate if an established, defensible cut-point is available. Inappropriate choice of a cut-point can induce bias, particularly if it is chosen to maximize the difference between two intervention arms in a clinical trial.

Where ordinal scales are summarized using methods for dichotomous data, one of the two sets of grouped categories is defined to be the event and intervention effects are described using risk ratios, odds ratios or risk differences (see Section 9.2.2). When ordinal scales are summarized using methods for continuous data, the intervention effect is expressed as a difference in means or standardized difference in means (see Section 9.2.3). Difficulties will be encountered if studies have summarized their results using medians (see Chapter 7, Section 7.7.3.5).

Unless individual patient data are available, the analyses reported by the investigators in the clinical trials typically determine the approach that is used in the meta-analysis.

## 9.2.5    Effect measures for counts and rates

Some types of event can happen to a person more than once, for example, a myocardial infarction, fracture, an adverse reaction or a hospitalization. It may be preferable, or necessary, to address the number of times these events occur rather than simply whether each person experienced any event (that is, rather than treating them as dichotomous data). We refer to this type of data as **count data**. For practical purposes, count data may be conveniently divided into counts of rare events and counts of common events.

Counts of rare events are often referred to as 'Poisson data' in statistics. Analyses of rare events often focus on **rates**. Rates relate the counts to the amount of time during which they could have happened. For example, the result of one arm of a clinical trial could be that 18 myocardial infarctions (MIs) were experienced, across all participants in that arm, during a period of 314 person-years of follow-up, the rate is 0.057 per person-year or 5.7 per 100 person-years. The summary statistic usually used in meta-analysis is the **rate ratio** (also abbreviated to RR), which compares the rate of events in the two groups by dividing one by the other. It is also possible to use a difference in rates as a summary statistic, although this is much less common.

Counts of more common events, such as counts of decayed, missing or filled teeth, may often be treated in the same way as continuous outcome data. The intervention effect used will be the mean difference which will compare the difference in the mean number of events (possibly standardized to a unit time period) experienced by participants in the intervention group compared with participants in the control group.

### 9.2.5.1    Warning: counting events or counting participants?

A common error is to attempt to treat count data as dichotomous data. Suppose that in the example just presented, the 314 person-years arose from 157 patients observed on average for 2 years. One may be tempted to quote the results as 18/157. This is inappropriate if multiple MIs from the same patient could have contributed to the total of 18 (say if the 18 arose through 12 patients having single MIs and 3 patients each having 2 MIs). The total number of events could theoretically exceed the number of patients, making the results nonsensical. For example, over the course of one year, 35 epileptic participants in a study may experience 63 seizures among them.

## 9.2.6 Effect measures for time-to-event (survival) outcomes

**Time-to-event data** arise when interest is focused on the time elapsing before an event is experienced. They are known generically as **survival data** in statistics, since death is often the event of interest, particularly in cancer and heart disease. Time-to-event data consist of pairs of observations for each individual: (i) a length of time during which no event was observed, and (ii) an indicator of whether the end of that time period corresponds to an event or just the end of observation. Participants who contribute some period of time that does not end in an event are said to be 'censored'. Their event-free time contributes information and they are included in the analysis. Time-to-event data may be based on events other than death, such as recurrence of a disease event (for example, time to the end of a period free of epileptic fits) or discharge from hospital.

Time-to-event data can sometimes be analysed as dichotomous data. This requires the status of all patients in a study to be known at a fixed time-point. For example, if all patients have been followed for at least 12 months, and the proportion who have incurred the event before 12 months is known for both groups, then a 2 × 2 table can be constructed (see Box 9.2.a) and intervention effects expressed as risk ratios, odds ratios or risk differences.

It is not appropriate to analyse time-to-event data using methods for continuous outcomes (e.g. using mean times-to-event) as the relevant times are only known for the subset of participants who have had the event. Censored participants must be excluded, which almost certainly will introduce bias.

The most appropriate way of summarizing time-to-event data is to use methods of survival analysis and express the intervention effect as a **hazard ratio**. Hazard is similar in notion to risk, but is subtly different in that it measures instantaneous risk and may change continuously (for example, your hazard of death changes as you cross a busy road). A hazard ratio is interpreted in a similar way to a risk ratio, as it describes how many times more (or less) likely a participant is to suffer the event at a particular point in time if they receive the experimental rather than the control intervention. When comparing interventions in a study or meta-analysis a simplifying assumption is often made that the hazard ratio is constant across the follow-up period, even though hazards themselves may vary continuously. This is known as the proportional hazards assumption.

## 9.2.7 Expressing intervention effects on log scales

The values of ratio intervention effects (such as the odds ratio, risk ratio, rate ratio and hazard ratio) usually undergo log transformations before being analysed, and they may occasionally be referred to in terms of their log transformed values. Typically the *natural* log transformation (log base *e*, written 'ln') is used.

Ratio summary statistics all have the common feature that the lowest value that they can take is 0, that the value 1 corresponds with no intervention effect, and the highest value that an odds ratio can ever take is infinity. This number scale is not symmetric.

For example, whilst an odds ratio of 0.5 (a halving) and an OR of 2 (a doubling) are opposites such that they should average to no effect, the average of 0.5 and 2 is not an OR of 1 but an OR of 1.25. The log transformation makes the scale symmetric: the log of 0 is minus infinity, the log of 1 is 0, and the log of infinity is infinity. In the example, the log of the OR of 0.5 is −0.69 and the log of the OR of 2 is 0.69. The average of −0.69 and 0.69 is 0 which is the log transformed value of an OR of 1, correctly implying no average intervention effect.

Graphical displays for meta-analysis performed on ratio scales usually use a log scale. This has the effect of making the confidence intervals appear symmetric, for the same reasons.

## 9.3    Study designs and identifying the unit of analysis

### 9.3.1    Unit-of-analysis issues

An important principle in clinical trials is that the analysis must take into account the level at which randomization occurred. In most circumstances the number of observations in the analysis should match the number of 'units' that were randomized. In a simple parallel group design for a clinical trial, participants are individually randomized to one of two intervention groups, and a single measurement for each outcome from each participant is collected and analysed. However, there are numerous variations on this design. Authors should consider whether in each study:

- groups of individuals were randomized together to the same intervention (i.e. cluster-randomized trials);

- individuals undergo more than one intervention (e.g. in a cross-over trial, or simultaneous treatment of multiple sites on each individual); and

- there are multiple observations for the same outcome (e.g. repeated measurements, recurring events, measurements on different body parts).

There follows a more detailed list of situations in which unit-of-analysis issues commonly arise, together with directions to relevant discussions elsewhere in the *Handbook*.

### 9.3.2    Cluster-randomized trials

In a cluster-randomized trial, groups of participants are randomized to different interventions. For example, the groups may be schools, villages, medical practices, patients of a single doctor or families. See Chapter 16 (Section 16.3).

### 9.3.3  Cross-over trials

In a cross-over trial, all participants receive all interventions in sequence: they are randomized to an ordering of interventions, and participants act as their own control. See Chapter 16 (Section 16.4).

### 9.3.4  Repeated observations on participants

In studies of long duration, results may be presented for several periods of follow-up (for example, at 6 months, 1 year and 2 years). Results from more than one time-point for each study cannot be combined in a standard meta-analysis without a unit-of-analysis error. Some options are as follows.

- Obtain individual patient data and perform an analysis (such as time-to-event analysis) that uses the whole follow-up for each participant. Alternatively, compute an effect measure for each individual participant which incorporates all time-points, such as total number of events, an overall mean, or a trend over time. Occasionally, such analyses are available in published reports.

- Define several different outcomes, based on different periods of follow-up, and to perform separate analyses. For example, time frames might be defined to reflect short-term, medium-term and long-term follow-up.

- Select a single time-point and analyse only data at this time for studies in which it is presented. Ideally this should be a clinically important time-point. Sometimes it might be chosen to maximize the data available, although authors should be aware of the possibility of reporting biases.

- Select the longest follow-up from each study. This may induce a lack of consistency across studies, giving rise to heterogeneity.

### 9.3.5  Events that may re-occur

If the outcome of interest is an event that can occur more than once, then care must be taken to avoid a unit-of-analysis error. Count data should not be treated as if they are dichotomous data. See Section 9.2.5.

### 9.3.6  Multiple treatment attempts

Similarly, multiple treatment attempts per participant can cause a unit-of-analysis error. Care must be taken to ensure that the number of participants randomized, and not the number of treatment attempts, is used to calculate confidence intervals. For example, in subfertility studies, women may undergo multiple cycles, and authors might erroneously use cycles as the denominator rather than women. This is similar to the situation in cluster-randomized trials, except that each participant is the 'cluster'. See methods described in Chapter 16 (Section 16.3).

### 9.3.7   Multiple body parts I: body parts receive the same intervention

In some studies, people are randomized, but multiple parts (or sites) of the body receive the same intervention, a separate outcome judgement being made for each body part, and the number of body parts is used as the denominator in the analysis. For example, eyes may be mistakenly used as the denominator without adjustment for the non-independence between eyes. This is similar to the situation in cluster-randomized trials, except that participants are the 'clusters'. See methods described in Chapter 16 (Section 16.3).

### 9.3.8   Multiple body parts II: body parts receive different interventions

A different situation is that in which different parts of the body are randomized to *different* interventions. 'Split-mouth' designs in oral health are of this sort, in which different areas of the mouth are assigned different interventions. These trials have similarities to cross-over trials: whereas in cross-over trials individuals receive multiple treatments at different times, in these trials they receive multiple treatments at different sites. See methods described in Chapter 16 (Section 16.4). It is important to distinguish these studies from those in which participants receive the same intervention at multiple sites (Section 9.3.7).

### 9.3.9   Multiple intervention groups

Studies that compare more than two intervention groups need to be treated with care. Such studies are often included in meta-analysis by making multiple pair-wise comparisons between all possible pairs of intervention groups. A serious unit-of-analysis problem arises if the same group of participants is included twice in the same meta-analysis (for example, if 'Dose 1 vs Placebo' and 'Dose 2 vs Placebo' are both included in the same meta-analysis, with the same placebo patients in both comparisons). See Chapter 16 (Section 16.5).

# 9.4    Summarizing effects across studies

## 9.4.1    Meta-analysis

An important step in a systematic review is the thoughtful consideration of whether it is appropriate to combine the numerical results of all, or perhaps some, of the studies. Such a **meta-analysis** yields an overall statistic (together with its confidence interval) that summarizes the effectiveness of the experimental intervention compared with a control intervention (see Section 9.1.2). This section describes the principles and methods used to carry out a meta-analysis for the main types of data encountered.

Formulae for all the methods described are provided in a supplementary document *Statistical Algorithms in Review Manager 5* (available on the *Handbook* web site), and a longer discussion of the issues discussed in this section appear in Deeks et al. (Deeks 2001).

## 9.4.2    Principles of meta-analysis

All commonly-used methods for meta-analysis follow the following basic principles:

1. Meta-analysis is typically a two-stage process. In the first stage, a summary statistic is calculated for each study, to describe the observed intervention effect. For example, the summary statistic may be a risk ratio if the data are dichotomous or a difference between means if the data are continuous.

2. In the second stage, a summary (pooled) intervention effect estimate is calculated as a weighted average of the intervention effects estimated in the individual studies. A weighted average is defined as

$$\text{weighted average} = \frac{\text{sum of (estimate} \times \text{weight)}}{\text{sum of weights}} = \frac{\sum Y_i W_i}{\sum W_i}$$

   where $Y_i$ is the intervention effect estimated in the $i$th study, $W_i$ is the weight given to the $i$th study, and the summation is across all studies. Note that if all the weights are the same then the weighted average is equal to the mean intervention effect. The bigger the weight given to the $i$th study, the more it will contribute to the weighted average. The weights are therefore chosen to reflect the amount of information that each study contains. For ratio measures (OR, RR, etc), $Y_i$ is the natural logarithm of the measure.

3. The combination of intervention effect estimates across studies may optionally incorporate an assumption that the studies are not all estimating the same intervention effect, but estimate intervention effects that follow a distribution across studies. This is the basis of a **random-effects meta-analysis** (see Section 9.5.4). Alternatively, if

it is assumed that each study is estimating exactly the same quantity a **fixed-effect meta-analysis** is performed.

4. The standard error of the summary (pooled) intervention effect can be used to derive a confidence interval, which communicates the precision (or uncertainty) of the summary estimate, and to derive a P value, which communicates the strength of the evidence against the null hypothesis of no intervention effect.

5. As well as yielding a summary quantification of the pooled effect, all methods of meta-analysis can incorporate an assessment of whether the variation among the results of the separate studies is compatible with random variation, or whether it is large enough to indicate inconsistency of intervention effects across studies (see Section 9.5).

## 9.4.3    A generic inverse-variance approach to meta-analysis

A very common and simple version of the meta-analysis procedure is commonly referred to as the **inverse-variance method**. This approach is implemented in its most basic form in RevMan, and is used behind the scenes in certain meta-analyses of both dichotomous and continuous data.

The inverse variance method is so named because the weight given to each study is chosen to be the inverse of the variance of the effect estimate (i.e. one over the square of its standard error). Thus larger studies, which have smaller standard errors, are given more weight than smaller studies, which have larger standard errors. This choice of weight minimizes the imprecision (uncertainty) of the pooled effect estimate.

A fixed-effect meta-analysis using the inverse-variance method calculates a weighted average as

$$\text{generic inverse-variance weighted average} = \frac{\sum Y_i \left(1/\text{SE}_i^2\right)}{\sum \left(1/\text{SE}_i^2\right)},$$

where $Y_i$ is the intervention effect estimated in the $i$th study, $\text{SE}_i$ is the standard error of that estimate, and the summation is across all studies. The basic data required for the analysis are therefore an estimate of the intervention effect and its standard error from each study.

### 9.4.3.1    Random-effects (DerSimonian and Laird) method for meta-analysis

A variation on the inverse-variance method is to incorporate an assumption that the different studies are estimating different, yet related, intervention effects. This produces a random-effects meta-analysis, and the simplest version is known as the DerSimonian and Laird method (DerSimonian 1986). Random-effects meta-analysis is discussed in

Section 9.5.4. To undertake a random-effects meta-analysis, the standard errors of the study-specific estimates ($SE_i$ above) are adjusted to incorporate a measure of the extent of variation, or heterogeneity, among the intervention effects observed in different studies (this variation is often referred to as tau-squared ($\tau^2$, or $Tau^2$)). The amount of variation, and hence the adjustment, can be estimated from the intervention effects and standard errors of the studies included in the meta-analysis.

### 9.4.3.2 *The generic inverse variance outcome type in RevMan*

Estimates and their standard errors may be entered directly into RevMan under the 'Generic inverse variance' outcome. The software will undertake fixed-effect meta-analyses and random-effects (DerSimonian and Laird) meta-analyses, along with assessments of heterogeneity. For ratio measures of intervention effect, the data should be entered as natural logarithms (for example as a log odds ratio and the standard error of the log odds ratio). However, it is straightforward to instruct the software to display results on the original (e.g. odds ratio) scale. Rather than displaying summary data separately for the treatment groups, the forest plot will display the estimates and standard errors as they were entered beside the study identifiers. It is possible to supplement or replace this with a column providing the sample sizes in the two groups.

Note that the ability to enter estimates and standard errors directly into RevMan creates a high degree of flexibility in meta-analysis. For example, it facilitates the analysis of properly analysed cross-over trials, cluster-randomized trials and non-randomized studies, as well as outcome data that are ordinal, time-to-event or rates. However, in most situations for analyses of continuous and dichotomous outcome data it is preferable to enter more detailed data into RevMan (i.e. specifically as simple summaries of dichotomous or continuous data for each group). This avoids the need for the author to calculate effect estimates, and allows the use of methods targeted specifically at different types of data (see Sections 9.4.4 and 9.4.5). Also, it is helpful for the readers of the review to see the summary statistics for each intervention group in each study.

## 9.4.4 Meta-analysis of dichotomous outcomes

There are four widely used methods of meta-analysis for dichotomous outcomes, three fixed-effect methods (Mantel-Haenszel, Peto and inverse variance) and one random-effects method (DerSimonian and Laird). All of these methods are available as analysis options in RevMan. The Peto method can only pool odds ratios whilst the other three methods can pool odds ratios, risk ratios and risk differences. Formulae for all of the meta-analysis methods are given by Deeks et al. (Deeks 2001).

Note that zero cells (e.g. no events in one group) cause problems with computation of estimates and standard errors with some methods. The RevMan software automatically adds 0.5 to each cell of the $2 \times 2$ table for any such study.

### 9.4.4.1    Mantel-Haenszel methods

The Mantel-Haenszel methods (Mantel 1959, Greenland 1985) are the default fixed-effect methods of meta-analysis programmed in RevMan. When data are sparse, either in terms of event rates being low or study size being small, the estimates of the standard errors of the effect estimates that are used in the inverse variance methods may be poor. Mantel-Haenszel methods use a different weighting scheme that depends upon which effect measure (e.g. risk ratio, odds ratio, risk difference) is being used. They have been shown to have better statistical properties when there are few events. As this is a common situation in Cochrane reviews, the Mantel-Haenszel method is generally preferable to the inverse variance method. In other situations the two methods give similar estimates.

### 9.4.4.2    Peto odds ratio method

Peto's method (Yusuf 1985) can only be used to pool odds ratios. It uses an inverse variance approach but utilizes an approximate method of estimating the log odds ratio, and uses different weights. An alternative way of viewing the Peto method is as a sum of 'O − E' statistics. Here, O is the observed number of events and E is an expected number of events in the experimental intervention group of each study.

The approximation used in the computation of the log odds ratio works well when intervention effects are small (odds ratios are close to 1), events are not particularly common and the studies have similar numbers in experimental and control groups. In other situations it has been shown to give biased answers. As these criteria are not always fulfilled, Peto's method is not recommended as a default approach for meta-analysis.

Corrections for zero cell counts are not necessary when using Peto's method. Perhaps for this reason, this method performs well when events are very rare (Bradburn 2007) (see Chapter 16, Section 16.9). Also, Peto's method can be used to combine studies with dichotomous outcome data with studies using time-to-event analyses where log-rank tests have been used (see Section 9.4.9).

### 9.4.4.3    Random-effects method

The random-effects method (DerSimonian 1986) incorporates an assumption that the different studies are estimating different, yet related, intervention effects. As described in Section 9.4.3.1, the method is based on the inverse-variance approach, making an adjustment to the study weights according to the extent of variation, or heterogeneity, among the varying intervention effects. The random-effects method and the fixed-effect method will give identical results when there is no heterogeneity among the studies. Where there is heterogeneity, confidence intervals for the average intervention effect will be wider if the random-effects method is used rather than a fixed-effect method, and corresponding claims of statistical significance will be more conservative. It is also possible that the central estimate of the intervention effect will change if there are relationships between observed intervention effects and sample sizes. See Section 9.5.4 for further discussion of these issues.

RevMan implements two random-effects methods for dichotomous data: a Mantel-Haenszel method and an inverse-variance method. The difference between the two is subtle: the former estimates the amount of between-study variation by comparing each study's result with a Mantel-Haenszel fixed-effect meta-analysis result, whereas the latter estimates the amount of variation across studies by comparing each study's result with an inverse-variance fixed-effect meta-analysis result. In practice, the difference is likely to be trivial. The inverse-variance method was added in RevMan version 5.

### 9.4.4.4 *Which measure for dichotomous outcomes?*

Summary statistics for dichotomous data are described in Section 9.2.2. The effect of intervention can be expressed as either a relative or an absolute effect. The risk ratio (relative risk) and odds ratio are relative measures, while the risk difference and number needed to treat are absolute measures. A further complication is that there are in fact two risk ratios. We can calculate the risk ratio of an event occurring or the risk ratio of no event occurring. These give different pooled results in a meta-analysis, sometimes dramatically so.

The selection of a summary statistic for use in meta-analysis depends on balancing three criteria (Deeks 2002). First, we desire a summary statistic that gives values that are similar for all the studies in the meta-analysis and subdivisions of the population to which the interventions will be applied. The more consistent the summary statistic the greater is the justification for expressing the intervention effect as a single summary number. Second, the summary statistic must have the mathematical properties required for performing a valid meta-analysis. Third, the summary statistic should be easily understood and applied by those using the review. It should present a summary of the effect of the intervention in a way that helps readers to interpret and apply the results appropriately. Among effect measures for dichotomous data, no single measure is uniformly best, so the choice inevitably involves a compromise.

*Consistency*: Empirical evidence suggests that relative effect measures are, on average, more consistent than absolute measures (Engels 2000, Deeks 2002). For this reason it is wise to avoid performing meta-analyses of risk differences, unless there is a clear reason to suspect that risk differences will be consistent in a particular clinical situation. On average there is little difference between the odds ratio and risk ratio in terms of consistency (Deeks 2002). When the study aims to reduce the incidence of an adverse outcome (see Section 9.2.2.5) there is empirical evidence that risk ratios of the adverse outcome are more consistent than risk ratios of the non-event (Deeks 2002). Selecting an effect measure on the basis of what is the most consistent in a *particular* situation is not a generally recommended strategy, since it may lead to a selection that spuriously maximizes the precision of a meta-analysis estimate.

*Mathematical properties*: The most important mathematical criterion is the availability of a reliable variance estimate. The number needed to treat does not have a simple variance estimator and cannot easily be used directly in meta-analysis, although it can be computed from the other summary statistics (see Chapter 12, Section 12.5). There is no consensus as to the importance of two other often cited mathematical properties: the fact that the behaviour of the odds ratio and the risk difference do not rely on which of the two outcome states is coded as the event, and the odds ratio being the only statistic which is unbounded (see Section 9.2.2).

*Ease of interpretation*: The odds ratio is the hardest summary statistic to understand and to apply in practice, and many practising clinicians report difficulties in using them. There are many published examples where authors have misinterpreted odds ratios from meta-analyses as if they were risk ratios. There must be some concern that routine presentation of the results of systematic reviews as odds ratios will lead to frequent overestimation of the benefits and harms of treatments when the results are applied in clinical practice. Absolute measures of effect are also thought to be more easily interpreted by clinicians than relative effects (Sinclair 1994), and allow trade-offs to be made between likely benefits and likely harms of interventions. However, they are less likely to be generalizable.

It seems important to avoid using summary statistics for which there is empirical evidence that they are unlikely to give consistent estimates of intervention effects (the risk difference) and it is impossible to use statistics for which meta-analysis cannot be performed (the number needed to treat). Thus it is generally recommended that analysis proceeds using risk ratios (taking care to make a sensible choice over which category of outcome is classified as the event) or odds ratios. It may be wise to plan to undertake a sensitivity analysis to investigate whether choice of summary statistic (and selection of the event category) is critical to the conclusions of the meta-analysis (see Section 9.7).

It is often sensible to use one statistic for meta-analysis and re-express the results using a second, more easily interpretable statistic. For example, meta-analysis may often be best performed using relative effect measures (risk ratios or odds ratio) and the results re-expressed using absolute effect measures (risk differences or numbers needed to treat – see Chapter 12, Section 12.5). This is one of the key motivations for 'Summary of findings' tables in Cochrane reviews: see Chapter 11 (Section 11.5). If odds ratios are used for meta-analysis they can also be re-expressed as risk ratios (see Chapter 12, Section 12.5.4). In all cases the same formulae can be used to convert upper and lower confidence limits. However, it is important to note that all of these transformations require specification of a value of baseline risk indicating the likely risk of the outcome in the 'control' population to which the experimental intervention will be applied. Where the chosen value for this assumed control risk is close to the typical observed control group risks across the studies, similar estimates of absolute effect will be obtained regardless of whether odds ratios or risk ratios are used for meta-analysis. Where the assumed control risk differs from the typical observed control group risk, the predictions of absolute benefit will differ according to which summary statistic was used for meta-analysis.

## 9.4.5 Meta-analysis of continuous outcomes

Two methods of analysis are available in RevMan for meta-analysis of continuous data: the inverse-variance fixed-effect method and the inverse-variance random-effects method. The methods will give exactly the same answers when there is no heterogeneity.

Where there is heterogeneity, confidence intervals for the average intervention effect will be wider if the random-effects method is used rather than a fixed-effect method, and corresponding P values will be less significant. It is also possible that the central estimate of the intervention effect will change if there are relationships between observed intervention effects and sample sizes. See Section 9.5.4 for further discussion of these issues.

Authors should be aware that an assumption underlying methods for meta-analysis of continuous data is that the outcomes have a normal distribution in each intervention arm in each study. This assumption may not always be met, although it is unimportant in very large studies. It is useful to consider the possibility of skewed data (see Section 9.4.5.3).

### 9.4.5.1    *Which measure for continuous outcomes?*

There are two summary statistics used for meta-analysis of continuous data: the mean difference (MD) and the standardized mean difference (SMD) (see Section 9.2.3). Selection of summary statistics for continuous data is principally determined by whether studies all report the outcome using the same scale (when the mean difference can be used) or using different scales (when the standardized mean difference has to be used).

The different roles played in the two approaches by the standard deviations of outcomes observed in the two groups should be understood.

- For the mean difference approach, the standard deviations are used together with the sample sizes to compute the weight given to each study. Studies with small standard deviations are given relatively higher weight whilst studies with larger standard deviations are given relatively smaller weights. This is appropriate if variation in standard deviations between studies reflects differences in the reliability of outcome measurements, but is probably not appropriate if the differences in standard deviation reflect real differences in the variability of outcomes in the study populations.

- For the standardized mean difference approach, the standard deviations are used to standardize the mean differences to a single scale (see Section 9.2.3.2), as well as in the computation of study weights. It is assumed that between-study variation in standard deviations reflects only differences in measurement scales and not differences in the reliability of outcome measures or variability among study populations.

These limitations of the methods should be borne in mind where unexpected variation of standard deviations across studies is observed.

### 9.4.5.2    *Meta-analysis of change scores*

In some circumstances an analysis based on changes from baseline will be more efficient and powerful than comparison of final values, as it removes a component of between-person variability from the analysis. However, calculation of a change score requires measurement of the outcome twice and in practice may be less efficient for outcomes which are unstable or difficult to measure precisely, where the measurement error may be larger than true between-person baseline variability. Change-from-baseline outcomes may also be preferred if they have a less skewed distribution than final measurement outcomes. Although sometimes used as a device to 'correct' for unlucky randomization, this practice is not recommended.

The preferred statistical approach to accounting for baseline measurements of the outcome variable is to include the baseline outcome measurements as a covariate in a regression model or analysis of covariance (ANCOVA). These analyses produce an 'adjusted' estimate of the treatment effect together with its standard error. These analyses are the least frequently encountered, but as they give the most precise and least biased estimates of treatment effects they should be included in the analysis when they are available. However, they can only be included in a meta-analysis using the generic inverse-variance method, since means and standard deviations are not available for each intervention group separately.

In practice an author is likely to discover that the studies included in a review may include a mixture of change-from-baseline and final value scores. However, mixing of outcomes is not a problem when it comes to meta-analysis of mean differences. There is no statistical reason why studies with change-from-baseline outcomes should not be combined in a meta-analysis with studies with final measurement outcomes when using the (unstandardized) mean difference method in RevMan. In a randomized trial, mean differences based on changes from baseline can usually be assumed to be addressing exactly the same underlying intervention effects as analyses based on final measurements. That is to say, the difference in mean final values will on average be the same as the difference in mean change scores. If the use of change scores does increase precision, the studies presenting change scores will appropriately be given higher weights in the analysis than they would have received if final values had been used, as they will have smaller standard deviations.

When combining the data authors must be careful to use the appropriate means and standard deviations (either of final measurements or of changes from baseline) for each study. Since the mean values and standard deviations for the two types of outcome may differ substantially it may be advisable to place them in separate subgroups to avoid confusion for the reader, but the results of the subgroups can legitimately be pooled together.

However, final value and change scores should not be combined together as standardized mean differences, since the difference in standard deviation reflects not differences in measurement scale, but differences in the reliability of the measurements.

A common practical problem associated with including change-from-baseline measures is that the standard deviation of changes is not reported. Imputations of standard deviations is discussed in Chapter 16 (Section 16.1.3).

### 9.4.5.3   Meta-analysis of skewed data

Analyses based on means are appropriate for data that are at least approximately normally distributed, and for data from very large trials. If the true distribution of outcomes is asymmetrical then the data are said to be skewed. Skew can sometimes be diagnosed from the means and standard deviations of the outcomes. A rough check is available, but it is only valid if a lowest or highest possible value for an outcome is known to exist. Thus the check may be used for outcomes such as weight, volume and blood concentrations, which have lowest possible values of 0, or for scale outcomes with minimum or maximum scores, but it may not be appropriate for change from baseline measures. The check involves calculating the observed mean minus the lowest possible value (or the highest possible value minus the observed mean), and dividing this by the standard deviation. A ratio less than 2 suggests skew (Altman 1996). If the ratio is less than 1 there is strong evidence of a skewed distribution.

Transformation of the original outcome data may substantially reduce skew. Reports of trials may present results on a transformed scale, usually a log scale. Collection of appropriate data summaries from the trialists, or acquisition of individual patient data, is currently the approach of choice. Appropriate data summaries and analysis strategies for the individual patient data will depend on the situation. Consultation with a knowledgeable statistician is advised.

Where data have been analysed on a log scale, results are commonly presented as geometric means and ratios of geometric means. A meta-analysis may be then performed on the scale of the log-transformed data; an example of the calculation of the required means and standard deviation is given in Chapter 7 (Section 7.7.3.4). This approach depends on being able to obtain transformed data for all studies; methods for transforming from one scale to the other are available (Higgins 2008a). Log-transformed and untransformed data can not be mixed in a meta-analysis.

## 9.4.6  Combining dichotomous and continuous outcomes

Occasionally authors encounter a situation where data for the same outcome are presented in some studies as dichotomous data and in other studies as continuous data. For example, scores on depression scales can be reported as means or as the percentage of patients who were depressed at some point after an intervention (i.e. with a score above a specified cut-point). This type of information is often easier to understand and more helpful when it is dichotomized. However, deciding on a cut-point may be arbitrary and information is lost when continuous data are transformed to dichotomous data.

There are several options for handling combinations of dichotomous and continuous data. Generally, it is useful to summarize results from all the relevant, valid studies in a similar way, but this is not always possible. It may be possible to collect missing data from investigators so that this can be done. If not, it may be useful to summarize the data in three ways: by entering the means and standard deviations as continuous outcomes, by entering the counts as dichotomous outcomes and by entering all of the data in text form as 'Other data' outcomes.

There are statistical approaches available which will re-express odds ratios as standardized mean differences (and *vice versa*), allowing dichotomous and continuous data to be pooled together. Based on an assumption that the underlying continuous measurements in each intervention group follow a logistic distribution (which is a symmetrical distribution similar in shape to the normal distribution but with more data in the distributional tails), and that the variability of the outcomes is the same in both treated and control participants, the odds ratios can be re-expressed as a standardized mean difference according to the following simple formula (Chinn 2000):

$$SMD = \frac{\sqrt{3}}{\pi} \ln OR.$$

The standard error of the log odds ratio can be converted to the standard error of a standardized mean difference by multiplying by the same constant ($\sqrt{3}/\pi = 0.5513$). Alternatively standardized mean differences can be re-expressed as log odds ratios by multiplying by $\pi/\sqrt{3} = 1.814$. Once standardized mean differences (or log odds ratios) and their standard errors have been computed for all studies in the meta-analysis, they can be combined using the generic inverse-variance method in RevMan. Standard errors can be computed for all studies by entering the data in RevMan as dichotomous and continuous outcome type data, as appropriate, and converting the confidence intervals for the resulting log odds ratios and standardized mean differences into standard errors (see Chapter 7, Section 7.7.7.2).

## 9.4.7   Meta-analysis of ordinal outcomes and measurement scales

Ordinal and measurement scale outcomes are most commonly meta-analysed as dichotomous data (if so see Section 9.4.4) or continuous data (if so see Section 9.4.5) depending on the way that the study authors performed the original analyses.

Occasionally it is possible to analyse the data using proportional odds models where ordinal scales have a small number of categories, the numbers falling into each category for each intervention group can be obtained, and the same ordinal scale has been used in all studies. This approach may make more efficient use of all available data than dichotomization, but requires access to statistical software and results in a summary statistic for which it is challenging to find a clinical meaning.

The proportional odds model uses the proportional odds ratio as the measure of intervention effect (Agresti 1996). Suppose that there are three categories, which are ordered in terms of desirability such that 1 is the best and 3 the worst. The data could be dichotomized in two ways. That is, category 1 constitutes a success and categories 2–3 a failure, or categories 1–2 constitute a success and category 3 a failure. A proportional odds model would assume that there is an equal odds ratio for both dichotomies of the data. Therefore, the odds ratio calculated from the proportional odds model can be interpreted as the odds of success on the experimental intervention relative to control, irrespective of how the ordered categories might be divided into success or failure. Methods (specifically polychotomous logistic regression models) are available for calculating study estimates of the log odds ratio and its standard error and for conducting a meta-analysis in advanced statistical software packages (Whitehead 1994).

Estimates of log odds ratios and their standard errors from a proportional odds model may be meta-analysed using the generic inverse-variance method in RevMan (see Section 9.4.3.2). Both fixed-effect and random-effects methods of analysis are available. If the same ordinal scale has been used in all studies, but has in some reports been presented as a dichotomous outcome, it may still be possible to include all studies in the meta-analysis. In the context of the three-category model, this might mean that for some studies category 1 constitutes a success, while for others both categories 1 and 2 constitute a success. Methods are available for dealing with this, and for combining data from scales that are related but have different definitions for their categories (Whitehead 1994).

## 9.4.8   Meta-analysis of counts and rates

Results may be expressed as **count data** when each participant may experience an event, and may experience it more than once (see Section 9.2.5). For example, 'number of strokes', or 'number of hospital visits' are counts. These events may not happen at all, but if they do happen there is no theoretical maximum number of occurrences for an individual.

As described in Chapter 7 (Section 7.7.5), count data may be analysed using methods for dichotomous (see Section 9.4.4), continuous (see Section 9.4.5) and time-to-event data (see Section 9.4.9) as well as being analysed as rate data.

Rate data occur if counts are measured for each participant along with the time over which they are observed. This is particularly appropriate when the events being counted are rare. For example, a woman may experience two strokes during a follow-up period of two years. Her rate of strokes is one per year of follow-up (or, equivalently 0.083 per month of follow-up). Rates are conventionally summarized at the group level. For example, participants in the control group of a clinical trial may experience 85 strokes during a total of 2836 person-years of follow-up. An underlying assumption associated with the use of rates is that the risk of an event is constant across participants and over time. This assumption should be carefully considered for each situation. For example, in contraception studies, rates have been used (known as Pearl indices) to describe the number of pregnancies per 100 women-years of follow-up. This is now considered inappropriate since couples have different risks of conception, and the risk for each woman changes over time. Pregnancies are now analysed more often using life tables or time-to-event methods that investigate the time elapsing before the first pregnancy.

Analysing count data as rates is not always the most appropriate approach and is uncommon in practice. This is because:

1. the assumption of a constant underlying risk may not be suitable; and

2. statistical methods are not as well developed as they are for other types of data.

The results of a study may be expressed as a **rate ratio**, that is the ratio of the rate in the experimental intervention group to the rate in the control group. Suppose $E_E$ events occurred during $T_E$ participant-years of follow-up in the experimental intervention group, and $E_C$ events during $T_C$ participant-years in the control intervention group. The rate ratio is

$$\text{rate ratio} = \frac{E_E/T_E}{E_C/T_C} = \frac{E_E T_C}{E_C T_E}.$$

The (natural) logarithms of the rate ratios may be combined across studies using the generic inverse-variance method (see Section 9.4.3.2). An approximate standard error of the log rate ratio is given by

$$\text{SE of ln rate ratio} = \sqrt{\frac{1}{E_E} + \frac{1}{E_C}}.$$

A correction of 0.5 may be added to each count in the case of zero events. Note that the choice of time unit (i.e. patient-months, women-years, etc) is irrelevant since it is cancelled out of the rate ratio and does not figure in the standard error. However the units should still be displayed when presenting the study results. An alternative means of estimating the rate ratio is through the approach of Whitehead and Whitehead (Whitehead 1991).

In a randomized trial, rate ratios may often be very similar to relative risks obtained after dichotomizing the participants, since the average period of follow-up should be similar in all intervention groups. Rate ratios and relative risks will differ, however, if an intervention affects the likelihood of some participants experiencing multiple events.

It is possible also to focus attention on the rate difference,

$$\text{rate difference} = \frac{E_E}{T_E} - \frac{E_C}{T_C}.$$

An approximate standard error for the rate difference is

$$\text{SE of rate difference} = \sqrt{\frac{E_E}{T_E^2} + \frac{E_C}{T_C^2}}.$$

The analysis again requires use of the generic inverse-variance method in RevMan. One of the only discussions of meta-analysis of rates, which is still rather short, is that by Hasselblad and McCrory (Hasselblad 1995).

## 9.4.9   Meta-analysis of time-to-event outcomes

Two approaches to meta-analysis of time-to-event outcomes are available in RevMan. Which is used will depend on what data have been extracted from the primary studies, or obtained from re-analysis of individual patient data.

If 'O − E' and 'V' statistics have been obtained, either through re-analysis of individual patient data or from aggregate statistics presented in the study reports, then these statistics may be entered directly into RevMan using the 'O − E and Variance' outcome type. There are several ways to calculate 'O − E' and 'V' statistics. Peto's method applied to dichotomous data (Section 9.4.4.2) gives rise to an odds ratio; a log-rank approach gives rise to a hazard ratio, and a variation of the Peto method for analysing time-to-event data gives rise to something in between. The appropriate effect measure should be specified in RevMan. Only fixed-effect meta-analysis methods are available in RevMan for 'O − E and Variance' outcomes.

Alternatively if estimates of log hazard ratios and standard errors have been obtained from results of Cox proportional hazards regression models, study results can be combined using the generic inverse-variance method (see Section 9.4.3.2). Both fixed-effect and random-effects analyses are available.

If a mixture of log-rank and Cox model estimates are obtained from the studies, all results can be combined using the generic inverse-variance method, as the log-rank estimates can be converted into log hazard ratios and standard errors using the formulae given in Chapter 7 (Section 7.7.6).

## 9.4.10   A summary of meta-analysis methods available in RevMan

Table 9.4.a lists the options for statistical analysis that are available in RevMan. RevMan requires the author to select one preferred method for each outcome. If these are not specified then the software defaults to the fixed-effect Mantel-Haenszel odds ratio for dichotomous outcomes, the fixed-effect mean difference for continuous outcomes and the fixed-effect model for generic inverse-variance outcomes. It is important that authors

**Table 9.4.a**   Summary of meta-analysis methods available in RevMan

| Type of data | Effect measure | Fixed-effect methods | Random-effects methods |
|---|---|---|---|
| Dichotomous | Odds ratio (OR) | Mantel-Haenszel (M-H) Inverse variance (IV) Peto | Mantel-Haenszel (M-H) Inverse variance (IV) |
| | Risk ratio (RR) | Mantel-Haenszel (M-H) Inverse variance (IV) | Mantel-Haenszel (M-H) Inverse variance (IV) |
| | Risk difference (RD) | Mantel-Haenszel (M-H) Inverse variance (IV) | Mantel-Haenszel (M-H) Inverse variance (IV) |
| Continuous | Mean difference (MD) | Inverse variance (IV) | Inverse variance (IV) |
| | Standardized mean difference (SMD) | Inverse variance (IV) | Inverse variance (IV) |
| O − E and Variance | *User-specified* (default 'Peto odds ratio') | Peto | *None* |
| Generic inverse variance | *User-specified* | Inverse variance (IV) | Inverse variance (IV) |
| Other data | *User-specified* | *None* | *None* |

make it clear which method they are using when results are presented in the text of a review, since it cannot be guaranteed that a meta-analysis displayed to the user will coincide with the selected preferred method.

### 9.4.11    Use of vote counting for meta-analysis

Occasionally meta-analyses use 'vote counting' to compare the number of positive studies with the number of negative studies. Vote counting is limited to answering the simple question "is there any evidence of an effect?" Two problems can occur with vote-counting, which suggest that it should be avoided whenever possible. Firstly, problems occur if subjective decisions or statistical significance are used to define 'positive' and 'negative' studies (Cooper 1980, Antman 1992). To undertake vote counting properly the number of studies showing harm should be compared with the number showing benefit, regardless of the statistical significance or size of their results. A sign test can be used to assess the significance of evidence for the existence of an effect in either direction (if there is no effect the studies will be distributed evenly around the null hypothesis of no difference). Secondly, vote counting takes no account of the differential weights given to each study. Vote counting might be considered as a last resort in situations when standard meta-analytical methods cannot be applied (such as when there is no consistent outcome measure).

## 9.5    Heterogeneity

### 9.5.1    What is heterogeneity?

Inevitably, studies brought together in a systematic review will differ. Any kind of variability among studies in a systematic review may be termed heterogeneity. It can be helpful to distinguish between different types of heterogeneity. Variability in the participants, interventions and outcomes studied may be described as **clinical diversity** (sometimes called clinical heterogeneity), and variability in study design and risk of bias may be described as **methodological diversity** (sometimes called methodological heterogeneity). Variability in the intervention effects being evaluated in the different studies is known as **statistical heterogeneity**, and is a consequence of clinical or methodological diversity, or both, among the studies. Statistical heterogeneity manifests itself in the observed intervention effects being more different from each other than one would expect due to random error (chance) alone. We will follow convention and refer to **statistical heterogeneity** simply as **heterogeneity**.

Clinical variation will lead to heterogeneity if the intervention effect is affected by the factors that vary across studies; most obviously, the specific interventions or patient characteristics. In other words, the true intervention effect will be different in different studies.

Differences between studies in terms of methodological factors, such as use of blinding and concealment of allocation, or if there are differences between studies in the way the outcomes are defined and measured, may be expected to lead to differences in the observed intervention effects. Significant statistical heterogeneity arising from methodological diversity or differences in outcome assessments suggests that the studies are not all estimating the same quantity, but does not necessarily suggest that the true intervention effect varies. In particular, heterogeneity associated solely with methodological diversity would indicate the studies suffer from different degrees of bias. Empirical evidence suggests that some aspects of design can affect the result of clinical trials, although this is not always the case. Further discussion appears in Chapter 8.

The scope of a review will largely determine the extent to which studies included in a review are diverse. Sometimes a review will include studies addressing a variety of questions, for example when several different interventions for the same condition are of interest (see also Chapter 5, Section 5.6). Studies of each intervention should be analysed and presented separately. Meta-analysis should only be considered when a group of studies is sufficiently homogeneous in terms of participants, interventions and outcomes to provide a meaningful summary. It is often appropriate to take a broader perspective in a meta-analysis than in a single clinical trial. A common analogy is that systematic reviews bring together apples and oranges, and that combining these can yield a meaningless result. This is true if apples and oranges are of intrinsic interest on their own, but may not be if they are used to contribute to a wider question about fruit. For example, a meta-analysis may reasonably evaluate the average effect of a class of drugs by combining results from trials where each evaluates the effect of a different drug from the class.

There may be specific interest in a review in investigating how clinical and methodological aspects of studies relate to their results. Where possible these investigations should be specified *a priori*, i.e. in the systematic review protocol. It is legitimate for a systematic review to focus on examining the relationship between some clinical characteristic(s) of the studies and the size of intervention effect, rather than on obtaining a summary effect estimate across a series of studies (see Section 9.6). Meta-regression may best be used for this purpose, although it is not implemented in RevMan (see Section 9.6.4).

## 9.5.2 Identifying and measuring heterogeneity

It is important to consider to what extent the results of studies are consistent. If confidence intervals for the results of individual studies (generally depicted graphically using horizontal lines) have poor overlap, this generally indicates the presence of statistical heterogeneity. More formally, a statistical test for heterogeneity is available. This chi-squared ($\chi^2$, or Chi$^2$) test is included in the forest plots in Cochrane reviews. It assesses whether observed differences in results are compatible with chance alone. A low P value (or a large chi-squared statistic relative to its degree of freedom) provides evidence of heterogeneity of intervention effects (variation in effect estimates beyond chance).

Care must be taken in the interpretation of the chi-squared test, since it has low power in the (common) situation of a meta-analysis when studies have small sample size or are few in number. This means that while a statistically significant result may indicate a problem with heterogeneity, a non-significant result must not be taken as evidence of no heterogeneity. This is also why a P value of 0.10, rather than the conventional level of 0.05, is sometimes used to determine statistical significance. A further problem with the test, which seldom occurs in Cochrane reviews, is that when there are many studies in a meta-analysis, the test has high power to detect a small amount of heterogeneity that may be clinically unimportant

Some argue that, since clinical and methodological diversity always occur in a meta-analysis, statistical heterogeneity is inevitable (Higgins 2003). Thus the test for heterogeneity is irrelevant to the choice of analysis; heterogeneity will always exist whether or not we happen to be able to detect it using a statistical test. Methods have been developed for quantifying inconsistency across studies that move the focus away from testing whether heterogeneity is present to assessing its impact on the meta-analysis. A useful statistic for quantifying inconsistency is

$$I^2 = \left(\frac{Q - df}{Q}\right) \times 100\%,$$

where Q is the chi-squared statistic and df is its degrees of freedom (Higgins 2002, Higgins 2003). This describes the percentage of the variability in effect estimates that is due to heterogeneity rather than sampling error (chance).

Thresholds for the interpretation of $I^2$ can be misleading, since the importance of inconsistency depends on several factors. A rough guide to interpretation is as follows:

- 0% to 40%: might not be important;

- 30% to 60%: may represent moderate heterogeneity*;

- 50% to 90%: may represent substantial heterogeneity*;

- 75% to 100%: considerable heterogeneity*.

*The importance of the observed value of $I^2$ depends on (i) magnitude and direction of effects and (ii) strength of evidence for heterogeneity (e.g. P value from the chi-squared test, or a confidence interval for $I^2$).

## 9.5.3    Strategies for addressing heterogeneity

A number of options are available if (statistical) heterogeneity is identified among a group of studies that would otherwise be considered suitable for a meta-analysis.

1. Check again that the data are correct
   Severe heterogeneity can indicate that data have been incorrectly extracted or entered into RevMan. For example, if standard errors have mistakenly been entered as standard deviations for continuous outcomes, this could manifest itself in overly

narrow confidence intervals with poor overlap and hence substantial heterogeneity. Unit-of-analysis errors may also be causes of heterogeneity (see Section 9.3).

2. Do not do a meta-analysis

   A systematic review need not contain any meta-analyses (O'Rourke 1989). If there is considerable variation in results, and particularly if there is inconsistency in the direction of effect, it may be misleading to quote an average value for the intervention effect.

3. Explore heterogeneity

   It is clearly of interest to determine the causes of heterogeneity among results of studies. This process is problematic since there are often many characteristics that vary across studies from which one may choose. Heterogeneity may be explored by conducting subgroup analyses (see Section 9.6.3) or meta-regression (see Section 9.6.4), though this latter method is not implemented in RevMan. Ideally, investigations of characteristics of studies that may be associated with heterogeneity should be pre-specified in the protocol of a review (see Section 9.1.7). Reliable conclusions can only be drawn from analyses that are truly pre-specified before inspecting the studies' results, and even these conclusions should be interpreted with caution. In practice, authors will often be familiar with some study results when writing the protocol, so true pre-specification is not possible. Explorations of heterogeneity that are devised after heterogeneity is identified can at best lead to the generation of hypotheses. They should be interpreted with even more caution and should generally not be listed among the conclusions of a review. Also, investigations of heterogeneity when there are very few studies are of questionable value.

4. Ignore heterogeneity

   Fixed-effect meta-analyses ignore heterogeneity. The pooled effect estimate from a fixed-effect meta-analysis is normally interpreted as being the best estimate of the intervention effect. However, the existence of heterogeneity suggests that there may not be a single intervention effect but a distribution of intervention effects. Thus the pooled fixed-effect estimate may be an intervention effect that does not actually exist in any population, and therefore have a confidence interval that is meaningless as well as being too narrow, (see Section 9.5.4). The P value obtained from a fixed-effect meta-analysis does however provide a meaningful test of the null hypothesis that there is no effect in every study.

5. Perform a random-effects meta-analysis

   A random-effects meta-analysis may be used to incorporate heterogeneity among studies. This is not a substitute for a thorough investigation of heterogeneity. It is intended primarily for heterogeneity that cannot be explained. An extended discussion of this option appears in Section 9.5.4.

6. Change the effect measure

   Heterogeneity may be an artificial consequence of an inappropriate choice of effect measure. For example, when studies collect continuous outcome data using different scales or different units, extreme heterogeneity may be apparent when using the mean difference but not when the more appropriate standardized mean difference is used. Furthermore, choice of effect measure for dichotomous outcomes (odds ratio, relative risk, or risk difference) may affect the degree of heterogeneity among results. In particular, when control group risks vary, homogeneous odds ratios or risk ratios will necessarily lead to heterogeneous risk differences, and *vice versa*. However, it remains unclear whether homogeneity of intervention effect in a particular meta-analysis is a suitable criterion for choosing between these measures (see also Section 9.4.4.4).

7. Exclude studies
   Heterogeneity may be due to the presence of one or two outlying studies with results that conflict with the rest of the studies. In general it is unwise to exclude studies from a meta-analysis on the basis of their results as this may introduce bias. However, if an obvious reason for the outlying result is apparent, the study might be removed with more confidence. Since usually at least one characteristic can be found for any study in any meta-analysis which makes it different from the others, this criterion is unreliable because it is all too easy to fulfil. It is advisable to perform analyses both with and without outlying studies as part of a sensitivity analysis (see Section 9.7). Whenever possible, potential sources of clinical diversity that might lead to such situations should be specified in the protocol.

## 9.5.4  Incorporating heterogeneity into random-effects models

A fixed-effect meta-analysis provides a result that may be viewed as a 'typical intervention effect' from the studies included in the analysis. In order to calculate a confidence interval for a fixed-effect meta-analysis the assumption is made that the true effect of intervention (in both magnitude and direction) is the same value in every study (that is, fixed across studies). This assumption implies that the observed differences among study results are due solely to the play of chance, i.e. that there is no statistical heterogeneity.

When there is heterogeneity that cannot readily be explained, one analytical approach is to incorporate it into a random-effects model. A random-effects meta-analysis model involves an assumption that the effects being estimated in the different studies are not identical, but follow some distribution. The model represents our lack of knowledge about why real, or apparent, intervention effects differ by considering the differences as if they were random. The centre of this distribution describes the average of the effects, while its width describes the degree of heterogeneity. The conventional choice of distribution is a normal distribution. It is difficult to establish the validity of any distributional assumption, and this is a common criticism of random-effects meta-analyses. The importance of the particular assumed shape for this distribution is not known.

Note that a random-effects model does not 'take account' of the heterogeneity, in the sense that it is no longer an issue. It is always advisable to explore possible causes of heterogeneity, although there may be too few studies to do this adequately (see Section 9.6).

For random-effects analyses in RevMan, the pooled estimate and confidence interval refer to the centre of the distribution of intervention effects, but do not describe the width of the distribution. Often the pooled estimate and its confidence interval are quoted in isolation as an alternative estimate of the quantity evaluated in a fixed-effect meta-analysis, which is inappropriate. The confidence interval from a random-effects meta-analysis describes uncertainty in the location of the mean of systematically different effects in the different studies. It does not describe the degree of heterogeneity among studies as may be commonly believed. For example, when there are many studies in a meta-analysis, one may obtain a tight confidence interval around the random-effects estimate of the mean effect even when there is a large amount of heterogeneity.

In common with other meta-analysis software, RevMan presents an estimate of the between-study variance in a random-effects meta-analysis (known as tau-squared ($\tau^2$ or Tau$^2$)). The square root of this number (i.e. tau) is the estimated standard deviation of underlying effects across studies. For absolute measures of effect (e.g. risk difference, mean difference, standardized mean difference), an approximate 95% range of underlying effects can be obtained by creating an interval from $2 \times$ tau below the random-effects pooled estimate, to $2 \times$ tau above it. For relative measures (e.g. odds ratio, risk ratio), the interval needs to be centred on the natural logarithm of the pooled estimate, and the limits anti-logged (exponentiated) to obtain an interval on the ratio scale. Alternative intervals, for the predicted effect in a new study, have been proposed (Higgins 2008b). The range of the intervention effects observed in the studies may be thought to give a rough idea of the spread of the distribution of true intervention effects, but in fact it will be slightly too wide as it also describes the random error in the observed effect estimates.

If variation in effects (statistical heterogeneity) is believed to be due to clinical diversity, the random-effects pooled estimate should be interpreted differently from the fixed-effect estimate since it relates to a different question. The random-effects estimate and its confidence interval address the question 'what is the average intervention effect?' while the fixed-effect estimate and its confidence interval addresses the question 'what is the best estimate of the intervention effect?' The answers to these questions coincide either when no heterogeneity is present, or when the distribution of the intervention effects is roughly symmetrical. When the answers do not coincide, the random-effects estimate may not reflect the actual effect in any particular population being studied.

Methodological diversity creates heterogeneity through biases variably affecting the results of different studies. The random-effects pooled estimate will only estimate the average treatment effect if the biases are symmetrically distributed, leading to a mixture of over- and under-estimates of effect, which is unlikely to be the case. In practice it can be very difficult to distinguish whether heterogeneity results from clinical or methodological diversity, and in most cases it is likely to be due to both, so these distinctions in the interpretation are hard to draw.

For any particular set of studies in which heterogeneity is present, a confidence interval around the random-effects pooled estimate is wider than a confidence interval around a fixed-effect pooled estimate. This will happen if the $I^2$ statistic is greater than zero, even if the heterogeneity is not detected by the chi-squared test for heterogeneity (Higgins 2003) (see Section 9.5.2). The choice between a fixed-effect and a random-effects meta-analysis should never be made on the basis of a statistical test for heterogeneity.

In a heterogeneous set of studies, a random-effects meta-analysis will award relatively more weight to smaller studies than such studies would receive in a fixed-effect meta-analysis. This is because small studies are more informative for learning about the distribution of effects across studies than for learning about an assumed common intervention effect. Care must be taken that random-effects analyses are applied only when the idea of a 'random' distribution of intervention effects can be justified. In particular, if results of smaller studies are systematically different from results of larger ones, which can happen as a result of publication bias or within-study bias in smaller studies (Egger 1997, Poole 1999, Kjaergard 2001), then a random-effects meta-analysis will exacerbate the effects of the bias (see also Chapter 10, Section 10.4.4.1). A fixed-effect analysis will be affected less, although strictly it will also be inappropriate. In this situation it may be wise to present neither type of meta-analysis, or to perform a sensitivity analysis in which small studies are excluded.

Similarly, when there is little information, either because there are few studies or if the studies are small with few events, a random-effects analysis will provide poor estimates of the width of the distribution of intervention effects. The Mantel-Haenszel method will provide more robust estimates of the average intervention effect, but at the cost of ignoring the observed heterogeneity.

RevMan implements a version of random-effects meta-analysis that is described by DerSimonian and Laird (DerSimonian 1986). The attraction of this method is that the calculations are straightforward, but it has a theoretical disadvantage that the confidence intervals are slightly too narrow to encompass full uncertainty resulting from having estimated the degree of heterogeneity. Alternative methods exist that encompass full uncertainty, but they require more advanced statistical software (see also Chapter 16, Section 16.8). In practice, the difference in the results is likely to be small unless there are few studies. For dichotomous data, RevMan implements two versions of the DerSimonian and Laird random-effects model (see Section 9.4.4.3).

# 9.6   Investigating heterogeneity

## 9.6.1   Interaction and effect modification

Does the intervention effect vary with different populations or intervention characteristics (such as dose or duration)? Such variation is known as interaction by statisticians and as effect modification by epidemiologists. Methods to search for such interactions include subgroup analyses and meta-regression. All methods have considerable pitfalls.

## 9.6.2   What are subgroup analyses?

Subgroup analyses involve splitting all the participant data into subgroups, often so as to make comparisons between them. Subgroup analyses may be done for subsets of participants (such as males and females), or for subsets of studies (such as different geographical locations). Subgroup analyses may be done as a means of investigating heterogeneous results, or to answer specific questions about particular patient groups, types of intervention or types of study.

Subgroup analyses of subsets of participants within studies are uncommon in systematic reviews of the literature because sufficient details to extract data about separate participant types are seldom published in reports. By contrast, such subsets of participants are easily analysed when individual patient data have been collected (see Chapter 18). The methods we describe in Section 9.6.3 are for subgroups of trials.

Findings from multiple subgroup analyses may be misleading. Subgroup analyses are observational by nature and are not based on randomized comparisons. False negative and false positive significance tests increase in likelihood rapidly as more subgroup analyses are performed. If their findings are presented as definitive conclusions there is clearly a risk of patients being denied an effective intervention or treated with an ineffective (or even harmful) intervention. Subgroup analyses can also generate misleading recommendations about directions for future research that, if followed, would waste scarce resources.

It is useful to distinguish between the notions of 'qualitative interaction' and 'quantitative interaction' (Yusuf 1991). Qualitative interaction exists if the direction of effect is reversed, that is if an intervention is beneficial in one subgroup but is harmful in another. Qualitative interaction is rare. This may be used as an argument that the most appropriate result of a meta-analysis is the overall effect across all subgroups. Quantitative interaction exists when the size of the effect varies but not the direction, that is if an intervention is beneficial to different degrees in different subgroups.

Authors will find useful advice concerning subgroup analyses in Oxman and Guyatt (Oxman 1992) and Yusuf et al. (Yusuf 1991). See also Section 9.6.6.

### 9.6.3    Undertaking subgroup analyses

Subgroup analyses may be undertaken within RevMan. Meta-analyses within subgroups and meta-analyses that combine several subgroups are both permitted. It is tempting to compare effect estimates in different subgroups by considering the meta-analysis results from each subgroup separately. This should only be done informally by comparing the magnitudes of effect. Noting that either the effect or the test for heterogeneity in one subgroup is statistically significant whilst that in the other subgroup is not statistically significant does not indicate that the subgroup factor explains heterogeneity. Since different subgroups are likely to contain different amounts of information and thus have different abilities to detect effects, it is extremely misleading simply to compare the statistical significance of the results.

#### 9.6.3.1    *Is the effect different in different subgroups?*

Valid investigations of whether an intervention works differently in different subgroups involve comparing the subgroups with each other. When there are only two subgroups the overlap of the confidence intervals of the summary estimates in the two groups can be considered. Non-overlap of the confidence intervals indicates statistical significance, but note that the confidence intervals can overlap to a small degree and the difference still be statistically significant.

A simple approach for a significance test that can be used to investigate differences between two or more subgroups is described by Deeks et al. (Deeks 2001). This method is implemented in RevMan for fixed-effect analyses based on the inverse-variance method. If Mantel-Haenszel methods for the dichotomous data type are used, then the test would include a slight inaccuracy due to the way in which the heterogeneity chi-squared statistic is calculated. The procedure is based on the test for heterogeneity chi-squared statistics that appear in the bottom left hand corner of the forest plots, and proceeds as follows. Suppose a chi-squared heterogeneity statistic, $Q_{tot}$, is available for all of the studies, and that chi-squared heterogeneity statistics $Q_1$ up to $Q_J$ are available for J subgroups (such that every study is in one and only one subgroup). Then the new statistic $Q_{int} = Q_{tot} - (Q_1 + \cdots + Q_J)$, compared with a chi-squared distribution with $J - 1$ degrees of freedom, tests for a difference among the subgroups. A more flexible alternative to testing for differences between subgroups is to use meta-regression techniques, in which residual heterogeneity (that is, heterogeneity not explained by the subgrouping) is allowed (see Section 9.6.4). This approach may be regarded as preferable due to the high risk of false-positive results when comparing subgroups in a fixed-effect model (Higgins 2004).

## 9.6.4   Meta-regression

If studies are divided into subgroups (see Section 9.6.2), this may be viewed as an investigation of how a categorical study characteristic is associated with the intervention effects in the meta-analysis. For example, studies in which allocation sequence concealment was adequate may yield different results from those in which it was inadequate. Here, allocation sequence concealment, being either adequate or inadequate, is a categorical characteristic at the study level. Meta-regression is an extension to subgroup analyses that allows the effect of continuous, as well as categorical, characteristics to be investigated, and in principle allows the effects of multiple factors to be investigated simultaneously (although this is rarely possible due to inadequate numbers of studies) (Thompson 2002). Meta-regression should generally not be considered when there are fewer than ten studies in a meta-analysis.

Meta-regressions are similar in essence to simple regressions, in which an **outcome variable** is predicted according to the values of one or more **explanatory variables**. In meta-regression, the outcome variable is the effect estimate (for example, a mean difference, a risk difference, a log odds ratio or a log risk ratio). The explanatory variables are characteristics of studies that might influence the size of intervention effect. These are often called 'potential effect modifiers' or covariates. Meta-regressions usually differ from simple regressions in two ways. First, larger studies have more influence on the relationship than smaller studies, since studies are weighted by the precision of their respective effect estimate. Second, it is wise to allow for the residual heterogeneity among intervention effects not modelled by the explanatory variables. This gives rise to the term 'random-effects meta-regression', since the extra variability is incorporated in the same way as in a random-effects meta-analysis (Thompson 1999).

The regression coefficient obtained from a meta-regression analysis will describe how the outcome variable (the intervention effect) changes with a unit increase in the explanatory variable (the potential effect modifier). The statistical significance of the regression coefficient is a test of whether there is a linear relationship between intervention effect and the explanatory variable. If the intervention effect is a ratio measure, the log-transformed value of the intervention effect should always be used in the regression model (see Section 9.2.7), and the exponential of the regression coefficient will give an estimate of the relative change in intervention effect with a unit increase in the explanatory variable.

Meta-regression can also be used to investigate differences for categorical explanatory variables as done in subgroup analyses. If there are J subgroups membership of particular subgroups is indicated by using $J - 1$ dummy variables (which can only take values of zero or one) in the meta-regression model (as in standard linear regression modelling). The regression coefficients will estimate how the intervention effect in each subgroup differs from a nominated reference subgroup. The P value of each regression coefficient will indicate whether this difference is statistically significant.

Meta-regression may be performed using the 'metareg' macro available for the Stata statistical package.

## 9.6.5 Selection of study characteristics for subgroup analyses and meta-regression

Authors need to be cautious about undertaking subgroup analyses, and interpreting any that they do. Some considerations are outlined here for selecting characteristics (also called explanatory variables, potential effect modifiers or covariates) which will be investigated for their possible influence on the size of the intervention effect. These considerations apply similarly to subgroup analyses and to meta-regressions. Further details may be obtained from Oxman and Guyatt (Oxman 1992) and Berlin and Antman (Berlin 1994).

### 9.6.5.1    Ensure that there are adequate studies to justify subgroup analyses and meta-regressions

It is very unlikely that an investigation of heterogeneity will produce useful findings unless there is a substantial number of studies. It is worth noting the typical advice for undertaking simple regression analyses: that at least ten observations (i.e. ten studies in a meta-analysis) should be available for each characteristic modelled. However, even this will be too few when the covariates are unevenly distributed.

### 9.6.5.2    Specify characteristics in advance

Authors should, whenever possible, pre-specify characteristics in the protocol that later will be subject to subgroup analyses or meta-regression. Pre-specifying characteristics reduces the likelihood of spurious findings, first by limiting the number of subgroups investigated and second by preventing knowledge of the studies' results influencing which subgroups are analysed. True pre-specification is difficult in systematic reviews, because the results of some of the relevant studies are often known when the protocol is drafted. If a characteristic was overlooked in the protocol, but is clearly of major importance and justified by external evidence, then authors should not be reluctant to explore it. However, such *post hoc* analyses should be identified as such.

### 9.6.5.3    Select a small number of characteristics

The likelihood of a false positive result among subgroup analyses and meta-regression increases with the number of characteristics investigated. It is difficult to suggest a maximum number of characteristics to look at, especially since the number of available studies is unknown in advance. If more than one or two characteristics are investigated it may be sensible to adjust the level of significance to account for making multiple comparisons. The help of a statistician is recommended (see Chapter 16, Section 16.7).

### 9.6.5.4    Ensure there is scientific rationale for investigating each characteristic

Selection of characteristics should be motivated by biological and clinical hypotheses, ideally supported by evidence from sources other than the included studies. Subgroup analyses using characteristics that are implausible or clinically irrelevant are not likely to be useful and should be avoided. For example, a relationship between intervention effect and year of publication is seldom in itself clinically informative, and if statistically significant runs the risk of initiating a *post hoc* data dredge of factors that may have changed over time.

Prognostic factors are those that predict the outcome of a disease or condition, whereas effect modifiers are factors that influence how well an intervention works in affecting the outcome. Confusion between prognostic factors and effect modifiers is common in planning subgroup analyses, especially at the protocol stage. Prognostic factors are not good candidates for subgroup analyses unless they are also believed to modify the effect of intervention. For example, being a smoker may be a strong predictor of mortality within the next ten years, but there may not be reason for it to influence the effect of a drug therapy on mortality (Deeks 1998). Potential effect modifiers may include the precise interventions (dose of active treatment, choice of comparison treatment), how the study was done (length of follow-up) or methodology (design and quality).

### 9.6.5.5 Be aware that the effect of a characteristic may not always be identified

Many characteristics that might have important effects on how well an intervention works cannot be investigated using subgroup analysis or meta-regression. These are characteristics of participants that might vary substantially within studies, but which can only be summarized at the level of the study. An example is age. Consider a collection of clinical trials involving adults ranging from 18 to 60 years old. There may be a strong relationship between age and intervention effect that is apparent within each study. However, if the mean ages for the trials are similar, then no relationship will be apparent by looking at trial mean ages and trial-level effect estimates. The problem is one of aggregating individuals' results and is variously known as aggregation bias, ecological bias or the ecological fallacy (Morgenstern 1982, Greenland 1987, Berlin 2002). It is even possible for the differences between studies to display the opposite pattern to that observed within each study.

### 9.6.5.6 Think about whether the characteristic is closely related to another characteristic (confounded)

The problem of 'confounding' complicates interpretation of subgroup analyses and meta-regressions and can lead to incorrect conclusions. Two characteristics are confounded if their influences on the intervention effect cannot be disentangled. For example, if those studies implementing an intensive version of a therapy happened to be the studies that involved patients with more severe disease, then one cannot tell which aspect is the cause of any difference in effect estimates between these studies and others. In meta-regression, co-linearity between potential effect modifiers leads to similar difficulties as is discussed by Berlin and Antman (Berlin 1994). Computing correlations between study characteristics will give some information about which study characteristics may be confounded with each other.

## 9.6.6 Interpretation of subgroup analyses and meta-regressions

Appropriate interpretation of subgroup analyses and meta-regressions requires caution. For more detailed discussion see Oxman and Guyatt (Oxman 1992).

- Subgroup comparisons are observational
  It must be remembered that subgroup analyses and meta-regressions are entirely observational in their nature. These analyses investigate differences between studies. Even if individuals are randomized to one group or other within a clinical trial, they are not randomized to go in one trial or another. Hence, subgroup analyses suffer the limitations of any observational investigation, including possible bias through confounding by other study-level characteristics. Furthermore, even a genuine difference between subgroups is not necessarily due to the classification of the subgroups. As an example, a subgroup analysis of bone marrow transplantation for treating leukaemia

might show a strong association between the age of a sibling donor and the success of the transplant. However, this probably does not mean that the age of donor is important. In fact, the age of the recipient is probably a key factor and the subgroup finding would simply be due to the strong association between the age of the recipient and the age of their sibling.

- Was the analysis pre-specified or *post hoc*?
  Authors should state whether subgroup analyses were pre-specified or undertaken after the results of the studies had been compiled (*post hoc*). More reliance may be placed on a subgroup analysis if it was one of a small number of pre-specified analyses. Performing numerous *post hoc* subgroup analyses to explain heterogeneity is data dredging. Data dredging is condemned because it is usually possible to find an apparent, but false, explanation for heterogeneity by considering lots of different characteristics.

- Is there indirect evidence in support of the findings?
  Differences between subgroups should be clinically plausible and supported by other external or indirect evidence, if they are to be convincing.

- Is the magnitude of the difference practically important?
  If the magnitude of a difference between subgroups will not result in different recommendations for different subgroups, then it may be better to present only the overall analysis results.

- Is there a statistically significant difference between subgroups?
  To establish whether there is a different effect of an intervention in different situations, the magnitudes of effects in different subgroups should be compared directly with each other. In particular, statistical significance of the results within separate subgroup analyses should not be compared. See Section 9.6.3.1.

- Are analyses looking at within-study or between-study relationships?
  For patient and intervention characteristics, differences in subgroups that are observed within studies are more reliable than analyses of subsets of studies. If such within-study relationships are replicated across studies then this adds confidence to the findings.

## 9.6.7   Investigating the effect of baseline risk

One potentially important source of heterogeneity among a series of studies is when the underlying average risk of the outcome event varies between the studies. The baseline risk of a particular event may be viewed as an aggregate measure of case-mix factors such as age or disease severity. It is generally measured as the observed risk of the event in the control group of each study (the control group risk (CGR)). The notion is controversial in its relevance to clinical practice since baseline risk represents a summary of both known and unknown risk factors. Problems also arise because baseline risk will depend on the length of follow-up, which often varies across studies. However, baseline risk has received particular attention in meta-analysis because the information is readily available once dichotomous data have been prepared for use in meta-analyses. Sharp provides a full discussion of the topic (Sharp 2000).

Intuition would suggest that participants are more or less likely to benefit from an effective intervention according to their risk status. However, the relationship between baseline risk and intervention effect is a complicated issue. For example, suppose an intervention is equally beneficial in the sense that for all patients it reduces the risk of an event, say a stroke, to 80% of the baseline risk. Then it is not equally beneficial in terms of absolute differences in risk in the sense that it reduces a 50% stroke rate by 10 percentage points to 40% (number needed to treat = 10), but a 20% stroke rate by 4 percentage points to 16% (number needed to treat = 25).

Use of different summary statistics (risk ratio, odds ratio and risk difference) will demonstrate different relationships with baseline risk. Summary statistics that show close to no relationship with baseline risk are generally preferred for use in meta-analysis (see Section 9.4.4.4).

Investigating any relationship between effect estimates and the control group risk is also complicated by a technical phenomenon known as regression to the mean. This arises because the control group risk forms an integral part of the effect estimate. A high risk in a control group, observed entirely by chance, will on average give rise to a higher than expected effect estimate, and *vice versa*. This phenomenon results in a false correlation between effect estimates and control group risks. Methods are available, requiring sophisticated software, that correct for regression to the mean (McIntosh 1996, Thompson 1997). These should be used for such analyses and statistical expertise is recommended.

### 9.6.8  Dose-response analyses

The principles of meta-regression can be applied to the relationships between intervention effect and dose (commonly termed dose-response), treatment intensity or treatment duration (Greenland 1992, Berlin 1993). Conclusions about differences in effect due to differences in dose (or similar factors) are on strongest ground if participants are randomized to one dose or another within a study and a consistent relationship is found across similar studies. While authors should consider these effects, particularly as a possible explanation for heterogeneity, they should be cautious about drawing conclusions based on between-study differences. Authors should be particularly cautious about claiming that a dose-response relationship does not exist, given the low power of many meta-regression analyses to detect genuine relationships.

## 9.7  Sensitivity analyses

The process of undertaking a systematic review involves a sequence of decisions. Whilst many of these decisions are clearly objective and non-contentious, some will be somewhat arbitrary or unclear. For instance, if inclusion criteria involve a numerical value, the choice of value is usually arbitrary: for example, defining groups of older people may reasonably have lower limits of 60, 65, 70 or 75 years, or any value in between. Other decisions may be unclear because a study report fails to include the required information. Some decisions are unclear because the included studies themselves never obtained the information required: for example, the outcomes of those who unfortunately were lost to follow-up. Further decisions are unclear because there is no consensus on the best statistical method to use for a particular problem.

It is desirable to prove that the findings from a systematic review are not dependent on such arbitrary or unclear decisions. A sensitivity analysis is a repeat of the the primary analysis or meta-analysis, substituting alternative decisions or ranges of values for decisions that were arbitrary or unclear. For example, if the eligibility of some studies in the meta-analysis is dubious because they do not contain full details, sensitivity analysis may involve undertaking the meta-analysis twice: first, including all studies and second, only including those that are definitely known to be eligible. A sensitivity analysis asks the question, "Are the findings robust to the decisions made in the process of obtaining them?".

There are many decision nodes within the systematic review process which can generate a need for a sensitivity analysis. Examples include:

*Searching for studies:*
• Should abstracts whose results cannot be confirmed in subsequent publications be included in the review?

*Eligibility criteria:*
• Characteristics of participants: where a majority but not all people in a study meet an age range, should the study be included?

• Characteristics of the intervention: what range of doses should be included in the meta-analysis?

• Characteristics of the comparator: what criteria are required to define usual care to be used as a comparator group?

• Characteristics of the outcome: what time-point or range of time-points are eligible for inclusion?

• Study design: should blinded and unblinded outcome assessment be included, or should study inclusion be restricted by other aspects of methodological criteria?

*What data should be analysed?*
• Time-to-event data: what assumptions of the distribution of censored data should be made?

• Continuous data: where standard deviations are missing, when and how should they be imputed? Should analyses be based on change scores or on final values?

- Ordinal scales: what cut-point should be used to dichotomize short ordinal scales into two groups?

- Cluster-randomized trials: what values of the intraclass correlation coefficient should be used when trial analyses have not been adjusted for clustering?

- Cross-over trials: what values of the within-subject correlation coefficient should be used when this is not available in primary reports?

- All analyses: what assumptions should be made about missing outcomes to facilitate intention-to-treat analyses? Should adjusted or unadjusted estimates of treatment effects used?

*Analysis methods:*

- Should fixed-effect or random-effects methods be used for the analysis?

- For dichotomous outcomes, should odds ratios, risk ratios or risk differences be used?

- And for continuous outcomes, where several scales have assessed the same dimension, should results be analysed as a standardized mean difference across all scales or as mean differences individually for each scale?

Some sensitivity analyses can be pre-specified in the study protocol, but many issues suitable for sensitivity analysis are only identified during the review process where the individual peculiarities of the studies under investigation are identified. When sensitivity analyses show that the overall result and conclusions are not affected by the different decisions that could be made during the review process, the results of the review can be regarded with a higher degree of certainty. Where sensitivity analyses identify particular decisions or missing information that greatly influence the findings of the review, greater resources can be deployed to try and resolve uncertainties and obtain extra information, possibly through contacting trial authors and obtained individual patient data. If this cannot be achieved, the results must be interpreted with an appropriate degree of caution. Such findings may generate proposals for further investigations and future research.

Reporting of sensitivity analyses in a systematic review may best be done by producing a summary table. Rarely is it informative to produce individual forest plots for each sensitivity analysis undertaken.

Sensitivity analyses are sometimes confused with subgroup analysis. Although some sensitivity analyses involve restricting the analysis to a subset of the totality of studies, the two methods differ in two ways. First, sensitivity analyses do not attempt to estimate the effect of the intervention in the group of studies removed from the analysis, whereas in subgroup analyses, estimates are produced for each subgroup. Second, in sensitivity analyses, informal comparisons are made between different ways of estimating the same thing, whereas in subgroup analyses, formal statistical comparisons are made across the subgroups.

## 9.8  Chapter information

**Editors:** Jonathan J Deeks, Julian PT Higgins and Douglas G Altman on behalf of the Cochrane Statistical Methods Group.

---

### Box 9.8.a   The Cochrane Statistical Methods Group

Statistical issues are a core aspect of much of the work of the Cochrane Collaboration. The Statistical Methods Group (SMG) is a forum where all statistical issues related to the work of The Cochrane Collaboration are discussed. It has a broad scope, covering issues relating to statistical methods, training, software and research. It also attempts to ensure that adequate statistical and technical support is available to review groups.

The SMG dates back to 1993. Membership of the SMG is currently through membership of the group's email discussion list. The list is used for discussing all issues of importance for the group, whether research, training, software or administration. The group has over 130 members from over around 20 countries. All statisticians working with Cochrane Review Groups (CRGs) are strongly encouraged to join the SMG.

Specifically, the aims of the group are:

1. To develop general policy advice for the Collaboration on all statistical issues relevant to systematic reviews of healthcare interventions.
2. To take responsibility for statistics-orientated chapters of this *Handbook*.
3. To co-ordinate practical statistical support for CRGs.
4. To conduct training workshops and workshops on emerging topics as necessary.
5. To contribute to and review the statistical content of training materials provided within the Collaboration.
6. To develop and validate the statistical software used within the Collaboration.
7. To generate and keep up to date a list of the Statistical Methods Group, detailing their areas of interest and expertise, and maintain an email discussion list as a forum for discussing relevant methodological issues.
8. To maintain a research agenda dictated by issues important to the present and future functioning of the Collaboration, and to encourage research that tackles the agenda.

Web site: www.cochrane-smg.org

**This chapter should be cited as**: Deeks JJ, Higgins JPT, Altman DG (editors). Chapter 9: Analysing data and undertaking meta-analyses. In: Higgins JPT, Green S (editors). *Cochrane Handbook for Systematic Reviews of Interventions*. Chichester (UK): John Wiley & Sons, 2008.

**Contributing authors:** Doug Altman, Deborah Ashby, Jacqueline Birks, Michael Borenstein, Marion Campbell, Jon Deeks, Matthias Egger, Julian Higgins, Joseph Lau, Keith O'Rourke, Rob Scholten, Jonathan Sterne, Simon Thompson and Anne Whitehead.

**Acknowledgements:** We are grateful to the following for commenting helpfully on earlier drafts: Bodil Als-Nielsen, Doug Altman, Deborah Ashby, Jesse Berlin, Joseph Beyene, Jacqueline Birks, Michael Bracken, Marion Campbell, Chris Cates, Wendong Chen, Mike Clarke, Albert Cobos, Esther Coren, Francois Curtin, Roberto D'Amico, Keith Dear, Jon Deeks, Heather Dickinson, Diana Elbourne, Simon Gates, Paul Glasziou, Christian Gluud, Peter Herbison, Julian Higgins, Sally Hollis, David Jones, Steff Lewis, Philippa Middleton, Nathan Pace, Craig Ramsey, Keith O'Rourke, Rob Scholten, Guido Schwarzer, Jack Sinclair, Jonathan Sterne, Simon Thompson, Andy Vail, Clarine van Oel, Paula Williamson and Fred Wolf.

# 9.9   References

**Adams 2005**
Adams NP, Bestall JB, Malouf R, Lasserson TJ, Jones PW. Beclomethasone versus placebo for chronic asthma. *Cochrane Database of Systematic Reviews* 2005, Issue 1. Art No: CD002738.

**Agresti 1996**
Agresti A. *An introduction to categorical data analysis*. New York (NY): John Wiley & Sons, 1996.

**Altman 1996**
Altman DG, Bland JM. Detecting skewness from summary information. *BMJ* 1996; 313: 1200–1200.

**Antman 1992**
Antman EM, Lau J, Kupelnick B, Mosteller F, Chalmers TC. A comparison of results of meta-analyses of randomized control trials and recommendations of clinical experts: Treatments for myocardial infarction. *JAMA* 1992; 268: 240–248.

**Berlin 1993**
Berlin JA, Longnecker MP, Greenland S. Meta-analysis of epidemiologic dose-response data. *Epidemiology* 1993; 4: 218–228.

**Berlin 1994**
Berlin JA, Antman EM. Advantages and limitations of metaanalytic regressions of clinical trials data. *Online Journal of Current Clinical Trials* 1994; Doc No 134.

**Berlin 2002**
Berlin JA, Santanna J, Schmid CH, Szczech LA, Feldman KA. Individual patient- versus group-level data meta-regressions for the investigation of treatment effect modifiers: ecological bias rears its ugly head. *Statistics in Medicine* 2002; 21: 371–387.

**Bradburn 2007**

Bradburn MJ, Deeks JJ, Berlin JA, Russell LA. Much ado about nothing: a comparison of the performance of meta-analytical methods with rare events. *Statistics in Medicine* 2007; 26: 53–77.

**Chinn 2000**

Chinn S. A simple method for converting an odds ratio to effect size for use in meta-analysis. *Statistics in Medicine* 2000; 19: 3127–3131.

**Cooper 1980**

Cooper HM, Rosenthal R. Statistical versus traditional procedures for summarizing research findings. *Psychological Bulletin* 1980; 87: 442–449.

**Crawford 2007**

Crawford F, Hollis S. Topical treatments for fungal infections of the skin and nails of the feet. *Cochrane Database of Systematic Reviews* 2007, Issue 3. Art No: CD001434.

**Deeks 1998**

Deeks JJ. Systematic reviews of published evidence: Miracles or minefields? *Annals of Oncology* 1998; 9: 703–709.

**Deeks 2001**

Deeks JJ, Altman DG, Bradburn MJ. Statistical methods for examining heterogeneity and combining results from several studies in meta-analysis. In: Egger M, Davey Smith G, Altman DG (editors). *Systematic Reviews in Health Care: Meta-analysis in Context* (2nd edition). London (UK): BMJ Publication Group, 2001.

**Deeks 2002**

Deeks JJ. Issues in the selection of a summary statistic for meta-analysis of clinical trials with binary outcomes. *Statistics in Medicine* 2002; 21: 1575–1600.

**DerSimonian 1986**

DerSimonian R, Laird N. Meta-analysis in clinical trials. *Controlled Clinical Trials* 1986; 7: 177–188.

**Egger 1997**

Egger M, Smith GD, Schneider M, Minder C. Bias in meta-analysis detected by a simple, graphical test. *BMJ* 1997; 315: 629–634.

**Engels 2000**

Engels EA, Schmid CH, Terrin N, Olkin I, Lau J. Heterogeneity and statistical significance in meta-analysis: an empirical study of 125 meta-analyses. *Statistics in Medicine* 2000; 19: 1707–1728.

**Greenland 1985**

Greenland S, Robins JM. Estimation of a common effect parameter from sparse follow-up data. *Biometrics* 1985; 41: 55–68.

**Greenland 1987**

Greenland S. Quantitative methods in the review of epidemiologic literature. *Epidemiologic Reviews* 1987; 9: 1–30.

**Greenland 1992**

Greenland S, Longnecker MP. Methods for trend estimation from summarized dose-response data, with applications to meta-analysis. *American Journal of Epidemiology* 1992; 135: 1301–1309.

**Hasselblad 1995**

Hasselblad VIC, Mccrory DC. Meta-analytic tools for medical decision making: A practical guide. *Medical Decision Making* 1995; 15: 81–96.

**Higgins 2002**

Higgins JPT, Thompson SG. Quantifying heterogeneity in a meta-analysis. *Statistics in Medicine* 2002; 21: 1539–1558.

**Higgins 2003**

Higgins JPT, Thompson SG, Deeks JJ, Altman DG. Measuring inconsistency in meta-analyses. *BMJ* 2003; 327: 557–560.

**Higgins 2004**

Higgins JPT, Thompson SG. Controlling the risk of spurious findings from meta-regression. *Statistics in Medicine* 2004; 23: 1663–1682.

**Higgins 2008a**

Higgins JPT, White IR, Anzures-Cabrera J. Meta-analysis of skewed data: combining results reported on log-transformed or raw scales. *Statistics in Medicine* (in press, 2008).

**Higgins 2008b**

Higgins JPT, Thompson SG, Spiegelhalter DJ. A re-evaluation of random-effects meta-analysis. *Journal of the Royal Statistical Society Series A* (in press, 2008).

**Kjaergard 2001**

Kjaergard LL, Villumsen J, Gluud C. Reported methodologic quality and discrepancies between large and small randomized trials in meta-analyses. *Annals of Internal Medicine* 2001; 135: 982–989.

**Laupacis 1988**

Laupacis A, Sackett DL, Roberts RS. An assessment of clinically useful measures of the consequences of treatment. *New England Journal of Medicine* 1988; 318: 1728–1733.

**Mantel 1959**

Mantel N, Haenszel W. Statistical aspects of the analysis of data from retrospective studies of disease. *Journal of the National Cancer Institute* 1959; 22: 719–748.

**McIntosh 1996**

McIntosh MW. The population risk as an explanatory variable in research synthesis of clinical trials. *Statistics in Medicine* 1996; 15: 1713–1728.

**Moher 2005**

Moher M, Hey K, Lancaster T. Workplace interventions for smoking cessation. *Cochrane Database of Systematic Reviews* 2005, Issue 2. Art No: CD003440.

**Morgenstern 1982**

Morgenstern H. Uses of ecologic analysis in epidemiologic research. *American Journal of Public Health* 1982; 72: 1336–1344.

**O'Rourke 1989**

O'Rourke K, Detsky AS. Meta-analysis in medical research: strong encouragement for higher quality in individual research efforts. *Journal of Clinical Epidemiology* 1989; 42: 1021–1026.

**Oxman 1992**

Oxman AD, Guyatt GH. A consumers guide to subgroup analyses. *Annals of Internal Medicine* 1992; 116: 78–84.

**Pittler 2003**

Pittler MH, Ernst E. Kava extract versus placebo for treating anxiety. *Cochrane Database of Systematic Reviews* 2003, Issue 1. Art No: CD003383.

**Poole 1999**

Poole C, Greenland S. Random-effects meta-analyses are not always conservative. *American Journal of Epidemiology* 1999; 150: 469–475.

**Sackett 1996**

Sackett DL, Deeks JJ, Altman DG. Down with odds ratios! *Evidence Based Medicine* 1996; 1: 164–166.

**Sackett 1997**

Sackett DL, Richardson WS, Rosenberg W, Haynes BR. *Evidence-Based Medicine: How to Practice and Teach EBM*. Edinburgh (UK): Churchill Livingstone, 1997.

**Sharp 2000**

Sharp SJ. Analysing the relationship between treatment benefit and underlying risk: precautions and practical recommendations. In: Egger M, Davey Smith G, Altman DG (editors). *Systematic Reviews in Health Care: Meta-analysis in Context* (2nd edition). London (UK): BMJ Publication Group, 2000.

**Sinclair 1994**

Sinclair JC, Bracken MB. Clinically useful measures of effect in binary analyses of randomized trials. *Journal of Clinical Epidemiology* 1994; 47: 881–889.

**Thompson 1997**

Thompson SG, Smith TC, Sharp SJ. Investigating underlying risk as a source of heterogeneity in meta-analysis. *Statistics in Medicine* 1997; 16: 2741–2758.

**Thompson 1999**

Thompson SG, Sharp SJ. Explaining heterogeneity in meta-analysis: a comparison of methods. *Statistics in Medicine* 1999; 18: 2693–2708.

**Thompson 2002**

Thompson SG, Higgins JPT. How should meta-regression analyses be undertaken and interpreted? *Statistics in Medicine* 2002; 21: 1559–1574.

**Whitehead 1991**

Whitehead A, Whitehead J. A general parametric approach to the meta-analysis of randomised clinical trials. *Statistics in Medicine* 1991; 10: 1665–1677.

**Whitehead 1994**

Whitehead A, Jones NMB. A meta-analysis of clinical trials involving different classifications of response into ordered categories. *Statistics in Medicine* 1994; 13: 2503–2515.

**Yusuf 1985**

Yusuf S, Peto R, Lewis J, Collins R, Sleight P. Beta blockade during and after myocardial infarction: an overview of the randomised trials. *Progress in Cardiovascular Diseases* 1985; 27: 335–371.

**Yusuf 1991**

Yusuf S, Wittes J, Probstfield J, Tyroler HA. Analysis and interpretation of treatment effects in subgroups of patients in randomized clinical trials. *JAMA* 1991; 266: 93–98.

# 10 Addressing reporting biases

**Edited by Jonathan AC Sterne, Matthias Egger and David Moher on behalf of the Cochrane Bias Methods Group**

## Key Points

- Only a proportion of research projects will be published in sources easily identifiable by authors of systematic reviews. Reporting biases arise when the dissemination of research findings is influenced by the nature and direction of results.

- The contribution made to the totality of the evidence in systematic reviews by studies with statistically non-significant results is as important as that from studies with statistically significant results.

- The convincing evidence for the presence of several types of reporting biases (outlined in this chapter) demonstrates the need to search comprehensively for studies that meet the eligibility criteria for a Cochrane review.

- Prospective trial registration, now a requirement for publication in many journals, has the potential to substantially reduce the effects of publication bias.

- Funnel plots can be used for reviews with sufficient numbers of included studies, but an asymmetrical funnel plot should not be equated with publication bias.

- Several methods are available to test for asymmetry in a funnel plot and recommendations are included in the chapter for selecting an appropriate test.

# 10.1   Introduction

The dissemination of research findings is not a division into published or unpublished, but a continuum ranging from the sharing of draft papers among colleagues, through presentations at meetings and published abstracts, to papers in journals that are indexed in the major bibliographic databases (Smith 1999). It has long been recognized that only a proportion of research projects ultimately reach publication in an indexed journal and thus become easily identifiable for systematic reviews.

**Reporting biases** arise when the dissemination of research findings is influenced by the nature and direction of results. Statistically significant, 'positive' results that indicate that an intervention works are more likely to be published, more likely to be published rapidly, more likely to be published in English, more likely to be published more than once, more likely to be published in high impact journals and, related to the last point, more likely to be cited by others. The contribution made to the totality of the evidence in systematic reviews by studies with non-significant results is as important as that from studies with statistically significant results.

Table 10.1.a summarizes some different types of reporting biases. We consider these in more detail in Section 10.2, highlighting in particular the evidence supporting the presence of each bias. We discuss approaches for avoiding reporting biases in Cochrane reviews in Section 10.3, and address funnel plots and statistical methods for detecting potential biases in Section 10.4. Although for the purpose of discussing these biases we will sometimes denote statistically significant ($P < 0.05$) results as 'positive' results and statistically non-significant or null results as 'negative' results, such labels should not be used by Cochrane reviews authors.

**Table 10.1.a**   Definitions of some types of reporting biases

| Type of reporting bias | Definition |
| --- | --- |
| Publication bias | The *publication* or *non-publication* of research findings, depending on the nature and direction of the results |
| Time lag bias | The *rapid* or *delayed* publication of research findings, depending on the nature and direction of the results |
| Multiple (duplicate) publication bias | The *multiple* or *singular* publication of research findings, depending on the nature and direction of the results |
| Location bias | The publication of research findings in journals with different *ease of access* or *levels of indexing* in standard databases, depending on the nature and direction of results. |
| Citation bias | The *citation* or *non-citation* of research findings, depending on the nature and direction of the results |
| Language bias | The publication of research findings *in a particular language*, depending on the nature and direction of the results |
| Outcome reporting bias | The *selective reporting* of some outcomes but not others, depending on the nature and direction of the results |

## 10.2 Types of reporting biases and the supporting evidence

### 10.2.1 Publication bias

In a 1979 article, "The 'file drawer problem' and tolerance for null results", Rosenthal described a gloomy scenario where "the journals are filled with the 5% of the studies that show Type I errors, while the file drawers back at the lab are filled with the 95% of the studies that show non-significant (e.g. p>0.05) results" (Rosenthal 1979). The file drawer problem has long been suspected in the social sciences: a review of psychology journals found that of 294 studies published in the 1950s, 97.3% rejected the null hypothesis at the 5% level ($P < 0.05$) (Sterling 1959). The study was updated and complemented with three other journals (*New England Journal of Medicine, American Journal of Epidemiology, American Journal of Public Health*) (Sterling 1995). Little had changed in the psychology journals (95.6% reported significant results) and a high proportion of statistically significant results (85.4%) was also found in the general medical and public health journals. Similar results have been reported in many different areas such as emergency medicine (Moscati 1994), alternative and complementary medicine (Vickers 1998, Pittler 2000) and acute stroke trials (Liebeskind 2006).

It is possible that studies suggesting a beneficial intervention effect or a larger effect size are published, while a similar amount of data pointing in the other direction remains unpublished. In this situation, a systematic review of the published studies could identify a spurious beneficial intervention effect, or miss an important adverse effect of an intervention. In cardiovascular medicine, investigators who, in 1980, found an increased death rate among patients with acute myocardial infarction treated with a class I anti-arrhythmic dismissed it as a chance finding and did not publish their trial at the time (Cowley 1993). Their findings would have contributed to a more timely detection of the increased mortality that has since become known to be associated with the use of class I anti-arrhythmic agents (Teo 1993, CLASP Collaborative Group 1994).

Studies empirically examining the existence of publication bias can be viewed in two categories: indirect and direct evidence. Surveys of published results, such as those described above, can provide only indirect evidence of publication bias, as the proportion of all hypotheses tested for which the null hypothesis is truly false is unknown. There is also substantial direct evidence of publication bias. Roberta Scherer and colleagues recently updated a systematic review which summarizes 79 studies describing subsequent full publication of research initially presented in abstract or short report form (Scherer 2007). The data from 45 studies that included data on time to publication are summarized in Figure 10.2.a. Only about half of abstracts presented at conferences were later published in full (63% for randomized trials), and subsequent publication was associated with positive results, (Scherer 2007).

Additional direct evidence is available from a number of cohort studies of proposals submitted to ethics committees and institutional review boards (Easterbrook 1991, Dickersin 1992, Stern 1997, Decullier 2005, Decullier 2007), trials submitted to licensing authorities (Bardy 1998), analyses of trials registries (Simes 1987) or from

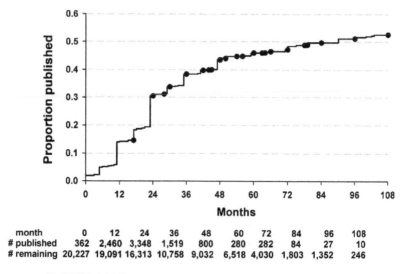

| month | 0 | 12 | 24 | 36 | 48 | 60 | 72 | 84 | 96 | 108 |
|---|---|---|---|---|---|---|---|---|---|---|
| # published | 362 | 2,460 | 3,348 | 1,519 | 800 | 280 | 282 | 84 | 27 | 10 |
| # remaining | 20,227 | 19,091 | 16,313 | 10,758 | 9,032 | 6,518 | 4,030 | 1,803 | 1,352 | 246 |

N = 20,227 abstracts
Circles show points where data censored because reports stopped follow-up.

**Figure 10.2.a**  Cumulative full publication of results initially presented as abstracts from 45 studies reporting time to publication that followed up research presented at meetings and conferences

cohorts of trials funded by specific funding agencies (Dickersin 1993). For each cohort of research proposals the principal investigators were contacted several years later to determine the publication status of each completed study. In all these studies publication was more likely if the intervention effects were large and statistically significant.

Hopewell et al. recently completed a methodology review of such studies, limited to those that considered clinical trials separately (Hopewell 2008). The percentages of full publication as journal articles in the five studies included in the review ranged from 36% to 94% (Table 10.2.a). Positive results were consistently more likely to have been published than negative results; the odds of publication were approximately four times greater if results were statistically significant (OR = 3.90, 95% CI 2.68 to 5.68) as shown in Figure 10.2.b. Other factors such as the study size, funding source, and academic rank and sex of primary investigator were not consistently associated with the probability of publication or were not possible to assess separately for clinical trials (Hopewell 2008).

### 10.2.1.1   Time lag bias

Studies continue to appear in print many years after approval by ethics committees. Hopewell and colleagues reviewed studies examining time to publication for results of clinical trials (Hopewell 2007a). The two studies included in this review (Stern 1997, Ioannidis 1998) found that about half of all trials were published and that those with

**Table 10.2.a**  Publication status of five cohorts of research projects approved by ethics committees or institutional review boards which had been completed and analysed at the time of follow-up. (Adapted from Hopewell et al. (Hopewell 2008).)

|  | Johns Hopkins University, Baltimore | National Institutes of Health, U.S.A. | Royal Prince Alfred Hospital, Sydney | National Agency for Medicine, Finland | National Institutes of Health, U.S.A., Multi-centre trials in HIV/AIDS |
|---|---|---|---|---|---|
| Reference | Dickersin 1992 | Dickersin 1993 | Stern 1997 | Bardy 1998 | Ioannidis 1998 |
| Period of approval | 1980 | 1979 | 1979–88 | 1987 | 1986–1996 |
| Year of follow-up | 1988 | 1988 | 1992 | 1995 | 1996 |
| Number approved | 168 | 198 | 130 | 188 | 66 |
| Published | 136 (81%) | 184 (93%) | 73 (56%) | 68 (36%) | 36 (54%) |
| Positive* | 84/96 (87%) | 121/124 (98%) | 55/76 (72%) | 52/111 (47%) | 20/27 (75%) |
| Negative* | 52/72 (72%) | 63/74 (85%) | 3/15 (20%) | 5/44 (11%) | 16/39 (41%) |
| Inconclusive/ null (if assessed separately) | Not assessed | Not assessed | 15/39 (38%) | 11/33 (33%) | Not assessed |

*Definitions differed by study.

positive results were published, on average, approximately 2–3 years earlier than trials with null or negative results.

Among proposals submitted to the Royal Prince Alfred Hospital Ethics Committee in Sydney, Australia, an estimated 85% of studies with significant results as compared to 65% of studies with null results had been published after 10 years (Stern 1997). The median time to publication was 4.7 years for studies with significant results and 8.0 years for studies with negative/null results. Similarly, trials conducted by multi-centre trial groups in the field of HIV infection in the United States appeared on average 4.3 years after the start of patient enrolment if results were statistically significant but took 6.5 years to be published if the results were negative (Ioannidis 1998). A recent study has found similar results (Decullier 2005). The fact that a substantial proportion of studies remain unpublished even a decade after the study had been completed and analysed is troubling as potentially important information remains hidden from systematic reviewers and consumers.

Ioannidis and colleagues also found that trials with positive and negative results differed little in the time they took to complete follow-up (Ioannidis 1998). Rather, the time lag was attributable to differences in the time from completion to publication (Ioannidis 1998). These findings indicate that time lag bias may be introduced in systematic reviews even in situations when most or all studies will eventually be

Review: Publication bias in clinical trials due to statistical significance or direction of trial results
Comparison: 01 Rate of publication and significance of trial result
Outcome: 01 Total number of trials published

| Study or sub-category | Positive n/N | Negative n/N | OR (fixed) 95% CI | Weight % | OR (fixed) 95% CI |
|---|---|---|---|---|---|
| **01 Positive versus negative or no difference** | | | | | |
| Bardy 1998 | 52/111 | 16/77 | | 35.13 | 3.36 [1.73, 6.53] |
| Subtotal (95% CI) | 111 | 77 | | 35.13 | 3.63 [1.73, 6.53] |
| Total events: 52 (Positive), 16 (Negative) | | | | | |
| Test for heterogeneity: not applicable | | | | | |
| Test for overall effect: Z = 3.57 (P = 0.0004) | | | | | |
| **02 Significant versus not significant** | | | | | |
| Dickersin 1992 | 84/96 | 52/72 | | 25.98 | 2.69 [1.22, 5.96] |
| Dickersin 1993 | 121/124 | 63/74 | | 6.68 | 7.04 [1.90, 26.16] |
| Subtotal (95% CI) | 220 | 146 | | 32.66 | 3.58 [1.84, 6.99] |
| Total events: 205 (Positive), 115 (Negative) | | | | | |
| Test for heterogeneity: Chi² = 1.51, df = 1 (P = 0.22), I² = 34.0% | | | | | |
| Test for overall effect: Z = 3.74 (P = 0.0002) | | | | | |
| **03 Positive (or favours experimental arm) versus negative (or favours control arm)** | | | | | |
| Ioannidis 1998 | 20/27 | 16/39 | | 11.87 | 4.11 [1.41, 11.99] |
| Subtotal (95% CI) | 27 | 39 | | 11.87 | 4.11 [1.41, 11.99] |
| Total events: 20 (Positive), 16 (Negative) | | | | | |
| Test for heterogeneity: not applicable | | | | | |
| Test for overall effect: Z = 2.58 (P = 0.010) | | | | | |
| **04 Significant versus non-significant trend or no difference** | | | | | |
| Stern 1997 | 55/76 | 18/54 | | 20.34 | 5.24 [2.46, 11.17] |
| Subtotal (95% CI) | 76 | 54 | | 20.34 | 5.24 [2.46, 11.17] |
| Total events: 55 (Positive), 18 (Negative) | | | | | |
| Test for heterogeneity: not applicable | | | | | |
| Test for overall effect: Z = 4.29 (P < 0.0001) | | | | | |
| Total (95% CI) | 434 | 316 | | 100.00 | 3.90 [2.68, 5.68] |
| Total events: 332 (Positive), 165 (Negative) | | | | | |
| Test for heterogeneity: Chi² = 2.40, df = 4 (P=0.66), I² = 0% | | | | | |
| Test for overall effect: Z = 7.12 (P < 0.0001) | | | | | |

0.01   0.1   1   10   100

Unpublished   Published

**Figure 10.2.b** Publication bias in clinical trials due to statistical significance or direction of trial results (adapted from Hopewell et al. (Hopewell 2008)).

published. Studies with positive results will dominate the literature and introduce bias for several years until the negative, but equally important, results finally appear. Furthermore, rare adverse events are likely to be found later in the research process than short-term beneficial effects.

### 10.2.1.2   Who is responsible for publication bias?

Studies with negative results could remain unpublished because authors fail to write manuscripts and submit them to journals, because such studies are peer reviewed less favourably, or because editors simply do not want to publish negative results. The peer review process is sometimes unreliable and susceptible to subjectivity, bias and conflict of interest (Peters 1982, Godlee 1999). Experimental studies in which test manuscripts were submitted to peer reviewers or journals showed that peer reviewers are more likely to referee favourably if results were in accordance with their own views (Mahoney 1977, Epstein 1990, Ernst 1994). For example, when a selected group of authors was asked to peer review a fictitious paper on transcutaneous electrical nerve stimulation (TENS) they were influenced by their own findings and preconceptions . Other studies have shown no association between publication of submitted manuscripts and study outcomes (Abbot 1998, Olson 2002), suggesting that although peer reviewers may hold strong beliefs which will influence their assessments, there is no general bias for or against positive findings.

A number of studies have directly asked authors why they had not published their findings. The most frequent answer was that they were not interesting enough to merit publication (e.g. journals would be unlikely to accept the manuscripts) (Easterbrook 1991, Dickersin 1992, Stern 1997, Weber 1998, Decullier 2005) or the investigators did not have enough time to prepare a manuscript (Weber 1998, Hartling 2004). Rejection of a manuscript by a journal was rarely mentioned as a reason for not publishing. Selective submission of papers by authors rather than selective recommendation by peer reviewers and selective acceptance by editors thus appears to be the dominant contributor to publication bias. In addition, Dickersin et al. examined the time from manuscript submission (to the journal *JAMA*) to full publication and found no association between this time and any study characteristics examined, including statistical significance of the study results (Dickersin 2002). Thus, time-lag bias may also be the result of delayed submission of manuscripts for publication by authors rather than by delayed publication by journals.

### 10.2.1.3   The influence of external funding and commercial interests

External funding has been found to be associated with publication independently of the statistical significance of the results (Dickersin 1997). Funding by government agencies was significantly associated with publication in three cohorts of proposals submitted to ethics committees (Easterbrook 1991, Dickersin 1992, Stern 1997) whereas

pharmaceutical industry sponsored studies were less likely to be published in two studies (Easterbrook 1991, Dickersin 1992). Indeed, a large proportion of clinical trials
submitted by drug companies to licensing authorities remain unpublished (Hemminki
1980, Bardy 1998).

In a systematic review, Lexchin et al. identified 30 studies published between 1966
and 2002 that examined whether funding of drug studies by the pharmaceutical industry
was associated with outcomes that are favourable to the funder. They found that research
funded by drug companies was less likely to be published than research funded by
other sources, and that studies sponsored by pharmaceutical companies were more
likely to have outcomes favouring the sponsor than were studies with other sponsors
(Lexchin 2003). Other studies have since examined these associations and have found
similar results (Bhandari 2004, Heres 2006). Heres et al., in a study of head-to-head
comparisons of antipsychotics, found that the overall outcome of the trials favoured
the drug manufactured by the industry sponsor in 90% of studies considered, and that
some similar studies reported opposing conclusions, each supporting the product of the
study sponsor (Heres 2006).

The implication is that the pharmaceutical industry tends to discourage the publication of negative studies that it has funded. For example, a manuscript reporting on a trial
comparing the bioequivalence of generic and brand levothyroxine products, which had
failed to produce the results desired by the sponsor of the study, Boots Pharmaceuticals,
was withdrawn because Boots took legal action against the university and the investigators. The actions of Boots, recounted in detail by one of the editors of *JAMA*, Drummond
Rennie (Rennie 1997), meant that publication of the paper (Dong 1997) was delayed
by about seven years. In a national survey of life-science faculty members in the United
States, 20% reported that they had experienced delays of more than six months in publication of their work and reasons for not publishing included "to delay the dissemination
of undesired results" (Blumenthal 1997). Delays in publication were associated with
involvement in commercialization and academic-industry research relationship, as well
as with male sex and higher academic rank of the investigator (Blumenthal 1997).

## 10.2.2   Other reporting biases

While publication bias has long been recognized and much discussed, other factors
can contribute to biased inclusion of studies in meta-analyses. Indeed, among published studies, the probability of identifying relevant studies for meta-analysis is also
influenced by their results. These biases have received much less consideration than
publication bias, but their consequences could be of equal importance.

### 10.2.2.1   Duplicate (multiple) publication bias

In 1989, Gøtzsche found that, among 244 reports of trials comparing non-steroidal anti-
inflammatory drugs in rheumatoid arthritis, 44 (18%) were redundant, multiple publications, which overlapped substantially with a previously published article. Twenty

trials were published twice, ten trials three times and one trial four times (Gøtzsche 1989). The production of multiple publications from single studies can lead to bias in a number of ways (Huston 1996). Most importantly, studies with significant results are more likely to lead to multiple publications and presentations (Easterbrook 1991), which makes it more likely that they will be located and included in a meta-analysis. It is not always obvious that multiple publications come from a single study, and one set of study participants may be included in an analysis twice. The inclusion of duplicated data may therefore lead to overestimation of intervention effects, as was demonstrated for trials of the efficacy of ondansetron to prevent postoperative nausea and vomiting (Tramèr 1997).

Other authors have described the difficulties and frustration caused by redundancy and the 'disaggregation' of medical research when results from a multi-centre trial are presented in several publications (Huston 1996, Johansen 1999). Redundant publications often fail to cross-reference each other (Bailey 2002, Barden 2003) and there are examples where two articles reporting the same trial do not share a single common author (Gøtzsche 1989, Tramèr 1997). Thus, it may be difficult or impossible for review authors to determine whether two papers represent duplicate publications of one study or two separate studies without contacting the authors, which may result in biasing a meta-analysis of this data.

### 10.2.2.2   *Location bias*

Research suggests that various factors related to the accessibility of study results are associated with effect sizes in trials. For example, in a series of trials in the field of complementary and alternative medicine, Pittler and colleagues examined the relationship between trial outcome, methodological quality and sample size with characteristics of the journals of publication of these trials (Pittler 2000). They found that trials published in low or non-impact factor journals were more likely to report significant results than those published in high-impact mainstream medical journals and that the quality of the trials was also associated with the journal of publication. Similarly, some studies suggest that trials published in English language journals are more likely to show strong significant effects than those published in non-English language journals (Egger 1997b), however this has not been shown consistently (Moher 2000, Jüni 2002, Pham 2005); see Section 10.2.2.4.

The term 'location bias' is also used to refer to the accessibility of studies based on variable indexing in electronic databases. Depending on the clinical question, choices regarding which databases to search may bias the effect estimate in a meta-analysis. For example, one study found that trials published in journals that were not indexed in MEDLINE might show a more beneficial effect than trials published in MEDLINE-indexed journals (Egger 2003). Another study of 61 meta-analyses found that, in general, trials published in journals indexed in EMBASE but not in MEDLINE reported smaller estimates of effect than those indexed in MEDLINE, but that the risk of bias may be minor, given the lower prevalence of the EMBASE unique trials (Sampson 2003). As above, these findings may vary substantially with the clinical topic being examined.

A final form of location bias is regional or developed country bias. Research supporting the evidence of this bias suggests that studies published in certain countries may be more likely than others to produce research showing significant effects of interventions. Vickers and colleagues demonstrated the potential existence of this bias (Vickers 1998).

### 10.2.2.3   Citation bias

The perusal of the reference lists of articles is widely used to identify additional articles that may be relevant although there is little evidence to support this methodology. The problem with this approach is that the act of citing previous work is far from objective and retrieving literature by scanning reference lists may thus produce a biased sample of studies. There are many possible motivations for citing an article. Brooks interviewed academic authors from various faculties at the University of Iowa and asked for the reasons for citing each reference in one of the authors' recent articles (Brooks 1985). Persuasiveness, i.e. the desire to convince peers and substantiate their own point of view, emerged as the most important reason for citing articles. Brooks concluded that authors advocate their own opinions and use the literature to justify their point of view: "Authors can be pictured as intellectual partisans of their own opinions, scouring the literature for justification" (Brooks 1985).

In Gøtzsche's analysis of trials of non-steroidal anti-inflammatory drugs in rheumatoid arthritis, trials demonstrating a superior effect of the new drug were more likely to be cited than trials with negative results (Gøtzsche 1987). Similar results were shown in an analysis of randomized trials of hepato-biliary diseases (Kjaergard 2002). Similarly, trials of cholesterol lowering to prevent coronary heart disease were cited almost six times more often if they were supportive of cholesterol lowering (Ravnskov 1992). Over-citation of unsupportive studies can also occur. Hutchison et al. examined reviews of the effectiveness of pneumococcal vaccines and found that unsupportive trials were more likely to be cited than trials showing that vaccines worked (Hutchison 1995).

Citation bias may affect the 'secondary' literature. For example, the *ACP Journal Club* aims to summarize original and review articles so that physicians can keep abreast of the latest evidence. However, Carter et al. found that trials with a positive outcome were more likely to be summarized, after controlling for other reasons for selection (Carter 2006). If positive studies are more likely to be cited, they may be more likely to be located and, thus, more likely to be included in a systematic review, thus biasing the findings of the review.

### 10.2.2.4   Language bias

Reviews have often been exclusively based on studies published in English. For example, among 36 meta-analyses reported in leading English-language general medicine journals from 1991 to 1993, 26 (72%) had restricted their search to studies reported in English (Grégoire 1995). This trend may be changing, with a recent review of 300 systematic reviews finding approximately 16% of reviews limited to trials published in English; systematic reviews published in paper-based journals were more likely than Cochrane reviews to report limiting their search to trials published in English (Moher 2007). In addition, of reviews with a therapeutic focus, Cochrane reviews were more likely than non-Cochrane reviews to report having no language restrictions (62% vs. 26%) (Moher 2007).

Investigators working in a non-English speaking country will publish some of their work in local journals (Dickersin 1994). It is conceivable that authors are more likely to report in an international, English-language journal if results are positive whereas negative findings are published in a local journal. This was demonstrated for the German-language literature (Egger 1997b).

Bias could thus be introduced in reviews exclusively based on English-language reports (Grégoire 1995, Moher 1996). However, the research examining this issue is conflicting. In a study of 50 reviews that employed comprehensive literature searches and included both English and non-English-language trials, Jüni et al. reported that non-English trials were more likely to produce significant results at $P < 0.05$, while estimates of intervention effects were, on average, 16% (95% CI 3% to 26%) more beneficial in non-English-language trials than in English-language trials (Jüni 2002). Conversely, Moher and colleagues examined the effect of inclusion or exclusion of English-language trials in two studies of meta-analyses and found, overall, that the exclusion of trials reported in a language other than English did not significantly affect the results of the meta-analyses (Moher 2003). These results were similar when the analysis was limited to meta-analyses of trials of conventional medicines. When the analyses were conducted separately for meta-analyses of trials of complementary and alternative medicines, however, the effect size of meta-analyses was significantly decreased by excluding reports in languages other than English (Moher 2003).

The extent and effects of language bias may have diminished recently because of the shift towards publication of studies in English. In 2006, Galandi et al. reported a dramatic decline in the number of randomized trials published in German-language healthcare journals: with fewer than two randomized trials published per journal and year after 1999 (Galandi 2006). While the potential impact of studies published in languages other than English in a meta-analysis may be minimal, it is difficult to predict in which cases this exclusion may bias a systematic review. Review authors may want to search without language restrictions and decisions about including reports from languages other than English may need to be taken on a case-by-case basis.

### 10.2.2.5  *Outcome reporting bias*

In many studies, a range of outcome measures is recorded but not all are reported (Pocock 1987, Tannock 1996). The choice of outcomes that are reported can be influenced by the results, potentially making published results misleading. For example, two separate analyses (Mandel 1987, Cantekin 1991) of a double-blind placebo-controlled trial assessing the efficacy of amoxicillin in children with non-suppurative otitis media reached opposite conclusions mainly because different 'weight' was given to the various outcome measures that were assessed in the study. This disagreement was conducted in the public arena, since it was accompanied by accusations of impropriety against the team producing the findings favourable to amoxicillin. The leader of this team had received substantial fiscal support, both in research grants and as personal honoraria, from the manufacturers of amoxicillin (Rennie 1991). It is a good example of how reliance upon the data chosen to be presented by the investigators can lead to distortion (Anonymous 1991). Such 'outcome reporting bias' may be particularly important for adverse effects. Hemminki examined reports of clinical trials submitted by drug companies to licensing authorities in Finland and Sweden and found that unpublished trials gave information on adverse effects more often than published trials (Hemminki 1980). Since then several other studies have shown that the reporting of adverse events and safety outcomes in clinical trials is often inadequate and selective (Ioannidis 2001, Melander 2003, Heres 2006). A group from Canada, Denmark and the UK recently pioneered empirical research into the selective reporting of study outcomes (Chan 2004a, Chan 2004b, Chan 2005). These studies are described in Chapter 8 (Section 8.13), along with a more detailed discussion of outcome reporting bias.

## 10.3 Avoiding reporting biases

### 10.3.1 Implications of the evidence concerning reporting biases

The convincing evidence for the presence of reporting biases, described in Section 10.2, demonstrates the need to search comprehensively for studies that meet the eligibility criteria for a Cochrane review. Review authors should ensure that multiple sources are searched; for example, a search of MEDLINE alone would not be considered sufficient. Sources and methods for searching are described in detail in Chapter 6. Comprehensive searches do not necessarily remove bias, however. Review authors should bear in mind, for example, that study reports may selectively present results; that reference lists may selectively cite sources; and that duplicate publication of results can be difficult to spot. Furthermore, the availability of study information may be subject to time-lag bias, particularly in fast-moving research areas. We now discuss two further means of reducing, or potentially avoiding, reporting biases: the inclusion of unpublished studies, and the use of trial registries.

### 10.3.2 Including unpublished studies in systematic reviews

Publication bias clearly is a major threat to the validity of any type of review, but particularly of unsystematic, narrative reviews. Obtaining and including data from unpublished trials appears to be one obvious way of avoiding this problem. Hopewell and colleagues conducted a review of studies comparing the effect of the inclusion or exclusion of 'grey' literature (defined here as reports that are produced by all levels of government, academics, business and industry in print and electronic formats but that are not controlled by commercial publishers) in meta-analyses of randomized trials (Hopewell 2007b). They included five studies (Fergusson 2000, McAuley 2000, Burdett 2003, Hopewell 2004), all of which showed that published trials had an overall greater intervention effect than grey trials. A meta-analysis of three of these studies suggested that, on average, published trials showed a 9% larger intervention effect than grey trials (Hopewell 2007b).

The inclusion of data from unpublished studies can itself introduce bias. The studies that can be located may be an unrepresentative sample of all unpublished studies. Unpublished studies may be of lower methodological quality than published studies: a study of 60 meta-analyses that included published and unpublished trials found that unpublished trials were less likely to conceal intervention allocation adequately and to blind outcome assessments (Egger 2003). In contrast, Hopewell and colleagues found no difference in the quality of reporting of this information (Hopewell 2004).

A further problem relates to the willingness of investigators of located unpublished studies to provide data. This may depend upon the findings of the study, more favourable results being provided more readily. This could again bias the findings of a systematic review. Interestingly, when Hetherington et al., in a massive effort to obtain information about unpublished trials in perinatal medicine, approached 42,000 obstetricians and paediatricians in 18 countries they identified only 18 unpublished trials that had been completed for more than two years (Hetherington 1989).

A questionnaire assessing the attitudes toward inclusion of unpublished data was sent to the authors of 150 meta-analyses and to the editors of the journals that published them (Cook 1993). Researchers and editors differed in their views about including unpublished data in meta-analyses. Support for the use of unpublished material was evident among a clear majority (78%) of meta-analysts while journal editors were less convinced (47%) (Cook 1993). This study was recently repeated, with a focus on the inclusion of grey literature in systematic reviews, and it was found that acceptance of inclusion of grey literature has increased and, although differences between groups remain (systematic review authors: 86%, editors: 69%), they may have decreased compared with the data presented by Cook et al. (Tetzlaff 2006).

Reasons for reluctance to include grey literature included the absence of peer-review of unpublished literature. It should be kept in mind, however, that the refereeing process has not always been a successful way of ensuring that published results are valid (Godlee 1999). The team involved in preparing a Cochrane review should have at least a similar level of expertise with which to appraise unpublished studies as a peer reviewer for a journal. On the other hand, meta-analyses of unpublished data from interested sources are clearly a cause for concern.

## 10.3.3 Trial registries and publication bias

In September 2004 a number of major medical journals belonging to the International Committee of Medical Journal Editors (ICMJE) announced they would no longer publish trials that were not registered at inception (Abbasi 2004). All trials that began enrolment of participants after September 2005 had to be registered in a public trials registry at or before the onset of enrolment to be considered for publication in those journals. The ICMJE described 'acceptable' registers: electronically searchable, freely accessible to the public, open to all registrants, and managed by a non-profit organization. Similarly, the ICMJE asks clinical trialists to adhere to a minimum dataset proposed by the World Health Organization.

If this long-overdue initiative is successful, it has the potential to substantially reduce the effects of publication bias. However this would depend on review authors identifying all relevant trials by searching online trial registries, and also on the results of unpublished trials identified via registries being made available to them. Initiatives to mandate the registration of trial results are currently in the early stages, are evolving quickly, and should have an impact on the accessibility of these data. While there is emerging evidence suggesting that some of the data fields requested in the registries are incomplete (Zarin 2005), this is likely to improve over time. The extent to which trial registration will facilitate the work of Cochrane review authors is unclear at present. For advice on searching trial registries, see Chapter 6 (Section 6.2.3).

## 10.4   Detecting reporting biases

### 10.4.1   Funnel plots

A funnel plot is a simple scatter plot of the intervention effect estimates from individual studies against some measure of each study's size or precision. In common with forest plots, it is most common to plot the effect estimates on the horizontal scale, and thus the measure of study size on the vertical axis. This is the opposite of conventional graphical displays for scatter plots, in which the outcome (e.g. intervention effect) is plotted on the vertical axis and the covariate (e.g. study size) is plotted on the horizontal axis.

The name 'funnel plot' arises from the fact that precision of the estimated intervention effect increases as the size of the study increases. Effect estimates from small studies will therefore scatter more widely at the bottom of the graph, with the spread narrowing among larger studies. In the absence of bias the plot should approximately resemble a symmetrical (inverted) funnel. This is illustrated in Panel A of Figure 10.4.a, in which the effect estimates in the larger studies are close to the true intervention odds ratio of 0.4.

If there is bias, for example because smaller studies without statistically significant effects (shown as open circles in Figure 10.4.a, Panel A) remain unpublished, this will lead to an asymmetrical appearance of the funnel plot with a gap in a bottom corner of the graph (Panel B). In this situation the effect calculated in a meta-analysis will tend to overestimate the intervention effect (Egger 1997a, Villar 1997). The more pronounced the asymmetry, the more likely it is that the amount of bias will be substantial.

Funnel plots were first used in educational research and psychology, with effect estimates plotted against total sample size (Light 1984). It is now usually recommended that the standard error of the intervention effect estimate be plotted, rather than the

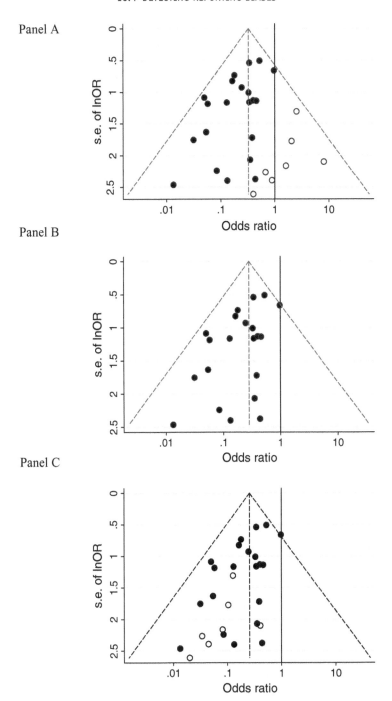

**Figure 10.4.a**  Hypothetical funnel plots
Panel A: symmetrical plot in the absence of bias. Panel B: asymmetrical plot in the presence of reporting bias. Panel C: asymmetrical plot in the presence of bias because some smaller studies (open circles) are of lower methodological quality and therefore produce exaggerated intervention effect estimates.

total sample size, on the vertical axis (Sterne 2001). This is because statistical power of a trial is determined by factors in addition to sample size, such as the number of participants experiencing the event for dichotomous outcomes, and the standard deviation of responses for continuous outcomes. For example, a study with 100,000 participants and 10 events is less likely to show a statistically significant intervention effect than a study with 1000 participants and 100 events. The standard error summarizes these other factors. Plotting standard errors on a reversed scale places the larger, or most powerful, studies towards the top of the plot. Another potential advantage of using standard errors is that a simple triangular region can be plotted, within which 95% of studies would be expected to lie in the absence of both biases and heterogeneity. These regions are included in Figure 10.4.a. Funnel plots of effect estimates against their standard errors (on a reversed scale) can be created using RevMan. A triangular 95% confidence region based on a fixed-effect meta-analysis can be included in the plot, and different plotting symbols allow studies in different subgroups to be identified.

Publication bias need not lead to asymmetry in funnel plots. In the absence of any intervention effect, selective publication based on the P value alone will lead to a symmetrical funnel plot in which studies on the extreme left or right are more likely to be published than those in the middle. This could bias the estimated between-study heterogeneity variance.

Ratio measures of intervention effect (such as odds ratios and risk ratios) should be plotted on a logarithmic scale. This ensures that effects of the same magnitude but opposite directions (for example odds ratios of 0.5 and 2) are equidistant from 1.0. For outcomes measured on a continuous (numerical) scale (e.g. blood pressure, depression score) intervention effects are measured as mean differences or standardized mean differences, which should therefore be used as the horizontal axis in funnel plots. So far as we are aware, no empirical investigations have examined choice of axes for funnel plots for continuous outcomes. For mean differences, the standard error is approximately proportional to the inverse of the square root of the number of participants, and therefore seems an uncontroversial choice for the vertical axis.

Some authors have argued that visual interpretation of funnel plots is too subjective to be useful. In particular, Terrin et al. found that researchers had only a limited ability to correctly identify funnel plots from meta-analyses subject to publication bias (Terrin 2005).

A further, important, problem with funnel plots is that some effect estimates (e.g. odds ratios and standardized mean differences) are naturally correlated with their standard errors, and can produce spurious asymmetry in a funnel plot. We discuss this problem in more detail in Section 10.4.3.

## 10.4.2  Different reasons for funnel plot asymmetry

Although funnel plot asymmetry has long been equated with publication bias (Light 1984, Begg 1988), the funnel plot should be seen as a generic means of displaying *small-study effects* – a tendency for the intervention effects estimated in smaller studies to differ from those estimated in larger studies (Sterne 2000). Small-study effects may

**Table 10.4.a** Possible sources of asymmetry in funnel plots

Adapted from Egger et al. (Egger 1997a).

---

1. **Selection biases**:
   - Publication bias:
     - Delayed publication (also known as 'time-lag' or 'pipeline') bias.
     - Location biases:
       - Language bias;
       - Citation bias;
       - Multiple publication bias.
   - Selective outcome reporting.
2. **Poor methodological quality leading to spuriously inflated effects in smaller studies**:
   - Poor methodological design;
   - Inadequate analysis;
   - Fraud.
3. **True heterogeneity**:
   - Size of effect differs according to study size (for example, due to differences in the intensity of interventions or differences in underlying risk between studies of different sizes).
4. **Artefactual**:
   - In some circumstances (see Section 10.4.3), sampling variation can lead to an association between the intervention effect and its standard error.
5. **Chance**.

---

be due to reasons other than publication bias (Egger 1997a, Sterne 2000). Some of these are shown in Table 10.4.a.

Differences in methodological quality are an important potential source of funnel plot asymmetry. Smaller studies tend to be conducted and analysed with less methodological rigour than larger studies (Egger 2003). Trials of lower quality also tend to show larger intervention effects (Schulz 1995). Therefore trials that would have been 'negative', if conducted and analysed properly, may become 'positive' (Figure 10.4.a, Panel C).

True heterogeneity in intervention effects may also lead to funnel plot asymmetry. For example, substantial benefit may be seen only in patients at high risk for the outcome which is affected by the intervention and these high risk patients are usually more likely to be included in early, small studies (Davey Smith 1994, Glasziou 1995). In addition, small trials are generally conducted before larger trials are established and in the intervening years standard treatment may have improved (resulting in smaller intervention effects in the larger trials). Furthermore, some interventions may have been implemented less thoroughly in larger trials and may, therefore, have resulted in smaller estimates of the intervention effect (Stuck 1998). Finally, it is of course possible that an asymmetrical funnel plot arises merely by the play of chance. Terrin et al. have suggested that the funnel plot is inappropriate for heterogeneous meta-analyses, drawing attention to the premise that the studies come from a single underlying population given by the originators of the funnel plot (Light 1984, Terrin 2003).

A proposed enhancement (Peters 2008) to the funnel plot is to include contour lines corresponding to perceived 'milestones' of statistical significance ($P = 0.01, 0.05, 0.1$

etc). This allows the statistical significance of study estimates, and areas in which studies are perceived to be missing, to be considered. Such 'contour-enhanced' funnel plots may help review authors to differentiate asymmetry due to publication bias from that due to other factors. For example if studies appear to be missing in areas of statistical non-significance (see Figure 10.4.b, Panel A for an example) then this adds credence to the possibility that the asymmetry is due to publication bias. Conversely, if the supposed missing studies are in areas of higher statistical significance (see Figure 10.4.b, Panel B for an example), this would suggest the cause of the asymmetry may be more likely to be due to factors other than publication bias (see Table 10.4.a). If there are no statistically significant studies then publication bias may not be a plausible explanation for funnel plot asymmetry (Ioannidis 2007b).

In interpreting funnel plots, systematic review authors thus need to distinguish the different possible reasons for funnel plot asymmetry listed in Table 10.4.a. Knowledge of the particular intervention, and the circumstances in which it was implemented in different studies, can help identify true heterogeneity as a cause of funnel plot asymmetry. There remains a concern that visual interpretation of funnel plots is inherently subjective. Therefore, we now discuss statistical tests for funnel plot asymmetry, and the extent to which they may assist in the objective interpretation of funnel plots. When review authors are concerned that small study effects are influencing the results of a meta-analysis, they may want to conduct sensitivity analyses in order to explore the robustness of the meta-analysis' conclusions to different assumptions about the causes of funnel plot asymmetry: these are discussed in Section 10.4.4.

## 10.4.3  Tests for funnel plot asymmetry

A test for funnel plot asymmetry (small study effects) formally examines whether the association between estimated intervention effects and a measure of study size (such as the standard error of the intervention effect) is greater than might be expected to occur by chance. For outcomes measured on a continuous (numerical) scale this is reasonably straightforward. Using an approach proposed by Egger et al. (Egger 1997a), we can perform a linear regression of the intervention effect estimates on their standard errors, weighting by 1/(variance of the intervention effect estimate). This looks for a straight-line relationship between intervention effect and its standard error. Under the null hypothesis of no small study effects (e.g. Panel A in Figure 10.4.a) such a line would be vertical. The greater the association between intervention effect and standard error (e.g. as in Panel B in Figure 10.4.a), the more the slope would move away from vertical. Note that the weighting is important to ensure the regression estimates are not dominated by the smaller studies.

When outcomes are dichotomous, and intervention effects are expressed as odds ratios, the approach proposed by Egger et al. (Egger 1997a) corresponds to a linear regression of the log odds ratio on its standard error, weighted by the inverse of the variance of the log odds ratio (Sterne 2000). This has been by far the most widely used and cited approach to testing for funnel plot asymmetry. Unfortunately, there are statistical problems with this approach, because the standard error of the log odds ratio

Panel A

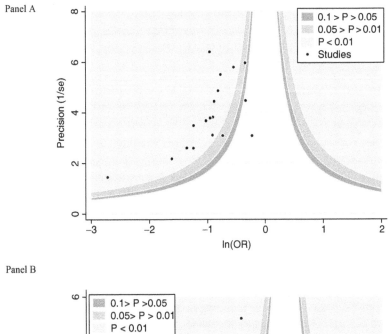

Panel B

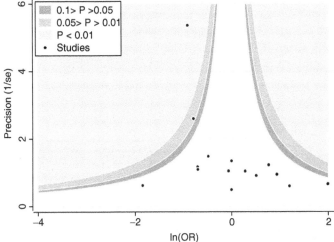

**Figure 10.4.b**   Contour-enhanced funnel plots
Panel A: there is a suggestion of missing studies on the right-hand-side of the plot, broadly in the area of non-significance (i.e. the white area where P > 0.1) for which publication bias is a plausible explanation. Panel B: there is a suggestion of missing studies on the bottom left-hand-side of the plot. Since the majority of this area contains regions of high statistical significance (i.e. indicated by darker shading), this reduces the plausibility that publication bias is the underlying cause of this funnel asymmetry.

is mathematically linked to the size of the odds ratio, even in the absence of small study effects (Irwig 1998) (see Deeks et al. for an algebraic explanation of this phenomenon (Deeks 2005)). This can cause funnel plots plotted using log odds ratios (or odds ratios on a log scale) to appear asymmetric and can mean that P values from the test of

**Table 10.4.b**   Proposed tests for funnel plot asymmetry

$N_{tot}$ is the total sample size, $N_E$ and $N_C$ are the sizes of the experimental and control intervention groups, S is the total number of events across both groups and $F = N_{tot} - S$. Note that only the first three of these tests (Begg 1994, Egger 1997a, Tang 2000) can be used for continuous outcomes.

| Reference | Basis of test |
|---|---|
| (Begg 1994) | Rank correlation between standardized intervention effect and its standard error. |
| (Egger 1997a) | Linear regression of intervention effect estimate against its standard error, weighted by the inverse of the variance of the intervention effect estimate. |
| (Tang 2000) | Linear regression of intervention effect estimate on $1/\sqrt{N_{tot}}$, with weights $N_{tot}$. |
| (Macaskill 2001)* | Linear regression of intervention effect estimate on $N_{tot}$, with weights $S \times F/N_{tot}$. |
| (Deeks 2005)* | Linear regression of log odds ratio on $1/\sqrt{ESS}$ with weights ESS, where effective sample size $ESS = 4N_E \times N_C/N_{tot}$. |
| (Harbord 2006)* | Modified version of the test proposed by Egger et al., based on the 'score' (O–E) and 'score variance' (V) of the log odds ratio. |
| (Peters 2006)* | Linear regression of intervention effect estimate on $1/N_{tot}$, with weights $S \times F/N_{tot}$. |
| (Schwarzer 2007)* | Rank correlation test, using mean and variance of the non-central hypergeometric distribution. |
| (Rücker 2008) | Test based on arcsine transformation of observed risks, with explicit modelling of between-study heterogeneity. |

*Test formulated in terms of odds ratios, but may be applicable to other measures of intervention effect.

Egger et al. are too small, leading to false-positive test results. These problems are especially prone to occur when the intervention has a large effect, there is substantial between-study heterogeneity, there are few events per study, or when all studies are of similar sizes.

A number of authors have therefore proposed alternative tests for funnel plot asymmetry: these are summarized in Table 10.4.b. Because it is impossible to know the precise mechanism for publication bias, simulation studies (in which the tests are evaluated on a large number of computer-generated datasets) are required to evaluate the characteristics of the tests under a range of assumptions about the mechanism for publication bias (Sterne 2000, Macaskill 2001, Harbord 2006, Peters 2006, Schwarzer 2007). The most comprehensive study (in terms of scenarios examined, simulations carried out and the range of tests compared) was reported by Rücker et al. (Rücker 2008). Results of this and the other published simulation studies inform the recommendations on testing for funnel plot asymmetry below. Although simulation studies provide useful insights, they inevitably evaluate circumstances that differ from a particular meta-analysis of interest, so their results must be interpreted carefully.

Most of this methodological work has focused on intervention effects measured as odds ratios. While it seems plausible to expect that corresponding problems will arise for intervention effects measured as risk ratios or standardized mean differences, further investigations of these situations are required.

There is ongoing debate over the representativeness of the parameter values used in the simulation studies, and the mechanisms used to simulate publication bias and small study effects, which are often chosen with little explicit justification. Some potentially useful variations on the different tests remain unexamined. Therefore it is not possible to make definitive recommendations on choice of tests for funnel plot asymmetry. Nevertheless, we can identify three tests that should be considered by review authors wishing to test for funnel plot asymmetry.

None of the tests described here is implemented in RevMan, and consultation with a statistician is recommended for their implementation.

### 10.4.3.1 Recommendations on testing for funnel plot asymmetry

For **all types of outcome**:

- As a rule of thumb, tests for funnel plot asymmetry should be used only when there are at least 10 studies included in the meta-analysis, because when there are fewer studies the power of the tests is too low to distinguish chance from real asymmetry.

- Tests for funnel plot asymmetry should not be used if all studies are of similar sizes (similar standard errors of intervention effect estimates). However, we are not aware of evidence from simulation studies that provides specific guidance on when study sizes should be considered 'too similar'.

- Results of tests for funnel plot asymmetry should be interpreted in the light of visual inspection of the funnel plot. For example, do small studies tend to lead to more or less beneficial intervention effect estimates? Are there studies with markedly different intervention effect estimates (outliers), or studies that are highly influential in the meta-analysis? Is a small P value caused by one study alone? Examining a contour-enhanced funnel plot, as outlined in Section 10.4.1, may further help interpretation of a test result.

- When there is evidence of small-study effects, publication bias should be considered as only one of a number of possible explanations (see Table 10.4.a). Although funnel plots, and tests for funnel plot asymmetry, may alert review authors to a problem which needs considering, they do not provide a solution to this problem.

- Finally, review authors should remember that, because the tests typically have relatively low power, even when a test does not provide evidence of funnel plot asymmetry, bias (including publication bias) cannot be excluded.

For **continuous outcomes with intervention effects measured as mean differences**:

- The test proposed by (Egger 1997a) may be used to test for funnel plot asymmetry. There is currently no reason to prefer any of the more recently proposed tests in this situation, although their relative advantages and disadvantages have not been formally examined. While we know of no research specifically on the power of the approach in the continuous case, general considerations suggest that the power will be greater than for dichotomous outcomes, but that use of the method with substantially fewer than 10 studies would be unwise.

## For **dichotomous outcomes with intervention effects measured as odds ratios:**

- The tests proposed by Harbord et al. (Harbord 2006) and Peters et al. (Peters 2006) avoid the mathematical association between the log odds ratio and its standard error (and hence false-positive test results) that occurs for the test proposed by Egger at al. when there is a substantial intervention effect, while retaining power compared with alternative tests. However, false-positive results may still occur in the presence of substantial between-study heterogeneity.

- The test proposed by Rücker et al. (Rücker 2008) avoids false-positive results both when there is a substantial intervention effect and in the presence of substantial between-study heterogeneity. As a rule of thumb, when the estimated between-study heterogeneity variance of log odds ratios, tau-squared, is more than 0.1, only the version of the arcsine test including random-effects (referred to as 'AS+RE' by Rücker et al.) has been shown to work reasonably well. However it is slightly conservative in the absence of heterogeneity, and its interpretation is less familiar because it is based on an arcsine transformation. (Note that although this recommendation is based on the magnitude of tau-squared other factors, including the sizes of the different studies and their distribution, influence a test's performance. We are not currently able to incorporate these other factors in our recommendations).

- When the heterogeneity variance tau-squared is less than 0.1, one of the tests proposed by Harbord 2006, Peters 2006 or Rücker 2008 can be used. (Test performance generally deteriorates as tau-squared increases).

- As far as possible, review authors should specify their testing strategy in advance (noting that test choice may be dependent on the degree of heterogeneity observed). They should apply only one test, appropriate to the context of the particular meta-analysis, from the above-recommended list and report only the result from their chosen test. Application of two or more tests is undesirable since the most extreme (largest or smallest) P value from a set of tests does not have a well-characterized interpretation.

## For **dichotomous outcomes with intervention effects measured as risk ratios or risk differences, and continuous outcomes with intervention effects measured as standardized mean differences:**

- Potential problems in funnel plots have been less extensively studied for these effect measures than for odds ratios, and firm guidance is not yet available.

- Meta-analyses of risk differences are generally considered less appropriate than meta-analyses using a ratio measure of effect (see Chapter 9, Section 9.4.4.4). For similar reasons, funnel plots using risk differences should seldom be of interest. If the risk ratio (or odds ratio) is constant across studies, then a funnel plot using risk differences will be asymmetrical if smaller studies have higher (or lower) baseline risk.

Based on a survey of meta-analyses published in the *Cochrane Database of Systematic Reviews*, these criteria imply that tests for funnel plot asymmetry should be used in only a minority of meta-analyses (Ioannidis 2007b).

*Tests for which there is insufficient evidence to recommend use*    The following comments apply to all intervention measures. The test proposed by Begg and Mazumdar (Begg 1994) has the same statistical problems but lower power than the test of Egger et al., and is therefore not recommended. The test proposed by Tang and Liu (Tang 2000) has not been evaluated in simulation studies, while the test proposed by Macaskill et al. (Macaskill 2001) has lower power than more recently proposed alternatives. The test proposed by Schwarzer et al. (Schwarzer 2007) avoids the mathematical association between the log odds ratio and its standard error, but has low power relative to the tests discussed above.

   In the context of meta-analyses of intervention studies considered in this chapter, the test proposed by Deeks et al. (Deeks 2005) is likely to have lower power than more recently proposed alternatives. This test was not designed as a test for publication bias in systematic reviews of randomized trials: rather it is aimed at meta-analyses of diagnostic test accuracy studies, where very large odds ratios and very imbalanced studies cause problems for other tests.

## 10.4.4   Sensitivity analyses

When review authors find evidence of small-study effects, they should consider sensitivity analyses examining how the results of the meta-analysis change under different assumptions relating to the reasons for these effects. We stress the exploratory nature of such analysis, due to the inherent difficulty in adjusting for publication bias and lack of research into the performance of such methods applied conditionally based on the results of tests for publication bias considered in Section 10.4.3. This area is relatively underdeveloped; the following approaches have been suggested.

### 10.4.4.1   *Comparing fixed and random-effects estimates*

In the presence of heterogeneity, a random-effects meta-analysis weights the studies relatively more equally than a fixed-effect analysis. It follows that in the presence of small-study effects such as those displayed in Figure 10.2.a, in which the intervention effect is more beneficial in the smaller studies, the random-effects estimate of the intervention effect will be more beneficial than the fixed-effect estimate. Poole and

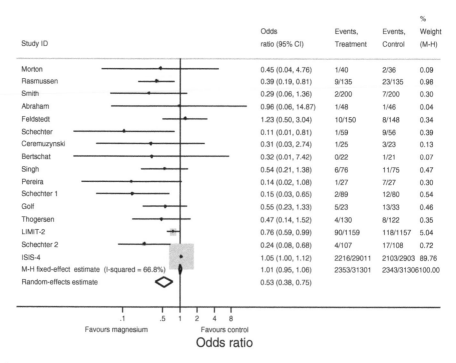

| Study ID | Odds ratio (95% CI) | Events, Treatment | Events, Control | % Weight (M-H) |
|---|---|---|---|---|
| Morton | 0.45 (0.04, 4.76) | 1/40 | 2/36 | 0.09 |
| Rasmussen | 0.39 (0.19, 0.81) | 9/135 | 23/135 | 0.98 |
| Smith | 0.29 (0.06, 1.36) | 2/200 | 7/200 | 0.30 |
| Abraham | 0.96 (0.06, 14.87) | 1/48 | 1/46 | 0.04 |
| Feldstedt | 1.23 (0.50, 3.04) | 10/150 | 8/148 | 0.34 |
| Schechter | 0.11 (0.01, 0.81) | 1/59 | 9/56 | 0.39 |
| Ceremuzynski | 0.31 (0.03, 2.74) | 1/25 | 3/23 | 0.13 |
| Bertschat | 0.32 (0.01, 7.42) | 0/22 | 1/21 | 0.07 |
| Singh | 0.54 (0.21, 1.38) | 6/76 | 11/75 | 0.47 |
| Pereira | 0.14 (0.02, 1.08) | 1/27 | 7/27 | 0.30 |
| Schechter 1 | 0.15 (0.03, 0.65) | 2/89 | 12/80 | 0.54 |
| Golf | 0.55 (0.23, 1.33) | 5/23 | 13/33 | 0.46 |
| Thogersen | 0.47 (0.14, 1.52) | 4/130 | 8/122 | 0.35 |
| LIMIT-2 | 0.76 (0.59, 0.99) | 90/1159 | 118/1157 | 5.04 |
| Schechter 2 | 0.24 (0.08, 0.68) | 4/107 | 17/108 | 0.72 |
| ISIS-4 | 1.05 (1.00, 1.12) | 2216/29011 | 2103/2903 | 89.76 |
| M-H fixed-effect estimate (I-squared = 66.8%) | 1.01 (0.95, 1.06) | 2353/31301 | 2343/31306 | 100.00 |
| Random-effects estimate | 0.53 (0.38, 0.75) | | | |

.1    .5    1    2    4    8

Favours magnesium          Favours control

Odds ratio

**Figure 10.4.c**  Comparison of fixed- and random-effects meta-analytic estimates of the effect of intravenous magnesium on mortality following myocardial infarction

Greenland summarized this by noting that "random-effects meta-analyses are not always conservative" (Poole 1999). This issue is also discussed in Chapter 9 (Section 9.5.4).

An extreme example of the differences between fixed- and random-effects analyses that can arise in the presence of small-study effects is shown in Figure 10.4.c, which displays both fixed- and random-effects estimates of the effect of intravenous magnesium on mortality following myocardial infarction. This is a well-known example in which beneficial effects of intervention were found in a meta-analysis of small studies, subsequently contradicted when the very large ISIS-4 study found no evidence that magnesium affected mortality.

Because there is substantial between-trial heterogeneity, the studies are weighted much more equally in the random-effects analysis than in the fixed-effect analysis. In the fixed-effect analysis the ISIS-4 trial gets 90% of the weight and so there is no evidence of a beneficial intervention effect. In the random-effects analysis the small studies dominate, and there appears to be clear evidence of a beneficial effect of intervention. To interpret the accumulated evidence, it is necessary to make a judgement about the likely validity of the combined evidence from the smaller studies, compared with that from the ISIS-4 trial.

We recommend that when review authors are concerned about the influence of small-study effects on the results of a meta-analysis in which there is evidence of between-study heterogeneity ($I^2>0$), they compare the fixed- and random-effects estimates of the intervention effect. If the estimates are similar, then any small-study effects have little effect on the intervention effect estimate. If the random-effects estimate is more beneficial, review authors should consider whether it is reasonable to conclude that the intervention was more effective in the smaller studies. If the larger studies tend to be those conducted with more methodological rigour, or conducted in circumstances more typical of the use of the intervention in practice, then review authors should consider reporting the results of meta-analyses restricted to the larger, more rigorous studies. Formal evaluation of such strategies in simulation studies would be desirable. Note that formal statistical comparisons of the fixed- and random-effects estimates of intervention effect are not possible, and that it is still possible for small-study effects to bias the results of a meta-analysis in which there is no evidence of heterogeneity, even though the fixed- and random-effects estimates of intervention effect will be identical in this situation.

### 10.4.4.2    Trim and fill

The 'trim and fill' method aims both to identify and correct for funnel plot asymmetry arising from publication bias (Taylor 1998, Duval 2000). The basis of the method is to (1) 'trim' (remove) the smaller studies causing funnel plot asymmetry, (2) use the trimmed funnel plot to estimate the true 'centre' of the funnel, then (3) replace the omitted studies and their missing 'counterparts' around the centre (filling). As well as providing an estimate of the number of missing studies, an adjusted intervention effect is derived by performing a meta-analysis including the filled studies.

The trim and fill method requires no assumptions about the mechanism leading to publication bias, provides an estimate of the number of missing studies, and also provides an estimated intervention effect 'adjusted' for the publication bias (based on the filled studies). However, it is built on the strong assumption that there should be a symmetric funnel plot, and there is no guarantee that the adjusted intervention effect matches what would have been observed in the absence of publication bias, since we cannot know the true mechanism for publication bias. Equally importantly, the trim and fill method does not take into account reasons for funnel plot asymmetry other than publication bias. Therefore, 'corrected' intervention effect estimates from this method should be interpreted with great caution. The method is known to perform poorly in the presence of substantial between-study heterogeneity (Terrin 2003, Peters 2007). Additionally, estimation and inferences are based on a dataset containing imputed intervention effect estimates. Such estimates, it can be argued, inappropriately contribute information that reduces the uncertainty in the summary intervention effect.

### 10.4.4.3    Fail-safe N

Rosenthal suggested assessing the potential for publication bias to have influenced the results of a meta-analysis by calculating the 'fail-safe N', the number of additional 'negative' studies (studies in which the intervention effect was zero) that would be needed to increase the P value for the meta-analysis to above 0.05 (Rosenthal 1979). However the estimate of fail-safe N is highly dependent on the mean intervention effect that is assumed for the unpublished studies (Iyengar 1988), and available methods lead to widely varying estimates of the number of additional studies (Becker 2005). The method also runs against the principle that in medical research in general, and systematic reviews in particular, one should concentrate on the size of the estimated intervention effect and the associated confidence intervals, rather than on whether the P value reaches a particular, arbitrary threshold, although related methods for effect sizes have also been proposed (Orwin 1983). Therefore this and related methods are not recommended for use in Cochrane reviews.

### 10.4.4.4    Other selection models

Other authors have proposed more sophisticated methods that avoid strong assumptions about the association between study P value and publication probability (Dear 1992, Hedges 1992). These methods can be extended to estimate intervention effects, corrected for the estimated publication bias (Vevea 1995). However they require a large number of studies so that a sufficient range of study P values is included. A Bayesian approach in which the number and outcomes of unobserved studies are simulated has also been proposed as a means of correcting intervention effect estimates for publication bias (Givens 1997). Recent work has examined the possibility of assessing robustness over a range of weight functions, thus avoiding the need for large numbers of studies (Vevea 2005). The complexity of the statistical methods, and the large number of studies needed, probably explain why selection models have not been widely used in practice.

### 10.4.4.5    Sensitivity analyses based on selection models

Copas developed a model in which the probability that a study is included in a meta-analysis depends on its standard error. Because it is not possible to estimate all model parameters precisely, he advocates sensitivity analyses in which the value of the estimated intervention effect is computed under a range of assumptions about the severity of the selection bias (Copas 1999). Rather than a single intervention effect estimated 'corrected' for publication bias, the reader can see how the estimated effect (and confidence interval) varies as the assumed amount of selection bias increases. Application of the method to epidemiological studies of environmental tobacco smoke and lung cancer suggests that publication bias may explain some of the association observed in meta-analyses of these studies (Copas 2000).

### 10.4.4.6    Testing for excess of studies with significant results

Ioannidis and Trikalinos propose a simple test that aims to evaluate whether there is an excess of studies that have formally statistically significant results (Ioannidis 2007a).

The test compares the number of studies that have formally statistically significant results with the number of statistically significant results expected under different assumptions about the magnitude of the effect size. The simplest assumption is that the effect size is equal to the observed summary effect in the meta-analysis (but this may introduce an element of circularity). Other values for the underlying effect size, and different thresholds of significance, may be used. Hence, like the contour funnel plots described in Section 10.4.1, but unlike the regression tests, this method considers the distribution of the significance of study results. However, unlike either the regression tests or contour funnel plots, the test does not make any assumption about small-study effects. An excess of significant results can reflect either suppression of whole studies or related selective/manipulative analysis and reporting practices that would cause similar excess.

The test has limited power, as do most other tests, when there are few studies and when there are few studies with significant results. Because the test has not been rigorously evaluated through simulation in comparison with alternative tests and under different scenarios, we currently do not recommend the test as an alternative to those described in Section 10.4.3.

A novel feature of the test is that it can be applied across a large number of meta-analyses on the same research field to examine the extent of publication and selective reporting biases across a whole domain of clinical research. Again, further evaluation of this approach would be welcome.

## 10.4.5 Summary

Although there is clear evidence that publication and other reporting biases lead to over-optimistic estimates of intervention effects, overcoming, detecting and correcting for publication bias is problematic. Comprehensive searches are important, particularly to identify studies as well defined as randomized trials. However, comprehensive searching is not sufficient to prevent some substantial potential biases.

Publication bias should be seen as one of a number of possible causes of 'small-study effects' – a tendency for estimates of the intervention effect to be more beneficial in smaller studies. Funnel plots allow review authors to make a visual assessment of whether small-study effects may be present in a meta-analysis. For continuous (numerical) outcomes with intervention effects measured as mean differences, funnel plots and statistical tests for funnel plot asymmetry are valid. However for dichotomous outcomes with intervention effects expressed as odds ratios, the standard error of the log odds ratio is mathematically linked to the size of the odds ratio, even in the absence of small-study effects. This can cause funnel plots plotted using log odds ratios (or odds ratios on a log scale) to appear asymmetric and can mean that P values from the test of Egger et al. are too small. For other effect measures, firm guidance is not yet offered. Three statistical tests for small-study effects are recommended for use in Cochrane reviews, provided that there are at least 10 studies. However, none is implemented in RevMan and statistical support is usually required. Only one test has been shown to work when the between-study heterogeneity variance exceeds 0.1. Results from tests for funnel plot asymmetry should be interpreted cautiously. When there is evidence of small-study effects, publication bias should be considered as only one of a number of possible explanations. In these circumstances, review authors should attempt to understand the source of the small-study effects, and consider their implications in sensitivity analyses.

## 10.5 Chapter information

**Editors:** Jonathan AC Sterne, Matthias Egger and David Moher on behalf of the Cochrane Bias Methods Group.

---

### Box 10.5.a   The Cochrane Bias Methods Group

The Bias Methods Group (BMG), previously the Reporting Bias Methods Group, was formally registered as a Methods Group in 2000. The BMG addresses a range of different forms of bias, such as publication bias, language bias, selective outcome reporting bias and biases arising from study design and conduct. A major initiative of the group, in collaboration with the Statistical Methods Group, was the development of the new guidance for assessing risk of bias of included studies in Cochrane reviews.

   Activities of BMG members include:

- undertaking empirical research to examine whether, and in which circumstances, various biases may have a substantial impact on systematic reviews, including the preparation of Cochrane Methodology reviews;
- undertaking methodological research on how to identify and address potential biases in systematic reviews and meta-analyses;
- helping to complete and co-ordinate Methods systematic reviews pertinent to the Group's remit;
- providing advice to Cochrane entities; and
- offering training to both Cochrane and non-Cochrane systematic reviewers via formal and informal opportunities.

The BMG membership emailing list is used as a forum for discussion and dissemination of information. Cochrane newsletters and email distribution lists, such as the Cochrane Methods Group newsletter, *Cochrane News* and CCInfo, are also used for dissemination of group activities.

*Funding*: The BMG receives infrastructure funding as part of a commitment by the Canadian Institutes of Health Research (CIHR) and the Canadian Agency for Drugs and Technologies in Health (CADTH) to fund Canadian-based Cochrane entities. This supports dissemination activities, web hosting, travel, training, workshops and a full time Co-ordinator position.

*Web site*: www.chalmersresearch.com\bmg

**This chapter should be cited as:** Sterne JAC, Egger M, Moher D (editors). Chapter 10: Addressing reporting biases. In: Higgins JPT, Green S (editors). *Cochrane Handbook for Systematic Reviews of Interventions*. Chichester (UK): John Wiley & Sons, 2008.

**Contributing authors:** James Carpenter, Matthias Egger, Roger Harbord, Julian Higgins, David Jones, David Moher, Jonathan Sterne, Alex Sutton and Jennifer Tetzlaff.

**Acknowledgements:** We thank Doug Altman, Jon Deeks, John Ioannidis, Jaime Peters and Gerta Rücker for helpful comments.

**Declarations of interest:** James Carpenter, Jon Deeks, Matthias Egger, Roger Harbord, David Jones, Jaime Peters, Gerta Rücker, Jonathan Sterne and Alex Sutton are all authors on papers proposing tests for funnel plot asymmetry.

# 10.6 References

**Abbasi 2004**
Abbasi K. Compulsory registration of clinical trials. *BMJ* 2004; 329: 637–638.
**Abbot 1998**
Abbot NC, Ernst E. Publication bias: direction of outcome is less important than scientific quality. *Perfusion* 1998; 11: 182–182.
**Anonymous 1991**
Anonymous. Subjectivity in data analysis. *The Lancet* 1991; 337: 401–402.
**Bailey 2002**
Bailey BJ. Duplicate publication in the field of otolaryngology-head and neck surgery. *Archives of Otolaryngology* 2002; 126: 211–216.
**Barden 2003**
Barden J, Edwards JE, McQuay HJ, Moore RA. Oral valdecoxib and injected parecoxib for acute postoperative pain: a quantitative systematic review. *BMC Anesthesiology* 2003; 3: 1.
**Bardy 1998**
Bardy AH. Bias in reporting clinical trials. *British Journal of Clinical Pharmacology* 1998; 46: 147–150.
**Becker 2005**
Becker BJ. Failsafe *N* or file-drawer number. In: Rothstein HR, Sutton AJ, Borenstein M (editors). *Publication Bias in Meta-Analysis* (1). Chichester (UK): John Wiley & Sons, 2005.
**Begg 1988**
Begg CB, Berlin JA. Publication bias: a problem in interpreting medical data. *Journal of the Royal Statistical Society Series A* 1988; 151: 419–463.
**Begg 1994**
Begg CB, Mazumdar M. Operating characteristics of a rank correlation test for publication bias. *Biometrics* 1994; 50: 1088–1101.
**Bhandari 2004**
Bhandari M, Busse JW, Jackowski D, Montori VM, Schünemann H, Sprague S, Mears D, Schemitsch EH, Heels-Ansdell D, Devereaux PJ. Association between industry funding and statistically significant pro-industry findings in medical and surgical randomized trials. *Canadian Medical Association Journal* 2004; 170: 477–480.

**Blumenthal 1997**

Blumenthal D, Campbell EG, Anderson MS, Causino N, Louis KS. Withholding research results in academic life science. Evidence from a national survey of faculty. *JAMA* 1997; 277: 1224–1228.

**Brooks 1985**

Brooks TA. Private acts and public objects: an investigation of citer motivations. *Journal of the American Society for Information Science* 1985; 36: 223–229.

**Burdett 2003**

Burdett S, Stewart LA, Tierney JF. Publication bias and meta-analyses: a practical example. *International Journal of Technology Assessment in Health Care* 2003; 19: 129–134.

**Cantekin 1991**

Cantekin EI, McGuire TW, Griffith TL. Antimicrobial therapy for otitits media with effusion ('secretory' otitits media). *JAMA* 1991; 266: 3309–3317.

**Carter 2006**

Carter AO, Griffin GH, Carter TP. A survey identified publication bias in the secondary literature. *Journal of Clinical Epidemiology* 2006; 59: 241–245.

**Chan 2004a**

Chan AW, Hróbjartsson A, Haahr MT, Gøtzsche PC, Altman DG. Empirical evidence for selective reporting of outcomes in randomized trials: comparison of protocols to published articles. *JAMA* 2004; 291: 2457–2465.

**Chan 2004b**

Chan AW, Krleža-Jeric K, Schmid I, Altman DG. Outcome reporting bias in randomized trials funded by the Canadian Institutes of Health Research. *Canadian Medical Association Journal* 2004; 171: 735–740.

**Chan 2005**

Chan AW, Altman DG. Identifying outcome reporting bias in randomised trials on PubMed: review of publications and survey of authors. *BMJ* 2005; 330: 753.

**CLASP Collaborative Group 1994**

CLASP Collaborative Group. CLASP: a randomized trial of low-dose aspirin for the prevention and treatment of pre-eclampsia among 9364 pregnant women. *The Lancet* 1994; 343: 619–629.

**Cook 1993**

Cook DJ, Guyatt GH, Ryan G, Clifton J, Buckingham L, Willan A, McIlroy W, Oxman AD. Should unpublished data be included in meta-analyses? Current convictions and controversies. *JAMA* 1993; 269: 2749–2753.

**Copas 1999**

Copas J. What works?: selectivity models and meta-analysis. *Journal of the Royal Statistical Society Series A* 1999; 162: 95–109.

**Copas 2000**

Copas JB, Shi JQ. Reanalysis of epidemiological evidence on lung cancer and passive smoking. *BMJ* 2000; 320: 417–418.

**Cowley 1993**

Cowley AJ, Skene A, Stainer K, Hampton JR. The effect of lorcainide on arrhythmias and survival in patients with acute myocardial infarction: an example of publication bias. *International Journal of Cardiology* 1993; 40: 161–166.

**Davey Smith 1994**

Davey Smith G, Egger M. Who benefits from medical interventions? Treating low risk patients can be a high risk strategy. *BMJ* 1994; 308: 72–74.

**Dear 1992**

Dear KBG, Begg CB. An approach to assessing publication bias prior to performing a meta-analysis. *Statistical Science* 1992; 7: 237–245.

**Decullier 2005**

Decullier E, Lheritier V, Chapuis F. Fate of biomedical research protocols and publication bias in France: retrospective cohort study. *BMJ* 2005; 331: 19.

**Decullier 2007**

Decullier E, Chapuis F. Oral presentation bias: a retrospective cohort study. *Journal of Epidemiology and Community Health* 2007; 61: 190–193.

**Deeks 2005**

Deeks JJ, Macaskill P, Irwig L. The performance of tests of publication bias and other sample size effects in systematic reviews of diagnostic test accuracy was assessed. *Journal of Clinical Epidemiology* 2005; 58: 882–893.

**Dickersin 1992**

Dickersin K, Min YI, Meinert CL. Factors influencing publication of research results: follow-up of applications submitted to two institutional review boards. *JAMA* 1992; 263: 374–378.

**Dickersin 1993**

Dickersin K, Min YI. NIH clinical trials and publication bias. *Online Journal of Current Clinical Trials* 1993; Doc No 50.

**Dickersin 1994**

Dickersin K, Scherer R, Lefebvre C. Identifying relevant studies for systematic reviews. *BMJ* 1994; 309: 1286–1291.

**Dickersin 1997**

Dickersin K. How important is publication bias? A synthesis of available data. *AIDS Education and Prevention* 1997; 9: 15–21.

**Dickersin 2002**

Dickersin K, Olson CM, Rennie D, Cook D, Flanagin A, Zhu Q, Reiling J, Pace B. Association between time interval to publication and statistical significance. *JAMA* 2002; 287: 2829–2831.

**Dong 1997**

Dong BJ, Hauck WW, Gambertoglio JG, Gee L, White JR, Bubp JL, Greenspan FS. Bioequivalence of generic and brand-name levothyroxine products in the treatment of hypothyroidism [see comments]. *JAMA* 1997; 277: 1205–1213.

**Duval 2000**

Duval S, Tweedie R. Trim and fill: A simple funnel-plot-based method of testing and adjusting for publication bias in meta-analysis. *Biometrics* 2000; 56: 455–463.

**Easterbrook 1991**

Easterbrook PJ, Berlin JA, Gopalan R, Matthews DR. Publication bias in clinical research. *The Lancet* 1991; 337: 867–872.

**Egger 1997a**

Egger M, Smith GD, Schneider M, Minder C. Bias in meta-analysis detected by a simple, graphical test. *BMJ* 1997; 315: 629–634.

**Egger 1997b**

Egger M, Zellweger Z, Schneider M, Junker C, Lengeler C, Antes G. Language bias in randomised controlled trials published in English and German. *The Lancet* 1997; 350: 326–329.

**Egger 2003**

Egger M, Jüni P, Bartlett C, Holenstein F, Sterne J. How important are comprehensive literature searches and the assessment of trial quality in systematic reviews? Empirical study. *Health Technology Assessment* 2003; 7: 1.

**Epstein 1990**

Epstein WM. Confirmational response bias among social work journals. *Science, Technology and Human Values* 1990; 15: 9–37.

**Ernst 1994**

Ernst E, Resch KL. Reviewer bias: A blinded experimental study. *Journal of Laboratory and Clinical Medicine* 1994; 124: 178–182.

**Fergusson 2000**

Fergusson D, Laupacis A, Salmi LR, McAlister FA, Huet C. What should be included in meta-analyses? An exploration of methodological issues using the ISPOT meta-analyses. *International Journal of Technology Assessment in Health Care* 2000; 16: 1109–1119.

**Galandi 2006**

Galandi D, Schwarzer G, Antes G. The demise of the randomised controlled trial: bibliometric study of the German-language health care literature, 1948 to 2004. *BMC Medical Research Methodology* 2006; 6: 30.

**Givens 1997**

Givens GH, Smith DD, Tweedie RL. Publication bias in meta-analysis:a Bayesian data-augmentation approach to account for issues exemplified in the passive smoking debate. *Statistical Science* 1997; 12: 221–250.

**Glasziou 1995**

Glasziou PP, Iriwg LM. An evidence based approach to individualising treatment. *BMJ* 1995; 311: 1356–1359.

**Godlee 1999**

Godlee F, Dickersin K. Bias, subjectivity, chance, and conflict of interest in editorial decisions. In: Godlee F, Jefferson T (editors). *Peer Review in Health Sciences*. London (UK): BMJ Books, 1999.

**Gøtzsche 1987**

Gøtzsche PC. Reference bias in reports of drug trials. *British Medical Journal (Clinical Research Edition)* 1987; 295: 654–656.

**Gøtzsche 1989**

Gøtzsche PC. Multiple publication of reports of drug trials. *European Journal of Clinical Pharmacology* 1989; 36: 429–432.

**Grégoire 1995**

Grégoire G, Derderian F, LeLorier J. Selecting the language of the publications included in a meta-analysis: is there a Tower of Babel bias? *Journal of Clinical Epidemiology* 1995; 48: 159–163.

**Harbord 2006**

Harbord RM, Egger M, Sterne JA. A modified test for small-study effects in meta-analyses of controlled trials with binary endpoints. *Statistics in Medicine* 2006; 25: 3443–3457.

**Hartling 2004**

Hartling L, Craig WR, Russell K, Stevens K, Klassen TP. Factors influencing the publication of randomized controlled trials in child health research. *Archives of Pediatrics and Adolescent Medicine* 2004; 158: 983–987.

**Hedges 1992**

Hedges LV. Modeling publication selection effects in meta-analysis. *Statistical Science* 1992; 7: 246–255.

**Hemminki 1980**

Hemminki E. Study of information submitted by drug companies to licensing authorities. *British Medical Journal* 1980; 280: 833–836.

**Heres 2006**
Heres S, Davis J, Maino K, Jetzinger E, Kissling W, Leucht S. Why olanzapine beats risperidone, risperidone beats quetiapine, and quetiapine beats olanzapine: an exploratory analysis of head-to-head comparison studies of second-generation antipsychotics. *American Journal of Psychiatry* 2006; 163: 185–194.

**Hetherington 1989**
Hetherington J, Dickersin K, Chalmers I, Meinert CL. Retrospective and prospective identification of unpublished controlled trials: lessons from a survey of obstetricians and pediatricians. *Pediatrics* 1989; 84: 374–380.

**Hopewell 2004**
Hopewell S. *Impact of grey literature on systematic reviews of randomized trials* (PhD thesis). University of Oxford, 2004.

**Hopewell 2007a**
Hopewell S, Clarke M, Stewart L, Tierney J. Time to publication for results of clinical trials. *Cochrane Database of Systematic Reviews* 2007, Issue 2. Art No: MR000011.

**Hopewell 2007b**
Hopewell S, McDonald S, Clarke M, Egger M. Grey literature in meta-analyses of randomized trials of health care interventions. *Cochrane Database of Systematic Reviews* 2007, Issue 2. Art No: MR000010.

**Hopewell 2008**
Hopewell S, Loudon K, Clarke M, Oxman AD, Dickersin K. Publication bias in clinical trials due to statistical significance or direction of trial results. *Cochrane Database of Systematic Reviews* (to appear).

**Huston 1996**
Huston P, Moher D. Redundancy, disaggregation, and the integrity of medical research. *The Lancet* 1996; 347: 1024–1026.

**Hutchison 1995**
Hutchison BG, Oxman AD, Lloyd S. Comprehensiveness and bias in reporting clinical trials. *Canadian Family Physician* 1995; 41: 1356–1360.

**Ioannidis 1998**
Ioannidis JP. Effect of the statistical significance of results on the time to completion and publication of randomized efficacy trials. *JAMA* 1998; 279: 281–286.

**Ioannidis 2001**
Ioannidis JP, Lau J. Completeness of safety reporting in randomized trials: an evaluation of 7 medical areas. *JAMA* 2001; 285: 437–443.

**Ioannidis 2007a**
Ioannidis JP, Trikalinos TA. An exploratory test for an excess of significant findings. *Clinical Trials* 2007; 4: 245–253.

**Ioannidis 2007b**
Ioannidis JP, Trikalinos TA. The appropriateness of asymmetry tests for publication bias in meta-analyses: a large survey. *Canadian Medical Association Journal* 2007; 176: 1091–1096.

**Irwig 1998**
Irwig L, Macaskill P, Berry G, Glasziou P. Bias in meta-analysis detected by a simple, graphical test. Graphical test is itself biased. *BMJ* 1998; 316: 470–471.

**Iyengar 1988**
Iyengar S, Greenhouse JB. Selection problems and the file drawer problem. *Statistical Science* 1988: 109–135.

**Johansen 1999**
Johansen HK, Gøtzsche PC. Problems in the design and reporting of trials of antifungal agents encountered during meta-analysis [see comments]. *JAMA* 1999; 282: 1752–1759.

**Jüni 2002**
Jüni P, Holenstein F, Sterne J, Bartlett C, Egger M. Direction and impact of language bias in meta-analyses of controlled trials: empirical study. *International Journal of Epidemiology* 2002; 31: 115–123.

**Kjaergard 2002**
Kjaergard LL, Gluud C. Citation bias of hepato-biliary randomized clinical trials. *Journal of Clinical Epidemiology* 2002; 55: 407–410.

**Lexchin 2003**
Lexchin J, Bero LA, Djulbegovic B, Clark O. Pharmaceutical industry sponsorship and research outcome and quality: systematic review. *BMJ* 2003; 326: 1167–1170.

**Liebeskind 2006**
Liebeskind DS, Kidwell CS, Sayre JW, Saver JL. Evidence of publication bias in reporting acute stroke clinical trials. *Neurology* 2006; 67: 973–979.

**Light 1984**
Light RJ, Pillemer DB. *Summing Up. The Science of Reviewing Research* (1). Cambridge (MA): Harvard University Press, 1984.

**Macaskill 2001**
Macaskill P, Walter SD, Irwig L. A comparison of methods to detect publication bias in meta-analysis. *Statistics in Medicine* 2001; 20: 641–654.

**Mahoney 1977**
Mahoney MJ. Publication prejudices: An experimental study of confirmatory bias in the peer review system. *Cognitive Therapy and Research* 1977; 1: 161–175.

**Mandel 1987**
Mandel EH, Rockette HE, Bluestone CD, Paradise JL, Nozza RJ. Efficacy of amoxicillin with and without decongestant-antihistamine for otitis media with effusion in children. *New England Journal of Medicine* 1987; 316: 432–437.

**McAuley 2000**
McAuley L, Pham B, Tugwell P, Moher D. Does the inclusion of grey literature influence estimates of intervention effectiveness reported in meta-analyses? *The Lancet* 2000; 356: 1228–1231.

**Melander 2003**
Melander H, Ahlqvist-Rastad J, Meijer G, Beermann B. Evidence b(i)ased medicine – selective reporting from studies sponsored by pharmaceutical industry: review of studies in new drug applications. *BMJ* 2003; 326: 1171–1173.

**Moher 1996**
Moher D, Fortin P, Jadad AR, Jüni P, Klassen T, Le Lorier J, Liberati A, Linde K, Penna A. Completeness of reporting of trials published in languages other than English: implications for conduct and reporting of systematic reviews. *The Lancet* 1996; 347: 363–366.

**Moher 2000**
Moher D, Pham B, Klassen TP, Schulz KF, Berlin JA, Jadad AR, Liberati A. What contributions do languages other than English make on the results of meta-analyses? *Journal of Clinical Epidemiology* 2000; 53: 964–972.

**Moher 2003**
Moher D, Pham B, Lawson ML, Klassen TP. The inclusion of reports of randomised trials published in languages other than English in systematic reviews. *Health Technology Assessment* 2003; 7: 1–90.

**Moher 2007**
Moher D, Tetzlaff J, Tricco AC, Sampson M, Altman DG. Epidemiology and reporting characteristics of systematic reviews. *PLoS Medicine* 2007; 4: e78.

**Moscati 1994**

Moscati R, Jehle D, Ellis D, Fiorello A, Landi M. Positive-outcome bias: comparison of emergency medicine and general medicine literatures. *Academic Emergency Medicine* 1994; 1: 267–271.

**Olson 2002**

Olson CM, Rennie D, Cook D, Dickersin K, Flanagin A, Hogan JW, Zhu Q, Reiling J, Pace B. Publication bias in editorial decision making. *JAMA* 2002; 287: 2825–2828.

**Orwin 1983**

Orwin RG. A fail-safe *N* for effect size in meta-analysis. *Journal of Educational Statistics* 1983; 8: 157–159.

**Peters 1982**

Peters DP, Ceci SJ. Peer review practices of psychology journals: The fate of published articles, submitted again. *Behavioral and Brain Sciences* 1982; 5: 187–255.

**Peters 2006**

Peters JL, Sutton AJ, Jones DR, Abrams KR, Rushton L. Comparison of two methods to detect publication bias in meta-analysis. *JAMA* 2006; 295: 676–680.

**Peters 2007**

Peters JL, Sutton AJ, Jones DR, Abrams KR, Rushton L. Performance of the trim and fill method in the presence of publication bias and between-study heterogeneity. *Statistics in Medicine* 2007; 26: 4544–4562.

**Peters 2008**

Peters J, Sutton AJ, Jones DR, Abrams KR, Rushton L. The contour enhanced funnel plot: an aid to interpreting funnel asymmetry. *Journal of Clinical Epidemiology* (in press, 2008).

**Pham 2005**

Pham B, Klassen TP, Lawson ML, Moher D. Language of publication restrictions in systematic reviews gave different results depending on whether the intervention was conventional or complementary. *Journal of Clinical Epidemiology* 2005; 58: 769–776.

**Pittler 2000**

Pittler MH, Abbot NC, Harkness EF, Ernst E. Location bias in controlled clinical trials of complementary/alternative therapies. *Journal of Clinical Epidemiology* 2000; 53: 485–489.

**Pocock 1987**

Pocock S, Hughes MD, Lee RJ. Statistical problems in the reporting of clinical trials. A survey of three medical journals. *New England Journal of Medicine* 1987; 317: 426–432.

**Poole 1999**

Poole C, Greenland S. Random-effects meta-analyses are not always conservative. *American Journal of Epidemiology* 1999; 150: 469–475.

**Ravnskov 1992**

Ravnskov U. Cholesterol lowering trials in coronary heart disease: frequency of citation and outcome. *BMJ* 1992; 305: 15–19.

**Rennie 1991**

Rennie D. The Cantekin affair. *JAMA* 1991; 266: 3333–3337.

**Rennie 1997**

Rennie D. Thyroid Storms. *JAMA* 1997; 277: 1238–1243.

**Rosenthal 1979**

Rosenthal R. The 'file drawer problem' and tolerance for null results. *Psychological Bulletin* 1979; 86: 638–641.

**Rücker 2008**

Rücker G, Schwarzer G, Carpenter J. Arcsine test for publication bias in meta-analyses with binary outcomes. *Statistics in Medicine* 2008; 27: 746–763.

**Sampson 2003**

Sampson M, Barrowman NJ, Moher D, Klassen TP, Pham B, Platt R, St JP, Viola R, Raina P. Should meta-analysts search Embase in addition to Medline? *Journal of Clinical Epidemiology* 2003; 56: 943–955.

**Scherer 2007**

Scherer RW, Langenberg P, von EE. Full publication of results initially presented in abstracts. *Cochrane Database of Systematic Reviews* 2007, Issue 2. Art No: MR000005.

**Schulz 1995**

Schulz KF, Chalmers I, Hayes RJ, Altman DG. Empirical evidence of bias. Dimensions of methodological quality associated with estimates of treatment effects in controlled trials. *JAMA* 1995; 273: 408–412.

**Schwarzer 2007**

Schwarzer G, Antes G, Schumacher M. A test for publication bias in meta-analysis with sparse binary data. *Statistics in Medicine* 2006.

**Simes 1987**

Simes RJ. Confronting publication bias: a cohort design for meta-analysis. *Statistics in Medicine* 1987; 6: 11–29.

**Smith 1999**

Smith R. What is publication? A continuum. *BMJ* 1999; 318: 142.

**Sterling 1959**

Sterling TD. Publication decisions and their possible effects on inferences drawn from tests of significance – or vice versa. *Journal of the American Statistical Association* 1959; 54: 30–34.

**Sterling 1995**

Sterling TD, Rosenbaum WL, Weinkam JJ. Publication decisions revisted: The effect of the outcome of statistical tests on the decision to publish and vice versa. *American Statatistician* 1995; 49: 108–112.

**Stern 1997**

Stern JM, Simes RJ. Publication bias: evidence of delayed publication in a cohort study of clinical research projects. *BMJ* 1997; 315: 640–645.

**Sterne 2000**

Sterne JAC, Gavaghan D, Egger M. Publication and related bias in meta-analysis: Power of statistical tests and prevalence in the literature. *Journal of Clinical Epidemiology* 2000; 53: 1119–1129.

**Sterne 2001**

Sterne JAC, Egger M. Funnel plots for detecting bias in meta-analysis: Guidelines on choice of axis. *Journal of Clinical Epidemiology* 2001; 54: 1046–1055.

**Stuck 1998**

Stuck AE, Rubenstein LZ, Wieland D. Bias in meta-analysis detected by a simple, graphical test. Asymmetry detected in funnel plot was probably due to true heterogeneity. Letter. *BMJ* 1998; 316: 469–471.

**Tang 2000**

Tang JL, Liu JL. Misleading funnel plot for detection of bias in meta-analysis. *Journal of Clinical Epidemiology* 2000; 53: 477–484.

**Tannock 1996**

Tannock IF. False-positive results in clinical trials: multiple significance tests and the problem of unreported comparisons. *Journal of the National Cancer Institute* 1996; 88: 206–207.

**Taylor 1998**

Taylor SJ, Tweedie RL. Practical estimates of the effect of publication bias in meta-analysis. *Australian Epidemiologist* 1998; 5: 14–17.

**Teo 1993**
Teo KK, Yusuf S, Furberg CD. Effects of prophylactic antiarrhythmic drug therapy in acute myocardial infarction. An overview of results from randomized controlled trials [see comments]. *JAMA* 1993; 270: 1589–1595.

**Terrin 2003**
Terrin N, Schmid CH, Lau J, Olkin I. Adjusting for publication bias in the presence of heterogeneity. *Statistics in Medicine* 2003; 22: 2113–2126.

**Terrin 2005**
Terrin N, Schmid CH, Lau J. In an empirical evaluation of the funnel plot, researchers could not visually identify publication bias. *Journal of Clinical Epidemiology* 2005; 58: 894–901.

**Tetzlaff 2006**
Tetzlaff J, Moher D, Pham B, Altman D. Survey of views on including grey literature in systematic reviews. *14th Cochrane Colloquium*, Dublin (Ireland), 2006.

**Tramèr 1997**
Tramèr MR, Reynolds DJ, Moore RA, McQuay HJ. Impact of covert duplicate publication on meta-analysis: a case study. *BMJ* 1997; 315: 635–640.

**Vevea 1995**
Vevea JL, Hedges LV. A general linear model for estimating effect size in the presence of publication bias. *Psychometrika* 1995; 60: 419–435.

**Vevea 2005**
Vevea JL, Woods CM. Publication bias in research synthesis: sensitivity analysis using a priori weight functions. *Psychological Methods* 2005; 10: 428–443.

**Vickers 1998**
Vickers A, Goyal N, Harland R, Rees R. Do certain countries produce only positive results? A systematic review of controlled trials. *Controlled Clinical Trials* 1998; 19: 159–166.

**Villar 1997**
Villar J, Piaggio G, Carroli G, Donner A. Factors affecting the comparability of meta-analyses and largest trials results in perinatology. *Journal of Clinical Epidemiology* 1997; 50: 997–1002.

**Weber 1998**
Weber EJ, Callaham ML, Wears RL, Barton C, Young G. Unpublished research from a medical specialty meeting: why investigators fail to publish. *JAMA* 1998; 280: 257–259.

**Zarin 2005**
Zarin DA, Tse T, Ide NC. Trial Registration at ClinicalTrials.gov between May and October 2005. *New England Journal of Medicine* 2005; 353: 2779–2787.

# 11 Presenting results and 'Summary of findings' tables

Holger J Schünemann, Andrew D Oxman, Julian PT Higgins, Gunn E Vist, Paul Glasziou and Gordon H Guyatt on behalf of the Cochrane Applicability and Recommendations Methods Group and the Cochrane Statistical Methods Group

## Key Points

- Tables and figures help to present included studies and their findings in a systematic and clear format.

- Forest plots are the standard way to illustrate results of individual studies and meta-analyses. These can be generated using Review Manager software, and a selection of them can be chosen for inclusion in the body of a Cochrane review.

- A 'Summary of findings' table provides key information concerning the quality of evidence, the magnitude of effect of the interventions examined, and the sum of available data on all important outcomes for a given comparison.

- The Abstract of a Cochrane review should be targeted primarily at healthcare decision makers (including clinicians, informed consumers and policy makers); and a 'Plain language summary' conveys the findings in a straightforward style that can be understood by consumers of health care.

## 11.1 Introduction

The Results section of a review should summarize the findings in a clear and logical order, and should explicitly address the objectives of the review. Review authors can use a variety of tables and figures to present information in a more convenient format:

- 'Characteristics of included studies' tables (including 'Risk of bias' tables).

- 'Data and analyses' (the full set of data tables and forest plots).

- Figures (a selection of forest plots, funnel plots, 'Risk of bias' plots and other figures).

- 'Summary of findings' tables.

- Additional tables.

'Characteristics of included studies' tables present information on individual studies; 'Data and analyses' tables and forest plots present outcome data from individual studies and may additionally include meta-analyses; 'Summary of findings' tables present the cumulative information, data and quality of evidence for the most important outcomes. The findings of a review also must be summarized for an abstract and for a plain language summary.

'Summary of findings' tables are key among these presentation tools, and a substantial part of this chapter is dedicated to them. We discuss the specification of the important outcomes that might be relevant to people considering the intervention(s) under study, a step that we believe is often neglected in Cochrane reviews. We then present examples of 'Summary of findings' tables, and describe the contents of those tables. Chapter 12 discusses issues in the interpretation of results.

## 11.2  'Characteristics of included studies' tables

Review authors must decide which characteristics of the studies are likely to be relevant to users of the review. Review authors should, as a minimum, include the following in the 'Characteristics of included studies' table:

**Methods:** study design (stating whether or not the study was randomized), including, where relevant, a clear indication of how the study differs from a standard parallel group design (e.g. a cross-over or cluster-randomized design); duration of the study (if not included under Intervention). Note: the 'Methods' entry should not include measures of risk of bias; these should appear in a 'Risk of bias' table (see Chapter 8, Section 8.5).

**Participants:** setting; relevant details of health status of participants; age; sex; country. Sufficient information should be provided to allow users of the review to determine the applicability of the study to their population, and to allow exploration of differences in participants across studies.

**Intervention:** a clear list of the intervention groups included in the study. If feasible, sufficient information should be provided for each intervention to be replicated in practice; for drug interventions, include details of drug name, dose, frequency, mode of administration (if not obvious), duration (if not included under Methods); for non-drug interventions, include relevant considerations and components related to the intervention.

**Outcomes:** a clear list of either (i) outcomes and time-points from the study that are considered in the review; or (ii) outcomes and time-points measured (or reported) in the study. Study results should not be included here (or elsewhere in this table).

**Notes:** further comments from the review authors on aspects of the study that are not covered by the categories above. Note that assessments of risk of bias should be made in a 'Risk of bias' table.

It is possible to add up to three extra fields in the 'Characteristics of included studies' table. Where appropriate, review authors are recommended to use an extra field to provide information about the funding of each study.

# 11.3 Data and analyses

## 11.3.1 The 'Data and analyses' section of a review

The 'Data and analyses' section of a Cochrane review is a detailed resource of results. It includes outcome data (numeric or text), forest plots and meta-analysis results. The root of the 'Data and analyses' resource is a table of comparisons, outcomes and (optionally) subgroups for which data are available. Analyses listed in this table comprise either a table of results ('other data' tables) or, more usually, a table of data accompanied by a forest plot. The 'Data and analyses' tables are included in the full publication of a Cochrane review. However, some formats of a published review may omit the forest plots and 'other data' tables (along with appendices), and so they should generally be considered as supplementary material, and key results should be included in the text of the review under 'Results'. The published review will always include a summary table of all analyses (including numbers of studies and meta-analysis results for each subgroup under each outcome for each comparison). The review should include the most important forest plots from the 'Data and analyses' resource as figures and these should be referenced in the 'Results' section (see Section 11.4.2).

## 11.3.2 Forest plots

A forest plot displays effect estimates and confidence intervals for both individual studies and meta-analyses (Lewis 2001). Each study is represented by a block at the point estimate of intervention effect with a horizontal line extending either side of the block. The area of the block indicates the weight assigned to that study in the meta-analysis while the horizontal line depicts the confidence interval (usually with a 95% level of confidence). The area of the block and the confidence interval convey similar information, but both make different contributions to the graphic. The confidence interval depicts the range of intervention effects compatible with the study's result and indicates whether each was individually statistically significant. The size of the block draws the eye towards the studies with larger weight (usually those with narrower confidence intervals), which dominate the calculation of the pooled result.

### *11.3.2.1   Forest plots in RevMan*

RevMan provides a flexible framework for producing forest plots in the 'Data and analyses' section of a Cochrane review. Components of a Cochrane forest plot are described in Box 11.3.a, and an example from RevMan is given in Figure 11.3.a, using results from a review of compression stockings to prevent deep vein thrombosis in airline passengers (Clarke 2006). A tutorial on the use of RevMan is available within RevMan (available from www.cc-ims.net).

---

**Box 11.3.a   Details provided in a Cochrane forest plot**

Forest plots for dichotomous outcomes and 'O–E and Variance' outcomes illustrate, by default:
1. the raw data (corresponding to the $2 \times 2$ tables) for each study;
2. point estimates and confidence intervals for the chosen effect measure, both as blocks and lines and as text;
3. a meta-analysis for each subgroup using the chosen effect measure and chosen method (fixed or random effects), both as a diamond and as text;
4. the total numbers of participants and total numbers with events in the experimental intervention and control intervention groups;
5. heterogeneity statistics (among-study variance (tau-squared, or $Tau^2$, or $\tau^2$) for random-effects meta-analyses, the chi-squared test, the $I^2$ statistic and a test for differences across subgroups if they are present and appropriate);
6. a test for overall effect (overall average effect for random-effects meta-analyses); and
7. percent weights given to each study.

Note that 3–7 are not displayed unless data are pooled. Furthermore, the test for differences across subgroups is not displayed for Mantel-Haenszel analyses. For 'O–E and Variance' outcomes it is also possible to enable display of the O–E and V statistics.

Forest plots for continuous outcomes illustrate, by default:

1. the raw data (means, standard deviations and sample sizes) for each arm in each study;

---

2. point estimates and confidence intervals for the chosen effect measure, both as blocks and lines and as text;
3. a meta-analysis for each subgroup using the chosen effect measure and chosen method (fixed or random effects), both as a diamond and as text;
4. the total numbers of participants in the experimental and control groups;
5. heterogeneity statistics (among-study variance (tau-squared) for random-effects meta-analyses, the chi-squared test, the $I^2$ statistic and a test for differences across subgroups if they are present);
6. a test for overall effect (overall average effect for random-effects meta-analyses); and
7. percent weights given to each study.

Note that 3–7 are not displayed unless the data are pooled.

Forest plots for the generic inverse variance method illustrate, by default:

1. the summary data for each study, as entered by the author (for ratio measures these will be on the natural log ('ln') scale);
2. point estimates and confidence intervals, both as blocks and lines and as text (for ratio measures these will be on the natural scale rather than the log scale);
3. a meta-analysis for each subgroup using the chosen method (fixed or random effects), both as a diamond and as text;
4. heterogeneity statistics (among-study variance (tau-squared) for random-effects meta-analyses, the chi-squared test, the $I^2$ statistic, and a test for differences across subgroups if they are present);
5. a test for overall effect (overall average effect for random-effects meta-analyses); and
6. percent weights given to each study.

Note that 3–6 are not shown unless data are pooled. It is possible additionally to enter sample sizes for experimental and control groups. These should be entered as appropriate for the design of the study. The sample sizes are not involved in the analysis, but if entered are displayed as:

7. numbers of participants in the experimental and control group for each study; and
8. the total numbers of participants in the experimental and control groups.

RevMan offers multiple options for changing the analysis methods (e.g. between fixed and random-effects meta-analyses, or using different measures of effect; see Chapter 9 (Section 9.4)) and graphics (e.g. scale of axes and ordering of studies). One forest plot for each dataset entered into RevMan is automatically incorporated into the full published version of the Cochrane review. Default analyses are displayed unless options are overridden. The defaults are Mantel-Haenszel odds ratios for dichotomous data, fixed-effect meta-analyses of mean differences for continuous data, Peto odds ratios for 'O–E and Variance' outcomes and fixed-effect meta-analyses for generic

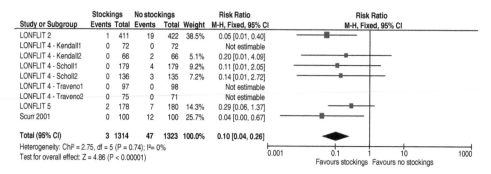

| Study or Subgroup | Stockings Events | Total | No stockings Events | Total | Weight | Risk Ratio M-H, Fixed, 95% CI |
|---|---|---|---|---|---|---|
| LONFLIT 2 | 1 | 411 | 19 | 422 | 38.5% | 0.05 [0.01, 0.40] |
| LONFLIT 4 - Kendall1 | 0 | 72 | 0 | 72 | | Not estimable |
| LONFLIT 4 - Kendall2 | 0 | 66 | 2 | 66 | 5.1% | 0.20 [0.01, 4.09] |
| LONFLIT 4 - Scholl1 | 0 | 179 | 4 | 179 | 9.2% | 0.11 [0.01, 2.05] |
| LONFLIT 4 - Scholl2 | 0 | 136 | 3 | 135 | 7.2% | 0.14 [0.01, 2.72] |
| LONFLIT 4 - Traveno1 | 0 | 97 | 0 | 98 | | Not estimable |
| LONFLIT 4 - Traveno2 | 0 | 75 | 0 | 71 | | Not estimable |
| LONFLIT 5 | 2 | 178 | 7 | 180 | 14.3% | 0.29 [0.06, 1.37] |
| Scurr 2001 | 0 | 100 | 12 | 100 | 25.7% | 0.04 [0.00, 0.67] |
| | | | | | | |
| Total (95% CI) | 3 | 1314 | 47 | 1323 | 100.0% | 0.10 [0.04, 0.26] |

Heterogeneity: Chi² = 2.75, df = 5 (P = 0.74); I² = 0%
Test for overall effect: Z = 4.86 (P < 0.00001)

0.001  0.1  1  10  1000
Favours stockings   Favours no stockings

**Figure 11.3.a**   Example of a RevMan forest plot

inverse variance outcomes (see Chapter 9, Section 9.4). The author should override any default settings that do not correspond with results reported in the text when setting up or editing outcomes in RevMan. This ensures that the results displayed are consistent with what is described in the text. In addition, the scale of the axis should be selected so that the point estimates (and most, if not all, of the confidence intervals) are visible in the plot.

A past convention in the *Cochrane Database of Systematic Reviews* (*CDSR*) has been that dichotomous outcomes have focused on unfavourable outcomes, so that risk ratios and odds ratios less than one (and risk differences less than zero) indicate that an experimental intervention is superior to a control intervention. This would result in effect estimates to the left of the vertical line in a forest plot implying a benefit of the experimental intervention. The convention is no longer encouraged since it is not universally appropriate. A much superior approach is to make it transparent which side of the line indicates benefit of which intervention by labelling the directions on the axis on the forest plots. RevMan allows authors to specify the labels used for 'experimental' and 'control' groups in each outcome. These labels are then used in the *CDSR*. Thus it is essential to know which way figures are constructed and should be interpreted. This is particularly important for measurement scale data where it is not always apparent to a reader which direction on a scale indicates worsening health.

Forest plots should not be generated that contain no studies, and are discouraged when only a single study is found for a particular outcome. To display outcomes that have been investigated only in single studies, authors can use a forest plot using a subgroup for each outcome (ensuring that the option to pool the data is disabled). Otherwise results of single studies may more conveniently be presented in an Additional table (see Section 11.6).

### 11.3.3   Other data tables

The 'Data and analyses' section allows an outcome type of 'Other data'. Results of individual trials may be entered here as plain text. This option is well suited for entering non-standard summary statistics such as median values, or for basic data underlying estimates and standard errors that have been entered under the Generic inverse variance outcome type (for example, means and standard deviations from cross-over trials).

## 11.4 Figures

### 11.4.1 Types of figures

Three sorts of figures may be included within the main content of a Cochrane review.

1. Forest plots (see Section 11.3.2) from among the full collection of 'Data and analyses' within RevMan.

2. Funnel plots (see Chapter 10, Section 10.4.1) from among the full collection of 'Data and analyses' within RevMan.

3. Additional figures.

Because the 'Data and analyses' section may not be included in some published formats of a Cochrane review, authors should incorporate the most important forest plots as figures within the main body of the review, and refer to them at relevant points in the text. Note, however, that the meta-analysis and subgroup analysis results from all 'Data and analyses' forest plots will be included as a table in all published formats of a Cochrane review.

As a general rule, figures offer a clear and systematic means of presenting results both from individual studies and from meta-analyses. However, reviews that contain large numbers of figures are often difficult to follow, especially when each figure contains very little information. Many scientific journals restrict the number of figures in a paper to around half a dozen, and similar considerations apply in most Cochrane Review Groups.

Important results from all figures should be overviewed in the Results section of the review text. Wherever numerical results taken from a figure are reported in the text of the review the authors should make their meaning and derivation clear, and provide a reference to the relevant figure.

### 11.4.2 Selecting RevMan analyses as figures

Forest plots and funnel plots from among the 'Data and analyses' may be selected as figures to appear as an integrated part of the published Cochrane review. Forest plots detailing all studies and study data for the primary outcomes would usually be included as figures. If there are sufficient studies, a funnel plot for one or more of the primary outcomes may be a useful supplement to these forest plots (see Chapter 10, Section 10.4.1).

### 11.4.3   Additional figures

Although RevMan can produce forest plots and funnel plots, it may be appropriate to include other types of figures in a review. Examples include:

1. 'overview' forest plots, where each line represents a meta-analysis rather than a study (for example, to illustrate multiple subgroup analyses or sensitivity analyses);

2. plots illustrating meta-regression analyses; and

3. L'Abbé plots.

Such plots may be produced in software other than RevMan and included as an 'additional' figure. Photographs and diagrams may be included in the same way for use in other parts of a Cochrane review.

Additional figures should seldom be required, and should not be used to draw forest plots that could be drawn using RevMan. Where possible, figures should be produced using statistical software packages that produce appropriate publication-quality graphics, such as Stata, SAS, SPSS, S-Plus or specialized meta-analysis software. General-purpose spreadsheet programs may not provide suitable flexibility nor produce output of adequate quality.

A separate document, *Considerations and recommendations for figures in Cochrane reviews: Graphs of statistical data*, provides extensive guidance on the content of additional figures that illustrate numerical data (available from www.cochrane.org/resources/handbook). The document includes descriptions and recommendations for the plots listed above and several others. Authors should refer to this document before submitting a review containing additional figures. All additional figures should be assessed by a statistical editor or advisor prior to submission of a Cochrane review to the *CDSR*. Authors should be aware that additional figures can often be large and take up valuable storage space on the Cochrane Library. Guidance on technical aspects of additional figures is available among the RevMan documentation at http://www.cc-ims.net.

The ability to incorporate additional figures in RevMan technically allows authors to attach tables as graphics files. Authors are discouraged from doing this due to the high volume of storage space taken up by graphics files. Authors are instead asked to use the Additional tables function, which is provided for this purpose.

## 11.5   'Summary of findings' tables

### 11.5.1   Introduction to 'Summary of findings' tables

'Summary of findings' tables present the main findings of a review in a transparent and simple tabular format. In particular, they provide key information concerning the quality of evidence, the magnitude of effect of the interventions examined, and the sum of available data on the main outcomes. Most reviews would be expected to have a single 'Summary of findings' table. Other reviews may include more than one, for example if the review addresses more than one major comparison, or substantially different populations. In the *CDSR,* the principal 'Summary of findings' table of a review will appear at the beginning, before the Background section. Other 'Summary of findings' tables will appear between the Results and Discussion sections.

The planning for the 'Summary of findings' table comes early in the systematic review, with the selection of the outcomes to be included in (i) the review and (ii) the 'Summary of findings' table. Because this is a crucial step, and one typically not formally addressed in traditional Cochrane reviews, we will review the issues in selecting outcomes here.

## 11.5.2  Selecting outcomes for 'Summary of findings' tables

Cochrane reviews begin by developing a review question and by listing all main outcomes that are important to patients and other decision makers (see Chapter 5, Section 5.4) to ensure production of optimally useful information. Consultation and feedback on the review protocol can enhance this process.

Important outcomes are likely to include widely familiar events such as mortality and major morbidity (such as strokes and myocardial infarction). However, they may also represent frequent minor and rare major side effects, symptoms and quality of life, burdens associated with treatment, and resource issues (costs). Burdens include the demands of adhering to an intervention that patients or caregivers (e.g. family) may dislike, such as having to undergo more frequent tests, or restrictions on lifestyle that certain interventions require.

Frequently, when formulating questions that include all patient-important outcomes for decision making, review authors will confront the fact that reports of randomized trials have not included all these outcomes. This is particularly true for adverse outcomes. For instance, randomized trials might contribute data on intended effects, and on frequent, relatively minor side effects, but not address the relative risk of rare adverse outcomes such as suicide attempts. Chapter 14 discusses strategies for adequately addressing adverse effects. To obtain data for all important outcomes it may be necessary to examine the results of observational studies.

If a review includes only randomized trials, addressing all important outcomes may not be possible within the constraints of the review. Review authors should acknowledge these limitations, and make them transparent to readers.

Review authors who take on the challenge of compiling and summarizing the best evidence for all relevant outcomes may face a number of challenges. These include the fact that the analysis of harm may be carried out in studies whose participants differ from those included in the studies used in the analysis of benefit. Thus, review authors will need to consider how much, if at all, the participants in observational studies differ from those in the randomized trials. This can influence the quality of evidence because of concerns about directness (see Chapter 12, Section 12.2). When review authors do not include information on these important outcomes in the review they should say so. Further discussion of these issues appears also in Chapter 13.

### 11.5.3 General template for 'Summary of findings' tables

While there may be good reasons for modifying the format of a 'Summary of findings' table for some reviews, a standard format for them has been developed with the aim of ensuring consistency and ease of use across reviews, inclusion of the most important information needed by decision makers, and optimal presentation of this information. Standard Cochrane 'Summary of findings' tables therefore include the following six elements using a fixed format (see Figure 11.5.a).

1. A list of all important outcomes, both desirable and undesirable.

2. A measure of the typical burden of these outcomes (e.g. illustrative risk, or illustrative mean, on control intervention).

3. Absolute and relative magnitude of effect (if both are appropriate).

4. Numbers of participants and studies addressing these outcomes.

5. A rating of the overall quality of evidence for each outcome (which may vary by outcome).

6. Space for comments.

As a measure of the magnitude of effect, for dichotomous outcomes the table will usually provide both a relative measure (e.g. risk ratio or odds ratio) and measures of absolute risk. For other types of data, either an absolute measure alone (such as difference in means for continuous data) or a relative measure alone (e.g. hazard ratio for time-to-event data) might be provided. Where possible, however, both relative and absolute measures of effect should be provided. Reviews with more than one main comparison require separate 'Summary of findings' tables for each comparison. Figure 11.5.a provides an example of a 'Summary of findings' table.

A detailed description of the contents of a 'Summary of findings' table appears in Section 11.5.6

### 11.5.4 Producing 'Summary of findings' tables

An additional piece of software, GRADEprofiler (GRADEpro), is available to assist review authors in the preparation of 'Summary of findings' tables. GRADEpro is able to retrieve data from RevMan and to combine this with user-entered control group risks to produce the relative effects and absolute risks associated with interventions. In

**Summary of findings:**

**Compression stockings compared with no compression stockings for people taking long flights**

**Patients or population:** Anyone taking a long flight (lasting more than 6 hours)

**Settings:** International air travel

**Intervention:** Compression stockings[1]

**Comparison:** Without stockings

| Outcomes | Illustrative comparative risks* (95% CI) | | Relative effect (95% CI) | Number of participants (studies) | Quality of the evidence (GRADE) | Comments |
|---|---|---|---|---|---|---|
| | Assumed risk | Corresponding risk | | | | |
| | Without stockings | With stockings | | | | |
| **Symptomatic deep vein thrombosis** (DVT) | See comment | See comment | Not estimable | 2821 (9 studies) | See comment | 0 participants developed symptomatic DVT in these studies. |
| **Symptom-less deep vein thrombosis** | **Low risk population** [2] | | **RR 0.10** (0.04 to 0.26) | 2637 (9 studies) | ⊕⊕⊕⊕ **High** | |
| | 10 per 1000 | 1 per 1000 (0 to 3) | | | | |
| | **High risk population** [2] | | | | | |
| | 30 per 1000 | 3 per 1000 (1 to 8) | | | | |
| **Superficial vein thrombosis** | 13 per 1000 | 6 per 1000 (2 to 15) | **RR 0.45** (0.18 to 1.13) | 1804 (8 studies) | ⊕⊕⊕◯ **Moderate**[3] | |
| **Oedema** Post-flight values measured on a scale from 0, no oedema, to 10, maximum oedema. | The mean oedema score ranged across control groups from **6 to 9**. | The mean oedema score in the intervention groups was on average **4.7 lower** (95% CI −4.9 to −4.5). | | 1246 (6 studies) | ⊕⊕◯◯ **Low**[4] | |
| **Pulmonary embolus** | See comment | See comment | Not estimable | 2821 (9 studies) | See comment | 0 participants developed pulmonary embolus in these studies.[5] |
| **Death** | See comment | See comment | Not estimable | 2821 (9 studies) | See comment | 0 participants died in these studies. |
| **Adverse effects** | See comment | See comment | Not estimable | 1182 (4 studies) | See comment | The tolerability of the stockings was described as very good with no complaints of side effects in 4 studies.[6] |

**Figure 11.5.a**   Example of a 'Summary of findings' table

| Adverse effects | See comment | See comment | Not estimable | 1182 (4 studies) | See comment | The tolerability of the stockings was described as very good with no complaints of side effects in 4 studies. [6] |
|---|---|---|---|---|---|---|

*The basis for the **assumed risk** is provided in footnotes. The **corresponding risk** (and its 95% confidence interval) is based on the assumed risk in the intervention group and the **relative effect** of the intervention (and its 95% CI).

CI: Confidence interval;   RR: Risk ratio     GRADE: GRADE Working Group grades of evidence (see explanations)

[1] 1 All the stockings in the 9 trials included in this review were below-knee compression stockings. In four trials the compression strength was 20-30 mm Hg at the ankle.  It was 10-20 mm Hg in the other four trials. Stockings come in different sizes.If a stocking is too tight around the knee it can prevent essential venous return causing the blood to pool around the knee. Compression stockings should be fitted properly. A stocking that is too tight could cut into the skin on a long flight and potentially cause ulceration and increased risk of DVT. Some stockings can be slightly thicker than normal leg covering and can be potentially restrictive with tight foot wear. It is a good idea to wear stockings around the house prior to travel to ensure a good, comfortable fitting. Stockings were put on 2 to 3 hours before the flight in most of the trials. The availability and cost of stockings can vary.

[2] Two trials recruited high risk participants defined as those with previous episodes of DVT, coagulation disorders, severe obesity, limited mobility due to bone or joint problems, neoplastic disease within the previous two years, large varicose veins or, in one of the studies, participants taller than 190 cm and heavier than 90 kg. The incidence for 7 trials that excluded high risk participants was 1.45% and the incidence for the 2 trials that recruited high-risk participants (with at least one risk factor) was 2.43%. We have rounded these off to 10 and 30 per 1,000 respectively.

[3] The confidence interval crosses no difference and does not rule out a small increase.

[4] The measurement  of oedema was not validated or blinded to the intervention. All of these studies were conducted by the same investigators.

[5] If there are very few or no events and the number of participants is large, judgement about the quality of evidence (particularly judgements about precision) may be based on the absolute effect. Here the quality rating may be considered "high" if the outcome was appropriately assessed and the event, in fact, did not occur in 2821 studied participants.

[6] None of the other trials reported adverse effects, apart from 4 cases of superficial vein thrombosis in varicose veins in the knee region that were compressed by the upper edge of the stocking in one trial.

**Figure 11.5.a**   *(Continued)*

addition, it leads the user through the process of a GRADE assessment, and produces a table that can be readily imported into RevMan as a 'Summary of findings' table. The table is imported as a special table (see Section 11.6) and cannot be modified in RevMan. Review authors can alternatively create their own table in RevMan.

## 11.5.5   Statistical considerations in 'Summary of findings' tables

Here we describe how absolute and relative measures of effect for dichotomous outcomes are obtained. Risk ratios, odds ratios and risk differences are different ways of comparing two groups with dichotomous outcome data (see Chapter 9, Section 9.2.2). Furthermore, there are two distinct risk ratios, depending on which event (e.g. 'yes' or 'no') is the focus of the analysis (see Chapter 9, Section 9.2.2.5). In the presence of a non-zero intervention effect, if there is variation in control group risks across studies, then it is impossible for more than one of these measures to be truly the same in every study. It has long been the expectation in epidemiology that relative measures of effect are more consistent than absolute measures of effect from one scenario to another. There is now empirical evidence to support this supposition (Engels 2000, Deeks 2001). For this reason, meta-analyses should generally use either a risk ratio or an odds ratio as a measure of effect (see Chapter 9, Section 9.4.4.4). Correspondingly, a single estimate of relative effect is likely to be a more appropriate summary than a single estimate of absolute effect. If a relative effect is indeed consistent across studies, then different control group risks will have different implications for absolute benefit. For instance, if the risk ratio is consistently 0.75, then treatment would reduce a control group risk of 80% to 60% in the intervention group (an absolute reduction of 20 percentage points) but would reduce a control group risk of 20% to 15% in the intervention group (an absolute reduction of 5 percentage points).

'Summary of findings' tables are built around the assumption of a consistent relative effect. It is then important to consider the implications of this effect for different control group risks. For any assumed control group risk, it is possible to estimate a corresponding intervention group risk from the meta-analytic risk ratio or odds ratio. Note that the numbers provided in the 'Corresponding risk' column are specific to the 'Assumed risks' in the adjacent column.

For meta-analytic risk ratio, RR, and assumed control risk, ACR, the corresponding intervention risk is obtained as:

$$\text{Corresponding intervention risk, per } 1000 = 1000 \times \text{ACR} \times \text{RR}.$$

As an example, in Figure 11.5.a, the meta-analytic risk ratio is RR = 0.10 (95% CI 0.04–0.26). Assuming a control risk of ACR = 10 per 1000 = 0.01, we obtain:

$$\text{Corresponding intervention risk, per } 1000 = 1000 \times 0.01 \times 0.10 = 1,$$

as indicated in Figure 11.5.a.

For meta-analytic odds ratio, OR, and assumed control risk, ACR, the corresponding intervention risk is obtained as:

$$\text{Corresponding intervention risk, per } 1000 = 1000 \times \left( \frac{\text{OR} \times \text{ACR}}{1 - \text{ACR} + (\text{OR} \times \text{ACR})} \right).$$

Upper and lower confidence limits for the corresponding intervention risk are obtained by replacing RR or OR by their upper and lower confidence limits, respectively (e.g. replacing 0.10 with 0.04, then with 0.26, in the example above). Such confidence intervals do not incorporate uncertainty in the assumed control risks.

When dealing with risk ratios, it is critical that the same definition of 'event' is used as was used for the meta-analysis. For example, if the meta-analysis focused on 'staying alive' rather than 'death' as the event, then assumed and corresponding risks in the 'Summary of findings' table must also refer to 'staying alive'.

In (rare) circumstances in which there is clear rationale to assume a consistent risk difference in the meta-analysis, it is in principle possible to present this for relevant 'assumed risks' and their corresponding risks, and to present the corresponding (different) relative effects for each assumed risk.

## 11.5.6  Detailed contents of a 'Summary of findings' table

### 11.5.6.1  Table title and header

The title of each 'Summary of findings' table should specify the clinical question, framed in terms of the population and making it clear exactly what comparison of interventions is being made. In Figure 11.5.a, the population is people taking very long plane flights, the intervention is compression stockings, and the control is no compression stockings.

The first rows of each 'Summary of findings' table should provide the following 'header' information:

**Patients or population:** This further clarifies the population (and possibly the sub-populations) of interest and ideally the magnitude of risk of the most crucial adverse outcome at which treatment is directed. For instance: patients on a long haul flight may be at different risks for DVT; or patients using SSRIs might be at different risk for side effects; or patients with atrial fibrillation may be at low ($<$ 1%), moderate (1% to 4%) or high ($>$ 4%) yearly risk of stroke.

**Setting:** This should specify any specific characteristics of the settings in which the studies were carried out that might limit the applicability of the summary of findings to other settings; e.g. primary care in Europe and North America.

**Intervention:** The experimental intervention.

**Comparison:** The control (comparison) intervention (including no specific treatment).

### 11.5.6.2  Outcomes

The rows of a 'Summary of findings' table should include all desirable and undesirable outcomes (listed in order of importance) that are essential for decision-making, up to a maximum of seven outcomes. If there is an excessive number of outcomes in the review, authors will need to omit the less important outcomes. Details of scales and time frames should be provided. Authors should aim to decide which outcomes are important for the 'Summary of findings' table during protocol development and before they undertake the review. However, review authors should be alert to the possibility that the importance of an outcome (e.g. a serious adverse effect) may only become known after the protocol was written or the analysis was carried out, and should take appropriate actions to include these in the 'Summary of findings' table. Note that authors should list these outcomes in the table *whether data are available or not.*

Serious adverse events should be included, but it might be possible to combine minor adverse events, and describe this in a footnote (note that it is not appropriate to add events together unless they are known to be independent). Multiple time points will be a particular problem. In general, to keep the table simple, only outcomes critical to decision making should be presented at multiple time points. The remainder should be presented at a common time point.

Continuous outcome measures can be shown in the 'Summary of findings' table; review authors should endeavour to make these interpretable to the target audience (see Chapter 12, Section 12.6). This requires that the units are clear and readily interpretable, for example, days of pain, or frequency of headache. However, many measurement instruments are not readily interpretable by non-specialist clinicians or patients, for example, points on a Beck Depression Inventory or quality of life score. For these, a more interpretable presentation might involve converting a continuous to a dichotomous outcome, such as > 50% improvement (see Chapter 12, Section 12.6).

### 11.5.6.3  *Illustrative comparative risks 1: Assumed risk (with control intervention)*

Authors should provide up to three typical risks for participants receiving the control intervention. It is recommended that these be presented in the form of a number of people experiencing the event per 1000 people (natural frequency). A suitable alternative greater than 1000 may be used for rare events, or 100 may be used for more frequent events. Assumed control intervention risks could be based on assessments of typical risks in different patient groups or at different lengths of follow-up. Ideally, risks would reflect groups that clinicians can easily identify on the basis of their presenting features. A footnote should specify the source or rationale for each control group risk, including the time period to which it corresponds where appropriate. In Figure 11.5.a, clinicians can easily differentiate individuals with risk factors for deep venous thrombosis from those without. If there is known to be little variation in baseline risk then review authors may use the median control group risk across studies.

### 11.5.6.4  *Illustrative comparative risks 2: Corresponding risk (with experimental intervention)*

For dichotomous outcomes, a corresponding absolute risk should be provided for each assumed risk in the preceding column, along with a confidence interval. This absolute risk with (experimental) intervention will usually be derived from the meta-analysis result presented as in the relative effect column (see Section 11.5.6.5). Formulae are provided in Section 11.5.5. Review authors should present the absolute effect in the same format as assumed risks with control intervention (see Section 11.5.6.3), e.g. as a number of people experiencing the event per 1000 people.

For continuous outcomes, a difference in means or standardized difference in means should be presented with its confidence interval. These will typically be obtained directly from a meta-analysis. Explanatory text should be used to clarify the meaning, as in Figure 11.5.a.

### 11.5.6.5 Relative effect (95% CI)

The relative effect will typically be a risk ratio or odds ratio (or occasionally a hazard ratio) with its accompanying 95% confidence interval, obtained from a meta-analysis performed on the basis of the same effect measure. Risk ratios and odds ratios are similar when the control intervention risks are low and effects are small, but differ considerably as these increase. The meta-analysis may involve an assumption of either fixed or random effects, depending on what the review authors consider appropriate.

### 11.5.6.6 Number of participants (studies)

This column should include the number of participants assessed in the included studies for each outcome and the corresponding number of studies that contributed these participants.

### 11.5.6.7 Quality of the evidence (GRADE)

Authors will comment on the quality of the body of evidence as 'High', 'Moderate', 'Low', or 'Very Low'. This is a matter of judgement, but the judgement process operates within a transparent structure and is described in Chapter 12 (Section 12.2). As an example, the quality would be 'High' if the summary is of several randomized trials with low risk of bias, but the rating of quality becomes lower if there are concerns about design or implementation, imprecision, inconsistency, indirectness, or reporting bias. Authors should use the specific evidence grading system developed by the GRADE collaboration .(GRADE Working Group 2004), which is described in detail in Chapter 12 (Section 12.2). Judgements other than of 'High' quality should be made transparent using footnotes or the Comments column in the 'Summary of findings' table (see Figure 11.5.a).

### 11.5.6.8 Comments

The aim of the Comments field is to provide additional comments to help interpret the information or data identified in the row. For example, this may be on the validity of the outcome measure or the presence of variables that are associated with the magnitude of effect. Important caveats about the results should be flagged here. Not all rows will need comments, so it is best to leave blank if there is nothing warranting a comment.

## 11.6 Additional tables

The Additional tables feature provides a flexible way of creating tables, allowing presentation of results of both trials and meta-analyses, and other meta-analytical investigations (such as meta-regression analyses). Important results from all Additional tables should be summarized in the Results section of the review text.

## 11.7 Presenting results in the text

### 11.7.1 Results of meta-analyses

The Results section should be organized to follow the order of comparisons and outcomes specified in the protocol so that it explicitly addresses the objectives of the review. The text should present the overall results in a logical and systematic way: it should not have to rely too heavily on the tables or figures, or constantly refer to them to get a clear picture of the review findings. Rather, tables should be used as an additional resource that might provide further details. However, excessive repetition of data in the text that are also provided in tables or figures should be avoided.

Answers to *post hoc* analyses and less important questions for which there happen to be plentiful data should not be overemphasized. *Post hoc* analyses should always be identified as such. Authors should make clear in the Results section the method of analysis used for each quoted result (in particular, the choice of effect measure, the direction of a beneficial effect and the meta-analysis model used), although the analytic methods themselves should be described in the Methods section. Results should always be accompanied by a measure of uncertainty, such as a 95% confidence interval. The abstract should summarize findings for only the most important comparisons and outcomes, and not selectively report those with the most significant results. It is helpful also to indicate the amount of information (numbers of studies and participants) on which analyses were based.

Each figure and Additional table should be referred to, explicitly, in the text. When referring to results in a figure, table or 'Data and analysis' forest plot that has not been selected as figures, the figure, table or analysis should be referenced in the text.

Authors should consider presenting results in formats that are easy to interpret. For example, odds ratios and standardized mean differences do not lend themselves to direct application in clinical practice but can be re-expressed in more accessible forms. See Chapter 12 (Sections 12.5 and 12.6).

### 11.7.2 Results without meta-analyses

Methods for meta-analysis allow quantification of direction of effect, size of effect and consistency of effect (see Chapter 9, Section 9.1). If suitable numerical data are not available for meta-analysis, or if meta-analyses are considered inappropriate, then these domains may often still be examined to provide a systematic assessment of the evidence available.

A narrative assessment of the evidence can be challenging, especially if the review includes a large number of studies; if the studies themselves examine complex interventions and outcomes; or if there is a lot of variation in the effects of the intervention. Patterns of effects, and similarities or differences between studies may therefore not be immediately obvious. Adopting a systematic approach to presentation is important to making sense of the results of a review. If a descriptive paragraph is provided for the results from each study, this should be done consistently, including the same elements of information for each study, presented in the same order. Organizing the studies into groupings or clusters is encouraged (e.g. by intervention type, population groups, setting etc) if a large number of studies (e.g. more than 20) have been included in the review, and can make the process of narratively describing the results more manageable. It can also enable identification of patterns in results, both within and between the groups that are formed.

## 11.8    Writing an abstract

All full reviews must include an abstract of not more than 400 words. The abstract should be kept as brief as possible without sacrificing important content. Abstracts to Cochrane reviews are published in MEDLINE and the Science Citation Index, and are made freely available on the internet. It is therefore important that they can be read as stand-alone documents.

The abstract should summarize the key methods, results and conclusions of the review and should not contain any information that is not in the review. Links to other parts of the review (such as references, studies, tables and figures) may not be included in the abstract. A hypothetical example of an abstract is included in Box 11.8.a.

---

**Box 11.8.a    Hypothetical example of an abstract**

(For the review 'A versus B for treating influenza in adults' by Peach A, Apricot D, Plum P.)

**Background**

A and B both have antiviral properties, but they are not widely used due to incomplete knowledge of their properties and concerns about possible adverse effects. This is an update of a Cochrane review first published in 1999, and previously updated in 2006.

**Objectives**

To assess the effects of A and B in adults with influenza.

**Search methods**

We searched the Cochrane Acute Respiratory Infections Group Trials Specialized Register (15 February 2007), the Cochrane Central Register of Controlled Trials (*The Cochrane Library* Issue 1, 2007), MEDLINE (January 1966 to January

---

2007), EMBASE (January 1985 to December 2006) and reference lists of articles. We also contacted manufacturers and researchers in the field.

**Selection criteria**

Randomized and quasi-randomized studies comparing A and/or B with placebo, or comparing doses or schedules of A and/or B in adults with influenza.

**Data collection**

Two authors independently assessed trial quality and extracted data. We contacted study authors for additional information. We collected adverse effects information from the trials.

**Main results**

Seventeen trials involving 689 people were included. Five trials involving 234 people compared A with placebo. Compared with placebo, A significantly shortened duration of fever by 23% (by 1.00 days, 95% confidence interval 0.73 to 1.29). Six trials involving 256 people compared B with placebo. B significantly shortened duration of fever by 33% compared with placebo (by 1.27 days, 95% confidence interval 0.77 to 1.77). The small amount of information available directly comparing A and B (two trials involving 53 people) did not indicate that the efficacy of the two drugs was different, although the confidence intervals were very wide. Based on four trials of 73 people, central nervous system effects were significantly more common with A than B (relative risk 2.58, 95% confidence interval 1.54 to 4.33).

**Authors' conclusions**

A and B both appear to be effective in the treatment of influenza. There is insufficient evidence to determine whether one is more effective than the other. Both drugs appear to be relatively well tolerated, although B may be safer.

---

Abstracts should be targeted primarily at healthcare decision makers (clinicians, informed consumers and policy makers) rather than just to researchers. Terminology should be reasonably comprehensible to a general rather than a specialist healthcare audience. Abbreviations should be avoided, except where they are widely understood (for example, HIV). Where essential, other abbreviations should be spelt out (with the abbreviations in brackets) on first use. Names of drugs and interventions that can be understood internationally should be used wherever possible. Trade names should not be used.

The content under each heading in the abstract should be as follows:

**Background:** This should be one or two sentences to explain the context or elaborate on the purpose and rationale of the review. If this version of the review is an update of an earlier one, it is helpful to include a sentence such as "This is an update of a Cochrane review first published in YEAR, and previously updated in YEAR".

**Objectives:** This should be a precise statement of the primary objective of the review, ideally in a single sentence, matching the Objectives in the main text of the review. Where possible the style should be of the form "To assess the effects of *[intervention or comparison]* for*[health problem]* for/in*[types of people, disease or problem and setting if specified]*".

**Search methods:** This should list the sources and the dates of the last search, for each source, using the active form 'We searched....' or, if there is only one author, the passive form can be used, for example, 'Database X, Y, Z were searched'. Search terms should not be listed here. If the CRG's Specialized Register was used, this should be listed first in the form 'Cochrane X Group Specialized Register'. The order for listing other databases should be the Cochrane Central Register of Controlled Trials, MEDLINE, EMBASE, other databases. The date range of the search for each database should be given. For the Cochrane Central Register of Controlled Trials this should be in the form 'Cochrane Central Register of Controlled Trials (*The Cochrane Library* 2007, Issue 1)'. For most other databases, such as MEDLINE, it should be in the form 'MEDLINE (January 1966 to December 2006)'. Searching of bibliographies for relevant citations can be covered in a generic phrase 'reference lists of articles'. If there were any constraints based on language or publication status, these should be listed. If individuals or organizations were contacted to locate studies this should be noted and it is preferable to use 'We contacted pharmaceutical companies' rather than a listing of all the pharmaceutical companies contacted. If journals were specifically handsearched for the review, this should be noted but handsearching to help build the Specialized Register of the CRG should not be listed.

**Selection criteria:** These should be given as '*[type of study]* of *[type of intervention or comparison]* in *[disease, problem or type of people]*'. Outcomes should only be listed here if the review was restricted to specific outcomes.

**Data collection and analysis:** This should be restricted to how data were extracted and assessed, and not include details of what data were extracted. This section should cover whether data extraction and assessments of risk of bias were done by more than one person. If the authors contacted investigators to obtain missing information, this should be noted here. What steps, if any, were taken to identify adverse effects should be noted.

**Main results:** This section should begin with the total number of studies and participants included in the review, and brief details pertinent to the interpretation of the results (for example, the risk of bias in the studies overall or a comment on the comparability of the studies, if appropriate). It should address the primary objective and be restricted to the main qualitative and quantitative results (generally including not more than six key results). The outcomes included should be selected on the basis of which are most likely to help someone making a decision about whether or not to use a particular intervention. Adverse effects should be included if these are covered in the review. If necessary, the number of studies and participants contributing to the separate outcomes should be noted, along with concerns over quality of evidence specific to these outcomes. The results should be expressed narratively as well as quantitatively if the numerical results are not clear or intuitive (such as those from a standardized mean differences analysis). The summary statistics in the abstract should be the same as those selected as the defaults for the review, and should be presented in a standard way, such as 'odds ratio 2.31 (95% confidence interval 1.13 to 3.45)'. Ideally, risks of events (percentage) or averages (for continuous data) should be reported for both comparison groups. If overall results are not calculated in the review, a qualitative assessment or a description of the range and pattern of the results can be given. However, 'vote counts' in which the numbers of 'positive' and 'negative' studies are reported should be avoided.

**Authors' conclusions:** The primary purpose of the review should be to present information, rather than to offer advice or recommendations. The Authors' conclusions should be succinct and drawn directly from the findings of the review so that they directly and obviously reflect the main results. Assumptions should generally not be made about practice circumstances, values, preferences, tradeoffs; and the giving of advice or recommendations should generally be avoided. Any important limitations of data and analyses should be noted. Important conclusions about the implications for research should be included if these are not obvious.

## 11.9 Writing a plain language summary

### 11.9.1 About plain language summaries

The plain language summary aims to summarize the review in a straightforward style that can be understood by consumers of health care. Plain language summaries are made freely available on the internet, so will often be read as stand-alone documents. Plain language summaries have two parts: a title and a body of text.

The first draft of the plain language summary should usually be written by the review authors and submitted with the review to the relevant CRG. This draft may be subject to alteration, and authors should anticipate one or more iterations. Many CRGs have plain language summary writing skills within their editorial team. Where this is not available, a central support service is available to assist CRGs in their writing and editing. This service is co-ordinated by the Cochrane Consumer Network, but review authors needing assistance with writing a plain language summary should contact their CRG.

Further information on the process of finalizing plain language summaries is available in the *Cochrane Manual* (available from www.cochrane.org/admin/manual.htm).

### 11.9.2 Plain language title

The first part of a plain language summary is a restatement of the review's title using plain language terms. It should include participants and intervention (and outcome, when included in the title of the review). As an example, a review title of 'Anticholinergic drugs versus other medications for overactive bladder syndrome in adults' might have a plain language title 'Drugs for overactive bladder syndrome'. Where the review title is easily understood, this should simply be restated as the plain language title, e.g. 'Interventions to reduce harm from continued tobacco use'.

The plain language title should not be declarative (it should not reflect the conclusions of the review). It should be written in sentence case (i.e. with a capital at the beginning of the title and for names, but the remainder in lower case; see examples above), should not be more than 256 characters in length, and should not end with a full stop.

### 11.9.3   Summary text

The second part, or body, of the plain language summary should be no more than 400 words in length and should include:

- A statement about why the review is important: for example definition of and background to the healthcare problem, signs and symptoms, prevalence, description of the intervention and the rationale for its use.

- The main findings of the review: this could include numerical summaries when the review has reported results in numerical form, but these should be given in a general and easily understood format. Results in the plain language summary should not be presented any differently from in the review (i.e. no new results should appear in the summary). Where possible an indication of the number of trials and participants on which the findings are based should be provided.

- A comment on any adverse effects.

- A brief comment on any limitations of the review (for example trials in very specific populations or poor methods of included trials).

At the end of the plain language summary authors may give web links (for example to other information or decision aids on CRG web sites, providing that these comply with The Cochrane Collaboration policy on web links. Graphs or pictures should not be included in the plain language summary. As with other components of a Cochrane review, plain language summaries should follow the format of the Cochrane Style Guide (available from www.cochrane.org/style).

## 11.10   Chapter information

**Authors:** Holger J Schünemann, Andrew D Oxman, Julian PT Higgins, Gunn E Vist, Paul Glasziou and Gordon H Guyatt on behalf of the Cochrane Applicability and Recommendations Methods Group and the Cochrane Statistical Methods Group.

**This chapter should be cited as:** Schünemann HJ, Oxman AD, Higgins JPT, Vist GE, Glasziou P, Guyatt GH. Chapter 11: Presenting results and 'Summary of findings' tables. In: Higgins JPT, Green S (editors), *Cochrane Handbook for Systematic Reviews of Interventions.* Chichester (UK): John Wiley & Sons, 2008.

**Acknowledgements:** Professor Penny Hawe contributed to the text on adverse effects. Jon Deeks provided helpful contributions. Sally Green, Janet Wale and Gill Gyte developed the guidance on plain language summaries, and we also drew on guidance for narrative synthesis by Rebecca Ryan and the Consumers and Communication Review Group. The material on writing abstracts builds on earlier versions of the *Handbook.* For details of previous authors and editors of the *Handbook*, please refer to Section 1.4. For details of the Cochrane Applicability and Recommendations Methods Group, see Chapter 12 (Box 12.8.a); for the Cochrane Statistical Methods Group, see Chapter 9 (Box 9.8.a).

**Conflict of interest:** Holger Schünemann, Andrew Oxman, Gunn Vist, Paul Glasziou and Gordon Guyatt have, to varying degrees, taken leadership roles in the GRADE Working Group from which many of the ideas around 'Summary of findings' tables have arisen.

# 11.11   References

**Clarke 2006**
Clarke M, Hopewell S, Juszczak E, Eisinga A, Kjeldstrøm M. Compression stockings for preventing deep vein thrombosis in airline passengers. *Cochrane Database of Systematic Reviews* 2006, Issue 2. Art No: CD004002.

**Deeks 2001**
Deeks JJ, Altman DG. Effect measures for meta-analysis of trials with binary outcomes. In: Egger M, Davey Smith G, Altman DG (editors). *Systematic Reviews in Health Care: Meta-analysis in Context* (2nd edition). London (UK): BMJ Publication Group, 2001.

**Engels 2000**
Engels EA, Schmid CH, Terrin N, Olkin I, Lau J. Heterogeneity and statistical significance in meta-analysis: an empirical study of 125 meta-analyses. *Statistics in Medicine* 2000; 19: 1707–1728.

**GRADE Working Group 2004**
GRADE Working Group. Grading quality of evidence and strength of recommendations. *BMJ* 2004; 328: 1490–1494.

**Lewis 2001**
Lewis S, Clarke M. Forest plots: trying to see the wood and the trees. *BMJ* 2001; 322: 1479–1480.

# 12 Interpreting results and drawing conclusions

Holger J Schünemann, Andrew D Oxman, Gunn E Vist,
Julian PT Higgins, Jonathan J Deeks, Paul Glasziou and
Gordon H Guyatt on behalf of the Cochrane Applicability
and Recommendations Methods Group

## Key Points

- The GRADE approach, adopted by The Cochrane Collaboration, specifies four levels
  of quality (high, moderate, low and very low) where the highest quality rating is
  for a body of evidence based on randomized trials. Review authors can downgrade
  randomized trial evidence depending on the presence of five factors and upgrade the
  quality of evidence of observational studies depending on three factors.

- Quality ratings are made separately for each outcome.

- Methods for computing, presenting and interpreting relative and absolute effects
  for dichotomous outcome data, including the number needed to treat (NNT), are
  described in this chapter.

- For continuous outcome measures, review authors can present pooled results for
  studies using the same units, the standardized mean difference and effect sizes when
  studies use the same construct but different scales, and odds ratios after transformation
  of the standardized mean differences.

- Review authors should not describe results as 'not statistically significant' or 'non-
  significant', but report the confidence interval together with the exact P value.

- Review authors should not make recommendations, but they can – after describing
  the quality of evidence and the balance of benefits and harms – highlight different
  actions that might be consistent with particular patterns of values and preferences.

## 12.1 Introduction

The purpose of Cochrane reviews is to facilitate healthcare decision-making by patients and the general public, clinicians, administrators, and policy makers. A clear statement of findings, a considered discussion and a clear presentation of the authors' conclusions are important parts of the review. In particular, the following issues can help people make better informed decisions and increase the usability of Cochrane reviews.

- Information on all important outcomes, including adverse outcomes.

- The quality of the evidence for each of these outcomes, as it applies to specific populations, and specific interventions.

- Clarification of the manner in which particular values and preferences may bear on the balance of benefits, harms, burden and costs of the intervention.

A 'Summary of findings' table, described in Chapter 11 (Section 11.5), provides key pieces of information in a quick and accessible format. Review authors are encouraged to include such tables in Cochrane reviews, and to ensure that there is sufficient description of the studies and meta-analyses to support their contents. The Discussion section of the text should provide complementary considerations. Authors should use five sub-headings to ensure they cover suitable material in the Discussion section and that they place the review in an appropriate context. These are 'Summary of main results (benefits and harms)'; 'Overall completeness and applicability of evidence'; 'Quality of the evidence'; 'Potential biases in the review process'; and 'Agreements and disagreements with other studies or reviews'. Authors' conclusions are divided into 'Implications for practice' and 'Implications for research'.

Because Cochrane reviews have an international audience, the discussion and authors' conclusions should, so far as possible, assume a broad international perspective and provide guidance for how the results could be applied in different settings, rather than being restricted to specific national or local circumstances. Cultural differences and economic differences may both play an important role in determining the best course of action. Furthermore, individuals within societies have widely varying values and preferences regarding health states, and use of societal resources to achieve particular health states. Even in the face of the same values and preferences, people may interpret the same research evidence differently. For all these reasons, different people will often make different decisions based on the same evidence.

Thus, the purpose of the review should be to present information and aid interpretation rather than to offer recommendations. The discussion and conclusions should help people understand the implications of the evidence in relation to practical decisions and apply the results to their specific situation. Authors should avoid specific recommendations that depend on assumptions about available resources and values. Authors can, however, aid decision-making by laying out different scenarios that describe certain value structures.

In this chapter we address first one of the key aspects of interpreting findings that is also fundamental in completing a 'Summary of findings' table: the quality of evidence related to each of the outcomes. We then provide a more detailed consideration of issues around applicability and around interpretation of numerical results, and provide suggestions for presenting authors' conclusions.

## 12.2   Assessing the quality of a body of evidence

### 12.2.1   The GRADE approach

The Grades of Recommendation, Assessment, Development and Evaluation Working Group (GRADE Working Group) has developed a system for grading the quality of evidence (GRADE Working Group 2004, Schünemann 2006b, Guyatt 2008a, Guyatt 2008b). Over 20 organizations including the World Health Organization (WHO), the American College of Physicians, the American College of Chest Physicians (ACCP), the American Endocrine Society, the American Thoracic Society (ATS), the Canadian Agency for Drugs and Technology in Health (CADTH), BMJ Clinical Evidence, the National Institutes of Health and Clinical Excellence (NICE) in the UK, and UpToDate® have adopted the GRADE system in its original format or with minor modifications (Schünemann 2006b, Guyatt 2006a, Guyatt 2006b). The BMJ encourages authors of clinical guidelines to use the GRADE system (www.bmj.com/advice/sections.shtml). The Cochrane Collaboration has adopted the principles of the GRADE system for evaluating the quality of evidence for outcomes reported in systematic reviews. This assessment is being phased in together with the introduction of the 'Summary of findings' table (see Chapter 11, Section 11.5).

For purposes of systematic reviews, the GRADE approach defines the quality of a body of evidence as the extent to which one can be confident that an estimate of effect or association is close to the quantity of specific interest. Quality of a body of evidence involves consideration of within-study risk of bias (methodological quality), directness of evidence, heterogeneity, precision of effect estimates and risk of publication bias, as described in Section 12.2.2. The GRADE system entails an assessment of the quality of a body of evidence for each individual outcome.

The GRADE approach specifies four levels of quality (Table 12.2.a). The highest quality rating is for randomized trial evidence. Review authors can, however, downgrade

**Table 12.2.a**   Levels of quality of a body of evidence in the GRADE approach

| Underlying methodology | Quality rating |
| --- | --- |
| Randomized trials; or double-upgraded observational studies. | High |
| Downgraded randomized trials; or upgraded observational studies. | Moderate |
| Double-downgraded randomized trials; or observational studies. | Low |
| Triple-downgraded randomized trials; or downgraded observational studies; or case series/case reports. | Very low |

**Table 12.2.b**   Factors that may decrease the quality level of a body of evidence

---

1. Limitations in the design and implementation of available studies suggesting high likelihood of bias.
2. Indirectness of evidence (indirect population, intervention, control, outcomes).
3. Unexplained heterogeneity or inconsistency of results (including problems with subgroup analyses).
4. Imprecision of results (wide confidence intervals).
5. High probability of publication bias.

---

randomized trial evidence to moderate, low, or even very low quality evidence, depending on the presence of the five factors in Table 12.2.b. Usually, quality rating will fall by one level for each factor, up to a maximum of three levels for all factors. If there are very severe problems for any one factor (e.g. when assessing limitations in design and implementation, all studies were unconcealed, unblinded, and lost over 50% of their patients to follow-up), randomized trial evidence may fall by two levels due to that factor alone.

Review authors will generally grade evidence from sound observational studies as low quality. If, however, such studies yield large effects and there is no obvious bias explaining those effects, review authors may rate the evidence as moderate or – if the effect is large enough – even high quality (Table 12.2.c). The very low quality level includes, but is not limited to, studies with critical problems and unsystematic clinical observations (e.g. case series or case reports).

## 12.2.2   Factors that decrease the quality level of a body of evidence

We now describe in more detail the five reasons for downgrading the quality of a body of evidence for a specific outcome (Table 12.2.b). In each case, if a reason is found for downgrading the evidence, it should be classified as 'serious' (downgrading the quality rating by one level) or 'very serious' (downgrading the quality grade by two levels).

1. **Limitations in the design and implementation**: Our confidence in an estimate of effect decreases if studies suffer from major limitations that are likely to result in a biased assessment of the intervention effect. For randomized trials, these methodological limitations include lack of allocation concealment, lack of blinding (particularly with subjective outcomes highly susceptible to biased assessment), a large

**Table 12.2.c**   Factors that may increase the quality level of a body of evidence

---

1. Large magnitude of effect.
2. All plausible confounding would reduce a demonstrated effect or suggest a spurious effect when results show no effect.
3. Dose-response gradient.

---

loss to follow-up, randomized trials stopped early for benefit or selective reporting of outcomes. Chapter 8 provides a detailed discussion of study-level assessments of risk of bias in the context of a Cochrane review, and proposes an approach to assessing the risk of bias for an outcome across studies as 'low risk of bias', 'unclear risk of bias' and 'high risk of bias' (Chapter 8, Section 8.7). These assessments should feed directly into this factor. In particular, 'low risk of bias' would indicate 'no limitation'; 'unclear risk of bias' would indicate either 'no limitation' or 'serious limitation'; and 'high risk of bias' would indicate either 'serious limitation' or 'very serious limitation'. Authors must use their judgement to decide between alternative categories, depending on the likely magnitude of the potential biases.

Every study addressing a particular outcome will differ, to some degree, in the risk of bias. Review authors must make an overall judgement on whether the quality of evidence for an outcome warrants downgrading on the basis of study limitations. The assessment of study limitations should apply to the studies contributing to the results in the 'Summary of findings' table, rather than to all studies that could potentially be included in the analysis. We have argued in Chapter 8 (Section 8.8.3) that the primary analysis should be restricted to studies at low (or low and unclear) risk of bias.

Table 12.2.d presents the judgements that must be made in going from assessments of the risk of bias to judgements about study limitations for each outcome included in a 'Summary of findings' table. A rating of high quality evidence can be achieved only when most evidence comes from studies that met the criteria for low risk of bias. For example, of the 22 trials addressing the impact of beta blockers on mortality in patients with heart failure, most probably or certainly used concealed allocation, all blinded at least some key groups and follow-up of randomized patients was almost complete (Brophy 2001). The quality of evidence might be downgraded by one level when most of the evidence comes from individual studies either with a crucial limitation for one criterion, or with some limitations for multiple criteria. For example, we cannot be confident that, in patients with falciparum malaria, amodiaquine and sulfadoxine-pyrimethamine together reduce treatment failures compared with sulfadoxine-pyrimethamine, because the apparent advantage of sulfadoxine-pyrimethamine was sensitive to assumptions regarding the event rate in those lost to follow-up (>20% loss to follow-up in two of three studies) (McIntosh 2005). An example of very serious limitations, warranting downgrading by two levels, is provided by evidence on surgery versus conservative treatment in the management of patients with lumbar disc prolapse (Gibson 2007). We are uncertain of the benefit of surgery in reducing symptoms after one year or longer, because the one trial included in the analysis had inadequate concealment of allocation and the outcome was assessed using a crude rating by the surgeon without blinding.

2. **Indirectness of evidence:** Two types of indirectness are relevant. First, a review comparing the effectiveness of alternative interventions (say A and B) may find that randomized trials are available, but they have compared A with placebo and B with placebo. Thus, the evidence is restricted to indirect comparisons between A and B. Second, a review may find randomized trials that meet eligibility criteria but which address a restricted version of the main review question in terms of population,

**Table 12.2.d** Further guidelines for factor 1 (of 5) in a GRADE assessment: Going from assessments of risk of bias to judgements about study limitations for main outcomes

| Risk of bias | Across studies | Interpretation | Considerations | GRADE assessment of study limitations |
|---|---|---|---|---|
| Low risk of bias. | Most information is from studies at low risk of bias. | Plausible bias unlikely to seriously alter the results. | No apparent limitations. | No serious limitations, do not downgrade. |
| Unclear risk of bias. | Most information is from studies at low or unclear risk of bias. | Plausible bias that raises some doubt about the results. | Potential limitations are unlikely to lower confidence in the estimate of effect. | No serious limitations, do not downgrade. |
| | | | Potential limitations are likely to lower confidence in the estimate of effect. | Serious limitations, downgrade one level. |
| High risk of bias. | The proportion of information from studies at high risk of bias is sufficient to affect the interpretation of results. | Plausible bias that seriously weakens confidence in the results. | Crucial limitation for one criterion, or some limitations for multiple criteria, sufficient to lower confidence in the estimate of effect. | Serious limitations, downgrade one level. |
| | | | Crucial limitation for one or more criteria sufficient to substantially lower confidence in the estimate of effect. | Very serious limitations, downgrade two levels. |

intervention, comparator or outcomes. For example, suppose that in a review addressing an intervention for secondary prevention of coronary heart disease, the majority of identified studies happened to be in people who also had diabetes. Then the evidence may be regarded as indirect in relation to the broader question of interest because the population is restricted to people with diabetes. The opposite scenario can equally apply: a review addressing the effect of a preventative strategy for coronary heart disease in people with diabetes may consider trials in people without diabetes to provide relevant, albeit indirect, evidence. This would be particularly likely if investigators had conducted few if any randomized trials in the target population (e.g. people with diabetes). Other sources of indirectness may arise from interventions studied (e.g. if in all included studies a technical intervention was implemented by expert, highly trained specialists in specialist centres, then evidence on the effects of the intervention outside these centres may be indirect), comparators used (e.g. if the control groups received an intervention that is less effective than standard treatment in most settings) and outcomes assessed (e.g. indirectness due to surrogate outcomes when data on patient-important outcomes are not available, or when investigators sought data on quality of life but only symptoms were reported). Review authors should make judgements transparent when they believe downgrading is justified based on differences in anticipated effects in the group of primary interest.

3. **Unexplained heterogeneity or inconsistency of results**: When studies yield widely differing estimates of effect (heterogeneity or variability in results), investigators should look for robust explanations for that heterogeneity. For instance, drugs may have larger relative effects in sicker populations or when given in larger doses. A detailed discussion of heterogeneity and its investigation is provided in Chapter 9 (Sections 9.5 and 9.6). If an important modifier exists, with strong evidence that important outcomes are different in different subgroups (which would ideally be pre-specified), then a separate 'Summary of findings' table may be considered for a separate population. For instance, a separate 'Summary of findings' table would be used for carotid endarterectomy in symptomatic patients with high grade stenosis in which the intervention is, in the hands of the right surgeons, beneficial (Cina 2000), and another (if they considered it worth it) for asymptomatic patients with moderate grade stenosis in which surgery is not beneficial (Chambers 2005). When heterogeneity exists and affects the interpretation of results, but authors fail to identify a plausible explanation, the quality of evidence decreases.

4. **Imprecision of results**: When studies include few participants and few events and thus have wide confidence intervals, authors can lower their rating of the quality of the evidence. The confidence intervals included in the 'Summary of findings' table will provide readers with information that allows them to make, to some extent, their own rating of precision.

5. **High probability of publication bias**: The quality of evidence level may be downgraded if investigators fail to report studies (typically those that show no effect: publication bias) or outcomes (typically those that may be harmful or for which no effect was observed: selective outcome reporting bias) on the basis of results. Selective reporting of outcomes is assessed at the study level as part of the assessment of risk of bias (see Chapter 8, Section 8.13), so for the studies contributing to the outcome in the 'Summary of findings' table this is addressed by factor 1 above (limitations in the design and implementation). If a large number of studies included in the review do not contribute to an outcome, or if there is evidence of publication bias, the quality of the evidence may be downgraded. Chapter 10 provides a detailed discussion of reporting biases, including publication bias, and how it may be tackled in a Cochrane review. A prototypical situation that may elicit suspicion of publication bias is when published evidence includes a number of small trials, all of which are industry funded (Bhandari 2004). For example, 14 trials of flavanoids in patients with haemorrhoids have shown apparent large benefits, but enrolled a total of only 1432 patients (that is, each trial enrolled relatively few

patients) (Alonso-Coello 2006). The heavy involvement of sponsors in most of these trials raises questions of whether unpublished trials suggesting no benefit exist.

A particular body of evidence can suffer from problems associated with more than one of the five factors above, and the greater the problems, the lower the quality of evidence rating that should result. One could imagine a situation in which randomized trials were available, but all or virtually all of these limitations would be present, and in serious form. A very low quality of evidence rating would result.

## 12.2.3   Factors that increase the quality level of a body of evidence

Although observational studies and downgraded randomized trials will generally yield a low rating for quality of evidence, there will be unusual circumstances in which authors could 'upgrade' such evidence to moderate or even high quality (Table 12.2.c).

1. On rare occasions when methodologically well-done observational studies yield large, consistent and precise estimates of the magnitude of an intervention effect, one may be particularly confident in the results. A large effect (e.g. RR > 2 or RR < 0.5) in the absence of plausible confounders, or a very large effect (e.g. RR > 5 or RR < 0.2) in studies with no major threats to validity, might qualify for this. In these situations, while the observational studies are likely to have provided an overestimate of the true effect, the weak study design may not explain all of the apparent observed benefit. Thus, despite reservations based on the observational study design, authors are confident that the effect exists. The magnitude of the effect in these studies may move the assigned quality of evidence from low to moderate (if the effect is large in the absence of other methodological limitations). For example, a meta-analysis of observational studies showed that bicycle helmets reduce the risk of head injuries in cyclists by a large margin (odds ratio [OR] 0.31, 95%CI 0.26–0.37) (Thompson 2000). This large effect, in the absence of obvious bias that could create the association, suggests a rating of moderate-quality evidence.

2. On occasion, all plausible biases from observational or randomized studies may be working to underestimate an apparent intervention effect. For example, if only sicker patients receive an experimental intervention or exposure, yet they still fare better, it is likely that the actual intervention or exposure effect is larger than the data suggest. For instance, a rigorous systematic review of observational studies including a total of 38 million patients demonstrated higher death rates in private for-profit versus private not-for-profit hospitals (Devereaux 2004). One possible bias relates to different disease severity in patients in the two hospital types. It is likely, however, that patients in the not-for-profit hospitals were sicker than those in the for-profit hospitals. Thus, to the extent that residual confounding existed, it would bias results against the not-for-profit hospitals. The second likely bias was the possibility that higher numbers of patients with excellent private insurance coverage could lead to a hospital having more resources and a spill-over effect that would benefit those without such

coverage. Since for-profit hospitals are likely to admit a larger proportion of such well-insured patients than not-for-profit hospitals, the bias is once again against the not-for-profit hospitals. Because the plausible biases would all diminish the demonstrated intervention effect, one might consider the evidence from these observational studies as moderate rather than low quality. A parallel situation exists when observational studies have failed to demonstrate an association but all plausible biases would have increased an intervention effect. This situation will usually arise in the exploration of apparent harmful effects. For example, because the hypoglycaemic drug phenformin causes lactic acidosis, the related agent metformin is under suspicion for the same toxicity. Nevertheless, very large observational studies have failed to demonstrate an association (Salpeter 2007). Given the likelihood that clinicians would be more alert to lactic acidosis in the presence of the agent and overreport its occurence, one might consider this moderate, or even high quality, evidence refuting a causal relationship between typical therapeutic doses of metformin and lactic acidosis.

3. The presence of a dose-response gradient may also increase our confidence in the findings of observational studies and thereby enhance the assigned quality of evidence. For example, our confidence in the result of observational studies that show an increased risk of bleeding in patients who have supratherapeutic anticoagulation levels is increased by the observation that there is a dose-response gradient between higher levels of the international normalized ratio (INR) and the increased risk of bleeding (Levine 2004).

## 12.3    Issues in applicability

### 12.3.1    The role of the review author

"A leap of faith is always required when applying any study findings to the population at large" or to a specific person. "In making that jump, one must always strike a balance between making justifiable broad generalizations and being too conservative in one's conclusions" (Friedman 1985).

To address adequately the extent to which a review is relevant for the purpose to which it is being put ('directness'), there are certain things the review author must do, and certain things the user of the review must do. We discuss here what the review author can do to help the user. Cochrane review authors must be extremely clear on the population, intervention, and outcomes that they are intending to address. Chapter 11 (Section 11.5.2) emphasizes a crucial step that has not traditionally been part of Cochrane reviews: the specification of all patient-important outcomes relevant to the intervention strategies under comparison.

With respect to participant and intervention factors, review authors need to make *a priori* hypotheses about possible effect modifiers, and then examine those hypotheses. If they find apparent subgroup effects, they must ultimately decide whether or not these effects are credible (Oxman 2002). Differences between subgroups, particularly those that correspond to differences between studies, need to be interpreted cautiously. Some chance variation between subgroups is inevitable, so unless there is strong evidence of an interaction authors should not assume that the subgroup effect exists. If, despite due caution, review authors judge subgroup effects as credible, they should conduct separate meta-analyses for the relevant subgroups, and produce separate 'Summary of findings' tables for those subgroups.

The user of the review will be challenged with 'individualization' of the findings. For example, even if relative effects are similar across subgroups, absolute effects will differ according to baseline risk. Review authors can help provide this information by identifying identifiable groups of people with varying risks in the 'Summary of findings' tables, as discussed in Chapter 11 (Section 11.5.5). Users can then identify the patients before them as belonging to a particular risk group, and assess their likely magnitude of benefit or harm accordingly.

Another decision users must make is whether the patients before them are so different from those included in the studies that they cannot use the results of the systematic review and meta-analysis at all. Review authors can point out that, rather than rigidly applying the inclusion and exclusion criteria of studies, it is better to ask whether there are compelling reasons why the evidence should not be applied to a particular patient (Guyatt 1994). Authors can sometimes help clinical decision makers by identifying important variation where divergence might limit the applicability of results (Schünemann 2006a), including: biologic and cultural variation, and variation in adherence to an intervention.

In addressing these issues, authors cannot be aware of, or address, the myriad of differences in circumstances around the world. They can, however, address differences of known importance to many people and, importantly, they should avoid assuming that other people's circumstances are the same as their own in discussing the results and drawing conclusions.

## 12.3.2   Biologic variation

Issues of biologic variation that authors should consider include divergence in pathophysiology (e.g. biologic differences between women and men that are likely to affect responsiveness to a treatment) and divergence in a causative agent (e.g. for infectious diseases such as malaria).

## 12.3.3   Variation in context and culture

Some interventions, particularly non-pharamcological interventions, may work in some contexts but not in others; the situation has been described as program by context interaction (Hawe 2004). Context factors might pertain to the host organization in which an intervention is offered, such as the expertise, experience and morale of the staff expected to carry out the intervention, the competing priorities for the staff's attention, the local resources such as service and facilities made available to the program and the status or importance given to the program by the host organization. Broader context issues might include aspects of the system within which the host organization operates, such as the fee or payment structure for healthcare providers. Context factors may also pertain to the characteristics of the target group or population services (such aspects include the cultural and linguistic diversity, socioeconomic position, rural/urban setting), which may mean that a particular style of care or relationship evolves between service providers and consumers that may or may not match the values and technology of the program. For many years these aspects have been acknowledged (but not clearly specified) when decision makers have argued that results of evidence reviews from other countries do not apply in their own country.

Whilst some programs/interventions have been transferred from one context to another and benefits have been observed, others have not (Resnicow 1993, Lumley 2004). Authors should take caution when making generalizations from one context to another. Authors should report on the presence (or otherwise) of context-related information in intervention studies, where this information is available (Hawe 2004).

### 12.3.4   Variation in adherence

Variation in the adherence of the recipients and providers of care can limit the applicability of results. Predictable differences in adherence can be due to divergence in economic conditions or attitudes that make some forms of care not accessible or not feasible in some settings, such as in developing countries (Dans 2007). It should not be assumed that high levels of adherence in closely monitored randomized trials will translate into similar levels of adherence in normal practice.

### 12.3.5   Variation in values and preferences

Management decisions involve trading off benefits and downsides of proposed management strategies. The right choice may differ for people with different values and preferences, and it is up to the clinician to ensure that decisions are consistent with patients' values and preferences. We describe how the review author can help this process in Section 12.7.

## 12.4   Interpreting results of statistical analyses

### 12.4.1   Confidence intervals

Results for both individual studies and meta-analyses are reported with a point estimate together with an associated confidence interval. For example, "The odds ratio was 0.75 with a 95% confidence interval of 0.70 to 0.80". The point estimate (0.75) is the best guess of the magnitude and direction of the experimental intervention's effect compared with the control intervention. The confidence interval describes the uncertainty inherent in this estimate, and describes a range of values within which we can be reasonably sure that the true effect actually lies. If the confidence interval is relatively narrow (e.g. 0.70 to 0.80), the effect size is known precisely. If the interval is wider (e.g. 0.60 to 0.93) the uncertainty is greater, although there may still be enough precision to make decisions about the utility of the intervention. Intervals that are very wide (e.g. 0.50 to 1.10) indicate that we have little knowledge about the effect, and that further information is needed.

A 95% confidence interval is often interpreted as indicating a range within which we can be 95% certain that the true effect lies. This statement is a loose interpretation, but is useful as a rough guide. The strictly-correct interpretation of a confidence interval is based on the hypothetical notion of considering the results that would be obtained if the study were repeated many times. If a study were repeated infinitely often, and on each occasion a 95% confidence interval calculated, then 95% of these intervals would contain the true effect.

The width of the confidence interval for an individual study depends to a large extent on the sample size. Larger studies tend to give more precise estimates of effects (and hence have narrower confidence intervals) than smaller studies. For continuous outcomes, precision depends also on the variability in the outcome measurements (the standard deviation of measurements across individuals); for dichotomous outcomes it depends on the risk of the event, and for time-to-event outcomes it depends on the number of events observed. All these quantities are used in computation of the standard errors of effect estimates from which the confidence interval is derived.

The width of a confidence interval for a meta-analysis depends on the precision of the individual study estimates and on the number of studies combined. In addition, for random-effects models, precision will decrease with increasing heterogeneity and confidence intervals will widen correspondingly (see Chapter 9, Section 9.5.4). As more studies are added to a meta-analysis the width of the confidence interval usually decreases. However, if the additional studies increase the heterogeneity in the meta-analysis and a random-effects model is used, it is possible that the confidence interval width will increase.

Confidence intervals and point estimates have different interpretations in fixed-effect and random-effects models. While the fixed-effect estimate and its confidence interval address the question 'what is the best (single) estimate of the effect?', the random-effects estimate assumes there to be a distribution of effects, and the estimate and its confidence interval address the question 'what is the best estimate of the average effect?'

A confidence interval may be reported for any level of confidence (although they are most commonly reported for 95%, and sometimes 90% or 99%). For example, the odds ratio of 0.80 could be reported with an 80% confidence interval of 0.73 to 0.88; a 90% interval of 0.72 to 0.89; and a 95% interval of 0.70 to 0.92. As the confidence level increases, the confidence interval widens.

There is logical correspondence between the confidence interval and the P value (see Section 12.4.2). The 95% confidence interval for an effect will exclude the null value (such as an odds ratio of 1.0 or a risk difference of 0) if and only if the test of significance yields a P value of less than 0.05. If the P value is exactly 0.05, then either the upper or lower limit of the 95% confidence interval will be at the null value. Similarly, the 99%

confidence interval will exclude the null if and only if the test of significance yields a P value of less than 0.01.

Together, the point estimate and confidence interval provide information to assess the clinical usefulness of the intervention. For example, suppose that we are evaluating a treatment that reduces the risk of an event and we decide that it would be useful only if it reduced the risk of an event from 30% by at least 5 percentage points to 25% (these values will depend on the specific clinical scenario and outcome). If the meta-analysis yielded an effect estimate of a reduction of 10 percentage points with a tight 95% confidence interval, say, from 7% to 13%, we would be able to conclude that the treatment was useful since both the point estimate and the entire range of the interval exceed our criterion of a reduction of 5% for clinical usefulness. However, if the meta-analysis reported the same risk reduction of 10% but with a wider interval, say, from 2% to 18%, although we would still conclude that our best estimate of the effect of treatment is that it is useful, we could not be so confident as we have not excluded the possibility that the effect could be between 2% and 5%. If the confidence interval was wider still, and included the null value of a difference of 0%, we will not have excluded the possibility that the treatment has any effect whatsoever, and would need to be even more sceptical in our conclusions.

Confidence intervals with different levels of confidence can demonstrate that there is differential evidence for different degrees of benefit or harm. For example, it might be possible to report the same analysis results (i) with 95% confidence that the intervention does not cause harm; (ii) with 90% confidence that it has some effect; and (iii) with 80% confidence that it has a patient-important benefit. These elements may suggest both usefulness of the intervention and the need for additional research.

Review authors may use the same general approach to conclude that an intervention is *not* useful. Continuing with the above example where the criterion for a minimal patient-important difference is a 5% risk difference, an effect estimate of 2% with a confidence interval of 1% to 4% suggests that the intervention is not useful.

## 12.4.2   P values and statistical significance

A P value is the probability of obtaining the observed effect (or larger) under a 'null hypothesis', which in the context of Cochrane reviews is either an assumption of 'no effect of the intervention' or 'no differences in the effect of intervention between studies' (no heterogeneity). Thus, a P value that is very small indicates that the observed effect is very unlikely to have arisen purely by chance, and therefore provides evidence against the null hypothesis. It has been common practice to interpret a P value by examining whether it is smaller than particular threshold values. In particular, P values less than 0.05 are often reported as "statistically significant", and interpreted as being small enough to justify rejection of the null hypothesis. However, the 0.05 threshold is an arbitrary one that became commonly used in medical and psychological research largely because P values were determined by comparing the test statistic against tabulations of specific percentage points of statistical distributions. RevMan, like other statistical packages, reports precise P values. If review authors decide to present a P value with the results of a meta-analysis, they should report a precise P value, together with the 95% confidence interval.

In RevMan, two P values are provided. One relates to the summary effect in a meta-analysis and is from a Z test of the null hypothesis that there is no effect (or no effect on average in a random-effects meta-analysis). The other relates to heterogeneity between studies and is from a chi-squared test of the null hypothesis that there is no heterogeneity (see Chapter 9, Section 9.5.2).

For tests of a summary effect, the computation of P involves both the effect estimate and the sample size (or, more strictly, the precision of the effect estimate). As sample size increases, the range of plausible effects that could occur by chance is reduced. Correspondingly, the statistical significance of an effect of a particular magnitude will be greater (the P value will be smaller) in a larger study than in a smaller study.

P values are commonly misinterpreted in two ways. First, a moderate or large P value (e.g. greater than 0.05) may be misinterpreted as evidence that "the intervention has no effect". There is an important difference between this statement and the correct interpretation that "there is not strong evidence that the intervention has an effect". To avoid such a misinterpretation, review authors should always examine the effect estimate and its 95% confidence interval, together with the P value. In small studies or small meta-analyses it is common for the range of effects contained in the confidence interval to include both no intervention effect and a substantial effect. Review authors are advised not to describe results as 'not statistically significant' or 'non-significant'.

The second misinterpretation is to assume that a result with a small P value for the summary effect estimate implies that an intervention has an important benefit. Such a misinterpretation is more likely to occur in large studies, such as meta-analyses that accumulate data over dozens of studies and thousands of participants. The P value addresses the question of whether the intervention effect is precisely nil; it does not examine whether the effect is of a magnitude of importance to potential recipients of the intervention. In a large study, a small P value may represent the detection of a trivial effect. Again, inspection of the point estimate and confidence interval helps correct interpretations (see Section 12.4.1).

## 12.5    Interpreting results from dichotomous outcomes (including numbers needed to treat)

### 12.5.1    Relative and absolute risk reductions

Clinicians may be more inclined to prescribe an intervention that reduces the risk of death by 25% than one that reduces the risk of death by 1 percentage point, although both presentations of the evidence may relate to the same benefit (i.e. a reduction in risk from 4% to 3%). The former refers to the *relative* reduction in risk and the latter to the *absolute* reduction in risk. As described in Chapter 9 (Section 9.2.2), there are several measures for comparing dichotomous outcomes in two groups. Meta-analyses are usually undertaken using risk ratios (RR), odds ratios (OR) or risk differences (RD), but there are several alternative ways of expressing results.

**Relative risk reduction** (RRR) is a convenient way of re-expressing a risk ratio as a percentage reduction:

$$RRR = 100\% \times (1 - RR).$$

For example, a risk ratio of 0.75 translates to a relative risk reduction of 25%, as in the example above.

The risk difference is often referred to as the **absolute risk reduction** (ARR), and may be presented as a percentage (for example, 1%), as a decimal (for example, 0.01), or as counts (for example, 10 out of 1000). A simple transformation of the risk difference known as the number needed to treat (NNT) is a common alternative way of presenting the same information. We discuss NNTs in Section 12.5.2, and consider different choices for presenting absolute effects in Section 12.5.3. We then describe computations for obtaining these numbers from the results of individual studies and of meta-analyses.

## 12.5.2 More about the number needed to treat (NNT)

The **number needed to treat** (NNT) is defined as the expected number of people who need to receive the experimental rather than the comparator intervention for one additional person to either incur or avoid an event in a given time frame. Thus, for example, an NNT of 10 can be interpreted as 'it is expected that one additional (or less) person will incur an event for every 10 participants receiving the experimental intervention rather than control over a given time frame'. It is important to be clear that:

1. since the NNT is derived from the risk difference, it is still a *comparative* measure of effect (experimental versus a certain control) and not a general property of a single intervention; and

2. the NNT gives an 'expected value'. For example, NNT = 10 does not imply that one additional event *will* occur in each and every group of ten people.

NNTs can be computed for both beneficial and detrimental events, and for interventions that cause both improvements and deteriorations in outcomes. In all instances NNTs are expressed as positive whole numbers, all decimals being rounded up. Some authors use the term 'number needed to harm' (NNH) when an intervention leads to a deterioration rather than improvement in outcome. However, this phrase is unpleasant, misleading and inaccurate (most notably, it can easily be read to imply the number of people who will experience a harmful outcome if given the intervention), and it is strongly recommended that 'number needed to harm' and 'NNH' are avoided. The preferred alternative is to use phrases such as 'number needed to treat for an additional beneficial outcome' (NNTB) and 'number needed to treat for an additional harmful outcome' (NNTH) to indicate direction of effect.

As NNTs refer to events, their interpretation needs to be worded carefully when the binary outcome is a dichotomization of a scale-based outcome. For example, if the outcome is pain measured on a 'none, mild, moderate or severe' scale it may have been dichotomized as 'none or mild' versus 'moderate or severe'. It would be inappropriate for an NNT from these data to be referred to as an 'NNT for pain'. It is an 'NNT for moderate or severe pain'.

## 12.5.3   Expressing absolute risk reductions

Users of reviews are liable to be influenced by the choice of statistical presentations of the evidence. Hoffrage et al. suggest that physicians' inferences about statistical outcomes are more appropriate when they deal with 'natural frequencies' – whole numbers of people, both treated and untreated – (e.g. treatment results in a drop from 20 out of 1000 to 10 out of 1000 women having breast cancer), than when effects are presented as percentages (e.g. 1% absolute reduction in breast cancer risk) (Hoffrage 2000). Probabilities may be more difficult to understand than frequencies, particularly when events are rare. While standardization may be important in improving the presentation of research evidence (and participation in healthcare decisions), current evidence suggests that the presentation of natural frequencies for expressing differences in absolute risk is best understood by consumers of healthcare information. This evidence provides the rationale for presenting absolute risks in 'Summary of findings' tables as numbers of people with events per 1000 people receiving the intervention.

Risk ratios and relative risk reductions remain crucial because relative effect tends to be substantially more stable across risk groups than does absolute benefit. Review authors can use their own data to study this consistency (Cates 1999, Smeeth 1999). Risk differences are least likely to be consistent across baseline event rates; thus, they are rarely appropriate for computing numbers needed to treat in systematic reviews. If a relative effect measure (OR or RR) is chosen for meta-analysis, then a control group risk needs to be specified as part of the calculation of an ARR or NNT. It is crucial to express absolute benefit for each clinically identifiable risk group, clarifying the time period to which this applies. Studies in patients with differing severity of disease or studies with different lengths of follow-up will almost certainly have different control group risks. In these cases, different control group risks lead to different ARRs and NNTs (except when the intervention has no effect). A recommended approach is to re-express an odds ratio or a risk ratio as a variety of NNTs across a range of assumed control risks (ACRs) (McQuay 1997, Smeeth 1999, Sackett 2000). Review authors should bear these considerations in mind not only when constructing their 'Summary of findings' table, but also in the text of their review.

For example a review of oral anticoagulants to prevent stroke presented information to users by describing absolute benefits for various baseline risks (Aguilar 2005). They presented their principal findings as "The inherent risk of stroke should be considered in the decision to use oral anticoagulants in atrial fibrillation patients, selecting those who stand to benefit most for this therapy" (Aguilar 2005). Among high-risk atrial fibrillation patients with prior stroke or transient ischaemic attack who have stroke rates of about 12% (120 per 1000) per year, warfarin prevents about 70 strokes yearly per 1000 patients, whereas for low-risk atrial fibrillation patients (with a stroke rate of about 2% per year or 20 per 1000), warfarin prevents only 12 strokes. This presentation helps users to understand the important impact that typical baseline risks have on the absolute benefit that they can expect.

### 12.5.4  Computations

Direct computation of an absolute risk reduction (ARR) or a number needed to treat (NNT) depends on the summary statistic (odds ratio, risk ratio or risk differences) available from the study or meta-analysis. When expressing results of meta-analyses, authors should use, in the computations, whatever statistic they determined to be the most appropriate summary for pooling (see Chapter 9, Section 9.4.4.4). Here we present calculations to obtain ARR as a reduction in the number of participants per 1000. For example, a risk difference of −0.133 corresponds to 133 *fewer* participants with the event per 1000.

ARRs and NNTs should not be computed from the aggregated total numbers of participants and events across the trials. This approach ignores the randomization within studies, and may produce seriously misleading results if there is unbalanced randomization in any of the studies.

When computing NNTs, the values obtained are by convention always rounded up to the next whole number.

#### *12.5.4.1  Computing NNT from a risk difference (RD)*

NNTs can be calculated for single studies as follows. Note that this approach, although applicable, should only very rarely be used for the results of a meta-analysis of risk differences, because meta-analyses should usually be undertaken using a relative measure of effect (RR or OR).

A NNT may be computed from a risk difference as

$$\text{NNT} = \frac{1}{\text{absolute value of risk difference}} = \frac{1}{|\text{RD}|},$$

where the vertical bars ('absolute value of') in the denominator indicate that any minus sign should be ignored. It is convention to round the NNT up to the nearest whole number. For example, if the risk difference is −0.12 the NNT is 9; if the risk difference is −0.22 the NNT is 5.

### 12.5.4.2  Computing absolute risk reduction or NNT from a risk ratio (RR)

To aid interpretation, review authors may wish to compute an absolute risk reduction or NNT from the results of a meta-analysis of risk ratios. In order to do this, an assumed control risk (ACR) is required. It will usually be appropriate to do this for a range of different ACRs. The computation proceeds as follows:

$$\text{number fewer per } 1000 = 1000 \times \text{ACR} \times (1 - \text{RR}),$$

$$\text{NNT} = \left| \frac{1}{\text{ACR} \times (1 - \text{RR})} \right|$$

As an example, suppose the risk ratio is RR $= 0.92$, and an assumed control risk of ACR $= 0.3$ (300 per 1000) is assumed. Then the effect on risk is 24 fewer per 1000:

$$\text{number fewer per } 1000 = 1000 \times 0.3 \times (1 - 0.92) = 24$$

The NNT is 42:

$$\text{NNT} = \left| \frac{1}{0.3 \times (1 - 0.92)} \right| = \left| \frac{1}{0.3 \times 0.08} \right| = 41.67.$$

### 12.5.4.3  Computing absolute risk reduction or NNT from an odds ratio (OR)

Review authors may wish to compute an absolute risk reduction or NNT from the results of a meta-analysis of odds ratios. In order to do this, an assumed control risk (ACR) is required. It will usually be appropriate to do this for a range of different ACRs. The computation proceeds as follows:

$$\text{number fewer per } 1000 = 1000 \times \left( \text{ACR} - \frac{\text{OR} \times \text{ACR}}{1 - \text{ACR} + \text{OR} \times \text{ACR}} \right)$$

$$\text{NNT} = \frac{1}{\left| \text{ACR} - \dfrac{\text{OR} \times \text{ACR}}{1 - \text{ACR} + \text{OR} \times \text{ACR}} \right|}$$

As an example, suppose the odds ratio is OR $= 0.73$, and a control risk of ACR $= 0.3$ is assumed. Then the effect on risk is 62 fewer per 1000:

$$\text{number fewer per } 1000 = 1000 \times \left( 0.3 - \frac{0.73 \times 0.3}{1 - 0.3 + 0.73 \times 0.3} \right)$$

$$= 1000 \times \left( 0.3 - \frac{0.219}{1 - 0.3 + 0.219} \right) = 1000 \times (0.3 - 0.238)$$

$$= 61.7$$

The NNT is 17:

$$
\text{NNT} = \frac{1}{\left| \left( 0.3 - \dfrac{0.73 \times 0.3}{1 - 0.3 + 0.73 \times 0.3} \right) \right|} = \frac{1}{\left| 0.3 - \dfrac{0.219}{1 - 0.3 + 0.219} \right|}
$$

$$
= \frac{1}{|0.3 - 0.238|} = 16.2.
$$

### *12.5.4.4   Computing risk ratio from an odds ratio (OR)*

Because risk ratios are easier to interpret than odds ratios, but odds ratios have favourable mathematical properties, a review author may decide to undertake a meta-analysis based on odds ratios, but to express the result as a summary risk ratio (or relative risk reduction). This requires an assumed control risk (ACR). Then

$$
\text{RR} = \frac{\text{OR}}{1 - \text{ACR} \times (1 - \text{OR})}
$$

It will often be reasonable to perform this transformation using the median control group risk from the studies in the meta-analysis.

### *12.5.4.5   Computing confidence limits*

Confidence limits for ARRs and NNTs may be calculated by applying the above formulae to the upper and lower confidence limits for the summary statistic (RD, RR or OR) (Altman 1998). Note that this confidence interval does not incorporate uncertainty around the control group risk (CGR).

In the case of what conventionally are considered non-statistically significant results (for example, the 95% confidence interval of OR or RR includes the value 1) one of the confidence limits will indicate benefit and the other harm. Thus, appropriate use of the words 'fewer' and 'more' is required for each limit when presenting results in terms of events. For NNTs, the two confidence limits should be labelled as NNTB and NNTH to indicate the direction of effect in each case. The confidence interval for the NNT will include a 'discontinuity': within the interval there will be an infinitely large NNTB, which will switch to an infinitely large NNTH.

## 12.6   Interpreting results from continuous outcomes (including standardized mean differences)

### 12.6.1   Meta-analyses with continuous outcomes

When outcomes are continuous, review authors have a number of options in presenting pooled results. If all studies have used the same units, a meta-analysis may generate a pooled estimate in those units, as a difference in mean response (see, for instance, the row summarizing results for oedema in Chapter 11, Figure 11.5.a). The units of such outcomes may be difficult to interpret, particularly when they relate to rating scales. 'Summary of findings' tables should include the minimum and maximum of the scale of measurement, and the direction (again, see the Oedema column of Chapter 11, Figure 11.5.a). Knowledge of the smallest change in instrument score that patients perceive is important – the minimal important difference – and can greatly facilitate the interpretation of results. Knowing the minimal important difference allows authors and users to place results in context, and authors should state the minimal important difference – if known – in the Comments column of their 'Summary of findings' table.

When studies have used different instruments to measure the same construct, a standardized means difference (SMD) may be used in meta-analysis for combining continuous data (see Chapter 9, Section 9.2.3.2). For clinical interpretation, such an analysis may be less helpful than dichotomizing responses and presenting proportions of patients benefiting. Methods are available for creating dichotomous data out of reported means and standard deviations, but require assumptions that may not be met (Suissa 1991, Walter 2001).

The SMD expresses the intervention effect in standard units rather than the original units of measurement. The SMD is the difference in mean effects in the experimental and control groups divided by the pooled standard deviation of participants' outcomes (see Chapter 9, Section 9.2.3.2). The value of a SMD thus depends on both the size of the effect (the difference between means) and the standard deviation of the outcomes (the inherent variability among participants).

Without guidance, clinicians and patients may have little idea how to interpret results presented as SMDs. There are several possibilities for re-expressing such results in more helpful ways, as follows.

## 12.6.2    Re-expressing SMDs using rules of thumb for effect sizes

Rules of thumb exist for interpreting SMDs (or 'effect sizes'), which have arisen mainly from researchers in the social sciences. One example is as follows: 0.2 represents a small effect, 0.5 a moderate effect, and 0.8 a large effect (Cohen 1988). Variations exist (for example, <0.41 = small, 0.40 to 0.70 = moderate, >0.70 = large). Review authors might consider including a rule of thumb in the Comments column of a 'Summary of findings' table. However, some methodologists believe that such interpretations are problematic because *patient* importance of a finding is context-dependent and not amenable to generic statements.

## 12.6.3    Re-expressing SMDs by transformation to odds ratio

A transformation of a SMD to a (log) odds ratio is available, based on the assumption that an underlying continuous variable has a logistic distribution with equal standard deviation in the two intervention groups (Furukawa 1999, Chinn 2000). The assumption is unlikely to hold exactly and the results must be regarded as an approximation. The log odds ratio is estimated as

$$\ln OR = \frac{\pi}{\sqrt{3}} SMD,$$

(or approximately $1.81 \times SMD$) The resulting odds ratio can then be combined with an assumed control group risk to obtain an absolute risk reduction as in Section 12.5.4.3. These control group risks refer to proportions of people who have improved by some (unspecified) amount in the continuous outcome ('responders'). Table 12.6.a shows some illustrative results from this method. These NNTs may be converted to people per thousand by using the formula 1000/NNT.

## 12.6.4   Re-expressing SMDs using a familiar instrument

The final possibility for interpreting the SMD is to express it in the units of one or more of the specific measurement instruments. Multiplying a SMD by a typical among-person standard deviation for a particular scale yields an estimate of the difference in mean outcome scores (experimental versus control) on that scale. The standard deviation could be obtained as the pooled standard deviation of baseline scores in one of the studies. To better reflect among-person variation in practice, it may be preferable to use a standard deviation from a representative observational study. The pooled effect is thus re-expressed in the original units of that particular instrument and the clinical relevance and impact of the intervention effect can be interpreted. However, authors should be aware that such back-transformation of effect sizes can be misleading if it is applied to individual studies rather than for a summary measure of effect (Scholten 1999). Consider two studies that *did* use the same instrument and observed the same effect, but observed different among-participant variability (perhaps due to different inclusion criteria). Then back-transformations using the different standard deviations from these studies would yield different sizes of effect for *the same scale* and *the same effect*.

**Table 12.6.a**   NNTs equivalant to specific SMDs for various given 'proportions improved' in the control group

| Control group proportion improved | 10% | 20% | 30% | 40% | 50% | 60% | 70% | 80% | 90% |
|---|---|---|---|---|---|---|---|---|---|
| SMD = 0.1 | 57 | 33 | 26 | 23 | 23 | 24 | 28 | 37 | 66 |
| SMD = 0.2 | 27 | 16 | 13 | 12 | 12 | 13 | 15 | 20 | 36 |
| SMD = 0.5 | 9 | 6 | 5 | 5 | 5 | 6 | 7 | 10 | 18 |
| SMD = 0.8 | 5 | 4 | 3 | 3 | 4 | 4 | 5 | 7 | 14 |
| SMD = 1.0 | 4 | 3 | 3 | 3 | 3 | 4 | 5 | 7 | 13 |

## 12.7    Drawing conclusions

### 12.7.1    Conclusions sections of a Cochrane review

Authors' conclusions from a Cochrane review are divided into implications for practice and implications for research. In deciding what these implications are, it is useful to consider four factors: the quality of evidence, the balance of benefits and harms, values and preferences and resource utilization (Eddy 1990). Considering these factors involves judgements and effort that go beyond the work of most review authors.

### 12.7.2    Implications for practice

Drawing conclusions about the practical usefulness of an intervention entails making trade-offs, either implicitly or explicitly, between the estimated benefits, harms and the estimated costs. Making such trade-offs, and thus making specific recommendations for an action, goes beyond a systematic review and requires additional information and informed judgements that are typically the domain of clinical practice guideline developers. Authors of Cochrane reviews should not make recommendations.

If authors feel compelled to lay out actions that clinicians and patients could take, they should – after describing the quality of evidence and the balance of benefits and harms – highlight different actions that might be consistent with particular patterns of values and preferences. Other factors that might influence a decision should also be highlighted, including any known factors that would be expected to modify the effects of the intervention, the baseline risk or status of the patient, costs and who bears those costs, and the availability of resources. Authors should ensure they consider all patient-important outcomes, including those for which limited data may be available. This process implies a high level of explicitness about judgements about values or preferences attached to different outcomes. The highest level of explicitness would involve a formal economic analysis with sensitivity analysis involving different assumptions about values and preferences; this is beyond the scope of most Cochrane reviews (although they might well be used for such analyses) (Mugford 1989, Mugford 1991); this is discussed in Chapter 15.

A review on the use of anticoagulation in cancer patients to increase survival (Akl 2007) provides an example for laying out clinical implications for situations where there are important trade-offs between desirable and undesirable effects of the intervention: "The decision for a patient with cancer to start heparin therapy for survival benefit should balance the benefits and downsides and integrate the patient's values and preferences (Haynes 2002). Patients with a high preference for survival prolongation (even though that prolongation may be short) and limited aversion to bleeding who do not consider heparin therapy a burden may opt to use heparin, while those with aversion to bleeding and the related burden of heparin therapy may not."

## 12.7.3   Implications for research

Review conclusions should help people make well-informed decisions about future healthcare research. The 'Implications for research' should comment on the need for further research, and the nature of the further research that would be most desirable. A format has been proposed for reporting research recommendations ('EPICOT'), as follows (Brown 2006):

- E (Evidence): What is the current evidence?

- P (Population): Diagnosis, disease stage, co-morbidity, risk factor, sex, age, ethnic group, specific inclusion or exclusion criteria, clinical setting.

- I (Intervention): Type, frequency, dose, duration, prognostic factor.

- C (Comparison): Placebo, routine care, alternative treatment/management.

- O (Outcome): Which clinical or patient-related outcomes will the researcher need to measure, improve, influence or accomplish? Which methods of measurement should be used?

- T (Time stamp): Date of literature search or recommendation.

Other factors that might be considered in recommendations include the disease burden of the condition being addressed, the timeliness (e.g. length of follow-up, duration of intervention), and the study type that would best suit subsequent research (Brown 2006).

Cochrane review authors should ensure that they include the PICO aspects of this format. It is also helpful to note the study types, as well as any particular design features, that would best address the research question.

A review of compression stockings for prevention of deep vein thrombosis in airline passengers provides an example where there is some convincing evidence of a benefit of the intervention: "This review shows that the question of the effects on symptomless DVT of wearing versus not wearing compression stockings in the types of people studied in these trials should now be regarded as answered. Further research may be justified to investigate the relative effects of different strengths of stockings or of stockings compared to other preventative strategies. Further randomized trials to address the remaining uncertainty about the effects of wearing versus not wearing compression stockings on outcomes such as death, pulmonary embolus and symptomatic DVT would need to be large." (Clarke 2006).

A review of therapeutic touch for anxiety disorder provides an example of the implications for research when no eligible studies had been found: "This review highlights the need for randomised controlled trials to evaluate the effectiveness of therapeutic touch in reducing anxiety symptoms in people diagnosed with anxiety disorders.

Future trials need to be rigorous in design and delivery, with subsequent reporting to include high quality descriptions of all aspects of methodology to enable appraisal and interpretation of results." (Robinson 2007).

### 12.7.4   Common errors in reaching conclusions

A common mistake when there is inconclusive evidence is to confuse 'no evidence of an effect' with 'evidence of no effect'. When there is inconclusive evidence, it is wrong to claim that it shows that an intervention has 'no effect' or is 'no different' from the control intervention. It is safer to report the data, with a confidence interval, as being compatible with either a reduction or an increase in the outcome. When there is a 'positive' but statistically non-significant trend authors commonly describe this as 'promising', whereas a 'negative' effect of the same magnitude is not commonly described as a 'warning sign'; such language may be harmful.

Another mistake is to frame the conclusion in wishful terms. For example, authors might write "the included studies were too small to detect a reduction in mortality" when the included studies showed a reduction or even increase in mortality that failed to reach conventional levels of statistical significance. One way of avoiding errors such as these is to consider the results blinded; i.e. consider how the results would be presented and framed in the conclusions had the direction of the results been reversed. If the confidence interval for the estimate of the difference in the effects of the interventions overlaps the null value, the analysis is compatible with both a true beneficial effect and a true harmful effect. If one of the possibilities is mentioned in the conclusion, the other possibility should be mentioned as well.

Another common mistake is to reach conclusions that go beyond the evidence. Often this is done implicitly, without referring to the additional information or judgements that are used in reaching conclusions about the implications of a review for practice. Even when additional information and explicit judgements support conclusions about the implications of a review for practice, review authors rarely conduct systematic reviews of the additional information. Furthermore, implications for practice are often dependent on specific circumstances and values that must be taken into consideration. As we have noted, authors should always be cautious when drawing conclusions about implications for practice and they should not make recommendations.

## 12.8   Chapter information

**Authors:** Holger J Schünemann, Andrew D Oxman, Gunn E Vist, Julian PT Higgins, Jonathan J Deeks, Paul Glasziou and Gordon H Guyatt on behalf of the Cochrane Applicability and Recommendations Methods Group.

**This chapter should be cited as:** Schünemann HJ, Oxman AD, Vist GE, Higgins JPT, Deeks JJ, Glasziou P, Guyatt GH. Chapter 12: Interpreting results and drawing conclusions. In: Higgins JPT, Green S (editors), *Cochrane Handbook for Systematic Reviews of Interventions*. Chichester (UK): John Wiley & Sons, 2008.

**Acknowledgements:** Jonathan Sterne, Michael Borenstein and Rob JM Scholten contributed text.

**Declarations of interest:** Holger Schünemann, Andrew Oxman, Gunn Vist, Paul Glasziou and Gordon Guyatt have, to varying degrees, taken leadership roles in the GRADE Working Group from which many of the ideas in this chapter have arisen.

---

**Box 12.8.a The Cochrane Applicability and Recommendations Methods Group**

We anticipate continued evolution of the methodologies described in this chapter. The main arenas in which relevant discussions will take place are the Applicability and Recommendations Methods Group (ARMG) and the GRADE Working Group. Both discussion groups welcome new participants with an eagerness to learn more and to contribute to further developments in rating quality of evidence, and in framing issues in the application of Cochrane reviews.

The Applicability and Recommendations Methods Group (ARMG) is comprised of individuals with interest and expertise in the interpretation, applicability and transferability of the results of systematic reviews to individuals and groups. The ARMG's objective is to explore the process of going from evidence to health-care recommendations. The ultimate goals are to make this process as rigorous as possible.

Specific areas currently considered important include:
- evaluating the quality of evidence (www.gradeworkinggroup.org);
- variation of effect with baseline risk;
- prediction of benefit from the patient's expected event rate or severity;
- consideration of how the strength of evidence and the magnitude and precision of the effects bear on the implications; and
- consideration of how people's values bear on the implications when weighing benefits and harms based on individual clinical features.

---

# 12.9 References

**Aguilar 2005**

Aguilar MI, Hart R. Oral anticoagulants for preventing stroke in patients with non-valvular atrial fibrillation and no previous history of stroke or transient ischemic attacks. *Cochrane Database of Systematic Reviews* 2005, Issue 3. Art No: CD001927.

**Akl 2007**

Akl EA, Kamath G, Kim SY, Yosuico V, Barba M, Terrenato I, Sperati F, Schünemann HJ. Oral anticoagulation for prolonging survival in patients with cancer. *Cochrane Database of Systematic Reviews* 2007, Issue 2. Art No: CD006466.

**Alonso-Coello 2006**

Alonso-Coello P, Zhou Q, Martinez-Zapata MJ, Mills E, Heels-Ansdell D, Johanson JF, Guyatt G. Meta-analysis of flavonoids for the treatment of haemorrhoids. *British Journal of Surgery* 2006; 93: 909–920.

**Altman 1998**

Altman DG. Confidence intervals for the number needed to treat. *BMJ* 1998; 317: 1309–1312.

**Bhandari 2004**

Bhandari M, Busse JW, Jackowski D, Montori VM, Schünemann H, Sprague S, Mears D, Schemitsch EH, Heels-Ansdell D, Devereaux PJ. Association between industry funding and statistically significant pro-industry findings in medical and surgical randomized trials. *Canadian Medical Association Journal* 2004; 170: 477–480.

**Brophy 2001**

Brophy JM, Joseph L, Rouleau JL. Beta-blockers in congestive heart failure. A Bayesian meta-analysis. *Annals of Internal Medicine* 2001; 134: 550–560.

**Brown 2006**

Brown P, Brunnhuber K, Chalkidou K, Chalmers I, Clarke M, Fenton M, Forbes C, Glanville J, Hicks NJ, Moody J, Twaddle S, Timimi H, Young P. How to formulate research recommendations. *BMJ* 2006; 333: 804–806.

**Cates 1999**

Cates C. Confidence intervals for the number needed to treat: Pooling numbers needed to treat may not be reliable. *BMJ* 1999; 318: 1764–1765.

**Chambers 2005**

Chambers BR, Donnan GA. Carotid endarterectomy for asymptomatic carotid stenosis. *Cochrane Database of Systematic Reviews* 2005, Issue 4. Art No: CD001923.

**Chinn 2000**

Chinn S. A simple method for converting an odds ratio to effect size for use in meta-analysis. *Statistics in Medicine* 2000; 19: 3127–3131.

**Cina 2000**

Cina CS, Clase CM, Haynes RB. Carotid endarterectomy for symptomatic carotid stenosis. *Cochrane Database of Systematic Reviews* 2000, Issue 2. Art No: CD001081.

**Clarke 2006**

Clarke M, Hopewell S, Juszczak E, Eisinga A, Kjeldstrøm M. Compression stockings for preventing deep vein thrombosis in airline passengers. *Cochrane Database of Systematic Reviews* 2006, Issue 2. Art No: CD004002.

**Cohen 1988**

Cohen J. *Statistical Power Analysis in the Behavioral Sciences* (2nd edition). Hillsdale (NJ): Lawrence Erlbaum Associates, Inc., 1988.

**Dans 2007**

Dans AM, Dans L, Oxman AD, Robinson V, Acuin J, Tugwell P, Dennis R, Kang D. Assessing equity in clinical practice guidelines. *Journal of Clinical Epidemiology* 2007; 60: 540–546.

**Devereaux 2004**

Devereaux PJ, Choi PT, El-Dika S, Bhandari M, Montori VM, Schünemann HJ, Garg AX, Busse JW, Heels-Ansdell D, Ghali WA, Manns BJ, Guyatt GH. An observational study found that authors of randomized controlled trials frequently use concealment of randomization and blinding, despite the failure to report these methods. *Journal of Clinical Epidemiology* 2004; 57: 1232–1236.

**Eddy 1990**
Eddy DM. Clinical decision making: from theory to practice. Anatomy of a decision. *JAMA* 1990; 263: 441–443.

**Friedman 1985**
Friedman LM, Furberg CD, DeMets DL. *Fundamentals of Clinical Trials* (2nd edition). Littleton (MA): John Wright PSG, Inc., 1985.

**Furukawa 1999**
Furukawa TA. From effect size into number needed to treat. *The Lancet* 1999; 353: 1680.

**Gibson 2007**
Gibson JN, Waddell G. Surgical interventions for lumbar disc prolapse. *Cochrane Database of Systematic Reviews* 2007, Issue 2. Art No: CD001350.

**GRADE Working Group 2004**
GRADE Working Group. Grading quality of evidence and strength of recommendations. *BMJ* 2004; 328: 1490–1494.

**Guyatt 1994**
Guyatt GH, Sackett DL, Cook DJ. Users' guides to the medical literature. II. How to use an article about therapy or prevention. B. What were the results and will they help me in caring for my patients? Evidence-Based Medicine Working Group. *JAMA* 1994; 271: 59–63.

**Guyatt 2006a**
Guyatt G, Gutterman D, Baumann MH, Addrizzo-Harris D, Hylek EM, Phillips B, Raskob G, Lewis SZ, Schünemann H. Grading strength of recommendations and quality of evidence in clinical guidelines: report from an American College of Chest Physicians Task Force. *Chest* 2006; 129: 174–181.

**Guyatt 2006b**
Guyatt G, Vist G, Falck-Ytter Y, Kunz R, Magrini N, Schünemann H. An emerging consensus on grading recommendations? *ACP Journal Club* 2006; 144: A8–A9.

**Guyatt 2008a**
Guyatt GH, Oxman AD, Kunz R, Vist GE, Falck-Ytter Y, Schünemann HJ. What is 'quality of evidence' and why is it important to clinicians? *BMJ* 2008; 336: 995–998.

**Guyatt 2008b**
Guyatt GH, Oxman AD, Vist GE, Kunz R, Falck-Ytter Y, Alonso-Coello P, Schünemann HJ. GRADE: an emerging consensus on rating quality of evidence and strength of recommendations. *BMJ* 2008; 336: 924–926.

**Hawe 2004**
Hawe P, Shiell A, Riley T, Gold L. Methods for exploring implementation variation and local context within a cluster randomised community intervention trial. *Journal of Epidemiology and Community Health* 2004; 58: 788–793.

**Haynes 2002**
Haynes RB, Devereaux PJ, Guyatt GH. Clinical expertise in the era of evidence-based medicine and patient choice. *ACP Journal Club* 2002; 136: A11–A14.

**Hoffrage 2000**
Hoffrage U, Lindsey S, Hertwig R, Gigerenzer G. Medicine. Communicating statistical information. *Science* 2000; 290: 2261–2262.

**Levine 2004**
Levine MN, Raskob G, Beyth RJ, Kearon C, Schulman S. Hemorrhagic complications of anticoagulant treatment: the Seventh ACCP Conference on Antithrombotic and Thrombolytic Therapy. *Chest* 2004; 126: 287S–310S.

**Lumley 2004**

Lumley J, Oliver SS, Chamberlain C, Oakley L. Interventions for promoting smoking cessation during pregnancy. *Cochrane Database of Systematic Reviews* 2004, Issue 4. Art No: CD001055.

**McIntosh 2005**

McIntosh HM, Jones KL. Chloroquine or amodiaquine combined with sulfadoxine-pyrimethamine for treating uncomplicated malaria. *Cochrane Database of Systematic Reviews* 2005, Issue 4. Art No: CD000386.

**McQuay 1997**

McQuay HJ, Moore A. Using numerical results from systematic reviews in clinical practice. *Annals of Internal Medicine* 1997; 126: 712–720.

**Mugford 1989**

Mugford M, Kingston J, Chalmers I. Reducing the incidence of infection after caesarean section: implications of prophylaxis with antibiotics for hospital resources. *BMJ* 1989; 299: 1003–1006.

**Mugford 1991**

Mugford M, Piercy J, Chalmers I. Cost implications of different approaches to the prevention of respiratory distress syndrome. *Archives of Disease in Childhood* 1991; 66: 757–764.

**Oxman 2002**

Oxman A, Guyatt G. When to believe a subgroup analysis. In: Guyatt G, Rennie D (editors). *Users' Guides to the Medical Literature: A Manual for Evidence-Based Clinical Practice.* Chicago (IL): AMA Press, 2002.

**Resnicow 1993**

Resnicow K, Cross D, Wynder E. The Know Your Body program: a review of evaluation studies. *Bulletin of the New York Academy of Medicine* 1993; 70: 188–207.

**Robinson 2007**

Robinson J, Biley FC, Dolk H. Therapeutic touch for anxiety disorders. *Cochrane Database of Systematic Reviews* 2007, Issue 3. Art No: CD006240.

**Sackett 2000**

Sackett DL, Richardson WS, Rosenberg W, Haynes BR. *Evidence-Based Medicine: How to Practice and Teach EBM* (2nd edition). Edinburgh (UK): Churchill Livingstone, 2000.

**Salpeter 2007**

Salpeter S, Greyber E, Pasternak G, Salpeter E. Risk of fatal and nonfatal lactic acidosis with metformin use in type 2 diabetes mellitus. *Cochrane Database of Systematic Reviews* 2007, Issue 4. Art No: CD002967.

**Scholten 1999**

Scholten RJPM. From effect size into number needed to treat [letter]. *The Lancet* 1999; 453: 598.

**Schünemann 2006a**

Schünemann HJ, Fretheim A, Oxman AD. Improving the use of research evidence in guideline development: 13. Applicability, transferability and adaptation. *Health Research Policy and Systems* 2006; 4: 25.

**Schünemann 2006b**

Schünemann HJ, Jaeschke R, Cook DJ, Bria WF, El-Solh AA, Ernst A, Fahy BF, Gould MK, Horan KL, Krishnan JA, Manthous CA, Maurer JR, McNicholas WT, Oxman AD, Rubenfeld G, Turino GM, Guyatt G. An official ATS statement: grading the quality of evidence and strength of recommendations in ATS guidelines and recommendations. *American Journal of Respiratory and Critical Care Medicine* 2006; 174: 605–614.

**Smeeth 1999**

Smeeth L, Haines A, Ebrahim S. Numbers needed to treat derived from meta-analyses – sometimes informative, usually misleading. *BMJ* 1999; 318: 1548–1551.

**Suissa 1991**

Suissa S. Binary methods for continuous outcomes: a parametric alternative. *Journal of Clinical Epidemiology* 1991; 44: 241–248.

**Thompson 2000**

Thompson DC, Rivara FP, Thompson R. Helmets for preventing head and facial injuries in bicyclists. *Cochrane Database of Systematic Reviews* 2000, Issue 2. Art No: CD001855.

**Walter 2001**

Walter SD. Number needed to treat (NNT): estimation of a measure of clinical benefit. *Statistics in Medicine* 2001; 20: 3947–3962.

# PART 3: Special topics

# 13 Including non-randomized studies

**Barnaby C Reeves, Jonathan J Deeks, Julian PT Higgins and George A Wells on behalf of the Cochrane Non-Randomised Studies Methods Group**

## Key Points

- For some Cochrane reviews, the question of interest cannot be answered by randomized trials, and review authors may be justified in including non-randomized studies.

- Potential biases are likely to be greater for non-randomized studies compared with randomized trials, so results should always be interpreted with caution when they are included in reviews and meta-analyses. Particular concerns arise with respect to differences between people in different intervention groups (selection bias) and studies that do not explicitly report having had a protocol (reporting bias).

- We recommend that eligibility criteria, data collection and critical assessment of included studies place an emphasis on specific features of study design (e.g. which parts of the study were prospectively designed) rather than 'labels' for study designs (such as case-control versus cohort).

- Risk of bias in non-randomized studies can be assessed in a similar manner to that used for randomized trials, although more attention must be paid to the possibility of selection bias.

- Meta-analyses of non-randomized studies must consider how potential confounders are addressed, and consider the likelihood of increased heterogeneity resulting from residual confounding and from other biases that vary across studies.

## 13.1 Introduction

### 13.1.1 What this chapter is about

This chapter has been prepared by the Non-Randomised Studies Methods Group (NRSMG) of The Cochrane Collaboration (see Box 13.8.a). It is intended to support review authors who are considering including non-randomized studies in Cochrane reviews. **Non-randomized studies** (NRS) are defined here as any quantitative study estimating the effectiveness of an intervention (harm or benefit) that does not use randomization to allocate units to comparison groups. This includes studies where allocation occurs in the course of usual treatment decisions or peoples' choices, i.e. studies usually called *observational*. There are many types of non-randomized intervention study, including cohort studies, case-control studies, controlled before-and-after studies, interrupted-time-series studies and controlled trials that use inappropriate randomization strategies (sometimes called quasi-randomized studies). Box 13.1.a summarizes some commonly-used study design labels for non-randomized studies. We explain in Section 13.5.1 why we do not necessarily advise that these labels are used in Cochrane reviews.

This chapter aims to describe the particular challenges that arise if NRS are included in a Cochrane review, and is informed by theoretical or epidemiological considerations, empirical research, and discussions among members of the NRSMG. The chapter makes recommendations about what to do when it is possible to support the recommendations on the basis of evidence or established theory. When it is not possible to make any recommendations, the chapter aims to set out the pros and cons of alternative actions and to identify questions for further methodological research.

Review authors who are considering including NRS in a Cochrane review should not start with this chapter unless they are already familiar with the process of preparing a systematic review of randomized trials. The format and basic steps of a Cochrane review should be the same whether it includes only randomized trials or includes NRS. The reader is referred to Part 1 of the Handbook for a detailed description of these steps. Every step in carrying out a systematic review is more difficult when NRS are included and a review author should seek to include expert epidemiologists and methodologists in the review team. As an example of such collaboration, a review of NRS included nine authors, five of whom were methodologists (Siegfried 2003).

### 13.1.2 Why consider non-randomized studies?

The Cochrane Collaboration focuses particularly on systematic reviews of randomized trials because they are more likely to provide unbiased information than other study designs about the differential effects of alternative forms of health care. Reviews of NRS are only likely to be undertaken when the question of interest cannot be answered by a review of randomized trials. The NRSMG believes that review authors may be justified in including NRS which are moderately susceptible to bias. Broadly, the

## Box 13.1.a Some types of NRS design used for evaluating the effects of interventions

Designs are distinguished below by labels in common use and descriptions are intentionally non-specific because the labels are interpreted in different ways with respect to details. The NRSMG does not advocate using these labels for reasons explained in Section 13.5.1.

| | |
|---|---|
| Non-randomized controlled trial. | An experimental study in which people are allocated to different interventions using methods that are not random. |
| Controlled before-and-after study. | A study in which observations are made before and after the implementation of an intervention, both in a group that receives the intervention and in a control group that does not. |
| Interrupted-time-series study. | A study that uses observations at multiple time points before and after an intervention (the 'interruption'). The design attempts to detect whether the intervention has had an effect significantly greater than any underlying trend over time. |
| Historically controlled study. | A study that compares a group of participants receiving an intervention with a similar group from the past who did not. |
| Cohort study. | A study in which a defined group of people (the cohort) is followed over time, to examine associations between different interventions received and subsequent outcomes. A 'prospective' cohort study recruits participants before any intervention and follows them into the future. A 'retrospective' cohort study identifies subjects from past records describing the interventions received and follows them from the time of those records. |
| Case-control study. | A study that compares people with a specific outcome of interest ('cases') with people from the same source population but without that outcome ('controls'), to examine the association between the outcome and prior exposure (e.g. having an intervention). This design is particularly useful when the outcome is rare. |
| Cross-sectional study. | A study that collects information on interventions (past or present) and current health outcomes, i.e. restricted to health states, for a group of people at a particular point in time, to examine associations between the outcomes and exposure to interventions. |
| Case series (uncontrolled longitudinal study). | Observations are made on a series of individuals, usually all receiving the same intervention, before and after an intervention but with no control group. |

NRSMG considers that there are three main reasons for including NRS in a Cochrane review:

(a) To examine the case for undertaking a randomized trial by providing an explicit evaluation of the weaknesses of available NRS. The findings of a review of NRS may also be useful to inform the design of a subsequent randomized trial, e.g. through the identification of relevant subgroups.

(b) To provide evidence of the effects (benefit or harm) of interventions that cannot be randomized, or which are extremely unlikely to be studied in randomized trials. In these contexts, a disinterested (free from bias and partiality) review that systematically reports the findings and limitations of available NRS can be useful.

(c) To provide evidence of effects (benefit or harm) that cannot be adequately studied in randomized trials, such as long-term and rare outcomes, or outcomes that were not known to be important when existing, major randomized trials were conducted.

Three other reasons are often cited in support of systematic reviews of NRS but are poor justifications:

(d) Studying effects in patient groups not recruited to randomized trials (such as children, pregnant women, the elderly). Although it is important to consider whether the results of trials can be generalized to people who are excluded from them, it is not clear that this can be achieved by consideration of non-randomized studies. Regardless of whether estimates from NRS agree or disagree with those of randomized trials, there is always potential for bias in the results of the NRS, such that misleading conclusions are drawn.

(e) To supplement existing randomized trial evidence. Adding non-randomized to randomized evidence may change an imprecise but unbiased estimate into a precise but biased estimate, i.e. an exchange of undesirable uncertainty for unacceptable error.

(f) When an intervention effect is really large. Implicitly, this is a result-driven or *post-hoc* justification, since the review (or some other synthesis of the evidence) needs to be undertaken to observe the likely size of the effects. Whilst it is easier to argue that large effects are less likely to be completely explained by bias than small effects (Glasziou 2007), for the practice of health care it is still important to obtain unbiased estimates of the magnitude of large effects to make clinical and economic decisions (Reeves 2006). Thus randomized trials are still needed for large effects (and they need not be large if the effects are truly large). There may be ethical opposition to randomized trials of interventions already suspected to be associated with a large benefit as a result of a systematic review of NRS, making it difficult to randomize participants, and interventions postulated to have large effects may also be difficult to randomize for other reasons (e.g. surgery vs. no surgery). However, the justification for a systematic review of NRS in these circumstances should be classified as (b), i.e. interventions that are unlikely to be randomized, rather than as (f).

### 13.1.3 Key issues about the inclusion of non-randomized studies in a Cochrane review

Randomized trials are the preferred design for studying the effects of healthcare interventions because, in most circumstances, the randomized trial is the study design that is least likely to be biased. Any Cochrane review must consider the risk of bias in individual primary studies, including both the likely direction and magnitude of bias (see Chapter 8). A review that includes NRS also requires review authors to do this. The principle of considering risk of bias is exactly the same. However, potential biases are likely to be greater for NRS compared with randomized trials. Review authors need to consider (a) the weaknesses of the designs that have been used (such as noting their potential to ascertain causality), (b) the execution of the studies through a careful assessment of their risk of bias, especially (c) the potential for selection bias and confounding to which all NRS are suspect and (d) the potential for reporting biases, including selective reporting of outcomes.

Susceptibility to selection bias (understood in this *Handbook* to mean differences in the baseline characteristics of individuals in different intervention groups, rather than whether the selected sample is representative of the population) is widely regarded as the principal difference between randomized trials and NRS. Randomization with adequate allocation sequence concealment reduces the possibility of systematic selection bias in randomized trials so that differences in characteristics between groups can be attributed to chance. In NRS, allocation to groups depends on other factors, often unknown. Confounding occurs when selection bias gives rise to imbalances between intervention and control groups (or case and control groups in case-control studies) on prognostic factors, i.e. the distributions of the factors differ between groups *and* the factors are associated with outcome. Confounding can have two effects in a meta-analysis: (a) shifting the estimate of the intervention effect (systematic bias) and (b) increasing the variability of the observed effects, introducing excessive heterogeneity among studies (Deeks 2003). It is important to consider both of these possible effects (see Section 13.6.1). Section 13.5 provides a more detailed discussion of susceptibility to bias in NRS.

### 13.1.4 The importance of a protocol for a Cochrane review that includes non-randomized studies

Chapter 2 establishes the importance of writing a protocol for a Cochrane review before carrying out the review. As the methodological choices made during a review of NRS are complex and may affect the review findings, a protocol is even more important for a review that includes NRS. The rationale for doing a review that includes NRS (see Section 13.1.2) should be documented in the protocol. The protocol should include much more detail than for a review of randomized trials, pre-specifying key methodological decisions about the methods to be used and the analyses that are planned. The protocol needs to specify details that are not relevant for randomized trials (e.g. the methods planned to identify potential confounding factors and to assess the susceptibility of primary studies to confounding), as well as providing more detail about standard steps in the review process that are more difficult when including NRS (e.g. specification of eligibility criteria and the search strategy for identifying eligible studies).

The NRSMG recognizes that it may not be possible to pre-specify all decisions about the methods used in a review. Nevertheless, review authors should aim to make all decisions about the methods for the review without reference to the findings of primary studies, and report methodological decisions that had to be made or modified after collecting data about the study findings.

### 13.1.5   Structure of subsequent sections in the chapter

Each of the sections in this chapter, which focus in turn on different steps of the review process, is structured in the same way. First, for a particular step, we summarize what is different when NRS (compared with randomized trials) are included in Cochrane reviews and, where applicable, describe conceptual issues that need to be considered. This first part includes relevant evidence, where there is some. Second, we summarize our guidance and, where available, describe existing resources that are available to support review authors.

## 13.2   Developing criteria for including non-randomized studies

### 13.2.1   What is different when including non-randomized studies?

#### 13.2.1.1   Including both randomized and non-randomized studies

Review authors may want to include NRS in a review because only a small number of randomized trials can be identified, or because of perceived limitations of the randomized trials. In this chapter, we strongly recommend that review authors should not make any attempt to combine evidence from randomized trials and NRS. This recommendation means that criteria for included study designs should generally specify randomized or non-randomized studies when trying to evaluate the effect of an intervention on a particular outcome. (However, a single review might consist of 'component' reviews that include different study designs for different outcomes, for example, randomized trials for evaluating benefits and NRS to evaluate harms; see Chapter 14.)

Alternatively, where randomized trial evidence is desired but unlikely to be available, eligibility criteria could reasonably be structured to say that NRS would only be included where randomized trials are found not to be available. In time, as such a review is updated, the NRS may be dropped when randomized trials become available. Where both randomized trials and NRS of an intervention exist and, for one or more of the reasons given in Section 13.1.2, both are included in the review, these should be presented separately; alternatively, if there is an adequate number of randomized trials, comments about relevant NRS can be included in the Discussion section of a review although this is rarely particularly helpful.

### 13.2.1.2  *Evaluating benefits and harms*

Cochrane reviews aim to quantify the effects of healthcare interventions, both beneficial and harmful, and both expected and unexpected. Most reviews estimate the expected benefits of an intervention that are assessed in randomized trials. Randomized trials may report some of the harms of an intervention, either those which were expected and which the trial was designed to assess, or those which were not expected but which were collected in the trial as part of standard monitoring of safety. However, many serious harms of an intervention are too rare or do not appear during the follow-up period of randomized trials, and therefore will not be reported. Therefore, one of the most important roles for reviews of NRS is to assess potential unexpected or rare harms of interventions (reason (c) in Section 13.1.1). Criteria for selecting important and relevant studies for evaluating rare or long-term adverse and unexpected effects are difficult to set. Although the relative strengths and weaknesses of different study designs are the same as for beneficial outcomes, the choice of study designs to include may depend on both the frequency of an outcome and its importance. For example, for some rare adverse outcomes only case series or case-control studies may be available. Study designs that are more susceptible to bias may be acceptable for evaluation of serious events in the absence of better evidence.

Confounding may be less of a threat to the validity of a review when researching rare harms or unexpected effects of interventions than when researching expected effects, since it is argued that 'confounding by indication' mainly influences treatment decisions with respect to outcomes about which the clinicians are primarily concerned. However, confounding can never be ruled out because the same features that are confounders for the expected effects may also be direct confounders for the unexpected effects, or be correlated with features that are confounders.

A related issue is the need to distinguish between *quantifying* and *detecting* an effect of an intervention. Quantifying the intended benefits of an intervention – maximizing the precision of the estimate and minimizing susceptibility to bias – is critical when weighing up the relative merits of alternative interventions for the same condition. A review should also try to quantify the harms of an intervention, minimizing susceptibility to bias as far as possible. However, if a review can establish beyond reasonable doubt that an intervention causes a particular harm, the precision and susceptibility to bias of the estimated effect may not be critical. In other words, the seriousness of the harm may outweigh any benefit from the intervention. This situation is more likely to occur when there are competing interventions for a condition.

### 13.2.1.3   Determining which types of non-randomized study to include

A randomized trial is a prospective, experimental study design specifically involving random allocation of participants to interventions. Although there are variations in randomized trial design (including random allocation of individuals, clusters or body parts; multi-arm trials, factorial trials and cross-over trials) they constitute a distinctive study category. By contrast, NRS cover a number of fundamentally different designs, several of which were originally conceived in the context of aetiological epidemiology. Some of these are summarized in Box 13.1.a, although this is not an exhaustive list, and many studies combine ideas from different basic designs. As we discuss in 13.2.2 these labels are not consistently applied. The diversity of NRS designs raises two related questions. First, should all NRS designs of a particular effectiveness question be included in a review? Second, if review authors do not include all NRS designs, what criteria should be used to decide which study designs to include and which to exclude?

It is generally accepted that criteria should be set to limit the kinds of evidence included in a systematic review. The primary reason is that the risk of bias varies across studies. For this reason, many Cochrane reviews only include randomized trials (when available). For the same reason, it is argued that review authors should only include NRS that are least likely to be biased. It is not helpful to include primary studies in a review when the results of the studies are likely to be biased, even if there is no better evidence. This is because a misleading effect estimate may be more harmful to future patients than no estimate at all, particularly if the people using the evidence to make decisions are unaware of its limitations (Doll 1993, Peto 1995).

There is no agreement about the study design criteria that should be used to limit the inclusion of NRS in a Cochrane review. One strategy is to include only those study designs that will give reasonably valid effect estimates. Another strategy is to include the best available study designs which have been used to answer a question. The first strategy would mean that reviews are consistent and include the same types of NRS, but that some reviews include no studies at all. The second strategy leads to different reviews including different study designs according to what was available. For example, it might be entirely appropriate to use different criteria for inclusion when reviewing the harms, compared with the benefits, of an intervention. This approach is already evident in the *Cochrane Database of Systematic Reviews* (*CDSR*), with editors of some Cochrane Review Groups (CRGs) restricting reviews to randomized trials only and other CRG editors allowing specific types of NRS to be included in reviews (typically in healthcare areas where randomized trials are infrequent).

Whichever point of view is adopted, criteria can only be chosen with respect to a hierarchy of primary study designs, ranked in order of risk of bias according to study design features. Existing 'evidence hierarchies' for studies of effectiveness (Eccles 1996, National Health and Medical Research Council 1999, Oxford Centre for Evidence-based Medicine 2001) appear to have arisen largely by applying hierarchies for aetiological research questions to effectiveness questions. For example, cohort studies are conventionally regarded as providing better evidence than case-control studies. It is not clear that this is always appropriate since aetiological hierarchies place more emphasis on establishing causality (e.g. dose-response relationship, exposure preceding outcome) than on valid quantification of the effect size. Also, study designs used for studying the effects of interventions can be very much more diverse and complex (Shadish 2002) and may not be easily assimilated into existing evidence hierarchies (see the array of designs in Box 13.1.a, for example). Different designs are susceptible to different biases, and it is often unclear which biases have the greatest impact and how they vary between clinical situations.

### 13.2.1.4 *Distinguishing between aetiology and effectiveness research questions*

Including NRS in a Cochrane review allows, in principle, the inclusion of truly observational studies where the use of an intervention has occurred in the course of usual health care or daily life. For interventions that are not restricted to a medical setting, this may mean interventions that a study participant chooses to take, e.g. over-the-counter preparations. Including observational studies in a review also allows exposures to be studied that are not obviously 'interventions', e.g. nutritional choices, and other behaviours that may affect health. This introduces a 'grey area' between evidence about effectiveness and aetiology. It is important to distinguish carefully between different aetiological and effectiveness research questions related to a particular exposure. For example, nutritionists may be interested in the health-related effects of a diet that includes a minimum of five portions of fruit or vegetables per day ('five-a-day'), an aetiological question. On the other hand, public health professionals may be interested in the health-related effects of interventions to promote a change in diet to include 'five-a-day', an effectiveness question. Because of other differences between studies relevant to these two kinds of question (e.g. duration of follow-up and outcomes investigated), studies addressing the former type of question are often perceived as being 'better' or 'more relevant' without acknowledging or realizing that they are addressing different research questions. In other instances the health intervention being evaluated in the NRS will have been undertaken for a purpose other than improving health. For example, a review of circumcision for preventing transmission of HIV included NRS where circumcision had been undertaken for cultural or religious reasons (Siegfried 2003), and it was unclear whether using the intervention for health purposes would have the same effect.

## 13.2.2  Guidance and resources available to support review authors

Review authors should first check with the editors of the CRG under which they propose to register their protocol whether there is a CRG-specific policy in place about the inclusion of NRS in a review. Authors should also discuss with the editors the extent of methodological advice available in the CRG since they are likely to require more support than with a review that includes randomized trials only, and attempt to recruit informed methodologists to their review team. Regrettably, the NRSMG is not currently in a position to collaborate with authors on particular reviews, but encourages authors who include NRS in their reviews to feedback their experiences to the NRSMG, particularly where their experiences support, or contradict, the experiences described in this chapter.

Review authors intending to review the adverse effects (harms) of an intervention should read Chapter 14, which has been prepared by the Adverse Effects Methods Group.

We recommend that review authors use explicit study design features (NB: not study design labels) when deciding which types of NRS to include in a review. Members of the NRSMG have developed two lists that can be used for this purpose, although experience using them is limited. Tables 13.2.a and 13.2.b describe separate lists for individually-allocated and cluster-allocated studies. Sixteen (or fifteen) items are grouped under four headings:

1. Was there a comparison?

2. How were groups created?

3. Which parts of the study were prospective?

4. On which variables was comparability [between groups receiving different interventions] assessed?

The items are designed to characterize key features of studies which, on the basis of the experiences of NRSMG members and 'first principles' (rather than evidence), are suspected to define the major study design categories or to be associated with susceptibility to bias. The tables indicate which features are associated with different NRS designs, identified by labels that are more specific than those in Box 13.1.a. There is not total consensus about the use of these (column) labels. This disagreement does not mean that the row items are inappropriate or poorly described; the value of the lists depends on the agreement between review authors when classifying primary studies. We will also propose that these lists be used as checklists in the processes of data collection and as part of the critical assessment of the studies (Section 13.4.2 and Section 13.5.2). Instructions for using the items as checklists in Box 13.4.a provide further explanation of the terms.

A number of organizations are carrying out systematic reviews of NRS where there are no, or very few, randomized trials. Reviews are often commissioned on behalf of organizations responsible for issuing policy or guidance to healthcare professionals, e.g. the National Institute for Health and Clinical Excellence (NICE), the Canadian Agency for Drugs and Technologies in Health (CADTH), and carried out by teams of systematic reviewers in university departments of health sciences. In general, reviewers in these

**Table 13.2.a**  List of study design features (studies with allocation to interventions at the individual level)

| | RCT | Q-RCT | NRCT | CBA | PCS | RCS | HCT | NCC | CC | XS | BA | CR/CS |
|---|---|---|---|---|---|---|---|---|---|---|---|---|
| *Was there a comparison:* | | | | | | | | | | | | |
| Between two or more groups of participants receiving different interventions? | Y | Y | Y | Y | Y | Y | Y | Y | Y | Y | N | N |
| Within the same group of participants over time? | P | P | N | Y | N | N | N | N | N | N | Y | N |
| *Were participants allocated to groups by:* | | | | | | | | | | | | |
| Concealed randomization? | Y | N | N | N | N | N | N | N | N | N | na | na |
| Quasi-randomization? | N | Y | N | N | N | N | N | N | N | N | na | na |
| By other action of researchers? | N | N | Y | P | N | N | N | N | N | N | na | na |
| Time differences? | N | N | N | N | N | N | Y | N | N | N | na | na |
| Location differences? | N | N | P | P | P | P | P | na | na | na | na | na |
| Treatment decisions? | N | N | N | P | P | P | N | N | N | P | na | na |
| Participants' preferences? | N | N | N | P | P | P | N | N | N | P | na | na |
| On the basis of outcome? | N | N | N | N | N | N | N | Y | Y | P | na | na |
| Some other process? (specify) | | | | | | | | | | | | |
| *Which parts of the study were prospective:* | | | | | | | | | | | | |
| Identification of participants? | Y | Y | Y | P | Y | N | P* | Y | N | N | P | P |
| Assessment of baseline and allocation to intervention? | Y | Y | Y | P | Y | N | P* | Y | N | N | na | na |
| Assessment of outcomes? | Y | Y | Y | P | Y | P | P | Y | N | N | P | P |
| Generation of hypotheses? | Y | Y | Y | Y | Y | Y | Y | Y | P | P | P | na |
| *On what variables was comparability between groups assessed:* | | | | | | | | | | | | |
| Potential confounders? | P | P | P | P | P | P | P | P | P | P | N | na |
| Baseline assessment of outcome variables? | P | P | P | Y | P | P | P | N | N | N | N | na |

Y = Yes; P = Possible for one group only; N = No; na = not applicable. NB: Note that 'possibly' is used in the table to indicate cells where *either* 'Y' or 'N' may be the case. It should not be used as a response option when applying the checklist; if uncertain, the response should be 'can't tell' (see Box 13.4.a).
RCT = Randomized controlled trial; Q-RCT = Quasi-randomized controlled trial; NRCT = Non-randomized controlled trial; CBA = Controlled before-and-after study; PCS = Prospective cohort study; RCS = Retrospective cohort study; HCT = Historically controlled study; NCC = Nested case-control trial; CC = Case-control study; XS = Cross-sectional study; BA = Before-and-after comparison; CR/CS = Case report/Case series.

**Table 13.2.b** List of study design features (studies with allocation to interventions at the group level)

| | CIRCT | CIQ-RCT | CINRT | CITS | CChBA | ITS | ChBA | EcoXS |
|---|---|---|---|---|---|---|---|---|
| *Was there a comparison:* | | | | | | | | |
| Between two or more groups of clusters receiving different interventions? | Y | Y | Y | Y | Y | N | N | Y |
| Within the same group of clusters over time? | P | P | N | Y | N | Y | Y | N |
| *Were clusters allocated to groups by:* | | | | | | | | |
| Concealed randomization? | Y | N | N | N | N | N | N | N |
| Quasi-randomization? | N | Y | N | N | N | N | N | N |
| By other action of researchers? | N | N | Y | N | P | N | N | N |
| Time differences? | N | N | N | Y | Y | Y | Y | Y |
| Location differences? | N | N | P | P | P | N | N | P |
| Policy/public health decisions? | Na | na | P | P | P | P | na | na |
| Cluster preferences? | Na | na | P | P | P | P | na | na |
| Some other process? (specify) | | | | | | | | |
| *Which parts of the study were prospective:* | | | | | | | | |
| Identification of participating clusters? | Y | Y | Y | P | P | P | P | N |
| Assessment of baseline and allocation to intervention? | Y | Y | Y | P | P | P | P | N |
| Assessment of outcomes? | Y | Y | Y | P | P | P | P | N |
| Generation of hypotheses? | Y | Y | Y | Y | Y | Y | Y | P |
| *On what variables was comparability between groups assessed:* | | | | | | | | |
| Potential confounders? | P | P | P | P | P | P | P | P |
| Baseline assessment of outcome variables? | P | P | P | Y | Y | Y | Y | N |

Note that 'cluster' refers to an entity (e.g. an organization), not necessarily to a group of participants; 'group' refers to one or more clusters; see Box 13.4.a.
Note that 'possibly' is used in the table to indicate cells where *either* 'Y' or 'N' may be the case. It should not be used as a response option when applying the checklist; if uncertain, 'can't tell' should be used (see Box 13.4.a).
Y = Yes; P = Possibly; P* = Possible for one group only; N = No; NR = Not required. CIRCT = Cluster randomized controlled trial; CIQ-RCT = Cluster quasi-randomized controlled trial; CINRT = Cluster non-randomized controlled trial; CITS = Controlled interrupted time series (Shadish 2002); CChBA = Controlled cohort before-and-after study (Shadish 2002); ITS = Interrupted time series; ChBA = Cohort before-and-after study (Shadish 2002); EcoXS = Ecological cross-sectional study.

teams have sought to apply methods developed for systematic reviews of randomized trials to NRS. These groups include:

- Effective Practice and Organisation of Care (EPOC) Group (www.epoc.cochrane.org);

- The Centre for Reviews and Dissemination (www.york.ac.uk/inst/crd);

- EPPI centre, Institute of Education, University of London (eppi.ioe.ac.uk);

- The Effective Public Health Practice Project (EPHPP), Canadian Ministry of Health, Long-Term Care and the City of Hamilton, Public Health Services (link to list of EPHPP reviews: old.hamilton.ca/phcs/ephpp).

CRGs and Cochrane review authors have tended to limit inclusion of NRS by study design or methodological quality, acknowledging that NRS design influences susceptibility to bias. For example, the EPOC CRG accepts protocols that include interrupted time series and controlled before-and-after studies, but not other NRS designs. Other reviews have limited inclusion to studies with 'adequate methodological quality' (Taggart 2001).

## 13.2.3  Summary

- Review authors should carefully justify their rationale for including NRS in their systematic review.

- Review authors should consult the editorial policy of the CRG under which they propose to register their protocol concerning inclusion of NRS. Authors should consider the extent of methodological advice available in the CRG and the methodological support they have in their team.

- Review authors should specify eligibility criteria based on what researchers did (i.e. important aspects of study design), as well as factors relating to the specific review question of interest (i.e. intervention, population, health problem), to avoid ambiguity. We suggest that authors use the items in the NRSMG checklist, or a similar checklist, to do this.

- Review authors also need information about what researchers did in primary studies to categorize the studies identified. We suggest that authors use the NRSMG lists of study design features, or a similar tool, for these purposes, and record when important aspects of study design are unclear or not reported.

- Authors reviewing questions about the adverse effects (harms) of interventions should read Chapter 14.

## 13.3    Searching for non-randomized studies

### 13.3.1    What is different when including non-randomized studies?

#### 13.3.1.1    Comprehensiveness of search strategy

When a review aims to include randomized trials only, a key principle of searching for eligible studies is that review authors should try as hard as possible to identify all randomized trials of the review question that have ever been started. Therefore, review authors are recommended to search trial registers, conference abstracts, grey literature, etc, as well as standard bibliographic databases such as MEDLINE, PUBMED, EMBASE (see Chapter 6). It is argued that a systematic review needs to search comprehensively in order to avoid publication biases. It is easy to argue that authors of a review that includes NRS should do the same (Petticrew 2001). However, it is important to set out the premises underpinning the original rationale for a comprehensive search and to consider very carefully whether they apply to reviews of NRS. The premises are:

(a) A finite population exists of randomized trials that investigate the review question.

(b) All randomized trials in this population can be identified through a search that is sufficiently comprehensive because randomized trials are relatively easily identified, registers of them are available, and they are difficult to do without funding and ethics approval, which also create an 'audit trail' (Chan 2004).

(c) All randomized trials in this population, if well conducted, provide valuable information.

(d) Ease of access to information about these randomized trials is related to their findings, so that the most readily identified trials may be a biased subset. This is publication bias: studies with statistically significant and favourable findings are more likely to be published in accessible places (see Chapter 10, Section 10.2). Because smaller studies are less likely to produce such findings, failure to identify all studies may result in funnel plot asymmetry. An unbiased answer can in theory be reached by identifying all randomized trials, i.e. by a comprehensive search to uncover the small, non-significant or unfavourable studies. Smaller studies may also suffer differentially from other biases, giving rise to an alternative cause of funnel plot asymmetry. The risks of these biases are reasonably well understood and may be assessed (Chapter 10, Section 10.4).

It is not clear that these premises apply equally to NRS.

Section 13.2.1.3 points out that NRS include diverse designs, and that there is difficulty in categorizing them. Even if review authors are able to set specific study design criteria against which potential NRS should be assessed for inclusion, many of the potentially eligible NRS will report insufficient information to allow them to be classified.

There is a further problem in defining exactly when a NRS comes into existence. For example, is a cohort study that has collected data on the interventions and outcome of interest, but that has not examined their association, an eligible NRS? Is computer output in a filing cabinet that includes a calculated odds ratio for the relevant association an eligible NRS? Consequently, it is difficult to define a 'finite population of NRS' for a particular review question. Some NRS that have been done may not be traceable at all, i.e. they are not to be found even in the proverbial 'bottom drawer'.

Notwithstanding the problems in defining what constitutes an eligible NRS, the actual identification of NRS provides important challenges. This is not just to do with poor reporting but also to do with:

- the absence of registers of NRS;

- poor indexing of important study design characteristics, etc;

- NRS not always requiring ethical approval (at least in the past);

- NRS not always having a research sponsor or funder; and

- NRS not always having been executed according to a pre-specified protocol.

There is no evidence that reporting biases affect randomized trials and NRS differentially. However, it is difficult to believe that reporting biases could affect NRS *less* than randomized trials, given the increasing number of features associated with carrying out and reporting randomized trials that act to prevent reporting biases which are frequently absent in NRS (pre-specified protocol, ethical approval including progress and final reports, the CONSORT statement (Moher 2001), trial registers and indexing of publication type in bibliographic databases). Unlike the situation for randomized trials, the likely magnitude and determinants of publication bias are not known.

The benefits of comprehensive searching for NRS are unclear, and this is a topic that requires further research. It is possible that the studies which are the hardest to find may be the most biased, if being hard to identify relates to poor design and small size. With reviews of randomized trials, comprehensive searching offers potential protection against bias because a defined population of eligible studies exists, so small studies with non-significant findings should, ultimately, be identified. With reviews of NRS, even if a *theoretical* finite population of eligible studies can be defined, one does not have similar confidence that missing studies with non-significant findings can be identified.

### 13.3.1.2  Identifying NRS in searches

It is easy to design a search strategy that identifies all evidence about an intervention by creating search strings for the population and disease characteristics, the intervention, and possibly the comparator. When a review aims to include randomized trials only, various approaches are available to restrict the search strategy to randomized trials (see Chapter 6):

(a) Search for previous reviews of the review question.

(b) Use resources, such as CENTRAL or CRG-specific registers, that are 'rich' in randomized trials.

(c) Use methodological filters and indexing fields, such as publication type in MEDLINE, to limit searches to studies that are likely to be randomized trials.

(d) Search trial registers.

To restrict the search to particular non-randomized study designs is more difficult. Of the above approaches, only (a) and (b) are likely to be at all helpful. Review authors should certainly search CRG-specific registers for potentially relevant NRS. Some CRGs (e.g. the EPOC Group) include particular types of NRS in CRG-specific registers (authors should check with their CRG). The process of identifying studies for inclusion in CENTRAL means that some, but not all, NRS are included, so searches of this database will not be comprehensive, even for studies that use a particular design. There are no databases of NRS similar to CENTRAL.

As discussed in Section 13.2.1.3, study design labels are not used consistently by authors and are not indexed reliably by bibliographic databases. Strategy (c) is unlikely to be helpful because study design labels other than randomized trial are not reliably indexed by bibliographic databases and are often used inconsistently by authors of primary studies. Some review authors have tried to develop and 'validate' search strategies for NRS (Wieland 2005, Fraser 2006, Furlan 2006). Authors have also sought to optimize search strategies for adverse effects (see Chapter 14, Section 14.5) (Golder 2006b, Golder 2006c). Because of the time-consuming nature of systematic reviews that include NRS, attempts to develop search strategies for NRS have not investigated large numbers of review questions. Therefore, review authors should be cautious about assuming that previous strategies can necessarily be applied to new topics.

### 13.3.1.3   *Reviewing citations and abstracts*

Randomized trials can usually be identified in search results simply from the titles and abstracts, particularly since the implementation of reporting standards. Unfortunately, the design details of NRS that are required to assess eligibility are often not described in titles or abstracts and require access to the full study report.

## 13.3.2   Guidance and resources available to support review authors

The NRSMG does not recommend limiting search strategies by index terms relating to study design. However, review authors may wish to contact researchers who have reported some success in developing efficient search strategies for NRS (see Section 13.3.1) and other review authors who have carried out Cochrane reviews (or other systematic reviews) of NRS for review questions similar to their own.

When searching for NRS, review authors are recommended to search for studies investigating all effects of an intervention and not to limit search strategies to specific outcomes (Chapter 6). When searching for NRS of specific rare or long-term (usually adverse or unintended) outcomes of an intervention, including free text and MeSH terms for specific outcomes in the search strategy may be justified. Members of the Adverse Effects Methods Group have experience of doing this (see Chapter 14, Section 14.5).

Review authors should check with their CRG editors whether the CRG-specific register includes studies with particular study design features and should seek the advice of information retrieval experts within the CRG and in the Information Retrieval Methods Group (see Chapter 6, Box 6.7.a).

### 13.3.3  Summary

- To identify studies of the expected beneficial effects of interventions, search strategies should include search strings for the intervention and the population and health problem of interest. Currently, there are no recommended methods for restricting search strategies by study design;

- Review authors searching for evidence relating to 'suspected' adverse effects may want to consider searching for specific outcomes (i.e. adverse effects) of interest. This approach obviously cannot be used for more general searches of possible adverse effects of an intervention (see Chapter 14, Section 14.5);

- Exhaustive searching, which is recommended for randomized trials, may not be justified when reviewing NRS. However, there is no research at present to guide authors about this important issue.

## 13.4  Selecting studies and collecting data

### 13.4.1  What is different when including non-randomized studies?

Search results often contain large numbers of irrelevant citations, and abstracts often do not provide adequate detail about NRS design (which are likely to be required to judge eligibility). Therefore, unlike the situation when reviewing randomized trials, very many full reports of studies may need to be obtained and read in order to select eligible studies.

Review authors need to collect all of the data required for a systematic review of randomized trials (see Chapter 7) and also data to describe (a) the features of the design of a primary study (see Section 13.2.2), (b) confounding factors considered and the methods used to control for confounding (see Section 13.1.3), (c) aspects of risk of bias specific for NRS (see Section 13.5.1) and (d) the results (see Section 13.6.1).

Review authors normally collect 'raw' information about the results when reviewing randomized trials, e.g. for a dichotomous outcome, the total number of participants and the number experiencing the outcome in each group. If participants are randomized to groups, a comparison of these raw data is assumed to be unbiased. For a NRS, a comparison of the same raw data is 'unadjusted' and susceptible to confounding. Authors usually also report an 'adjusted' comparison estimated from a regression model which cannot be summarized in the same way. Review authors should still record the sample size recruited to each group, and the number analysed and the number of events, but also need to document any adjusted effect estimates and their standard errors or confidence intervals. These data can be used to display adjusted effect estimates and their precision in forest plots and, if appropriate, to pool data across studies.

Anecdotally, the experience of review authors is that NRS are poorly reported so that the required information is difficult to find, and different review authors may extract different information from the same paper. Data collection forms may need to be customized to the research question being investigated. Because of the diversity of potentially eligible studies and the ways in which they are reported, developing the data collection form can require several iterations in the course of reviewing a sample of primary studies. It is almost impossible to finalize these forms in advance.

Results in NRS may be presented using different measures of effect and uncertainty or statistical significance depending on the reporting style and analyses undertaken. Expert statistical advice may assist review authors to transform or 'work back' from the information provided in a paper to obtain a consistent effect measure across studies. Data collection sheets need to be able to handle the different kinds of information about study findings that authors may encounter.

## 13.4.2    Guidance and resources available to support review authors

As well as providing information for deciding about eligibility, the questions in Table 13.2.a and Table 13.2.b represent a convenient checklist for collecting relevant data from NRS about study design features. In using this checklist to collect information about the studies and to decide on eligibility, the intention should be to document what researchers did in the primary studies, rather than what researchers called their studies or think they did. Items should be recorded as 'Yes', 'No' or 'Can't tell'. Box 13.4.a provides guidance on using these tables as checklists.

Data collection forms have been developed for use in NRSMG workshops to illustrate data extraction from NRS. These include: the study design checklist, templates for collecting information about confounding factors, their comparability at baseline, methods used to adjust for confounding, and effect estimates. These resources (available from the *Handbook* resource web site, www.cochrane.org/resources/handbook) can be used as a guide to the types of data collection forms that review authors will need. However, review authors will need to customize the forms carefully for the review question being studied.

## Box 13.4.a   User guide for data collection/study assessment using checklist in Table 13.2.a or Table 13.2.b

Note: Users need to be very clear about the way in which the terms 'group' and 'cluster' are used in these tables. Table 13.2.a only refers to groups, which is used in its conventional sense to mean a number of individual participants. With the exception of allocation on the basis of outcome, 'group' can be interpreted synonymously with 'intervention group'. Table 13.2.b refers to both clusters and groups. In this table, 'clusters' are typically an organizational entity such as a family health practice, or administrative area, not an individual. As in Table 13.2.a, 'group' is synonymous with 'intervention group' and is used to describe a collection of allocated units, but in Table 13.2.b these units are clusters rather than individuals. Furthermore, although individuals are nested in clusters, a cluster does not necessarily represent a fixed collection of individuals. For instance, in cluster-allocated studies, clusters are often studied at two or more time-points (periods) with different collections of individuals contributing to the data collected at each time-point.

*Was there a comparison?*

Typically, researchers compare two or more groups that receive different interventions; the groups may be studied over the same time period, or over different time periods (see below). Sometimes researchers compare outcomes in just one group but at two time-points. It is also possible that researchers may have done both, i.e. studying two or more groups and measuring outcomes at more than one time-point.

*Were participants/clusters allocated to groups by?*

These items aim to describe how groups were formed. None will apply if the study does not compare two or more groups of subjects. The information is often not reported or is difficult to find in a paper. The items provided cover the main ways in which groups may be formed. More than one option may apply to a single study, although some options are mutually exclusive (i.e. a study is either randomized or not).

Randomization: Allocation was carried out on the basis of truly random sequence. Such studies are covered by the standard guidance elsewhere in this *Handbook*. Check carefully whether allocation was adequately concealed until subjects were definitively recruited.

Quasi-randomization: Allocation was done on the basis of a pseudo-random sequence, e.g. odd/even hospital number or date of birth, alternation. Note: when such methods are used, the problem is that allocation is rarely concealed. These studies are often included in systematic reviews that only include randomized trials, using assessment of the risk of bias to distinguish them from properly randomized trials.

By other action of researchers: This is a catch-all category and further details should be noted if the researchers report them. Allocation happened as the result of some decision or system applied by the researchers. For example, subjects managed in particular 'units' of provision (e.g. wards, general practices) were 'chosen' to receive the intervention and subjects managed in other units to receive the control intervention.

Time differences: Recruitment to groups did not occur contemporaneously. For example, in a historically controlled study subjects in the control group are typically recruited earlier in time than subjects in the intervention group; the intervention is then introduced and subjects receiving the intervention are recruited. Both groups are usually recruited in the same setting. If the design was under the control of the researchers, both this option and 'other action of researchers' must be ticked for a single study. If the design 'came about' by the introduction of a new intervention, both this option and 'treatment decisions' must be ticked for a single study.

Location differences: Two or more groups in different geographic areas were compared, and the choice of which area(s) received the intervention and control interventions was not made randomly. So, both this option and 'other action of researchers' could be ticked for a single study.

Treatment decisions: Intervention and control groups were formed by naturally occurring variation in treatment decisions. This option is intended to reflect treatment decisions taken mainly by the clinicians responsible; the following option is intended to reflect treatment decisions made mainly on the basis of subjects' preferences. If treatment preferences are uniform for particular provider 'units', or switch over time, both this option and 'location' or 'time' differences should be ticked.

Patient preferences: Intervention and control groups were formed by naturally occurring variation in patients' preferences. This option is intended to reflect treatment decisions made mainly on the basis of subjects' preferences; the previous option is intended to reflect treatment decisions taken mainly by the clinicians responsible.

On the basis of outcome: A group of people who experienced a particular outcome of interest were compared with a group of people who did not, i.e. a case-control study. Note: this option should be ticked for papers that report analyses of *multiple risk factors for a particular outcome* in a large series of subjects, i.e. in which the total study population is divided into those who experienced the outcome and those who did not. These studies are much closer to nested case-control studies than cohort studies, even when longitudinal data are collected prospectively for consecutive patients.

Additional options for cluster-allocated studies.

Location differences: see above.

Policy/public health decisions: Intervention and control groups were formed by decisions made by people with the responsibility for implementing policies about public health or service provision. Where such decisions are coincident with clusters, or where such people are the researchers themselves, this item overlaps with 'other action of researchers' and 'cluster preferences'.

Cluster preferences: Intervention and control groups were formed by naturally occurring variation in the preferences of clusters, e.g. preferences made collectively or individually at the level of the cluster entity.

*Which parts of the study were prospective?*

These items aim to describe which parts of the study were conducted prospectively. In a randomized controlled trial, all four of these items would be prospective. For NRS it is also possible that all four are prospective, although inadequate detail may be presented to discern this, particularly for generation of hypotheses. In some cohort studies, participants may be identified, and have been allocated to treatment retrospectively, but outcomes are ascertained prospectively.

*On what variables was comparability of groups assessed?*

These questions should identify 'before-and-after' studies. Baseline assessment of outcome variables is particularly useful when outcomes are measured on continuous scales, e.g. health status or quality of life.

*Response options*

Try to use only 'Yes', 'No' and 'Can't tell' response options. 'N/a' should be used if a study does not report a comparison between groups.

## 13.4.3 Summary

- Reviewing citations and abstracts identified by searching will be very time consuming, first because of the volume of citations identified and second because the information needed to judge eligibility may not be reported in the title or abstract.

- Collect data as for a randomized trial (i.e. details of study, study population, sample size recruited, sample size analysed, etc).

- Collect data about what researchers did (NRSMG checklist, or similar),

- Collect data about the confounding factors considered.

- Collect data about the comparability of groups on confounding factors considered.

- Collect data about the methods used to control for confounding.

- Collect data about multiple effect estimates (both unadjusted and adjusted estimates, if available).

# 13.5   Assessing risk of bias in non-randomized studies

## 13.5.1   What is different when including non-randomized studies?

### 13.5.1.1   Sources of bias in non-randomized studies

Bias may be present in findings from NRS in many of the same ways as in poorly designed or conducted randomized trials (see Chapter 8). For example, numbers of exclusions in NRS are frequently unclear, intervention and outcome assessment are often not conducted according to standardized protocols, and outcomes may not be assessed blind. The biases caused by these problems are likely to be similar to those that occur in randomized trials, and review authors should be familiar with Chapter 8 that describes these issues. None of these problems are any less difficult to overcome in a well-planned non-randomized prospective study than in a randomized trial.

In NRS, use of allocation mechanisms other than concealed randomization means that groups are unlikely to be comparable. These potential systematic differences between characteristics of participants in different intervention 'groups' are likely to be the issue of key concern in most NRS, and we refer to this as selection bias. When selection bias produces imbalances in prognostic factors associated with the outcome of interest then 'confounding' is said to occur. Statistical methods are sometimes used to counter bias introduced from confounding by producing 'adjusted' estimates of intervention effects, and part of the assessment of study quality may involve making judgements about the appropriateness of the analysis as well as the design and execution of the study.

The variety of study designs classified as NRS, and their varying susceptibility to different biases, makes it difficult to produce a generic robust tool that can be used to evaluate risk of bias. Within a review that includes NRS of different designs, several tools for assessment of risk of bias may need to be created. Inclusion of a knowledgeable methodologist in the review team is essential to identify the key areas of weakness in the included study designs.

With randomized trials, assessment of the risk of bias focuses on systematic bias, which is usually assumed to be 'optimistic' in direction. The tendency for researchers to design, execute, analyse and report their primary studies to give the findings that are expected, consciously or subconsciously, is also likely to apply to NRS where researchers have control over key decisions (e.g. allocation to intervention, or selection of centres). In truly observational NRS, bias arising from 'confounding by indication' may not be so consistent; healthcare professionals may have differing opinions about the appropriateness of alternative interventions for their patients, contingent on the patients' presenting severity of illness or co-morbidities. Differences in case-mix between locations that are being compared may be haphazard. Therefore, when reviewing NRS, the variability of biases and the between-study heterogeneity they induce is at least as important as systematic bias.

## *13.5.1.2   Evidence of risk of bias in non-randomized studies*

Some insight into the risk of bias in non-randomized studies can be obtained by comparing randomized trials at low risk of bias with randomized trials at high risk of bias. Controlled trials that allocate participants by quasi-randomization, or that fail to conceal allocation during recruitment, are at risk of selection bias, just like a prospectively conducted, overtly non-randomized, trial or cohort study. Chapter 8 reviews evidence on several aspects of risk of bias in randomized trials, and points out that methodological limitations in randomized trials tend to exaggerate the beneficial effects of interventions.

Researchers have also compared the findings of separate meta-analyses of randomized trials and NRS of the same research question, assuming that such methodological systematic reviews provide a way to investigate the risk of bias in NRS. Some reviews of this kind have reported discrepancies by study design but fair comparisons are very difficult to make (MacLehose 2000). There are at least two reasons for this:

- Randomized trials and NRS of precisely the same question are rare; for example, studies of the same intervention using different study designs usually differ systematically with respect to the population, intervention or outcome.

- Randomized trials and NRS may differ systematically in several ways with respect to their risk of bias (reporting biases as well as selection, performance, detection and attrition biases), and NRS are frequently of relatively poor quality.

These reasons may explain the inconsistent conclusions from methodological systematic reviews that have compared findings from randomized trials and NRS of the same research question. Deeks et al. reviewed eight such reviews (Deeks 2003), and found that:

- 5/8 concluded that there were differences between effects estimated by randomized trials and NRS for many but not all interventions, with no consistent pattern;

- 1/8 concluded that NRS overestimated the effect [benefit] for all interventions studied;

- 2/8 concluded that the effects estimated by randomized trials and NRS were "remarkably similar".

A similar methodological review compared the findings of randomized trials and patient preference studies (King 2005). The review concluded that there is little evidence that preferences "significantly affect validity", such that preferences did not appear to confound intervention effects.

Some considerations in the interpretation of these sorts of empirical studies are relevant. First, both the publication of primary studies and the selection of primary studies by review authors may be biased. There is also the possibility of bias in their classification of the review findings. Deeks et al. found that the same comparison was sometimes classified as discrepant in one review and comparable in a second. This highlights the difficulty of defining what represents a 'difference'.

Second, the observation that differences were not consistently optimistic remains an important one and is consistent with the principle that effect estimates from NRS are more heterogeneous than expected by chance (Greenland 2004). Some empirical evidence for this comes from innovative simulation studies (Deeks 2003). Deeks et al. pointed out that biases in NRS are highly variable, and may best be considered as introducing extra uncertainty in the results rather than an estimable systematic bias. This uncertainty acts over and above that accounted for in confidence intervals, and in large studies may easily be 5 to 10 times the magnitude of the 95% confidence interval.

Finally, methodological reviews are caught in a circular loop: they need to assume either that NRS are valid and hence differences between effect estimates from randomized trials and NRS are also valid and can be attributed to external factors, or that NRS are biased and hence differences between effect estimates from randomized trials and NRS can be explained by differential risk of bias. The truth may well lie somewhere in between these extremes, but the fact remains that methodological reviews cannot unequivocally partition discrepancies to different sources. Moreover, if multiple factors distinguish randomized trials and NRS and influence effect size, then observing no difference between the effect sizes estimated from randomized trials and NRS can also be explained as the consequence of effects of multiple factors influencing the effect of an intervention in different directions. It is not logical to assume that finding no difference means that NRS are valid and finding a difference means that NRS are not valid.

## 13.5.2   Guidance and resources available to support review authors

### 13.5.2.1   *General considerations in assessing risk of bias in non-randomized studies*

Reporting of randomized trials is relatively straightforward and, increasingly, guided by the CONSORT statement (Moher 2001). A similar consensus statement, STROBE, for the reporting of observational epidemiological studies has been developed, although much more recently (von Elm 2007, Vandenbroucke 2007). Therefore, the quality of reporting of information required to assess the risk of bias is likely to be less good for NRS. This is likely to hinder any assessment of risk of bias.

A protocol is a tool to protect against bias; when registered in advance of a study starting, it proves that aspects of study design and analysis were considered in advance of starting to recruit, and that data definitions and methods for standardizing data collection were defined. Because of the need for research ethics approval, all randomized trials must have a protocol, even if protocols vary in their quality and the items that they specify; many randomized trials, particularly those sponsored by industry, also have detailed study manuals. Historically, researchers have not had to obtain research ethics approval for many NRS, and primary NRS rarely report whether the methods are based on a protocol. Therefore, the protection offered by a protocol often does not exist for NRS. The implications of not having a protocol have not been researched. However, it means, for example, that there is no constraint on the tendency of researchers to 'cherry-pick' outcomes, subgroups and analyses to report, which happens to a greater or lesser extent even in randomized trials where protocols exist (Chan 2004).

In common with randomized trials, dimensions of bias to be assessed include selection bias (concerning comparability of groups, confounding and adjustment), performance bias (concerning the fidelity of the interventions, and quality of the information regarding who received what interventions, including blinding of participants and healthcare providers), detection bias (concerning unbiased and correct assessment of outcome, including blinding of assessors), attrition bias (concerning completeness of sample, follow-up and data) and reporting bias (concerning publication biases and selective reporting of results). Assessment of risk of bias in randomized trials has developed by identifying the design features which are used to prevent each of these dimensions, and noting whether each trial fulfils the requirements. Risk of bias assessments for NRS should proceed in the same way, with pre-specification of the features to be assessed in the protocol, recording what happened in the study, and a judgement of whether this was adequate, inadequate or unclear as a method to avoid risk of this particular bias. Determining these features is likely to require expert input from an epidemiologist, and will depend in part on the clinical question. Particular care should be given to the assessment of confounding (see Section 13.5.2.2).

The reason for careful attention to the design *features* of primary studies (such as how participants were allocated to groups, or which parts of the study were prospective) rather than design *labels* (such as 'cohort' or 'cross-sectional') is because it is hypothesized that the risk of bias is influenced by the specific features of a study rather than a broad categorization of the approach taken. Furthermore, terms such as 'cohort' and 'cross-sectional' are ambiguous and cover a diverse range of specific study designs. No empirically-derived list is available of study design features that are relevant to the risk of bias, although a shortlist can be constructed from evidence and theory about the risk of bias in aetiological studies and randomized trials (see Section 13.2.2 and 13.4.2).

Because of the diversity of NRS, different methods may be needed to assess NRS with different design features. One important distinction is between studies in which allocation to groups is by outcome (e.g. case-control studies) and studies in which allocation to groups is more directly related to interventions. In the former type of study, it is the exposure of interest, rather than the outcome, that is most susceptible to bias; review authors need to ask whether researchers assessing the exposure were masked to whether participants had experienced the outcome or not (i.e. were cases or controls). Case-control studies are well suited to investigating associations between rare outcomes and multiple exposures, so may have an important role in generating evidence about the potential adverse effects and unintended beneficial effects of interventions. They have also been used to evaluate large-scale public health interventions such as accident prevention and screening (MacLehose 2000), which are difficult or expensive to evaluate by randomized trials. However, review authors should familiarize themselves with epidemiological considerations that particularly apply to such studies (Rothman 1986). Note that some analyses of patient registries also have similarities with case-control studies: for example, if the entire database is divided into groups of patients who have or have not experienced a particular outcome and exposures associated with the outcome are investigated. Review authors require a deeper knowledge of epidemiology when assessing the risk of bias in NRS, compared with randomized trials.

### 13.5.2.2   Confounding and adjustment

Researchers do not always make the same decisions concerning confounding factors, so the method used to control for confounding is an important source of heterogeneity between studies. There may be differences in the confounding factors considered, the method used to control for confounding and the precise way in which confounding factors were measured and included in analyses. Many (but not all) NRS describe the confounding factors that were considered and whether confounding was taken into account by the study design or analysis; most also report the baseline characteristics of the groups being compared. However, assessing what researchers actually did to control for confounding may be difficult; far fewer studies describe precisely how confounding factors were measured or fitted as covariates in regression models (e.g. as a continuous, ordinal, or grouped categorical variable).

Some specific suggestions for assessing risk of selection bias are as follows.

• At the stage of writing the protocol, list potential confounding factors.

• Identify the confounding factors that the researchers have considered and those that have been omitted. Note the ways in which they have been measured (the ability to control for a confounding factor depends on the precision with which the factor is measured (Concato 1992)).

• Assess the balance between comparator groups at baseline with respect to the main prognostic or confounding factors.

• Identify what researchers did to control for selection bias, i.e. any design features used for this purpose (e.g. matching or restriction to particular subgroups) and the methods of analysis (e.g. stratification or regression modelling with propensity scores or covariates).

There is no established method for identifying a pre-specified set of important confounders. Listing potential confounding factors should certainly be done 'independently' and, one might argue, 'systematically'. The list should not be generated solely on the basis of factors considered in primary studies included in the review (at least, not without some form of independent validation), since the number of potential confounders is likely to increase over time (hence, older studies may be out of date) and researchers themselves may simply choose to measure confounders considered in previous studies (hence, such a list could be selective). (Researchers investigating aetiological associations often do not explain their choice of confounding factors (Pocock 2004).) Rather, the list should be based on evidence (although undertaking a systematic review to identify all potential prognostic factors is extreme) and expert opinion from members of the review team and advisors.

Reporting results of assessments of confounders in a Cochrane review may best be achieved by creating additional tables listing the pre-stated confounders as columns, the studies as rows, and indicating whether each study: (i) restricted participant selection so that all groups had the same value for the confounder (e.g. restricting the study to male participants only); (ii) demonstrated balance between groups for the confounder; (iii) matched on the confounder; or (iv) adjusted for the confounder in statistical analyses to quantify the effect size.

### 13.5.2.3    *Tools for assessing methodological quality or risk of bias in non-randomized studies*

Chapter 8 (Section 8.5) describes the 'Risk of bias' tool that review authors are expected to use for assessing risk of bias in randomized trials. This involves consideration of six features: sequence generation, allocation sequence concealment, blinding, incomplete outcome data, selective outcome reporting and 'other' potential sources of bias. Items are assessed by: (i) providing a description of what happened in the study; (ii) providing a judgement on the adequacy of the study with regard to the item. The judgement is formulated by answering a pre-specified question, such that an answer of 'Yes' indicates low risk of bias, an answer of 'No' indicates high risk of bias, and an answer of 'Unclear' indicates unclear or unknown risk of bias. The tool was not developed with NRS in mind, and the six domains are not necessarily appropriate for NRS. However, the general structure of the tool and the assessments seems useful to follow when creating risk of bias assessments for NRS.

For experimental and controlled studies, and for prospective cohort studies (see Box 13.1.a and Section 13.2.2), the six domains in the standard 'Risk of bias' tool could usefully be assessed, whether allocation is randomized or not. This is the minimum assessment review authors should carry out and more details will usually be required. An additional component is to assess the risk of bias due to confounding. The depth of this assessment is likely to depend on the heterogeneity between studies and whether the review authors propose a quantitative synthesis (see Section 13.6). If studies are heterogeneous and no quantitative synthesis is proposed, then a less detailed assessment can nevertheless serve the purposes of illustrating the heterogeneity and informing interpretation of the findings of the review.

Many instruments for assessing methodological quality of non-randomized studies of interventions have been created, and were reviewed systematically by Deeks et al. (Deeks 2003). In their review they located 182 tools, which they reduced to a shortlist of 14, and identified six as potentially useful for systematic reviews as they "force the reviewer to be systematic in their study assessments and attempt to ensure that quality judgements are made in the most objective manner possible". However, all six required a degree of adjustment as they neglected to elicit detailed information about how study participants were allocated to groups, which in terms of the risk of selection bias is likely to be critical. Not all of the six tools were suitable for different study designs. In common with some tools for assessing the quality of randomized trials, some did not distinguish items relating to the quality of the study and the quality of reporting of the study. The two most useful tools identified in this review are the Downs and Black instrument and the Newcastle-Ottawa Scale (Downs 1998, Wells 2008).

The Downs and Black instrument has been modified for use in a methodological systematic review (MacLehose 2000). The reviewers found that some of the 29 items were difficult to apply to case-control studies, that the instrument required considerable epidemiological expertise and that it was time consuming to use. The Newcastle-Ottawa Scale, which has been used in NRSMG workshops to illustrate issues in data extraction from primary NRS, contains only eight items and is simpler to apply (Wells 2008). However, the items may still need to be customized to the review question of interest. Review authors also need to be aware of differences in epidemiological terminology in different countries; for example, the Newcastle-Ottawa Scale uses the term 'selection bias' to describe what others may call 'applicability' or 'generalizability'.

Acknowledging the importance of distinguishing between 'what researchers do' and 'what researchers report', review authors may also find it helpful to consider items included in reporting statements for randomized trials (Moher 2001) and observational epidemiological studies (Vandenbroucke 2007) in order to highlight gaps in reporting (and execution) in NRS (Reeves 2004, Reeves 2007).

### 13.5.2.4    *Practical limitations in assessing risk of bias in non-randomized studies*

Two studies of systematic reviews that included NRS have commented that only a minority of reviews assessed the methodological quality of included studies (Audige 2004, Golder 2006a). Members of the NRSMG have gained experience of trying to assess risk of bias in non-randomized studies. Anecdotally, review authors have reported that NRS are generally of poor methodological quality, or are poorly reported so that assessing methodological quality and risk of bias consistently across primary studies is difficult or impossible (Kwan 2004). Even the Newcastle-Ottawa scale has been reported to be difficult to apply, so agreement between review authors is likely to be modest. Methodological information can be difficult to find in papers, making the task frustrating, especially when using some of the more detailed instruments; review authors may spend a long time searching for details of what researchers did, only to conclude that the information was not reported. Nevertheless, collecting some factual information (for example, the confounders considered and what researchers did about confounding) can still be useful since such information illustrates the extent of heterogeneity between studies.

## 13.5.3    Summary

- At the stage of writing the protocol for the review, compile a list of potential confounding factors and justify the choice.

- At the stage of writing the protocol for the review, decide how the risk of bias in primary studies will be assessed, including the extent of control for confounding.

- For NRS conducted entirely prospectively, apply the methods that the Collaboration recommends for randomized trials.

- There is no single recommended instrument, so review authors are likely to need to include supplementary risk of bias instruments or items.

- Issues such as confounding cannot easily be addressed within the format of the new risk of bias tool and require creation of additional tables for reporting assessments.

- Collecting some factual information (for example, the confounders considered and what researchers did about confounding) is useful since such information illustrates the extent of heterogeneity between studies.

- Review authors who choose to include case-control studies in a Cochrane review should ensure that they are familiar with common pitfalls that can affect such studies and that they assess their susceptibility to bias using an instrument designed for this purpose.

- Review authors may decide that collecting great detail about the risk of confounding and other biases is not warranted. However, if this approach is taken, review authors must acknowledge the potential extent of the heterogeneity between studies with respect to potential residual confounding and other biases and demonstrate that they have considered this source of heterogeneity in their interpretation of the findings of the primary NRS reviewed.

## 13.6 Synthesis of data from non-randomized studies

### 13.6.1 What is different when including non-randomized studies?

Review authors should expect greater heterogeneity in a systematic review of NRS than a systematic review of randomized trials. This is due to the increased potential for methodological diversity through variation between primary studies in their risk of selection bias, variation in the way in which confounding is considered in the analysis and greater risk of other biases through poor design and execution. There is no way of controlling for these biases in the analysis of primary studies and no established method for assessing how, or the extent to which, these biases affect primary studies (but see Chapter 8).

There is a body of opinion that it is appropriate to pool results of non-randomized studies when they have large effects, but the logic of this view can be questioned. NRS with large effects are as likely (perhaps more likely) to be biased and to be heterogeneous as NRS with small effects. Judgements about the risk of bias and heterogeneity should be based on critical appraisal of the characteristics and methods of included studies, not on their results.

When assessing similarity of studies prior to a meta-analysis, review authors should also keep in mind that some features of studies, for example assessment of outcome not masked to intervention allocation, may be relatively homogeneous across NRS but still leave all studies at risk of bias.

If authors judge that included NRS are both reasonably resistant to biases and relatively homogeneous in this respect, they may wish to combine data across studies using meta-analysis (Taggart 2001). Unlike for randomized trials, it will usually be appropriate to analyse adjusted, rather than unadjusted, effect estimates, i.e. analyses that attempt to 'control for confounding'. This may require authors to choose between alternative adjusted estimates reported for one study. Meta-analysis of adjusted estimates can be performed as an inverse-variance weighted average, for example using the 'Generic inverse-variance' outcome type in RevMan (see Chapter 9, Section 9.4.3). In principle, any effect measure used in meta-analysis of randomized trials can also be used in meta-analysis of non-randomized studies (see Chapter 9, Section 9.2), although the odds ratio will commonly be used as it is the only effect measure for dichotomous outcomes that can be estimated from case-control studies, and is estimated when logistic regression is used to adjust for confounders.

One danger is that a very large NRS of poor methodological quality (for example based on routinely collected data) may dominate the findings of other, smaller studies at less risk of bias (perhaps carried out using customized data collection). Authors need to remember that the confidence intervals for effect estimates from larger NRS are less likely to represent the true uncertainty of the observed effect than are the confidence intervals for smaller NRS (see Section 13.5.1.2), although there is no way of estimating or correcting for this.

## 13.6.2   Guidance and resources available to support review authors

### 13.6.2.1   *Controlling for confounding*

Imbalances in prognostic factors in NRS (e.g. 'confounding by indication' (Grobbee 1997)) must be accounted for in the statistical analysis. There are several methods to control for confounding. Matching, i.e. the generation of similar intervention groups with respect to important prognostic factors, can be used to lessen confounding at the study design stage. Stratification and regression modelling are statistical approaches to control for confounding, which result in an estimated intervention effect adjusted for imbalances in observed prognostic factors. Some analyses use propensity score methods as part of a two-stage analysis. The probability of an individual receiving the experimental intervention (the propensity score) is first estimated according to their characteristics using a logistic regression model. This single summary measure of case-mix is then used for matching, stratification or in a regression model.

***Matching***   The selection of patients with similar values for important prognostic factors results in more comparable groups. Therefore, matching can be seen as a type of confounder adjustment. Matching can be either at the level of individual patients (i.e. one or more control participants are selected who has a similar characteristics to an intervention participant) or at the level of participant strata (i.e. selecting participants so that there are roughly the same number of control participants in one stratum, for example 60 years or older, as in the intervention group). Where direct matching has been used, the paired nature of the data has to be considered in the statistical analysis of a single study in order to obtain appropriate confidence intervals for the estimated effect of the intervention. Matching on a single measure such as the propensity score is easier to achieve than matching individuals with a particular set of characteristics.

***Stratification***     Stratification involves the division of participants into subgroups with respect to categorical (or categorized quantitative) prognostic factors, for example classifying age into decades, or weight into quartiles. The intervention effect is then estimated in each stratum and a pooled estimate is calculated across strata. This procedure can be interpreted as a meta-analysis at the level of an individual study. For dichotomous outcomes, the Mantel-Haenszel method is often used to estimate the overall intervention effect, with versions available for the odds ratio, the risk ratio and the risk difference as measures of intervention effect. Again, the propensity score may be used as the stratification variable.

***Modelling***     In a modelling approach, information on intervention and prognostic factors is incorporated into a regression equation. Advantages of regression models include the possibility of incorporating quantitative factors without categorization and the possibility of modelling trends in confounders measured on an ordinal scale. For dichotomous outcomes, a logistic regression model is almost always used to estimate the adjusted intervention effect. Thus, the odds ratio is (implicitly) used as the measure of intervention effect. Regression models are also available for risk ratio and absolute risk reduction measures of effect but these models are rarely used in practice. A linear regression model is typically used for continuous outcomes (perhaps after transformation of one or more variables), and a proportional hazards regression (Cox regression) model is typically used for time-to-event data. Regression models may also use the propensity score alone or in combination with other participant characteristics as explanatory variables.

Review authors should acknowledge that in any non-randomized study, even when experimental and control groups appear comparable at baseline, the effect size estimate is still at risk of bias due to residual confounding. This is because all methods to control for confounding are imperfect, for example for the following reasons.

- Unknown, and consequently unmeasured, confounding factors, which cannot be controlled for.

- Poor resolution in the measurement of confounders, e.g. co-morbidity assessed on a simple ordinal scale (Concato 1992), which represents non-differential error misclassification with respect to confounders.

- Practical constraints on the resolution of matching, and the number of confounders on which participants can be matched, in matched analyses.

- Poor resolution in the way confounders are measured in stratified analyses, or handled in analyses, illustrated by the width of strata (e.g. decades of age); this limitation also applies to regression models when confounders are categorized and modelled discretely.

- Assumptions in the way confounders are modelled in regression analyses, because of imperfect knowledge of the shape of the association between confounder and outcome.

There is no established method for judging the likely extent of residual confounding. The direction of bias from confounding is unpredictable and may differ between studies.

### 13.6.2.2    Combining studies

Estimated intervention effects for different study designs can be expected to be influenced to varying degrees by different sources of bias (see Section 13.5). Results from different study designs should be expected to differ systematically, resulting in increased heterogeneity. Therefore, we recommend that NRS which used different study designs (or which have different design features), or randomized trials and NRS, should not be combined in a meta-analysis.

Because of the need to control for confounding as best as possible, the estimated intervention effect and its standard error (or confidence interval) are key pieces of information which should be used for pooling NRS in a meta-analysis. (Simple numerators and denominators, or means and standard errors, for intervention and control groups cannot control for confounding unless the groups have been matched at the design stage.) Consequently, meta-analysis methods based on estimates and standard errors, and in particular the generic inverse-variance method, will be suitable for NRS (see Chapter 9, Section 9.4.3).

It is straightforward to extract an adjusted effect estimate and its standard error for a meta-analysis if a single adjusted estimate is reported for a particular outcome in a primary NRS. However, many NRS report both unadjusted and adjusted effect estimates, and some NRS report multiple adjusted estimates from analyses including different sets of covariates. Review authors should record both unadjusted and adjusted effect estimates but it can be difficult to choose between alternative adjusted estimates. No general recommendation can be made for the selection of which adjusted estimate is preferable. Possible selection rules are:

- use the estimate from the model that adjusted for the maximum number of covariates;

- use the estimate that is identified as the primary adjusted model by the authors; and

- use the estimate from the model that includes the largest number of confounders considered important at the outset by the review authors.

Sensitivity analyses could be performed by pooling separately the most optimistic and pessimistic results from each included study.

There is a subtle statistical point regarding the different interpretation of adjusted and unadjusted effects when expressed as odds or hazard ratios. The unadjusted effect estimate is known as the population average effect, and if the estimate were unbiased would be the effect of intervention observed in a population with an average mixture of prognostic characteristics. When estimates are adjusted for prognostic characteristics, the estimated effects are known as conditional estimates and are the intervention effects that would be observed in groups with particular combinations of the adjusted covariates. Mathematical research has shown that conditional estimates are usually larger (further from an OR or HR of 1) than population average estimates. This phenomenon may not be observed in systematic reviews due to heterogeneity in the estimates of the studies.

### 13.6.2.3   *Analysis of heterogeneity*

The exploration of possible sources of heterogeneity between studies should be part of any Cochrane review, and is discussed in detail in Chapter 9 (Section 9.6). Non-randomized studies may be expected to be more heterogeneous than randomized trials, given the extra sources of methodological diversity and bias. The simplest way to show the variation in results of studies is by drawing a forest plot (see Chapter 11, Section 11.3.2).

It may be of value to undertake meta-regression analyses to identify important determinants of heterogeneity, even in reviews where studies are considered too heterogeneous to pool. Such analyses may help to identify methodological features which systematically relate to observed intervention effects, and help to identify the subgroups of studies most likely to yield valid estimates of intervention effects.

### 13.6.2.4   *When pooling is judged not to be appropriate*

Before undertaking a meta-analysis, review authors must ask themselves the standard question about whether primary studies are 'similar enough' to justify pooling (see Chapter 9). Forest plots in RevMan allow the presentation of estimates and standard errors for each study, using the 'Generic inverse-variance' outcome type. Meta-analyses can be suppressed, or included only for subgroups within a plot. Providing that effect estimates from the included studies can be expressed using consistent effect measures, we recommend that review authors display individual study results for NRS with similar study design features using forest plots, as a standard feature. If consistent effect measures are not available, then additional tables should be used to present results in a systematic format.

If included studies are not sufficiently homogeneous to combine in a meta-analysis (which is expected to be the norm for reviews that include NRS), the NRSMG recommends displaying the results of included studies in a forest plot but suppressing the pooled estimate. Studies may be sorted in the forest plot (or shown in separate forest plots) by study design feature, or some other feature believed to reflect susceptibility to bias (e.g. number of Newcastle-Ottawa Scale 'stars' (Wells 2008)). Heterogeneity diagnostics and investigations (e.g. a test for heterogeneity, the $I^2$ statistic and meta-regression analyses) are worthwhile even when a judgement has been made that calculating a pooled estimate of effect is not (Higgins 2003, Siegfried 2003).

Narrative syntheses are, however, problematic, because it is difficult to set out or describe results without being selective or emphasizing some findings over others. Ideally, authors should set out in the review protocol how they plan to use narrative synthesis to report the findings of primary studies.

### 13.6.3  Summary

- Heterogeneity will be greater in a systematic review of NRS than in a systematic review of randomized trials. Therefore, authors should consider very carefully the likely extent of heterogeneity between included studies when deciding whether to pool findings quantitatively (i.e. by meta-analysis). We expect pooling of effect estimates from NRS to be the exception, rather than the rule.

- Effect estimates from NRS should not be combined with effect estimates from randomized trials, or across NRS that use dissimilar study design features.

- Forest plots should be used to summarize the findings from included studies.

- Heterogeneity diagnostics and investigations may be used irrespective of whether or not a decision has been taken to pool effect estimates from different studies.

## 13.7   Interpretation and discussion

### 13.7.1   Challenges in interpreting Cochrane reviews of effectiveness that include non-randomized studies

Review authors face great challenges in demonstrating convincingly that the result of a Cochrane review of NRS can give anything close to a definitive answer about the likely effect of an intervention (Deeks 2003). In many situations, reviews of NRS are likely to conclude that calculating an 'average' effect is not helpful (Siegfried 2003), that evidence from NRS is inadequate to prove effectiveness or harm (Kwan 2004) and that randomized trials should be undertaken (Taggart 2001).

Challenges arise at all stages of conducting a review of NRS: deciding which study designs to include, searching for studies, assessing studies for potential bias, and deciding whether to pool results. A review author needs to satisfy the reader of the review that these challenges have been adequately addressed, or should discuss how and why they cannot be met. In this section, the challenges are illustrated with reference to issues raised in the different sections of this chapter. The Discussion section of the review should address the extent to which the challenges have been met.

### 13.7.1.1  *Have all important and relevant studies been included?*

Even if the choice of eligible study designs can be justified, it may be difficult to show that all relevant studies have been identified because of poor indexing and inconsistent use of study design labels by researchers. Comprehensive search strategies that focus only on the health condition and intervention of interest are likely to result in a very long list of citations including relatively few eligible studies; conversely, restrictive strategies will inevitably miss some eligible studies. In practice, available resources may make it impossible to process the results from a comprehensive search, especially since authors will often have to read full papers rather than abstracts to determine eligibility. The implications of using a more or less comprehensive search strategy are not known.

### 13.7.1.2  *Has the risk of bias to included studies been adequately assessed?*

Interpretation of the results of a review of NRS must include consideration of the likely direction and magnitude of bias. Biases that affect randomized trials also affect NRS but typically to a greater extent. For example, attrition in NRS is often worse (and poorly reported), intervention and outcome assessment are rarely conducted according to standardized protocols, and outcomes are rarely blind. Too often these limitations of NRS are seen as part of doing a NRS, and their implications for risk of bias are not properly considered. For example, some users of evidence may consider NRS that investigate long-term outcomes to have 'better quality' than randomized trials of short-term outcomes, simply on the basis of their relevance without appraising their risk of bias (see Section 13.2.1.4).

Assessing the magnitude of confounding in NRS is especially problematic. Review authors must not only have adequate methods for assessment but also collect and report adequate detail about the confounding factors considered by researchers and the methods used to control for confounding. The information may not be available from the reports of the primary studies, preventing the review authors from investigating differences in the methods of eligible studies and other sources of heterogeneity that were considered likely to be important when the protocol was written.

Authors must remember the following points about confounding:

- The direction of the bias introduced by confounding is unpredictable;

- Methods used by researchers to control for confounding are like to vary between studies;

- The extent of residual confounding in any particular study is unknown, and is likely to vary between studies;

- Residual confounding (and other biases) means that confidence intervals underestimate the true uncertainty around an effect estimate.

- It is important to identify the likely confounding factors that have not been adjusted for, as well as those that have been adjusted for.

The challenges described above affect all systematic reviews of NRS. However, challenges may be less extreme in some healthcare areas (e.g. confounding may be less of a problem in observational studies of long-term or adverse effects, or some public health primary prevention interventions).

One clue to the presence of bias is notable between-study heterogeneity. Although heterogeneity can arise through differences in participants, interventions and outcome assessments, the possibility that bias is the cause of heterogeneity in reviews of NRS must be considered seriously. However, lack of heterogeneity does not indicate lack of bias, since it is possible that a consistent bias applies in all studies.

Can the magnitude and direction of bias be predicted? This is a subject of ongoing research which is attempting to gather empirical evidence on factors (such as study design and intervention type) that determine the size and direction of these biases. The ability to predict both the likely magnitude of bias and the likely direction of bias would greatly improve the usefulness of evidence from systematic reviews of NRS. There is currently some evidence that in some limited circumstances the direction, at least, can be predicted (Henry 2001)

## 13.7.2    Evaluating the strength of evidence provided by reviews that include non-randomized studies

'Exposing' the evidence from NRS on a particular health question enables informed debate about its meaning and importance, and the certainty which can be attributed to it. Critically, there needs to be a debate about the chance that the observed findings could be misleading. Formal hierarchies of evidence all place NRS low down on the list, but above those of clinical opinion (Eccles 1996, National Health and Medical Research Council 1999, Oxford Centre for Evidence-based Medicine 2001). This emphasizes the general concern about biases in NRS, and the difficulties of attributing causality to the observed effects. The strength of evidence provided by a systematic review of NRS is likely to depend on meeting the challenges set out in Section 13.7.1. The ability to meet these challenges will vary with healthcare context and outcome. In some contexts little confounding is likely to occur. For example, little prognostic information may be known when infants are vaccinated, limiting possible confounding (Jefferson, 2005).

Whether the debate concludes that there is a need for randomized trials or that the evidence from NRS is adequate for informed decision-making will depend on the cost placed on the uncertainty arising through use of potentially biased study designs, and the collective value of the observed effects. This value may depend on the wider healthcare context. It may not be possible to include assessments of the value within the review itself, and it may become evident only as part of the wider debate following publication.

For example, is evidence from NRS of a rare serious adverse effect adequate to decide that an intervention should not be used? The evidence is uncertain (due to a lack of randomized trials) but the value of knowing that there is the possibility of a potentially serious harm is considerable, and may be judged sufficient to withdraw the intervention. (It is worth noting that the judgement about withdrawing an intervention may depend on whether equivalent benefits can be obtained from elsewhere without such a risk; if not, the intervention may still be offered but with full disclosure of the potential harm.) Where evidence of benefit is not based on randomized trials and is therefore equivocal, the value attached to a systematic review of NRS of harm may be even greater.

In contrast, evidence of a small benefit of a novel intervention from a systematic review of NRS may not be sufficient for decision makers to recommend widespread implementation in the face of the uncertainty of the evidence and the substantial costs arising from provision of the intervention. In these circumstances, decision makers are likely to conclude that randomized trials should be undertaken if practicable and if the investment in the trial is likely to be repaid in the future.

The GRADE scheme for assessing the quality of a body of evidence is recommended for use in 'Summary of findings' tables in Cochrane reviews, and is summarized in Chapter 12 (Section 12.2). There are four quality levels: 'high', 'moderate', 'low' and 'very low'. A collection of studies that can be crudely categorized as randomized trials starts at the highest level, and may be downgraded due to study limitations (risk of bias), indirectness of evidence, heterogeneity, imprecision or publication bias. Collections of observational studies start at a level of 'low', and may be upgraded due to a large magnitude of effect, lack of concern about confounders or a dose-response gradient. Review authors will need to make judgements about whether evidence from NRS should be upgraded from a low level or possibly (e.g. in the case of quasi-randomized trials) downgraded from a high level.

## 13.7.3    Guidance for potential review authors

Carrying out a systematic review of NRS is much more difficult than carrying out a systematic review of randomized trials. It is likely that complex decisions, requiring expert methodological or epidemiological advice, will need to be made at each stage of the review. Potential review authors should therefore seek to collaborate with epidemiologists or methodologists, irrespective of whether a review aims to investigate harms or benefits, short-term or long-term outcomes, frequent or rare events.

Healthcare professionals are keen to be involved in doing reviews of NRS in areas where there are few or no randomized trials because they have the ambition to improve the evidence base in their specialty areas (the motivation for most Cochrane reviews). Methodologists are keen for more systematic reviews of NRS to inform the many areas of uncertainty in methodology highlighted by these chapters. However, healthcare professionals should also recognize that (a) the resources required to do a systematic review of NRS are likely to be much greater than for a systematic review of randomized trials and (b) the conclusions are likely to be much weaker and may make a relatively small contribution to the topic. Therefore, authors and CRG editors need to decide at an early stage whether the investment of resources is likely to be justified by the priority of the research question.

Bringing together the required team of healthcare professionals and methodologists may be easier for systematic reviews of NRS to estimate the effects of an intervention on long-term and rare adverse outcomes, for example when considering the side effects of drugs. However, these reviews may require the input of additional specialist authors, for example with relevant pharmacological expertise. There is a pressing need in many health conditions to supplement traditional systematic reviews of randomized trials of effectiveness with systematic reviews of adverse (unintended) effects. It is likely that these systematic reviews will usually need to include NRS.

## 13.8   Chapter information

**Authors:** Barnaby C Reeves, Jonathan J Deeks, Julian PT Higgins and George A Wells on behalf of the Cochrane Non-Randomised Studies Methods Group.

---

### Box 13.8.a   The Cochrane Non-Randomised Studies Methods Group

The Non-Randomised Studies Methods Group (NRSMG) of the Cochrane Collaboration advises the Steering Group to set policy and formulate guidance about the inclusion of non-randomized studies (NRS) of the effectiveness of healthcare interventions in Cochrane reviews. Membership of the group is open to anyone who wishes to contribute actively to the work of group. The work of the group is primarily methodological, rather than focused on particular healthcare interventions.

Activities of NRSMG members include:

- Developing guidelines to help decide when to include non-randomized data in Cochrane reviews.
- Conducting methodological research in the use of non-randomized studies, including search methods, quality assessment, meta-analysis, pitfalls and misuse.
- Conducting empirical research to compare bias in systematic reviews using both randomized and non-randomized studies, and to identify conditions under which randomized and non-randomized studies have led to similar conclusions, and situations in which the conclusions have been clearly contradictory.
- Collating examples of healthcare questions that (a) have been studied using both non-randomized studies and randomized trials, and (b) have not been (or which for a long period have not been) studied adequately by means of randomized trials.
- Providing training at annual Cochrane Colloquia.

---

**This chapter should be cited as:** Reeves BC, Deeks JJ, Higgins JPT, Wells GA. Chapter 13: Including non-randomized studies. In: Higgins JPT, Green S (editors), *Cochrane Handbook for Systematic Reviews of Interventions.* Chichester (UK): John Wiley & Sons, 2008.

**Acknowledgements:** We gratefully acknowledge Ole Olsen, Peter Gøtzsche, Angela Harden, Mustafa Soomro, Guido Schwarzer and Bev Shea for their early drafts of different sections. We also thank Laurent Audigé, Duncan Saunders, Alex Sutton, Helen Thomas and Gro Jamtved for comments on previous drafts.

# 13.9   References

**Audige 2004**

Audige L, Bhandari M, Griffin D, Middleton P, Reeves BC. Systematic reviews of nonrandomized clinical studies in the orthopaedic literature. *Clinical Orthopaedics and Related Research* 2004: 249–257.

**Chan 2004**

Chan AW, Hróbjartsson A, Haahr MT, Gøtzsche PC, Altman DG. Empirical evidence for selective reporting of outcomes in randomized trials: comparison of protocols to published articles. *JAMA* 2004; 291: 2457–2465.

**Concato 1992**

Concato J, Horwitz RI, Feinstein AR, Elmore JG, Schiff SF. Problems of comorbidity in mortality after prostatectomy. *JAMA* 1992; 267: 1077–1082.

**Deeks 2003**

Deeks JJ, Dinnes J, D'Amico R, Sowden AJ, Sakarovitch C, Song F, Petticrew M, Altman DG. Evaluating non-randomised intervention studies. *Health Technology Assessment* 2003; 7: 27.

**Doll 1993**

Doll R. Doing more good than harm: The evaluation of health care interventions: Summation of the conference. *Annals of the New York Academy of Sciences* 1993; 703: 310–313.

**Downs 1998**

Downs SH, Black N. The feasibility of creating a checklist for the assessment of the methodological quality both of randomised and non-randomised studies of health care interventions. *Journal of Epidemiology and Community Health* 1998; 52: 377–384.

**Eccles 1996**

Eccles M, Clapp Z, Grimshaw J, Adams PC, Higgins B, Purves I, Russel I. North of England evidence based guidelines development project: methods of guideline development. *BMJ* 1996; 312: 760–762.

**Fraser 2006**

Fraser C, Murray A, Burr J. Identifying observational studies of surgical interventions in MEDLINE and EMBASE. *BMC Medical Research Methodology* 2006; 6: 41.

**Furlan 2006**

Furlan AD, Irvin E, Bombardier C. Limited search strategies were effective in finding relevant nonrandomized studies. *Journal of Clinical Epidemiology* 2006; 59: 1303–1311.

**Glasziou 2007**

Glasziou P, Chalmers I, Rawlins M, McCulloch P. When are randomised trials unnecessary? Picking signal from noise. *BMJ* 2007; 334: 349–351.

**Golder 2006a**

Golder S, Loke Y, McIntosh HM. Room for improvement? A survey of the methods used in systematic reviews of adverse effects. *BMC Medical Research Methodology* 2006; 6: 3.

**Golder 2006b**

Golder S, McIntosh HM, Duffy S, Glanville J, Centre for Reviews and Dissemination and UK Cochrane Centre Search Filters Design Group. Developing efficient search strategies to identify reports of adverse effects in MEDLINE and EMBASE. *Health Information and Libraries Journal* 2006; 23: 3–12.

**Golder 2006c**

Golder S, McIntosh HM, Loke Y. Identifying systematic reviews of the adverse effects of health care interventions. *BMC Medical Research Methodology* 2006; 6: 22.

**Greenland 2004**

Greenland S. Interval estimation by simulation as an alternative to and extension of confidence intervals. *International Journal of Epidemiology* 2004; 33: 1389–1397.

**Grobbee 1997**

Grobbee DE, Hoes AW. Confounding and indication for treatment in evaluation of drug treatment for hypertension. *BMJ* 1997; 315: 1151–1154.

**Henry 2001**

Henry D, Moxey A, O'Connell D. Agreement between randomized and non-randomized studies: the effects of bias and confounding. *9th Cochrane Colloquium*, Lyon (France), 2001.

**Higgins 2003**

Higgins JPT, Thompson SG, Deeks JJ, Altman DG. Measuring inconsistency in meta-analyses. *BMJ* 2003; 327: 557–560.

**Jefferson 2005**

Jefferson T, Smith S, Demicheli V, Harnden A, Rivetti A, Di PC. Assessment of the efficacy and effectiveness of influenza vaccines in healthy children: systematic review. *The Lancet* 2005; 365: 773–780.

**King 2005**

King M, Nazareth I, Lampe F, Bower P, Chandler M, Morou M, Sibbald B, Lai R. Impact of participant and physician intervention preferences on randomized trials: a systematic review. *JAMA* 2005; 293: 1089–1099.

**Kwan 2004**

Kwan J, Sandercock P. In-hospital care pathways for stroke. *Cochrane Database of Systematic Reviews* 2004, Issue 2. Art No: CD002924.

**MacLehose 2000**

MacLehose RR, Reeves BC, Harvey IM, Sheldon TA, Russell IT, Black AM. A systematic review of comparisons of effect sizes derived from randomised and non-randomised studies. *Health Technology Assessment* 2000; 4: 1–154.

**Moher 2001**

Moher D, Schulz KF, Altman DG. The CONSORT Statement: revised recommendations for improving the quality of reports of parallel-group randomised trials. *The Lancet* 2001; 357: 1191–1194. (Available from www.consort-statement.org.)

**National Health and Medical Research Council 1999**

National Health and Medical Research Council. *A Guide to the Development, Implementation and Evaluation of Clinical Practice Guidelines [Endorsed 16 November 1998]*. Canberra (Australia): Commonwealth of Australia, 1999.

**Oxford Centre for Evidence-based Medicine 2001**
Oxford Centre for Evidence-based Medicine. Levels of evidence [May 2001]. Available from: http://www.cebm.net/index.aspx?o=1047 (accessed 1 January 2008).

**Peto 1995**
Peto R, Collins R, Gray R. Large-scale randomized evidence: large, simple trials and overviews of trials. *Journal of Clinical Epidemiology* 1995; 48: 23–40.

**Petticrew 2001**
Petticrew M. Systematic reviews from astronomy to zoology: myths and misconceptions. *BMJ* 2001; 322: 98–101.

**Pocock 2004**
Pocock SJ, Collier TJ, Dandreo KJ, de Stavola BL, Goldman MB, Kalish LA, Kasten LE, McCormack VA. Issues in the reporting of epidemiological studies: a survey of recent practice. *BMJ* 2004; 329: 883.

**Reeves 2004**
Reeves BC, Gaus W. Guidelines for reporting non-randomised studies. *Forschende Komplementärmedizin und klassische Naturheilkunde* 2004; 11 Suppl 1: 46–52.

**Reeves 2006**
Reeves BC. Parachute approach to evidence based medicine: as obvious as ABC. *BMJ* 2006; 333: 807–808.

**Reeves 2007**
Reeves BC, Langham J, Lindsay KW, Molyneux AJ, Browne JP, Copley L, Shaw D, Gholkar A, Kirkpatrick PJ. Findings of the International Subarachnoid Aneurysm Trial and the National Study of Subarachnoid Haemorrhage in context. *British Journal of Neurosurgery* 2007; 21: 318–323.

**Rothman 1986**
Rothman KJ. *Modern Epidemiology*. Boston (MA): Little, Brown & Company, 1986.

**Shadish 2002**
Shadish WR, Cook TD, Campbell DT. *Experimental and Quasi-Experimental Designs for Generalized Causal Inference*. Boston (MA): Houghton Mifflin, 2002.

**Siegfried 2003**
Siegfried N, Muller M, Volmink J, Deeks J, Egger M, Low N, Weiss H, Walker S, Williamson P. Male circumcision for prevention of heterosexual acquisition of HIV in men. *Cochrane Database of Systematic Reviews* 2003, Issue 3. Art No: CD003362.

**Taggart 2001**
Taggart DP, D'Amico R, Altman DG. Effect of arterial revascularisation on survival: a systematic review of studies comparing bilateral and single internal mammary arteries. *The Lancet* 2001; 358: 870–875.

**Vandenbroucke 2007**
Vandenbroucke JP, von Elm E, Altman DG, Gøtzsche PC, Mulrow CD, Pocock SJ, Poole C, Schlesselman JJ, Egger M. Strengthening the Reporting of Observational Studies in Epidemiology (STROBE): explanation and elaboration. *PLoS Medicine* 2007; 4: e297.

**von Elm 2007**
von Elm E, Altman DG, Egger M, Pocock SJ, Gøtzsche PC, Vandenbroucke JP. The Strengthening the Reporting of Observational Studies in Epidemiology (STROBE) statement: Guidelines for reporting observational studies. *PLoS Medicine* 2007; 4: e296.

**Wells 2008**
Wells GA, Shea B, O'Connell D, Peterson J, Welch V, Losos M, Tugwell P. The Newcastle-Ottawa Scale (NOS) for assessing the quality of nonrandomised studies in meta-analyses.

Available from: http://www.ohri.ca/programs/clinical_epidemiology/oxford.htm (accessed 1 January 2008).

**Wieland 2005**

Wieland S, Dickersin K. Selective exposure reporting and Medline indexing limited the search sensitivity for observational studies of the adverse effects of oral contraceptives. *Journal of Clinical Epidemiology* 2005; 58: 560–567.

# 14 Adverse effects

## Yoon K Loke, Deirdre Price and Andrew Herxheimer on behalf of the Cochrane Adverse Effects Methods Group

## Key Points

- To achieve a balanced perspective, all reviews should try to consider the adverse aspects of the interventions;

- A detailed analysis of adverse effects is particularly relevant when evidence on the potential for harm has a major influence on treatment or policy decisions;

- Interventions may have many different adverse effects, and reviews may need to focus on a few important ones in detail, together with a broader, more general summary of other potential adverse effects;

- As adverse effects data are often handled with less rigour than the primary outcomes of a study, the intensity of the monitoring of adverse effects and the clarity of reporting them need careful scrutiny;

- Data on adverse effects are often sparse, but the absence of information does not mean that the intervention is safe.

## 14.1 Introduction

### 14.1.1 The need to consider adverse effects

Every healthcare intervention comes with the risk, great or small, of harmful or adverse effects. A Cochrane review that considers only the favourable outcomes of the interventions that it examines, without also assessing the adverse effects, will lack balance and may make the intervention look more favourable than it should. This source of bias, like others, should be minimized. All reviews should try to include some consideration of the adverse aspects of the interventions.

This chapter addresses special issues relating to adverse effects in Cochrane reviews, with an emphasis on reviews in which adverse effects might be addressed using methods differing from those for other outcomes. Although in principle adverse effects are most reliably assessed using randomized trials, in practice many adverse events are too uncommon or too long term to be observed within randomized trials, or may not have been known when the trials were planned. A Cochrane review may use one of several strategies for addressing adverse effects, which differ in the extent to which the same methods are used to evaluate intended (beneficial) and unintended (beneficial or adverse) effects. The present chapter focuses on adverse effects that are usually taken to be unintended (Miettinen 1983). The different strategies for a review are discussed in Section 14.2.

### 14.1.2   Concepts and terminology

Many terms are used to describe harms associated with healthcare interventions. This can confuse review authors, particularly as published papers often use terms loosely and interchangeably. Some common related terms include 'adverse event' (an unfavourable outcome that occurs during or after the use of a drug or other intervention but is not necessarily caused by it), 'adverse effect' (an adverse event for which the causal relation between the intervention and the event is at least a reasonable possibility), 'adverse drug reaction' (an adverse effect specific to a drug), 'side effect' (any unintended effect, adverse or beneficial, of a drug that occurs at doses normally used for treatment), and 'complications' (adverse events or effects following surgical and other invasive interventions).

### 14.1.3   When it is most important to consider adverse effects

The resources devoted to including adverse outcomes in reviews should be considered in relation to the importance of the intervention itself. If an intervention clearly does not work, or has little potential benefit and is not widely used, it may not be worth devoting resources towards a detailed evaluation of adverse effects. On the other hand, a detailed analysis of adverse effects would be warranted if the information on potential harm appears to be essential in guiding decisions of clinicians, consumers and policymakers.

Table 14.1.a exemplifies situations where analysis of adverse effects has an important role in treatment decisions.

## 14.2   Scope of a review addressing adverse effects

### 14.2.1   Identical methods for beneficial and adverse effects

In this section, and in Sections 14.2.2 and 14.2.3, we describe three broad strategies that a Cochrane review may use to address adverse effects. The first strategy is to assess intended (beneficial) and unintended (adverse) effects together using the same

**Table 14.1.a**   Contexts and examples warranting detailed examination of adverse effects

---

**When the margin between benefits and adverse effects is narrow**

| | |
|---|---|
| Treatment is of modest or uncertain benefit, with an important possibility of adverse effects. | • Aspirin for prevention of cardiovascular events in a healthy patient; increase in haemorrhage;<br>• Antibiotics for acute otitis media in children; risk of rash and diarrhoea;<br>• Urgent direct current cardioversion in patients with new atrial fibrillation who are cardiovascularly stable; risk of stroke from cardioversion. |
| Treatment is potentially highly beneficial, but there are major safety concerns. | • Aspirin for patient with a stroke, but who has a past history of gastrointestinal haemorrhage;<br>• Carotid endarterectomy in older patients with ischaemic heart disease who present with stroke. |
| Treatment is potentially beneficial in long term, or to community, but no immediate direct benefit to individual. | • Improving uptake of a vaccine to promote herd immunity, while trying to assuage fears about early serious neurological adverse effects. |

**When a number of efficacious treatments differ in their safety profiles**

| | |
|---|---|
| Treatments are of equivalent efficacy, but they have different safety profiles. | • Antiepileptic drugs for women of childbearing age with epilepsy;<br>• A new insulin injection device is thought to cause less pain than the existing device. |
| The balance of benefits and adverse effects differs substantially, e.g. the most efficacious intervention may have serious adverse effects, while the less effective intervention is potentially safer. | • Disease-modifying drug in erosive rheumatoid arthritis, e.g. using hydroxychloroquine (relatively safe) or methotrexate (potentially more effective, but less safe);<br>• Polychemotherapy versus sequential single agent chemotherapy for metastatic breast cancer. |

**When adverse effects deter a patient from continuing on an efficacious treatment**

| | |
|---|---|
| Treatment is of considerable benefit but adverse effects threaten patients' adherence, and evidence is needed to guide further management. | • An effective intervention has well-recognized adverse effects, which can make it difficult for the patient to continue therapy. Evidence is needed on whether reducing the intensity of the intervention (e.g. lower dose or duration) will help avoid the adverse effects, or whether there is a treatment strategy that can prevent adverse effects (e.g. proton pump inhibitor for peptic ulcers caused by aspirin). |

---

methodology, applying common eligibility criteria (in terms of types of studies, types of participants and types of interventions).

This approach implies that a single search strategy may be used. A critical issue is how review authors deal with the three datasets that may potentially arise:

(a) Studies that report both the beneficial effects and adverse effects of interest;

(b) Studies that report beneficial effects but not adverse effects;

(c) Studies that report adverse effects, but not the beneficial outcomes of interest.

Studies of type (a) have the important advantage that benefits and adverse effects can be compared directly, since the data are derived from the same population and setting. Furthermore, evidence on benefits and adverse effects arises from studies with similar designs and quality. However, data on adverse effects may be very limited and in particular may be restricted to short-term harms because of the relatively short duration of included studies.

Evaluation of benefits and adverse effects using some combination of the three types of study (rather than (a) alone) will increase the amount of information available. For instance, datasets (a) and (b) could be used to evaluate beneficial effects, while (a) and (c) could be used to assess adverse effects. However, as the studies addressing adverse effects differ from those addressing beneficial effects, authors should note that it is difficult to compare benefits and adverse effects directly.

## 14.2.2    Different methods for beneficial and adverse effects

The second strategy is to use different eligibility criteria for selecting studies that address unintended (adverse) effects compared with studies that address intended (beneficial) effects.

Different types of studies may be needed to evaluate different outcomes (Glasziou 2004). The use of different eligibility criteria specifically addresses the problem that most experimental studies (such as randomized trials) are insufficient to evaluate rare, long-term or previously unrecognized adverse effects (see Section 14.4). This approach allows a more rigorous evaluation of adverse effects, but takes more time and resources, and means that benefits and adverse effects can often not be compared directly. While randomized trials have the advantage that the allocation of interventions is made by the randomization process, non-randomized studies involve different mechanisms for allocating interventions, and these should be scrutinized during the review.

## 14.2.3    Separate review for adverse effects

The third strategy is to undertake a separate review of adverse effects alone. This might be appropriate for an intervention that is given for a variety of diseases or conditions, yet whose adverse effect profile might be expected to be similar in different populations and settings. For example, aspirin is used in a wide variety of patients, such as those with stroke, or peripheral vascular disease, and also in those with coronary artery disease. The main effects of aspirin on outcomes relevant to these different conditions would typically be addressed in separate Cochrane reviews, but adverse effects (such as bleeding into the brain or gut) are sufficiently similar within the different disease groups that an independent review might address them together. Indeed, unless trials exist on combined populations, such a question would be difficult to address in any other way.

Similarly, there may be limited adverse effects data for an intervention in a sub-population, such as children. It may be worth analysing all available data for this sub-population (e.g. adverse effects of selective serotonin reuptake inhibitors in children), even if the trials were aimed at different disease conditions.

Authors of reviews of adverse effects alone must aim to provide adequate cross referencing (preferably through electronic links) to related reviews of intended effects of the intervention. If new safety concerns are identified when an efficacy review is updated, then the adverse effects review should be updated as soon as possible.

## 14.3    Choosing which adverse effects to include

### 14.3.1    Narrow versus broad focus

The selection of adverse outcomes to include in a review can be difficult. Specific adverse effects associated with an intervention may be known in advance of the review; others will not. Which effects will be most relevant to the review may be uncertain beforehand. The following general strategies may be used depending on the study question and the therapeutic or preventive context.

***Narrow focus***    A detailed analysis of one or two known or a few of the most serious adverse effects that are of special concern to patients and health professionals.

*Advantages:*    Easiest approach, especially with regard to data collection. Can focus on important adverse effects and reach a meaningful conclusion on issues that have a major impact on the treatment decision (McIntosh 2004).

*Disadvantages:*    Scope may be too narrow. Method is only really suitable for adverse events that are known in advance.

***Broad focus***    To detect a variety of adverse effects, whether known or previously unrecognized.

*Advantages:*    Wider coverage, and can evaluate new adverse effects that we may not have previously been aware of.

*Disadvantages:*    Potentially large volume of work with particular difficulties in the data collection process. Some researchers have found broad, non-specific evaluations to be very resource-intensive, with little useful information to show for the effort expended (McIntosh 2004). These researchers also point out that previously unrecognized adverse effects may be best detected through primary surveillance, rather than in a systematic review.

In order to address adverse effects in a more organized manner, review authors may choose to narrow down the broad focus into some of the following areas:

* The five to ten most frequent adverse effects;

* **All** adverse effects that either the patient or the clinician considers to be serious;

- By category, for example:

  - Diagnosed by lab results (e.g. hypokalaemia);

  - Patient-reported symptoms (e.g. pain).

### 14.3.2   Withdrawal or drop-out as an outcome measure for adverse effects

Withdrawal or drop-out is often used as an outcome measure in trial reports. Review authors should hesitate to interpret such data as surrogate markers for safety or tolerability because of the potential for bias:

- The attribution of reason(s) for discontinuation is complex and may be due to mild but irritating side effects, toxicity, lack of efficacy, non-medical reasons, or a combination of causes (Ioannidis 2004);

- The pressures on patients and investigators under trial conditions to keep the number of withdrawals and drop-outs low can result in rates that do not reflect the experience of adverse events within the study population;

- Unblinding of intervention assignment often precedes the decision to withdraw. This can lead to an over-estimate of the intervention's effect on patient withdrawal. For example, symptoms of patients in the placebo arm are less likely to lead to discontinuation. Conversely, patients in the active intervention group who complained of symptoms suggesting adverse effects may have been more readily withdrawn.

## 14.4   Types of studies

Most Cochrane reviews focus on randomized trials, which provide the most reliable estimates of effect. However, rare adverse events or long-term adverse effects are unlikely to be observed in clinical trials, and a thorough investigation may require the inclusion of cohort studies, case-control studies and even case reports or case series. In particular, the strategies outlined in Sections 14.2.2 and 14.2.3 are likely to be chosen specifically so that different study designs are included to address adverse effects. For more detailed discussion of issues in the inclusion of non-randomized studies (including case-control and cohort studies) in a Cochrane review, see Chapter 13 (Section 13.2). Some issues to consider in the inclusion of case reports appear in Section 14.6.3.

# 14.5   Search methods for adverse effects

## 14.5.1   Sources of information on adverse effects of drugs

In addition to the usual sources of evidence, described in Chapter 6, review authors who are planning an exhaustive search for adverse effects of a drug may wish to consider checking the following sources:

- Standard reference books on adverse effects such as Meyler's Side Effects of Drugs, the Side Effects of Drugs Annuals (SEDA), Martindale: The Complete Drug Reference, Davies Textbook of Adverse Drug Reactions and the papers they summarize;

- Regulatory authorities may issue safety alerts for a variety of commercial products based on information submitted to them by the manufacturer (which have not been published or made available elsewhere). Examples of safety bulletins can be found:

  ○ In the UK: Current Problems in Pharmacovigilance (www.mhra.gov.uk);

  ○ In Australia: the Australian Adverse Drug Reactions Bulletin (www.tga.gov.au/adr/aadrb.htm);

  ○ In the European Public Assessment Reports from the European Medicines Evaluation Agency (www.emea.eu);

  ○ In the US: Food and Drug Administration FDA Medwatch (www.fda.gov/medwatch);

- Specialist drug information databases such as full-text databases (e.g. Pharmanewsfeed and Iowa Drug Information Service (IDIS), bibliographic databases (e.g. Derwent Drug File, TOXLINE, Pharmline) and referenced summary databases (e.g. Drugdex, XPhram). However, review authors will have to consider the subscription costs to these specialist databases, particularly as their usefulness or additional yield have yet to be formally evaluated in the systematic review setting.

Review authors can also apply (usually on payment of a fee) to the WHO Uppsala Monitoring Centre (UMC; www.who-umc.org) for special searches of their spontaneous reporting database (Vigibase); this was for example done for a Cochrane review on melatonin (Herxheimer 2002). However, the rank order of the most common adverse effects reported for one particular drug in the UMC database was found to differ from the data derived from a meta-analysis of double-blind, randomized trials (Loke 2004): the UMC data on amiodarone showed thyroid problems to have the highest frequency, with skin reactions coming second, whereas the meta-analysis showed heart problems to be most common, followed by thyroid disorders.

Primary surveillance data (in the form of spontaneous case reports) are also freely available via the web sites of the regulatory authorities in Canada, USA, UK, and The Netherlands. However, the format of the information varies considerably, and interpretation and analysis of these databases require specialist skills (see also Section 14.6.3).

## 14.5.2   Search strategy for adverse effects

The optimal search strategy for specifically identifying reports of adverse effects has yet to be established (Golder 2006). Two main approaches can be used: using index terms and free-text searching. Both of these have limitations; it is advisable to combine them to maximize sensitivity (the likelihood of not missing studies that might be relevant). The development of a search strategy is likely to require several iterations. For instance, it may be necessary to repeat the electronic search incorporating additional index terms, subheadings and free-text terms derived from the terms used to index and describe the studies initially identified as relevant. In deciding which combination of terms to use, authors will need to balance comprehensiveness (sensitivity) against precision. Some considerations in the use of index terms and free text terms follow.

### 14.5.2.1   *Searching electronic databases for adverse effects using index terms*

Index terms (also called controlled vocabulary or thesaurus terms) such as Medical Subject Headings (MeSH) in MEDLINE and EMTREE in EMBASE are assigned to records in electronic databases to describe the studies. MEDLINE and EMBASE employ few useful indexing terms for adverse effects; they include DRUG TOXICITY/ and ADVERSE DRUG REACTION SYSTEMS in MEDLINE and DRUG TOXICITY/ and ADVERSE DRUG REACTION/ in EMBASE. However, the most useful way to search for adverse effects is by using subheadings (Golder 2006). Subheadings can be attached to index terms to describe specific aspects, for example 'side effects' of drugs, or 'complications' of surgery, or they can be used where they are searched for attaching to any index term (floating subheadings). The subheadings used to denote data on adverse effects differ in the major databases MEDLINE and EMBASE, for example:

Aspirin/adverse effects (MEDLINE)

Acetylsalicylic-acid/adverse-drug-reaction (EMBASE)

In the above example, Aspirin is the MeSH term and adverse effects is the subheading; Acetylsalicylic-acid is the EMTREE term and adverse-drug-reaction is the subheading.

Within a database, studies may be (i) indexed under the name of the intervention together with a subheading to denote that adverse effects occurred, for example, Aspirin/

adverse effects or Mastectomy/complications; or (ii) the adverse event itself may be indexed, together with the nature of the intervention, for example, Gastrointestinal Hemorrhage/ and Aspirin/ , or Lymphedema/ and Surgery/; or (iii) occasionally, an article may be indexed only under the adverse event, for example, Hemorrhage/chemically-induced.

Thus, no single index or subheading search term can be relied on to identify all data on adverse effects, but a combination of index terms and subheadings is useful in detecting reports of major adverse effects which the indexers are likely to regard as significant (Derry 2001).

Subheadings that can be used with the intervention or with all interventions (floated) and which may prove useful in MEDLINE are:

/adverse effects (NB if this subheading is exploded it will include the subheadings /poisoning and /toxicity)

/poisoning

/toxicity

/contraindications

Subheadings that can be used with the adverse outcome or with all outcomes (floated) and which may prove useful in MEDLINE are:

/chemically induced

/complications

Subheadings that can be used with the intervention or with all interventions (floated) and which may prove useful in EMBASE are:

/adverse drug reaction

/drug toxicity

Subheadings that can be used with the adverse outcome or with all outcomes (floated) and which may prove useful in EMBASE are:

/complication

/side effect

### 14.5.2.2   Searching electronic databases for adverse effects using free-text terms

Free-text terms (also called text words) are used by authors in the title and abstract of their studies when published as journal articles; these terms are then searchable in the title and abstract of electronic records in databases. Two important problems severely limit the usefulness of free-text searching:

1. The wide range of terms authors use to describe adverse effects, both in a general sense (toxicity, side effect, adverse effects) and more specifically (for example, lethargy, tiredness, malaise may be used synonymously);

2. The free-text search does not detect adverse effects that are not mentioned in the title or abstract of the study and are, therefore, not included in the electronic record (even though the full report describes them) (Derry 2001).

A highly sensitive free-text search should incorporate the potentially wide variety of synonymous terms while also taking into account different conventions in spelling and variations in the endings of terms to include, for example, singular and plural terms. This should then be combined with free-text terms involving the intervention of interest, for example:

> *(aspirin or acetylsalicylic acid) and (adverse or side or hemorrhage or haemorrhage or bleed or bleeding or blood loss).*

# 14.6    Assessing risk of bias for adverse effects

## 14.6.1    Clinical trials

Although the general advice is to assess risk of bias in clinical trials as described in Chapter 8, authors must also consider other specific factors that may have a larger influence on the adverse effects data. Areas of special concern include methods for monitoring and detecting adverse effects, conflicting interests (Jüni 2004), selective outcome reporting (Chan 2004) and blinding (Schulz 2002).

The primary outcome measure of an intervention may have been studied in a placebo controlled, well-masked, adequately concealed randomized trial. In contrast, the adverse effects data may be collected retrospectively, for example via an end-of-study questionnaire sent out only to those who are known to have received the active intervention. Although a low risk of bias may be assigned to the primary outcomes, the way in which harmful effects of the interventions are monitored may not permit a similar rating. The recommended risk of bias tool, implemented in RevMan, allows for different assessments of blinding and of incomplete outcome data for each outcome, or for a class of outcomes as defined by the review author.

The methods used in monitoring or detecting adverse effects are known to have a major influence on adverse effect frequencies: studies in which adverse effects are carefully sought will report a higher frequency than studies in which they are sought less carefully. For example, in a group of hypertensive patients, passive monitoring based on spontaneous reports yielded rates of 16%, while active surveillance using specific questioning found a rate of 62% (Olsen 1999). As different methods of monitoring adverse effects will yield different results, it may be difficult to compare studies, and pointless to do a formal meta-analysis (Edwards 1999). Duration and frequency of monitoring should also be noted.

Studies with limited follow-up or infrequent monitoring may not reliably detect adverse effects; the absence of information must not be interpreted as indicating the intervention is safe. In contrast, studies with rigorous follow-up and active surveillance for pre-defined adverse effects may be able to generate evidence that the intervention genuinely has few adverse effects.

Finally, the age of an intervention and the evolution of its use are likely to be related to the types of adverse events detected and their number. This is obvious for long-term effects such as carcinogenicity, but also because some interventions, for example in surgery, change more or less subtly over time.

Examples of potentially useful questions to consider in assessing the quality of evidence on adverse effects are:
On conduct:

- Are definitions of reported adverse effects given?

- Were the methods used for monitoring adverse effects reported? Use of prospective or routine monitoring; spontaneous reporting; patient checklist, questionnaire or diary; systematic survey of patients?

On reporting:

- Were any patients excluded from the adverse effects analysis?

- Does the report provide numerical data by intervention group?

- Which categories of adverse effects were reported by the investigators?

## 14.6.2 Case-control and cohort studies

While the study of beneficial effects almost always necessitates randomized trials, adverse effects of treatment can often be effectively investigated in non-randomized studies (Miettinen 1983). Vandenbroucke has proposed that observational studies of adverse effects of medical interventions offer some of the best chances for unbiased observational studies (Vandenbroucke 2004). This idea was empirically verified by a comparison of randomized and observational studies of adverse effects, which found that, if anything, risk estimates from observational studies were lower (Papaniko-laou 2006)). In some instances where observational studies showed markedly higher risks, they better reflected actual patient care (Vandenbroucke 2006). Like any study, case-control and cohort studies are potentially susceptible to bias, and any limitations of the data should therefore be critically discussed. See Chapter 13 (Section 13.5) for further discussion of assessing risk of bias in such studies. Jick has drafted a taxonomy of the type of study that is most likely to detect an adverse effect, as well as the type of study that is necessary for verification (Jick 1977).

## 14.6.3   Case reports

Case reports of adverse events are widely found in the published literature, and are also collated by regulatory agencies. There are specific methodological problems with the evaluation of such case reports. Review authors who are potentially interested in such data will need to consider the following issues.

***Do the reports have good predictive value?***   Anecdotal reports may turn out to be false alarms on subsequent investigation, rather than genuine indicators of the link between the intervention and adverse effect. Although one study has claimed that three quarters of a collection of anecdotal case reports from 1963 were correct (Venning 1982), a more recent systematic survey of 63 suspected adverse reactions found that most (52 of 63, 82.5%) had not yet been evaluated in more detail (Loke 2006). Controlled study data supporting the postulated link between drug and adverse event were available in only three cases, while in two cases controlled studies failed to confirm the link. Nevertheless, product information sheets or drug monographs may have been amended to include listings of these adverse events. It is thus not easy to tell whether a case report is a genuine alert or a false alarm. Still, case reports remain the cornerstone of the initial detection of new adverse effects (Stricker 2004). The removal of drugs from the market is overwhelmingly based on case reports and case series, in the past as well as in the present (Venning 1983, Arnaiz 2001). Removal of a drug from the market due to a dramatic effect does not require formal control groups (Glasziou 2007).

***Determining causality***   There is usually uncertainty as to whether the adverse event was caused by the intervention (particularly in patients who are taking a wide variety of treatments). Review authors must decide on the likelihood of the intervention having a causative role, or whether the occurrence of the adverse event during the intervention period was simply a coincidence. However, two independent review authors might not reach the same judgement from the same case report. Several studies have evaluated the responses of review authors who were asked to appraise reports of adverse event. In one study, complete agreement was obtained only 35% of the time between two observers who used causality criteria in an algorithm for assessing suspected adverse reactions (Lanctot 1995). In another study, three clinical pharmacologists, who evaluated 500 reports of suspected reactions, failed to agree on the culprit drug in 36% of the cases (Koch-Weser 1977).

*Is there a plausible biological mechanism linking the intervention to the adverse event?* A reported adverse event is more plausible if it can be explained by a well-understood biological mechanism. For example, amiodarone has an iodine-like chemical structure, which explains the commonly seen adverse effects on thyroid function.

*Do the reports provide enough information to allow detailed appraisal of the evidence?* One study looked at 1520 published case reports of suspected adverse reactions, and found substantial differences in the information provided in these reports (Kelly 2003). With regard to details of patient characteristics, only three patient variables were reported more than 90% of the time, while 12 others were reported less than 25% of the time. In assessing the culprit drug, Kelly found that only one drug variable (for instance dose or duration or frequency or exact formulation) was reported more than 90% of the time; six others were reported 14 to 74% of the time. The substantial variation in the nature of the reporting means that detailed appraisal is difficult for review authors.

*Are there any potential problems from using data from the reports, which might outweigh the perceived benefit of being comprehensive?* There is a trade-off between the desire to be 'all-inclusive' and the need to avoid publicizing biased or unreliable information that may trigger a false alarm. The MMR vaccination programme was disrupted by anecdotal reports in a reputable journal, with scores of people in the UK harmed by measles outbreaks from decreased vaccine uptake (Asaria 2006). The inclusion of extra (but potentially unreliable) information on 'adverse events' can have harmful effects, and review authors will need to carefully consider the negative impact and legal ramifications of conveying such information.

## 14.7 Chapter information

**Authors**: Yoon K Loke, Deirdre Price and Andrew Herxheimer on behalf of the Cochrane Adverse Effects Methods Group.

**This chapter should be cited as**: Loke YK, Price D, Herxheimer A. Chapter 14: Adverse effects. In: Higgins JPT, Green S (editors), *Cochrane Handbook for Systematic Reviews of Interventions*. Chichester (UK): John Wiley & Sons, 2008.

**Acknowledgements**: The following colleagues (listed alphabetically) have contributed their expertise to the Cochrane Adverse Effects Methods Group, in helping develop this guidance: Jeff Aronson, Anne-Marie Bagnall, Andrea Clarke, Sheena Derry, Anne Eisinga, Su Golder, Tom Jefferson, Harriet MacLehose, Heather McIntosh and Nerys Woolacott.

## Box 14.7.a The Cochrane Adverse Effects Methods Group

The Adverse Effects Methods Group (AEMG) provides methodological guidance on the appropriate techniques for the identification and systematic assessment of adverse effects. The origins of the AEMG date back almost a decade to the informal meetings of a few individuals who were involved in systematically evaluating the harmful effects of interventions. This led, in January 2001, to the formation of the Adverse Effect Subgroup as part of the Non-Randomised Studies Methods Group. In June 2007, the Adverse Effects Methods Group (AEMG) was officially registered.

The fundamental tenet of the AEMG is that every healthcare intervention carries some risk of harm. In order to reach a fully-informed decision, treatment choices need to be supported by a systematic assessment of benefits and harms. Reviews that focus mainly on treatment benefit, together with lack of information on harmful effects, would create difficulties for people who are trying to make balanced decisions. The AEMG aims to redress this imbalance, and aims to collaborate with Review Groups and Methods Groups to improve the methodology and quality of adverse effects analyses. The AEMG will be happy to look into any areas of methodological uncertainty that require further research, and hopes to develop and disseminate appropriate ways of filling any gaps that are identified.

*Web site*: aemg.cochrane.org

# 14.8 References

**Arnaiz 2001**

Arnaiz JA, Carne X, Riba N, Codina C, Ribas J, Trilla A. The use of evidence in pharmacovigilance. Case reports as the reference source for drug withdrawals. *European Journal of Clinical Pharmacology* 2001; 57: 89–91.

**Asaria 2006**

Asaria P, MacMahon E. Measles in the United Kingdom: can we eradicate it by 2010? *BMJ* 2006; 333: 890–895.

**Chan 2004**

Chan AW, Hróbjartsson A, Haahr MT, Gøtzsche PC, Altman DG. Empirical evidence for selective reporting of outcomes in randomized trials: comparison of protocols to published articles. *JAMA* 2004; 291: 2457–2465.

**Derry 2001**

Derry S, Kong LY, Aronson JK. Incomplete evidence: the inadequacy of databases in tracing published adverse drug reactions in clinical trials. *BMC Medical Research Methodology* 2001; 1: 7.

**Edwards 1999**

Edwards JE, McQuay HJ, Moore RA, Collins SL. Reporting of adverse effects in clinical trials should be improved: lessons from acute postoperative pain. *Journal of Pain and Symptom Management* 1999; 18: 427–437.

**Glasziou 2004**

Glasziou P, Vandenbroucke JP, Chalmers I. Assessing the quality of research. *BMJ* 2004; 328: 39–41.

**Glasziou 2007**

Glasziou P, Chalmers I, Rawlins M, McCulloch P. When are randomised trials unnecessary? Picking signal from noise. *BMJ* 2007; 334: 349–351.

**Golder 2006**

Golder S, McIntosh HM, Duffy S, Glanville J, Centre for Reviews and Dissemination and UK Cochrane Centre Search Filters Design Group. Developing efficient search strategies to identify reports of adverse effects in MEDLINE and EMBASE. *Health Information and Libraries Journal* 2006; 23: 3–12.

**Herxheimer 2002**

Herxheimer A, Petrie KJ. Melatonin for the prevention and treatment of jet lag. *Cochrane Database of Systematic Reviews* 2002, Issue 2. Art No: CD001520.

**Ioannidis 2004**

Ioannidis JPA, Evans SJ, Gøtzsche PC, O'Neill RT, Altman DG, Schulz K, Moher D. Better reporting of harms in randomized trials: an extension of the CONSORT statement. *Annals of Internal Medicine* 2004; 141: 781–788.

**Jick 1977**

Jick H. The discovery of drug-induced illness. *New England Journal of Medicine* 1977; 296: 481–485.

**Jüni 2004**

Jüni P, Nartey L, Reichenbach S, Sterchi R, Dieppe PA, Egger M. Risk of cardio-vascular events and rofecoxib: cumulative meta-analysis. *The Lancet* 2004; 364: 2021–2029.

**Kelly 2003**

Kelly WN. The quality of published adverse drug event reports. *Annals of Pharmacotherapy* 2003; 37: 1774–1778.

**Koch-Weser 1977**

Koch-Weser J, Sellers EM, Zacest R. The ambiguity of adverse drug reactions. *European Journal of Clinical Pharmacology* 1977; 11: 75–78.

**Lanctot 1995**

Lanctot KL, Naranjo CA. Comparison of the Bayesian approach and a simple algorithm for assessment of adverse drug events. *Clinical Pharmacology and Therapeutics* 1995; 58: 692–698.

**Loke 2004**

Loke YK, Derry S, Aronson JK. A comparison of three different sources of data in assessing the frequencies of adverse reactions to amiodarone. *British Journal of Clinical Pharmacology* 2004; 57: 616–621.

**Loke 2006**

Loke YK, Price D, Derry S, Aronson JK. Case reports of suspected adverse drug reactions – systematic literature survey of follow-up. *BMJ* 2006; 332: 335–339.

**McIntosh 2004**

McIntosh HM, Woolacott NF, Bagnall AM. Assessing harmful effects in systematic reviews. *BMC Medical Research Methodology* 2004; 4: 19.

**Miettinen 1983**

Miettinen OS. The need for randomization in the study of intended effects. *Statistics in Medicine* 1983; 2: 267–271.

**Olsen 1999**

Olsen H, Klemetsrud T, Stokke HP, Tretli S, Westheim A. Adverse drug reactions in current antihypertensive therapy: a general practice survey of 2586 patients in Norway. *Blood Pressure* 1999; 8: 94–101.

**Papanikolaou 2006**

Papanikolaou PN, Christidi GD, Ioannidis JP. Comparison of evidence on harms of medical interventions in randomized and nonrandomized studies. *Canadian Medical Association Journal* 2006; 174: 635–641.

**Schulz 2002**

Schulz KF, Grimes DA. Blinding in randomised trials: hiding who got what. *The Lancet* 2002; 359: 696–700.

**Stricker 2004**

Stricker BH, Psaty BM. Detection, verification, and quantification of adverse drug reactions. *BMJ* 2004; 329: 44–47.

**Vandenbroucke 2004**

Vandenbroucke JP. When are observational studies as credible as randomised trials? *The Lancet* 2004; 363: 1728–1731.

**Vandenbroucke 2006**

Vandenbroucke JP. What is the best evidence for determining harms of medical treatment? *Canadian Medical Association Journal* 2006; 174: 645–646.

**Venning 1982**

Venning GR. Validity of anecdotal reports of suspected adverse drug reactions: the problem of false alarms. *British Medical Journal (Clinical Research Edition)* 1982; 284: 249–252.

**Venning 1983**

Venning GR. Identification of adverse reactions to new drugs. II (continued): How were 18 important adverse reactions discovered and with what delays? *British Medical Journal (Clinical Research Edition)* 1983; 286: 365–368.

# 15 Incorporating economics evidence

Ian Shemilt, Miranda Mugford, Sarah Byford, Michael
Drummond, Eric Eisenstein, Martin Knapp, Jacqueline
Mallender, David McDaid, Luke Vale and Damian Walker
on behalf of the Campbell and Cochrane Economics
Methods Group

## Key Points

- Economics is the study of the optimal allocation of limited resources for the production of benefit to society and is therefore relevant to any healthcare decision.

- Optimal decisions also require best evidence of effectiveness.

- This chapter describes methods for incorporating economics perspectives and evidence into Cochrane reviews, with a focus on critical review of health economics studies.

- Incorporating economics perspectives and evidence into Cochrane reviews can enhance their usefulness and applicability for healthcare decision-making and new economic analyses.

## 15.1 The role and relevance of economics evidence in Cochrane reviews

### 15.1.1 Introduction

Cochrane reviews assemble, select, critique and combine trustworthy data from multiple research studies on the effectiveness and other aspects of healthcare interventions. They can provide robust evidence on intervention effectiveness, resulting in less selectively biased, more statistically powerful information, which may be more likely to convince decision makers compared with evidence from single studies.

However, in the face of scarce resources, decision makers often need to consider not only whether an intervention works, but also whether its adoption will lead to a more efficient use of resources. The topics of Cochrane reviews cover a wide range of questions whose answers are important for the improvement of individual and public health and well-being in environments where resources are limited. Coverage of economic aspects of interventions can therefore enhance the usefulness and applicability of Cochrane reviews as a component of the basis for healthcare decision-making (Lavis 2005).

It has been argued for many years that promoting effective care without taking into account the cost of care and the value of any health gain can lead to inefficient use of public and private funds allocated to health care, which may indirectly result in harm for individuals and the public (Williams 1987). Indeed, the case can be made that Archie Cochrane, who inspired much of the systematic review movement (and of course The Cochrane Collaboration), was in favour of decision-making informed by evidence on economics aspects of interventions as well as evidence on their effectiveness. The title of Cochrane's most famous work, his book of Rock Carling lectures, is *Effectiveness and Efficiency* (Cochrane 1972). Box 15.1.a contains two quotations from that book, illustrating the importance that Cochrane placed on the role of economic evidence in healthcare decision-making.

---

**Box 15.1.a   Archie Cochrane on health economics (Cochrane 1972)**

"Allocations of funds and facilities are nearly always based on the opinions of senior consultants, but, more and more, requests for additional facilities will have to be based on detailed arguments with 'hard evidence' as to the gain to be expected from the patients' angle and the cost. Few can possibly object to this." (p.82).

"If we are ever going to get the 'optimum' results from our national expenditure on the NHS we must finally be able to express the results in the form of the benefit and the cost to the population of a particular type of activity, and the increased benefit that would be obtained if more money were made available." (p.2).

---

## 15.1.2   Economics and economic evaluation

Economics is the study of the optimal allocation of limited resources for the production of benefit to society (Samuelson 2005). Resources are human time and skills, equipment, premises, energy and any other inputs required to implement and sustain a given course of action (e.g. referral of an individual patient to a programme of healthcare treatment, and subsequent management of sequelae and complications). Health economics studies are defined here as full economic evaluation studies, partial economic evaluation studies, and single effectiveness studies that include more limited information relating to the description, measurement or valuation of resource use associated with interventions.

Full economic evaluation is the comparative analysis of alternative courses of action in terms of both costs (resource use) and consequences (outcomes, effects) (Drummond 2005). This definition distinguishes full economic evaluation from economic analyses which focus solely on costs and resource use, or partial economic evaluations. Full economic evaluation is not a single research method; it is a framework for structuring specific decision problems. This means that the appropriate type of full economic evaluation, and thus the approach to data collection and analysis, is determined primarily by the decision problem, or economic question, at issue and the viewpoint of the decision maker (see also Section 15.2.1). Full economic evaluation studies aim to describe, measure and value all relevant alternative courses of action (e.g. intervention X versus comparator Y), their resource inputs and consequences. Cost-benefit analysis (CBA) falls into this category. Some approaches fall short of full valuation of all consequences, but are still considered full economic evaluations, including cost-effectiveness analysis (CEA) and cost-utility analysis (CUA). All types of full economic evaluation use a marginal approach to analysis. In other words, they aim to produce measures of *incremental* resource use, costs and/or cost-effectiveness. Brief descriptions of CEA, CUA and CBA are provided in Box 15.1.b (see also Chapter 2 of Drummond (Drummond 2005)).

Other types of studies of the use of healthcare resources do not make explicit comparisons between alternative interventions in terms of both costs (resource use) and consequences (effects). Such studies are not considered to be full economic evaluations but are known instead as partial economic evaluations. Partial economic evaluations can contribute useful evidence to an understanding of economic aspects of interventions. Health economics studies considered to be partial economic evaluations include cost analyses, cost-description studies and cost-outcome descriptions. In addition to full and partial economic evaluations, randomized trials and other types of single effectiveness studies may include more limited information relating to the description, measurement or valuation of resource use associated with interventions. Whilst the inclusion of this type of information may not always constitute a full or partial economic evaluation approach, it may still nevertheless contribute useful evidence to an understanding of economic aspects of interventions.

Economic evaluation studies both use, and are used in, systematic reviews of the effects of interventions. First, systematic reviews may include an economic component that incorporates a critical review of published and unpublished health economics studies (see Section 15.1.3). Second, as well as the increasing numbers of full and partial economic evaluations conducted alongside (and incorporating) single effectiveness studies, such as randomized trials (Maynard 2000, Neumann 2005), full economic evaluations are also increasingly based upon evidence of effects compiled using systematic review methods. Indeed, all of the types of full economic evaluation described above (CEAs, CUAs, CBAs) can be conducted alongside, and incorporating, a systematic review of effects, including use of a decision-analysis approach for pooling or modelling the available evidence on intervention costs and effects (Briggs 2006). Economic evaluation can be seen in this context as a further layer of evidence synthesis building on the systematic review process.

Cochrane reviews and other systematic reviews can therefore provide a useful source of data to inform subsequent, or parallel, full economic evaluation modelling exercises whether or not the review incorporates further coverage of economic aspects of interventions. In particular, a well-conducted meta-analysis of data on effect-size, adverse effects and complications assembled using a systematic review of randomized trials has been proposed as the least-biased source of data to inform effect-size and adverse effects parameters in an economic model (Cooper 2005). This needs to be supplemented by additional systematic searches of appropriate data sources to inform ranges of

---

### Box 15.1.b   Types of full economic evaluation

All types of full economic evaluation compare the costs (resource use) associated with one or more alternative interventions (e.g. intervention X versus comparator Y) with their consequences (outcomes, effects). All types value resources in the same way (i.e. by applying unit costs to measured units of resource use). The types differ primarily in the way they itemize and value effects. These differences reflect the different aims and viewpoints of different decision problems (or economic questions).

*Cost-effectiveness analysis (CEA):* the effects of an intervention (and its comparators) are measured in identical units of outcome (e.g. mortality, myocardial infarctions, lung function, weight, bleeds, secondary infections, revisional surgeries). Alternative interventions are compared in terms of 'cost per unit of effect'.

*Cost-utility analysis (CUA):* when alternative interventions produce different levels of effect in terms of both quantity and quality of life (or different effects), the effects may be expressed in utilities. Utilities are measures which comprise both length of life and subjective levels of well-being. The best known utility measure is the quality-adjusted life year, or QALY. Alternative interventions are compared in terms of cost per unit of utility gained (e.g. cost per QALY).

*Cost-benefit analysis (CBA):* when both resource inputs and effects of alternative interventions are expressed in monetary units, so that they compare directly and across programmes within the healthcare system, or with programmes outside health care (e.g. healthcare intervention vs. criminal justice intervention).

values for the other key parameters in the cost-effectiveness formula or economic model (Weinstein 2003, Philips 2004, Cooper 2005)

### 15.1.3  Coverage of economics issues in Cochrane reviews

The overall aim of this chapter is to describe how authors of Cochrane and other systematic reviews might compile the best evidence on economics aspects of interventions in addition to the best evidence on their effectiveness.

There is currently no formal requirement for Cochrane reviews to include coverage of economic issues. This guidance is therefore presented as a series of optional methods to be considered by Cochrane review authors seeking to include coverage of economic issues. The principal element of the methodological framework outlined is a critical review of health economics studies, which can be conducted as a fully integrated component of a Cochrane review. This involves the assembly, selection, critical appraisal, summary and possibly synthesis of data from relevant health economics studies. Three core premises of the guidance are as follows:

1. Given the international audience of end-users of Cochrane reviews, the overall aim of economics components of reviews should be to summarize what is known from different settings about economic aspects of interventions, to help end-users understand key economic trade-offs between alternative healthcare treatments or tests;

2. Key secondary aims are to provide a framework for Cochrane reviews to present clinical and economic data in a format that facilitates their use in subsequent, or parallel, economic analyses;

3. Economic issues are relevant to decision-making even when evidence of intervention effectiveness is unclear. First, end-users often need to be aware of evidence regarding the incremental resource use and costs associated with an intervention, versus relevant comparators, as this can help to clarify the case for investing in future research on both effectiveness and cost-effectiveness. Second, it is important for end-users to be aware of whether or not existing full economic evaluations are based on robust evidence regarding effectiveness.

Authors of Cochrane reviews seeking to include coverage of economic aspects of interventions will need to consider in detail, and from the earliest stages of protocol development, how economic issues relate to their specific review topic. Use of the methods described in this chapter will also require at least some training in the use of health economics methods. Therefore, once a decision to include coverage of economic issues has been taken, it is advisable to consult with a health economist who has experience of systematic review methods as soon as possible.

Some Cochrane Review Groups (CRGs) already have access to one or more experienced health economists who regularly contribute work on economics components of reviews. The Campbell and Cochrane Economics Methods Group (CCEMG) will seek to help authors of Cochrane reviews identify health economists willing to contribute work, or to provide advice or peer review support (see Box 15.10.a).

## 15.2 Planning the economics component of a Cochrane review

### 15.2.1 Formulating an economic question

Following a decision to include coverage of economic aspects of interventions in a Cochrane review, the first stage of research is to formulate one or more questions, or objectives, that the economics component of the review will seek to address. Each economics question or objective will determine methodological decisions in subsequent stages of the critical review of health economics studies.

Formulating an economic question requires close consideration of the role and relevance of economic issues to the specific overall review topic. The *preliminary* questions below are intended to provide useful starting points to help authors and editors conceptualize the role and relevance of economic issues.

- What is the economic burden to society (e.g. health system, health or social care providers, individuals, families, employers) of the condition or illness that the intervention is seeking to affect?

- What types of incremental resource inputs are required to implement and sustain the intervention, versus comparators (e.g. staff, equipment, drugs, inpatient hospital care)?

- What are the incremental resource consequences of implementing the intervention, versus comparators? *or* How might the intervention impact on the subsequent (downstream) use of resources, versus comparators (e.g. complications, secondary procedures, outpatient visits, time-off-work)?

- What are the incremental costs associated with changes in resource use that may result from the intervention, versus comparators (e.g. direct and indirect medical costs, patient out-of-pocket expenses, income from employment)?

- What is the economic value associated with incremental beneficial or adverse effects (outcomes) that may result from the intervention, versus comparators (e.g. measures of willingness-to-pay, or utility)?

- What are the potential trade-offs between costs (resource use) and beneficial or adverse effects that may need to be considered in a decision to adopt or reject a given course of action?

In considering these preliminary questions, it is important to take the following key issues into account:

- *Magnitude*: What is the likely order of magnitude of different items of incremental resource use or incremental costs associated with the intervention, versus comparators? In other words, which items of resource use (resource inputs and resource consequences) and which costs are likely to be the most important when making choices between alternative interventions?

- *Time horizon*: What is the time horizon over which important costs (resource use) and effects (outcomes) are likely to accrue? Cochrane reviews implicitly establish a time horizon for effects by specifying intermediate and final endpoint measures of effects as target outcome measures. There is a parallel need to consider whether the same time horizon is applicable when all relevant costs (resource use) and effects are considered together.

- *Analytic viewpoint*: Who is likely to bear the incremental costs associated with an intervention, versus comparators, and who receives the incremental benefits (e.g. patient, patient's family, healthcare provider or third-party payer, healthcare system, society)? Some costs (resource use) are relevant from one analytic viewpoint, but not from another. For example, the cost of providing informal care may be relevant from a patient or a societal viewpoint, but may be excluded when a narrower perspective is selected, such as that of the healthcare system. A further complication is that some resource use or cost categories may overlap between perspectives. Given the range of end-users of Cochrane reviews, a pragmatic approach is to consider the full range of perspectives and then to report not only measures of resource use and cost, but also who bears the cost or incurs the resource use.

Clinical event pathways can provide a further useful tool to help conceptualize the role and relevance of economic issues to a specific review topic. A clinical event pathway provides a systematic, explicit method of representing different health and social care processes and outcomes. The method involves describing the main pathways of events that have distinct resource implications or outcome values associated with them, from the point of introduction of the interventions, through subsequent changes in management of participants, to final outcomes (see also Chapter 2 of Donaldson (Donaldson 2002)). Figure 15.2.a shows an example clinical event pathway for the clinical event 'stroke'. In developing a clinical event pathway, it is again important to consider the key issues of magnitude, time horizon and analytic viewpoint.

Once the role and relevance of economic issues has been considered carefully, one or more economic questions, or objectives, can be formulated. Review authors should avoid asking economic questions of the form 'What is the cost-effectiveness of intervention X (compared with Y or Z)?', since a critical review of health economics studies is unlikely to provide a credible answer to this type of question that is applicable across settings. Economic questions, or objectives, should be stated explicitly in the Objectives section of the protocol for a review, alongside other research questions and objectives.

| Event pathway | Example |
|---|---|
| Clinical event. | Stroke. |
| ↓ | ↓ |
| Clinical event management + subsequent clinical events. | Acute care and rehabilitation + sequelae and complications of treatment. |
| ↓ | ↓ |
| Resources used to manage events and outcomes of events. | Length of hospital stay, intensity of rehabilitation therapy, management of sequelae and complications (e.g. bleeding from secondary prophylaxis) and health outcomes associated with each stage. |
| ↓ | ↓ |
| Cost of resources used and utilities of outcomes. | Valuation of resources using healthcare (and other) pay and prices and valuation of outcomes, for example using quality-adjusted life years (QALYs ) or willingness-to-pay (WTP). |

**Figure 15.2.a**   Clinical event pathways

Considerations of the role and relevance of economic issues can also be used to inform a commentary on economic aspects of interventions, to be included in the Background section of the review.

An 'economics commentary' can be included whether or not the authors intend to incorporate a critical review of health economics studies. This is useful to help set the interventions being studied in an economics context by highlighting their potential economic consequences for consideration by end-users of the review. The 'economics commentary' may highlight the economic burden of the illness or medical condition being addressed by interventions, the types of resources required to implement and sustain interventions (resource inputs), the potential impacts of interventions on the subsequent, downstream use of resources (resource consequences) and issues of cost-effectiveness. The commentary should be supported by appropriate references to, and critical comment on, relevant literature wherever possible. Box 15.2.a shows some examples of this type of commentary, extracted from Background sections of current Cochrane reviews.

## 15.2.2   Including measures of resource use, costs and cost-effectiveness as outcomes

The process of formulating economic questions can also help to clarify the set of important measures of resource use, costs or cost-effectiveness (or a combination of these) to be included as target outcomes in a review. These outcomes should be included alongside other target outcomes in the 'Types of outcome measures' part of the 'Criteria for considering studies for this review' section of a review. Wherever possible, it is useful to break down measures of resource use and costs to the level of specific items or categories (e.g. length of hospital stay in days, duration of operation in minutes, number of outpatient attendances, bleeds from secondary prophylaxis at six-month follow-up, number of days off work, direct medical resource use, direct medical costs,

## Box 15.2.a Background commentary highlighting economics aspects of interventions

"Faecal incontinence... can be a debilitating problem with medical, social and economic implications... In the United States more than $400 million is spent each year on a range of both urinary and faecal incontinence products... During 1991 the direct costs of pads, appliances and other prescription items throughout hospitals and long term care settings in the UK for incontinence in general was estimated at £68 million... With the rise in numbers of elderly people in the world, this condition will be an increasing challenge to both healthcare services and home carers." (Brown 2007).

"If such a new and relatively expensive treatment [Lamotrigine] is to be available for routine use, a clear understanding as to how it compares with a standard antiepileptic drug (AED) such as carbamazepine is needed. The potential cost implications are highlighted by a survey of epilepsy services in the North West, UK, which showed that almost 40% of drug costs (the largest single contributor of the direct costs of epilepsy) was accounted for by the new AEDs lamotrigine and vigabatrin, despite the fact they were only taken by seven per cent of patients." (Gamble 2006).

"The cost of palliative chemotherapy treatment for advanced colorectal cancer includes not only the costs associated with the administration of chemotherapy, but also the provision of support to manage chemotherapy related complications. If palliative chemotherapy improves symptom control and quality of life this may reduce patient dependency and need for other symptomatic/supportive care measures offsetting the cost of this treatment. On the other hand, if the incidence of chemotherapy related toxicity is high and there is a decrease in quality of life as a result of treatment, then the cost of palliative chemotherapy will become much greater than that of supportive care alone." (Best 2000).

indirect medical resource use or costs, patient out-of-pocket expenses) and to avoid the use of general descriptive terms for outcomes (e.g. 'costs', 'resource utilization', 'health economics'). Measures of cost-effectiveness that may be included as target outcome measures in a review include incremental cost-effectiveness ratios (ICERs), incremental cost-per QALY and cost-benefit ratios (see also Section 15.1.2).

### 15.2.3 Specifying types of health economics studies and the scope of the economics component of a review

A critical review of health economics studies should specify at the outset which types of studies will be considered for inclusion (see also Section 15.1.2). This decision is driven primarily by the economic questions or objectives that have been formulated and the measures of resource use, costs and cost-effectiveness included as target outcome measures.

This decision should be made in consultation with a health economist, since it is not necessarily a straightforward exercise to map the analytic pathways between different forms of economic questions, 'economic' outcome measures and different types of health economics studies. For example, if a cost-effectiveness analysis includes reporting of results from all interim stages of analysis alongside final results, it may be possible to extract outcome data relating to measures of resource use, costs and cost-effectiveness; however if only final results are reported, it may only be possible to extract outcome data relating to measures of cost-effectiveness.

The types of health economics studies to be considered for inclusion in the review should be stated in the 'Types of studies' part of the 'Criteria for considering studies for this review' section. An illustrative statement featuring the full range of types of economics studies is as follows:

### Types of studies

The following types of studies will be considered for inclusion in the critical review of health economics studies:

Full economic evaluation studies (i.e. cost-effectiveness analyses, cost-utility analyses, cost-benefit analyses) of [intervention(s) versus comparator(s)]; partial economic evaluations (i.e. cost analyses, cost-description studies, cost-outcome descriptions) of [intervention(s) and comparator(s)]; and randomized trials reporting more limited information, such as estimates of resource use or costs associated with [intervention(s) and comparator(s)].

A final key methodological decision when planning a critical review of health economics studies is to set out the scope of this element of the review process. There are at least three options for the scope of a critical review of health economics studies:

1. Consider only relevant health economics studies conducted alongside effectiveness studies that meet eligibility criteria for the effectiveness component of the review;

2. Consider relevant health economics studies conducted alongside, and also those based upon data sourced from effectiveness studies that meet eligibility criteria for the effectiveness component of the review;

3. Consider all relevant health economics studies, whether or not conducted alongside, or based upon, effectiveness studies that meet eligibility criteria for the effectiveness component of the review.

The first option might typically allow only health economics studies conducted alongside high quality randomized trials to be considered for inclusion in the economics component of the review. The second option would *additionally* allow for consideration of economic modelling studies based on a meta-analysis of data from high quality randomized trials. A good example of a review of health economic models is the review of screening for abdominal aortic aneurysm conducted by Campbell and colleagues (Campbell 2007). The third option is clearly a more inclusive one that allows for consideration of all relevant health economics studies, including those based upon observational studies or analysis of large administrative databases, or regression-based cost and resource use analyses, for example.

Little is known about the impact of including these different types of health economics studies upon the results of a critical review. However, it is plausible that this type of decision regarding 'scope' at least has the potential impact on results, since different options may involve consideration of different sets of studies (see also Section 15.5.2). Also, where a review includes both economic evaluations based on single studies (e.g. randomized trials) and model-based economic evaluations, it may be optimal to consider each of these categories of studies separately, in order to retain comparability amongst studies.

In practice, a majority of current Cochrane reviews that set out to incorporate coverage of evidence from health economics studies restrict this coverage to economic studies conducted alongside effectiveness studies meeting eligibility criteria for the effectiveness component of the review (i.e. the first option), but do not state this explicitly (Shemilt 2007). Since the decision regarding scope has the potential to exclude some health economics studies without any recourse to critical appraisal of their methodological quality, the result of this decision should be stated in the 'Types of studies' part of the 'Criteria for considering studies for this review' section of a review, alongside details of the types of economic studies to be considered for inclusion, for example by appending "The review will consider only health economics studies conducted alongside effectiveness studies included in the effectiveness component of the review" to the illustrative statement above.

# 15.3 Locating studies

## 15.3.1 Use of electronic search filters

Search methods for locating relevant health economics studies will differ depending on the scope of a critical review of such studies and the types of studies to be considered for inclusion (see also Sections 15.2.3 and 15.1.2). However, in all cases the first stage of the search strategy will have the same objective: to identify effectiveness studies retrieved for initial screening and potential inclusion in a Cochrane review which include relevant health economics studies.

Electronic records of effectiveness studies retrieved from electronic literature databases can be filtered using search strategies designed to capture health economics studies. This can precede visual screening of abstracts and full texts of studies, acting as an aid to location of economic studies by limiting the number of records to be assessed. Electronic filtering is most useful in reviews where the number of records retrieved from electronic literature databases is large (i.e. where this number is relatively small, use of electronic filters may not be judged necessary, but explicit criteria would still need to be applied).

The Centre for Reviews and Dissemination (CRD) has developed a series of electronic search strategies designed to capture potential economic evaluation studies for inclusion in the NHS Economic Evaluation Database (NHS EED). MEDLINE (Ovid CD-ROM), CINAHL (Ovid CD-ROM), EMBASE (Ovid online) and PsychINFO (Ovid online) versions are published in the NHS EED Handbook (Craig 2007) and online at www.york.ac.uk/inst/crd/nfaq2.htm. Each of these search strategies can be appended to review-specific search strategies of the corresponding database using the 'AND' operator, to filter search results for records which also contain 'economics' search terms.

These NHS EED search strategies are very broad and will capture economics methods studies and reviews of economics studies, as well as the full range of types of health economics studies (see Section 15.1.2). For more specific searches, narrower adaptations of the search strategies and close reading of the scope notes of MeSH are advised. The search strategies can also be adapted, in consultation with information retrieval specialists, for use in other electronic literature databases. Adaptation of the search strategies will need to take into account variations across databases in the indexing or classification of health economics studies. A useful annotated list of electronic literature databases that include coverage of health economics literature and details of internet sites containing relevant grey literature is available (Napper 2005).

An important procedural consideration when considering use of electronic search filters designed to capture health economics studies is that Cochrane reviews also frequently utilize other search filters designed to capture other specific study designs, such as randomized trials. These 'study design search filters' are also appended to review-specific search strategies using the 'AND' operator. Therefore, if the scope of the critical review is not restricted to health economics studies conducted alongside effectiveness studies included in the effectiveness component of the review (e.g. will also include model-based economic evaluations: see Section 15.2.3), then the 'economics search filter' should be appended to any other 'study design search filter' using the 'OR' operator, to ensure that all types of health economics studies to be considered are retrieved. Alternatively, if the scope of the critical review is limited to health economics studies conducted alongside effectiveness studies included in the effectiveness component of the review, then use of the 'economics search filter' is not required, since most of the economic studies to be considered will be retrieved using the 'study design search filter' (although, it is possible that in this case the search results may still omit some relevant economics studies, such as economic evaluations based on randomized trials but published separately from and usually after the trial results).

## 15.3.2   Use of specialist databases

The NHS Economic Evaluation Database (NHS EED) is published as part of *The Cochrane Library* (www.thecochranelibrary.com). Therefore, whenever users search

*The Cochrane Library*, NHS EED records will be highlighted as well as Cochrane reviews. NHS EED is also available free online from the Centre for Reviews and Dissemination (CRD) web site (see www.york.ac.uk/inst/crd/crddatabases.htm). The version of NHS EED in *The Cochrane Library* is updated quarterly, whilst the CRD web site version is updated monthly.

A search of NHS EED and processing of these search results is recommended for all Cochrane reviews, especially those incorporating a critical review of health economics studies. NHS EED contains structured abstracts of full economic evaluations in health care, published in all languages, as well as bibliographic records of partial economic evaluations, methodology studies and reviews of economic studies. The NHS EED structured abstract format includes a critical commentary written by independent health economist peer reviewers and presents details of methods, results and other data in a summary format that is directly useful to inform critical appraisal and data collection in a critical review of health economics studies (see Sections 15.5.2 and 15.4.2).

It may sometimes be considered useful to include NHS EED abstracts of relevant full economic evaluation studies as an appendix to a published Cochrane review, as was done by Rodgers et al. and Fayter et al. (Rodgers 2006, Fayter 2007) (see also Section 15.6.2). If NHS EED does not contain a structured abstract of a full economic evaluation identified during searches conducted for a Cochrane review, it would be useful if the review authors could alert the Campbell and Cochrane Economics Methods Group (Box 15.10.a), so that NHS EED researchers can be made aware of the need to consider producing an abstract.

Searches of NHS EED and other specialist databases of health economics literature (see below) can be conducted using adaptations of review-specific search strategies, excluding both 'economics search filters' and other 'study design search filters'. When searching The Cochrane Library, NHS EED is searched by default (i.e. unless the database is specifically excluded from the search using advanced search options). Information on how to search the CRD web site version of NHS EED can be accessed in CRD help pages at www.crd.york.ac.uk/crdweb/html/help.htm.

The desire to extend the principles of the UK-based NHS EED database to other European countries has led to the establishment of the European Network of Health Economic Evaluation Databases (EURONHEED), which is also freely available online (see http://infodoc.inserm.fr/euronheed/). NHS EED provides links to EURONHEED full abstract records only (from 2000 forward), so although a search of NHS EED will retrieve all full abstract records from both databases, it will not retrieve bibliographic records of partial economic evaluations, methodology studies or reviews of economics studies that are held in EURONHEED only.

NHS EED, EURONHEED and other specialist databases of health economics literature that may be searched for Cochrane reviews (including The CEA Registry, the Health Economic Evaluations Database (HEED) and Econlit) are fully described in a paper published by the NHS EED project team (Aguiar-Ibanez 2005). CRD also publishes an annotated online list containing details of these databases, including links to each database web site, at www.york.ac.uk/inst/crd/econ4.htm, as part of their 'Information resources in health economics' pages (www.york.ac.uk/inst/crd/econ.htm).

This annotated list also includes details of selected general databases which include coverage of health economics literature (see also Section 15.3.1).

If the scope of the critical review of health economics studies is limited to those studies conducted alongside effectiveness studies that meet eligibility criteria for the effectiveness component of the review (see Section 15.2.3), then the sole aim of a supplementary search of NHS EED and other specialist databases is to check whether they include any structured abstracts of full economic evaluation studies conducted alongside included effectiveness studies. However, if the scope of the critical review of health economics studies is broader (see Section 15.2.3), then an *additional* aim is to identify *further* economic studies for potential inclusion in the review.

## 15.4   Selecting studies and collecting data

### 15.4.1   Assessing relevance to the review topic

Once full-text papers of potentially relevant health economics studies have been obtained (and structured abstracts of full economic evaluations, where available), the next step is to assess the relevance of each of these studies to the specific review topic, as a preliminary stage to addressing the issue of risk of bias. Decisions to either include or exclude health economics studies on grounds of relevance should be based on whether or not they meet eligibility criteria relating to the target populations, interventions, comparisons and outcomes that were specified in the protocol for the review. Reasons for excluding health economics studies at this stage should be reported in 'Characteristics of excluded studies' tables.

### 15.4.2   Collecting data

Precise data collection requirements for the economics components of Cochrane reviews will need to be specified for each individual review, depending on the specific economics question or objective and on the measures of *incremental* resource use, costs or cost-effectiveness included as target outcomes. In general terms, two types of data will need to be collected: details of the characteristics of included health economics studies and details of their results. The potential to extract data as suggested below from published reports may be constrained by the quality of reporting of the health economics studies (where information is missing, a further option is to contact study authors to request additional details).

Useful data to be collected regarding the characteristics of each economic study are likely to include: year of study; details of interventions and comparators; study design and source(s) of resource use, unit costs and (if applicable) effectiveness data (see also Sections 15.1.2 and 15.2.3); decision-making jurisdiction, geographical and organizational setting; analytic viewpoint; and time horizon for both costs and effects (see Section 15.2.1).

For results, estimates of specific items of resource use associated with interventions and comparators and estimates of their unit costs should be extracted separately, if reported, as well as estimates of costs of the resource use (i.e. number of units of resource X unit cost). The type and quantity of each resource used should be extracted in natural units (e.g. length of hospital stay in days, duration of operation in minutes, number of outpatient attendances at six-month follow-up, number of days of work). It is also important to collect information on the price year and currency used to calculate estimates of costs and incremental costs. Measures of incremental resource use and costs should be collected at the individual patient level (i.e. resource use per patient, cost per patient), wherever possible. Both a point estimate and a measure of uncertainty (e.g. standard error or confidence interval) should be extracted for measures of incremental resource use, costs and cost-effectiveness, if reported. Additionally, it is useful to collect details of any sensitivity analyses undertaken, and any information regarding the impact of varying assumptions on the magnitude and direction of results.

CRD Report 6 (Craig 2007) includes a template for producing structured abstracts of full economic evaluations for inclusion in NHS EED (see also Section 15.3.2), together with notes to guide data collection and critical appraisal. These materials can provide a useful template for the design of data collection forms for use in the economics components of Cochrane reviews.

If a full economic evaluation already has a corresponding NHS EED structured abstract, this *may* obviate the need for researchers to undertake further data collection from the study. In parallel, given that critical appraisal and data collection from economic evaluation studies with no completed NHS EED abstract will need to be undertaken for the Cochrane review, authors are encouraged to consider registering with NHS EED to produce an abstract, in order to avoid duplication of effort. Please contact CCEMG for further information, or to initiate a request that a structured abstract is produced by NHS EED (see also Section 15.3.2).

# 15.5 Addressing risk of bias

## 15.5.1 Classification of studies by study design

A preliminary stage to be undertaken before addressing risk of bias is to classify the included health economics studies by study design. Methods underpinning critical appraisal of the methodological quality of health economics studies will vary slightly depending on study design.

Classification should consist of two stages:

1. Classification of the design of the health economics study.

2. Classification of the design of the study generating the effectiveness data on which the health economics study is based, if applicable.

Each health economics study may be classified (stage 1) as a type of full economic evaluation, a type of partial economic evaluation, or a type of effectiveness study (e.g. a randomized trial) reporting more limited information on the resource use or costs associated with an intervention (see Section 15.1.2). Classifying the design of the study that generates the effectiveness data on which the health economics study is based (stage 2) is only applicable in the case of health economics studies classified as a full economic evaluation or as a cost-outcome description at the first stage of classification. The study generating the effectiveness data may be a single study design (e.g. a randomized trial, a non-randomized trial, an observational study) or a synthesis of several studies (e.g. a meta-analysis of randomized trials) (see also Section 15.1.2).

It is likely to be useful to consult with a health economist when undertaking classification of health economics studies. This is because health economics studies reported to use one type of study design (e.g. a cost-benefit analysis) may, on closer inspection, turn out to use another (e.g. a cost-effectiveness analysis). This means that particular care is required when classifying economic studies encountered during a review (Zarnke 1997).

Depending on the scope of the critical review of health economics studies and the types of studies that will be considered for inclusion (see Section 15.2.3), health economics studies may be excluded at this stage, based on classification by study design. Once again, reasons for excluding health economic studies at this stage should be reported in 'Characteristics of excluded studies' tables.

## 15.5.2   Critical appraisal of methodological quality

The next stage of research is to undertake critical appraisal of the methodological quality of the remaining health economics studies, in order to address risk of bias. Variability in the quality of the conduct and reporting in health economic analyses is well documented (Neumann 2005). The core objective of critical appraisal of health economics studies is to assess whether they describe methods, assumptions, models and possible biases in a way that is transparent and fully supported by available evidence, the strength of which is made easily accessible to any critical reader (Rennie 2000).

Critical appraisal of health economics studies can be informed by the use of checklists that have been developed to guide assessments of methodological quality. Where checklists are used to inform critical appraisal of health economics studies in a Cochrane review, bibliographic details of the checklist should be cited in the 'Data collection and analysis' section. Whichever checklists are used, it is also useful to consider including additional tables to summarize completed checklists for included health economics studies in the published review.

The reliability of a full economic evaluation (see Section 15.5.2) is in part predicated on its use of reliable effectiveness data, so part of the critical appraisal of a full economic evaluation conducted alongside a single effectiveness study (e.g. a randomized trial) involves considering all those sources of potential bias that may apply to the effectiveness study used (see Chapter 8). For this type of full economic evaluation study, the critical appraisal will therefore consist of the following two parts.

1. Assessment of the risk of bias in results of the single effectiveness study on which the full economic evaluation study is based, informed by a recognized checklist for effectiveness studies.

2. Assessment of the methodological quality of the full economic evaluation study, informed by a recognized checklist for economic evaluations conducted alongside single study designs.

A number of checklists have been developed to guide critical appraisal of health economics studies. Whilst no checklists have been formally validated, two have received more scrutiny than most:

- British Medical Journal Checklist for authors and peer reviewers of economic submissions (Drummond 1996);

- CHEC list for assessment of methodological quality of economic evaluations (Evers 2005).

These checklists are reproduced in Figures 15.5.a and 15.5.b. Use of the 'Drummond checklist' and the 'Evers checklist' is recommended in Cochrane reviews to inform appraisal of the methodological quality of full economic evaluations conducted alongside single effectiveness studies, and also to inform critical appraisal of partial economic evaluations using the subset of applicable checklist items (see also Section 15.1.2).

If the scope of the critical review of health economics studies encompasses relevant economic modelling studies (see Section 15.2.3), then assessments of the methodological quality of such studies will need to be informed by a different checklist, since the 'Drummond checklist' and 'Evers checklist' are relevant but not sufficient for modelling studies. The 'Phillips checklist' is recommended to inform critical appraisal of the methodological quality of economic modelling studies (Philips 2004). Use of this checklist can be supplemented by referring to a published hierarchy of data sources which sets out the sources of data that are recognized as the best available sources to inform each parameter in an economic model (Cooper 2005).

Critical appraisal of the methodological quality of all types of full economic evaluation can usefully be informed by a corresponding NHS EED structured abstract, if available, to supplement the use of checklists (see also Section 15.3.2). This is because NHS EED structured abstracts include critical appraisal of study quality based on the same dimensions of quality reflected in the checklists recommended above.

There are as yet no widely validated minimum methodological criteria to be applied to screening economic studies for inclusion in systematic reviews. Decisions to include or exclude such studies will therefore need to be made on the basis of an overall judgement regarding their methodological quality, as well as their relevance in terms of the economic questions, interventions, populations and outcomes being studied (see Section 15.4.1). Eligibility criteria relating to dimensions of the methodological quality

| Item | Yes | No | Not clear | Not appropriate |
|------|-----|-----|-----------|-----------------|
| **Study design** | | | | |
| 1. The research question is stated. | ☐ | ☐ | ☐ | |
| 2. The economic importance of the research question is stated. | ☐ | ☐ | ☐ | |
| 3. The viewpoint(s) of the analysis are clearly stated and justified. | ☐ | ☐ | ☐ | |
| 4. The rationale for choosing alternative programmes or interventions compared is stated. | ☐ | ☐ | ☐ | |
| 5. The alternatives being compared are clearly described. | ☐ | ☐ | ☐ | |
| 6. The form of economic evaluation used is stated. | ☐ | ☐ | ☐ | |
| 7. The choice of form of economic evaluation is justified in relation to the questions addressed. | ☐ | ☐ | ☐ | |
| **Data collection** | | | | |
| 8. The source(s) of effectiveness estimates used are stated. | ☐ | ☐ | ☐ | |
| 9. Details of the design and results of effectiveness study are given (if based on a single study). | ☐ | ☐ | ☐ | ☐ |
| 10. Details of the methods of synthesis or meta-analysis of estimates are given (if based on a synthesis of a number of effectiveness studies). | ☐ | ☐ | ☐ | ☐ |
| 11. The primary outcome measure(s) for the economic evaluation are clearly stated. | ☐ | ☐ | ☐ | |
| 12. Methods to value benefits are stated. | ☐ | ☐ | ☐ | ☐ |
| 13. Details of the subjects from whom valuations were obtained were given. | ☐ | ☐ | ☐ | ☐ |
| 14. Productivity changes (if included) are reported separately. | ☐ | ☐ | ☐ | ☐ |
| 15. The relevance of productivity changes to the study question is discussed. | ☐ | ☐ | ☐ | ☐ |
| 16. Quantities of resource use are reported separately from their unit costs. | ☐ | ☐ | ☐ | |
| 17. Methods for the estimation of quantities and unit costs are described. | ☐ | ☐ | ☐ | |
| 18. Currency and price data are recorded. | ☐ | ☐ | ☐ | |
| 19. Details of currency of price adjustments for inflation or currency conversion are given. | ☐ | ☐ | ☐ | |
| 20. Details of any model used are given. | ☐ | ☐ | ☐ | ☐ |
| 21. The choice of model used and the key parameters on which it is based are justified. | ☐ | ☐ | ☐ | ☐ |
| **Analysis and interpretation of results** | | | | |
| 22. Time horizon of costs and benefits is stated. | ☐ | ☐ | ☐ | |
| 23. The discount rate(s) is stated. | ☐ | ☐ | ☐ | ☐ |
| 24. The choice of discount rate(s) is justified. | ☐ | ☐ | ☐ | ☐ |
| 25. An explanation is given if costs and benefits are not discounted. | ☐ | ☐ | ☐ | ☐ |
| 26. Details of statistical tests and confidence intervals are given for stochastic data. | ☐ | ☐ | ☐ | ☐ |
| 27. The approach to sensitivity analysis is given. | ☐ | ☐ | ☐ | ☐ |
| 28. The choice of variables for sensitivity analysis is justified. | ☐ | ☐ | ☐ | ☐ |
| 29. The ranges over which the variables are varied are justified. | ☐ | ☐ | ☐ | ☐ |
| 30. Relevant alternatives are compared. | ☐ | ☐ | ☐ | ☐ |
| 31. Incremental analysis is reported. | ☐ | ☐ | ☐ | ☐ |
| 32. Major outcomes are presented in a disaggregated as well as aggregated form. | ☐ | ☐ | ☐ | |
| 33. The answer to the study question is given. | ☐ | ☐ | ☐ | |
| 34. Conclusions follow from the data reported. | ☐ | ☐ | ☐ | |
| 35. Conclusions are accompanied by the appropriate caveats. | ☐ | ☐ | ☐ | |

**Figure 15.5.a** Drummond checklist (Reproduced from Drummond MF, Jefferson TO. Guidelines for authors and peer reviewers of economic submissions to the BMJ. The BMJ Economic Evaluation Working Party. *BMJ* 1996; 313: 275–283. Copyright 1996, BMJ Publishing Group Ltd.)

| | Item | Yes | No |
|---|---|---|---|
| 1. | Is the study population clearly described? | ☐ | ☐ |
| 2. | Are competing alternatives clearly described? | ☐ | ☐ |
| 3. | Is a well-defined research question posed in answerable form? | ☐ | ☐ |
| 4. | Is the economic study design appropriate to the stated objective? | ☐ | ☐ |
| 5. | Is the chosen time horizon appropriate to include relevant costs and consequences? | ☐ | ☐ |
| 6. | Is the actual perspective chosen appropriate? | ☐ | ☐ |
| 7. | Are all important and relevant costs for each alternative identified? | ☐ | ☐ |
| 8. | Are all costs measured appropriately in physical units? | ☐ | ☐ |
| 9. | Are costs valued appropriately? | ☐ | ☐ |
| 10. | Are all important and relevant outcomes for each alternative identified? | ☐ | ☐ |
| 11. | Are all outcomes measured appropriately? | ☐ | ☐ |
| 12. | Are outcomes valued appropriately? | ☐ | ☐ |
| 13. | Is an incremental analysis of costs and outcomes of alternatives performed? | ☐ | ☐ |
| 14. | Are all future costs and outcomes discounted appropriately? | ☐ | ☐ |
| 15. | Are all important variables, whose values are uncertain, appropriately subjected to sensitivity analysis? | ☐ | ☐ |
| 16. | Do the conclusions follow from the data reported? | ☐ | ☐ |
| 17. | Does the study discuss the generalizability of the results to other settings and patient/client groups? | ☐ | ☐ |
| 18. | Does the article indicate that there is no potential conflict of interest of study researcher(s) and funder(s)? | ☐ | ☐ |
| 19. | Are ethical and distributional issues discussed appropriately | ☐ | ☐ |

**Figure 15.5.b** Evers checklist (Reproduced from Evers S, Goossens M, de Vet H, van Tulder M, Ament A. Criteria list for assessment of methodological quality of economic evaluations: Consensus on Health Economic Criteria. *International Journal of Technology Assessment in Health Care* 2005; 21: 240–245, by permission of Cambridge University Press.)

of health economics studies should be stated in the 'Data collection and analysis' section.

It is also important to highlight that, to date, there has been relatively little empirical research to investigate the impact upon the results of a critical review of health economics studies, of decisions to include economic studies that meet some but not all standards of methodological quality. However, as with choice of eligibility criteria relating to quality and design of effectiveness studies, and to the design of health economics studies (see also Section 15.2.3), it is plausible that use of different data sources for measures of resource use, cost and/or cost-effectiveness has at least the potential to impact on results (see also Section 15.7).

## 15.6    Analysing and presenting results

The emphasis of guidance on analytic methods for the economics components of Cochrane reviews is upon tabulation of the characteristics and results of included health economics studies. This can be supplemented by a narrative summary which focuses on critical appraisal of included studies and discussion of their principal findings. Additionally, in some circumstances, a meta-analysis of resource use or cost data, or development of an economic model, may be considered. These options are described in more detail in the sections that follow. Further options for analysing health economics studies and presenting the results of these analyses need to be evaluated through further methodological research (see Section 15.9).

### 15.6.1    Presenting results in tables

'Characteristics of included studies tables' provide a natural place in a Cochrane review to present details of the characteristics of included health economics studies, such as year of study; details of interventions and comparators; study design; data sources; jurisdiction and setting; analytic perspective and time horizon (see also Section 15.4.2). Authors may also consider including additional tables to summarize checklists completed to inform assessments of the methodological quality of included health economics studies (see also Section 15.5.2).

The results of included health economics studies can be summarized using either 'Characteristics of included studies' tables, Additional tables, or both. In either case, where possible, point estimates of measures of items of resource use or costs should be presented with associated measures of uncertainty for both the target intervention and each of its comparators, as well as point estimates of *incremental* costs and/or cost-effectiveness, again with associated measures of uncertainty. It is also important to state the currency and price year alongside estimates of costs and/or incremental costs (if reported).

It may be possible to convert cost estimates to a common currency and price year, in order to facilitate comparison of estimates collected from different studies. An international exchange rate based on Purchasing Power Parities (PPPs) should be used to convert cost estimates to a target currency, and gross domestic product (GDP) deflators (or implicit price deflators for GDP) should be used to convert cost estimates to a fixed price year. Data sets containing PPP conversion rates and GDP deflator values are available from the International Monetary Fund in the World Economic Outlook Database (updated biannually: see www.imf.org/external/data.htm). Conversion of cost estimates to a common currency and price year should only be performed in consultation with an experienced health economist. CCEMG will aim to issue further methods guidance on this topic in due course.

### 15.6.2    Narrative summary of results

Cochrane reviews may include narrative summaries of the main characteristics and results of included economic studies, including measures of incremental resource use, cost and cost-effectiveness, to supplement and provide a commentary on tabulated results. This can be located in the Results section, alongside narrative summary of the results of effectiveness studies (see Chapter 11, Section 11.7).

The central aim of this narrative summary is to make explicit, for the end-user, the extent to which cost and resource use estimates collected from multiple studies are homogeneous between studies. This can be accomplished by describing differences in methods for assessing, and patterns of resource use and costs between comparison groups, both within and across included studies, with potential explanations for any inconsistencies in results between studies. As discussed earlier in this chapter, economic evaluation studies are constructed differently and for different purposes (see also Section 15.1.2). This is one factor that may lead to heterogeneity between studies in their methods and results. Where there is heterogeneity between economics studies in their methods or results, drawing attention to these potential sources of *statistical* heterogeneity can help to summarize the international economics literature in an explicit way that is likely to be useful to the end-users of reviews (Gilbody 1999). It is important to avoid using this section as a form of analysis leading to recommendations regarding cost-effectiveness (see also Section 15.8).

Other features of good practice in a narrative summary of included health economics studies include the following.

- reporting the overall numbers of health economics studies selected for inclusion in the review, by study design;

- outlining the economic questions addressed within included studies;

- reporting the designs of included studies;

- reporting the analytic viewpoints adopted within included studies;

- reporting the time horizons adopted within included studies;

- discussion of measures of *incremental* resource use, costs and/or cost-effectiveness reported within included studies;

- reporting measures of uncertainty alongside measures of resource use, costs and/or cost-effectiveness extracted from reports of included studies;

- reporting currency and price year alongside estimates of costs extracted from included studies;

- adjusting cost estimates extracted from reports of each included study to a common currency and price year, if possible;

- highlighting key features of sensitivity analyses undertaken and consistency of results, both within sensitivity analyses and across included studies;

- discussion of the overall methodological quality and limitations of included studies;

- discussion of the relevance and generalizability of the results of included studies to other jurisdictions and settings; and

- discussion of the quality of effectiveness data used in included health economics studies and the relationship between outcomes used and those estimated in the effectiveness component of the Cochrane review.

A further option is to provide links to completed NHS EED or other structured abstracts of full economic evaluation studies, if available. NHS EED structured abstracts include information on both the characteristics and results of full health economic evaluations (see also Section 15.3.2). Some systematic reviews include NHS EED abstracts of included full economic evaluations in an appendix, as well as a narrative summary of the abstracts in the main text of the review (Rodgers 2006, Fayter 2007).

## 15.6.3  Meta-analysis of resource use and cost data

There are currently no agreed-upon methods for pooling combined estimates of cost-effectiveness (e.g. incremental cost-effectiveness, cost-utility or cost-benefit ratios), extracted from multiple economic evaluations, using meta-analysis or other quantitative synthesis methods. However, in principle, if estimates of measures of resource use and costs in a common metric (and associated measures of uncertainty) are available from two or more included studies, for an intervention and its comparator, these can be pooled using a meta-analysis. In practice, extreme caution is advised when considering whether to undertake a meta-analysis of resource use or cost data as part of a Cochrane review. Prior to any decision to pool estimates using a meta-analysis, particular attention should be given to whether the metric in question has equivalent meaning across studies.

Resource use and costs are sensitive to variability across settings, both *within* a country and *between* countries, in features of the local context, such as local prices or aspects of service organization and delivery (Drummond 2001, Sculpher 2004). This may limit the generalizability and transferability of estimates of cost, resource use and, by implication, estimates of cost-effectiveness, across settings. It is also the principal reason that resource use and cost data relating to specific target populations and jurisdictions of interest are regarded as the best available source of data for use in economic evaluations to be used in resource allocation decision processes in the specific setting (Cooper 2005). These issues have generated debate on whether meta-analysis of measures of resource use or costs across wider geographical and political boundaries is likely to generate meaningful results, how the results of such meta-analyses should be interpreted and what additional value the results may have for end-users of Cochrane reviews. (Further discussions around issues of applicability and transferability of health economic evaluations can also be found in texts by Hutubessy et al and Kumaranayake and Walker (Kumaranayake 2002, Hutubessy 2003).

On the other hand, whether specific estimates of resource use or costs are generalizable, or transferable, across settings may be regarded as an empirical question. In circumstances where there is evidence of little variation in resource or cost use between studies, it may be regarded as legitimate to present a pooled estimate. Otherwise it is important that the distribution of costs is clearly presented. Many completed Cochrane reviews include meta-analyses of resource use data. A small number of Cochrane reviews include meta-analyses of cost data, although these are not always accompanied by critical appraisal of the methods used to generate these data.

If meta-analyses of resource use or cost data are undertaken in a Cochrane review, this should always be supported by thorough critical appraisal of the methods used to derive such estimates within the corresponding health economics studies (see Sections 15.5.2, and 15.6.2), alongside use of statistical methods to investigate and incorporate between-study heterogeneity (e.g. $I^2$, chi-squared; random-effects models: see Chapter 9, Section 9.5). Cost estimates collected from multiple studies should be adjusted to a common currency and price year before these data are pooled (see also Section 15.6.1). Authors should consult Chapter 9 for further guidance on the statistical procedures underpinning meta-analysis.

If meta-analyses of resource use or cost data are conducted, a narrative summary should be included in the Results section to comment on the direction and magnitude of results and their precision. Similarly, if two or more health economics studies are included in a review, but a decision is taken not to pool (in a meta-analysis) resource use and/or cost data that have been collected from these studies, this can be stated in the Methods section (see Box 15.6.a for an example of this type of statement).

---

**Box 15.6.a   Statement of a decision not to conduct a meta-analysis of resource use or cost data**

"[Resource use and cost outcomes] were not pooled as the outcomes were not considered comparable across trials... The results are specific to the countries in which the studies were undertaken because of differences between the public health systems. The detailed reports show very different apportionment of costs between different items in different countries." (Birks 2006).

---

## 15.6.4   Developing an economic model

Cochrane reviews can contribute key components of the evidence required to develop a subsequent or parallel full economic evaluation, including use of a decision-analysis approach for pooling or modelling the available evidence on intervention costs and effects (see also Sections 15.1.2 and 15.1.3). This approach usually involves estimation of the point estimate, and description of the joint distribution, of incremental costs and effects resulting from an intervention (in terms of cost-effectiveness, cost-utility or cost-benefit), compared with a relevant alternative, in a defined population and setting, and with included costs and outcomes agreed to be relevant from a specific, stated analytic viewpoint (e.g. patient, healthcare provider or third-party payer, healthcare system, society).

Economic modelling methods are not covered in detail here, as their routine use as part of the Cochrane review process is not recommended. However, authors of Cochrane reviews wishing to pursue the 'in-depth' economics of interventions are encouraged to collaborate with researchers with expertise in developing economic models. It may sometimes be possible to develop a general structure for an economic model as part of a Cochrane review, where the basic model inputs and outputs are similar across different settings, but where some (or even all) of the data required to populate the model are specific to a local setting.

Also, notwithstanding issues already discussed regarding the generalizability and transferability of the results of economic evaluations across jurisdictions and settings (see Section 15.6.3), it cannot be ruled out that it may sometimes be considered worthwhile (although time, resource and expertise intensive) to develop one or more economic models for publication in a Cochrane review. For example, one motivation to develop an economic model as part of a Cochrane review may be an intention to use the review to inform directly the design of future research that will incorporate an economic evaluation component. In these circumstances, developing a model can help to clarify the structural assumptions and parameters that need to be considered in an economic evaluation, and the data that will need to be collected during the research. If this type of approach is pursued in a Cochrane review, it needs to be made clear that each example economic model aims to provide an illustrative assessment of the cost-effectiveness of the interventions being compared, in an example jurisdiction and at a given point in time.

Economic modellers are also encouraged to consider utilizing the evidence contained in Cochrane reviews to inform the development of economic models. Efforts to incorporate economics evidence into Cochrane reviews using the methods outlined in this chapter aim in part to increase the relevance and applicability of Cochrane reviews for use in subsequent, or parallel, full economic evaluation modelling exercises.

## 15.7    Addressing reporting biases

It is widely recognized that commercial and other pressures may affect the funding of studies and reporting of the results of studies which focus on the economic value of healthcare interventions (Drummond 1992). Despite this, until recently relatively little research attention has been focused on the issue of publication and related biases in economic evaluation studies, compared with coverage of this issue with respect to effectiveness studies. However, several recent studies have begun to examine this issue using systematic review and research synthesis methods.

Bell and colleagues undertook a systematic review of published cost-effectiveness studies in health care and found that studies sponsored by industry were more likely to report ratios that fall beneath, and cluster around, commonly proposed cost-effectiveness acceptability thresholds, when compared with studies sponsored by non-industry sources (Bell 2006). Miners and colleagues undertook a systematic review to compare evidence on cost-effectiveness submitted to the National Institute of Health and Clinical Excellence (NICE) by manufacturers of the relevant health-care technologies and by contracted university-based assessment groups respectively. (Miners 2005). This study found that estimated incremental cost-effectiveness ratios submitted by manufacturers were, on average, significantly lower than those provided by the assessment groups for the same technology. Friedberg and colleagues found that published economic analyses of new drugs used in oncology funded by pharmaceutical companies were one eighth as likely to reach unfavourable quantitative conclusions (and 1.4 times as likely to reach favourable qualitative conclusions) when compared to non-profit funded studies (Friedberg 1999). Other reviews focusing on this issue have reached broadly similar conclusions (Freemantle 1997, Azimi 1998, Lexchin 2003). A common theme of the discussion in these methodology review studies is the authors' suspicion that reporting or publication biases are likely to be instrumental in the observed patterns of results. The general hypothesis is that economic analyses with results that suggest an intervention may be economically unattractive are, consciously or unconsciously, not published by sponsors, authors, or journal editors.

However, all of the above methodology review studies are limited by their design (limitations are usually acknowledged and discussed by the authors). The ideal and most robust study design to investigate the presence of reporting and publication biases would involve direct comparison of published and unpublished findings within studies, or direct comparison of the findings of published and unpublished studies (Song 2000). As such, a systematic, comprehensive comparison is clearly difficult to achieve, due to the inherent difficulties of identifying all relevant unpublished economic analyses. In the absence of such data, it is not possible to rule out alternative explanations for the observed patterns of results (e.g. the results could reflect the true distributions of incremental cost-effectiveness ratios).

Methods for addressing publication bias in systematic reviews, which can be applied, with the same caveats, in systematic reviews of economic studies, are covered in Chapter 10. Proposals that have been suggested to help address publication and related biases in economic evaluation studies, such as those that may be encountered in Cochrane reviews, are:

1. To encourage a more transparent, consistent approach to the conduct and reporting of economic analyses, through the promulgation of good practice guidelines and checklists for use in critical appraisal of such studies – in particular review-based studies and modelling studies;

2. To increase scrutiny of journal submissions for potential conflicts of interest of study sponsors and authors;

3. To increase access to all the underlying data used in an economic evaluation in order to increase transparency of methods.

## 15.8    Interpreting results

Interpretation of the results of a review of health economics studies is dependent on the specific economic questions and context of relevance to a given decision regarding the provision of health care. In Cochrane reviews – intended for an international audience – there are clearly a large number of potential economic questions and contextual factors that different decision-making constituencies may need to take into account. Given this global context, it is simply not feasible to interpret the results of a critical review of multiple economic evaluation studies in order to draw conclusions about the adoption or rejection of a healthcare treatment or diagnostic test, for example. However, whilst in these circumstances the Cochrane review is unlikely to provide the central aspect of any policy evaluation, it can still help to refine an economic discussion and to set this in an international context (Gilbody 1999).

In a review topic area with few or no relevant, high-quality economic evaluation studies, the critical review of health economics studies can serve to highlight a lack of economics evidence that future research may need to address. The need for further economic evaluation studies should be stated within the 'Implications for research' part of the 'Authors' conclusions' section of the review. Box 15.8.a shows two examples of this type of statement. It should also be considered that since a full economic evaluation is predicated on the availability of reliable data on intervention effectiveness, a lack of robust effectiveness studies would clearly impact upon the feasibility and availability of full economic evaluation studies. Again, whilst Cochrane and other systematic reviews cannot overcome this limitation, they can draw attention to it within their conclusions sections.

---

**Box 15.8.a    Highlighting a need for further economics studies in conclusions**

"Most of the time, the cost of the intervention is not calculated [in included studies] . This information is crucial. In future studies, cost savings should be calculated and balanced against the potential costs of the intervention... The question of whether cost effective services can be delivered is a critical question for today's healthcare environment. Thus studies that measure the costs as well as the effects of pharmacist interventions are needed." (Beney 2000).

---

## 15.9    Conclusions

This chapter has outlined a methodological framework for incorporating evidence from health economics studies into the Cochrane review process. Whilst this exercise is extremely unlikely, and is not recommended, to produce statements about whether "intervention X is cost-effective", it can help decision makers to understand the structure of the resource allocation problem they are addressing, the main parameters that need to be considered, variation between settings in terms of resource use, costs and cost-effectiveness, and potential reasons for these variations (Drummond 2002). Incorporating economics evidence can also enhance the usefulness and applicability of Cochrane reviews as a source of data for subsequent (or parallel) full economic evaluations. It is anticipated that this guidance will continue to be refined and updated as a result of being subjected to further criticism from a wider audience, and as the methods continue to develop based on experience of their use in Cochrane reviews and further methodological research.

The process of developing this guidance has also helped to clarify key priorities for further research aiming to develop and test alternative methods for the identification, appraisal, analysis and presentation of evidence on economic aspects of interventions. Key research priorities include: further development of a balance-sheet approach to summarizing the results of economics components of reviews, evaluation of the impact on the results of economic reviews of applying different methodological quality criteria or thresholds for inclusion of economic evaluation studies, and evaluation of methods which utilize individual-level data to investigate and deal with heterogeneity between settings in resource use, costs and utilities (and other measures of preferences for health states). These and other methods research priorities are listed on the 'Research' pages of the CCEMG web site (see Box 15.10.a).

---

**Box 15.10.a  The Campbell and Cochrane Economics Methods Group**

The Campbell and Cochrane Economics Methods Group (CCEMG) was formally registered as a Cochrane Collaboration methods group in 1998 and has been jointly registered as a Campbell Collaboration methods group since 2004. Core aims of the group include, within available resources, include the following:

- to promote and support consideration of economics issues within systematic reviews;
- to develop economics methods for Cochrane reviews that are relevant to the consumers of reviews and appropriate, unbiased and objective in terms of their application; and
- to link review authors and editors with economists who can help with reviews or provide specialist advice and peer review.

Many Cochrane reviews already include coverage of economics aspects of interventions. However, this chapter is the first time that the *Handbook* has included detailed guidance on the use of economics methods in Cochrane reviews. Future versions of the chapter will be informed by an ongoing programme of methodological research and further experience of Cochrane reviews incorporating economics evidence.

*E-mail*: research@c-cemg.org

*Web site*: www.c-cemg.org

## 15.10   Chapter information

**Authors:** Ian Shemilt, Miranda Mugford, Sarah Byford, Michael Drummond, Eric Eisenstein, Martin Knapp, Jacqueline Mallender, David McDaid, Luke Vale and Damian Walker on behalf of the Campbell and Cochrane Economics Methods Group.

**This chapter should be cited as:** Shemilt I, Mugford M, Byford S, Drummond M, Eisenstein E, Knapp M, Mallender J, McDaid D, Vale L, Walker D. Chapter 15: Incorporating economics evidence. In: Higgins JPT, Green S (editors), *Cochrane Handbook for Systematic Reviews of Interventions*. Chichester (UK): John Wiley & Sons, 2008.

**Acknowledgements:** Dawn Craig, Julian Higgins, Kevin Marsh and John Nixon commented on drafts.

## 15.11   References

**Aguiar-Ibanez 2005**
Aguiar-Ibanez R, Nixon J, Glanville J, Craig D, Rice S, Christie J, Drummond MF. Economic evaluation databases as an aid to healthcare decision-makers and researchers. *Expert Review of Pharmacoeconomics and Outcomes Research* 2005; 5: 721–722.

**Azimi 1998**
Azimi NA, Welch HG. The effectiveness of cost-effectiveness analysis in containing costs. *Journal of General Internal Medicine* 1998; 13: 664–669.

**Bell 2006**
Bell CM, Urbach DR, Ray JG, Bayoumi A, Rosen AB, Greenberg D, Neumann PJ. Bias in published cost effectiveness studies: systematic review. *BMJ* 2006; 332: 699–703.

**Beney 2000**
Beney J, Bero LA, Bond C. Expanding the roles of outpatient pharmacists: effects on health services utilisation, costs, and patient outcomes. *Cochrane Database of Systematic Reviews* 2000, Issue 3. Art No: CD000336.

**Best 2000**
Best L, Simmonds P, Baughan C, Buchanan R, Davis C, Fentiman I, George S, Gosney M, Northover J, Williams C, Colorectal Meta-analysis Collaboration. Palliative chemotherapy for advanced or metastatic colorectal cancer. *Cochrane Database of Systematic Reviews* 2000, Issue 2. Art No: CD001545.

**Birks 2006**
Birks J, Harvey RJ. Donepezil for dementia due to Alzheimer's disease. *Cochrane Database of Systematic Reviews* 2006, Issue 1. Art No: CD001190.

**Briggs 2006**
Briggs A, Sculpher M, Claxton K. *Decision Modelling for Health Economic Evaluation*. Oxford (UK): Oxford University Press, 2006.

**Brown 2007**
Brown SR, Nelson RL. Surgery for faecal incontinence in adults. *Cochrane Database of Systematic Reviews* 2007, Issue 2. Art No: CD001757.

**Campbell 2007**
Campbell H, Briggs A, Buxton M, Kim L, Thompson S. The credibility of health economic models for health policy decision-making: the case of population screening for

abdominal aortic aneurysm. *Journal of Health Services Research and Policy* 2007; 12: 11–17.

**Cochrane 1972**

Cochrane AL. *Effectiveness and Efficiency: Random Reflections on Health Services*. London (UK): Nuffield Provincial Hospitals Trust, 1972.

**Cooper 2005**

Cooper N, Coyle D, Abrams K, Mugford M, Sutton A. Use of evidence in decision models: an appraisal of health technology assessments in the UK since 1997. *Journal of Health Services Research and Policy* 2005; 10: 245–250.

**Craig 2007**

Craig D, Rice S. *CRD Report 6: NHS Economic Evaluation Database Handbook* (3rd edition). York (UK): Centre for Reviews and Dissemination, University of York, 2007.

**Donaldson 2002**

Donaldson C, Mugford M, Vale L. From effectiveness to efficiency: an introduction to evidence-based health economics. In: Donaldson C, Mugford M, Vale L (editors). *Evidence-based Health Economics: From Effectiveness to Efficiency in Systematic Reviews*. London (UK): BMJ Books, 2002.

**Drummond 1992**

Drummond MF. Economic evaluation of pharmaceuticals: science or marketing? *Pharmacoeconomics* 1992; 1: 8–13.

**Drummond 1996**

Drummond MF, Jefferson TO. Guidelines for authors and peer reviewers of economic submissions to the BMJ. The BMJ Economic Evaluation Working Party. *BMJ* 1996; 313: 275–283.

**Drummond 2001**

Drummond M, Pang F. Transferability of economic evaluation results. In: Drummond M, McGuire A (editors). *Economic Evaluation in Health Care: Merging Theory with Practice*. New York (NY): Oxford University Press, 2001.

**Drummond 2002**

Drummond M. Evidence-based medicine meets economic evaluation – an agenda for research. In: Donaldson C, Mugford M, Vale L (editors). *Evidence-based Health Economics: From Effectiveness to Efficiency in Systematic Reviews*. London (UK): BMJ Books, 2002.

**Drummond 2005**

Drummond MF, Sculpher MJ, Torrance GW, O'Brien BJ, Stoddart GL. *Methods for the Economic Evaluation of Health Care Programmes* (3rd edition). Oxford (UK): Oxford University Press, 2005.

**Evers 2005**

Evers S, Goossens M, de Vet H, van Tulder M, Ament A. Criteria list for assessment of methodological quality of economic evaluations: Consensus on Health Economic Criteria. *International Journal of Technology Assessment in Health Care* 2005; 21: 240–245.

**Fayter 2007**

Fayter D, Nixon J, Hartley S, Rithalia A, Butler G, Rudolf M, Glasziou P, Bland M, Stirk L, Westwood M. A systematic review of the routine monitoring of growth in children of primary school age to identify growth-related conditions. *Health Technology Assessment* 2007; 11: 22.

**Freemantle 1997**

Freemantle N, Mason J. Publication bias in clinical trials and economic analyses. *Pharmacoeconomics* 1997; 12: 10–16.

**Friedberg 1999**

Friedberg M, Saffran B, Stinson TJ, Nelson W, Bennett CL. Evaluation of conflict of interest in economic analyses of new drugs used in oncology. *JAMA* 1999; 282: 1453–1457.

**Gamble 2006**

Gamble CL, Williamson PR, Marson AG. Lamotrigine versus carbamazepine monotherapy for epilepsy. *Cochrane Database of Systematic Reviews* 2006, Issue 1. Art No: CD001031.

**Gilbody 1999**

Gilbody SM, Petticrew M. Rational decision-making in mental health: the role of systematic reviews. *Journal of Mental Health Policy and Economics* 1999; 2: 99–106.

**Hutubessy 2003**

Hutubessy R, Chisholm D, Edejer TT. Generalized cost-effectiveness analysis for national-level priority-setting in the health sector. *Cost Effectiveness and Resource Allocation* 2003; 1: 8.

**Kumaranayake 2002**

Kumaranayake L, Walker D. Cost-effectiveness analysis and priority setting: Global approach without local meaning? In: Lee K, Buse K, Fustukian S (editors). *Health Policy in a Globalising World*. Cambridge (UK): Cambridge University Press, 2002.

**Lavis 2005**

Lavis J, Davies H, Oxman A, Denis JL, Golden-Biddle K, Ferlie E. Towards systematic reviews that inform health care management and policy-making. *Journal of Health Services Research and Policy* 2005; 10 Suppl 1: 35–48.

**Lexchin 2003**

Lexchin J, Bero LA, Djulbegovic B, Clark O. Pharmaceutical industry sponsorship and research outcome and quality: systematic review. *BMJ* 2003; 326: 1167–1170.

**Maynard 2000**

Maynard A, Kanavos P. Health economics: an evolving paradigm. *Health Economics* 2000; 9: 183–190.

**Miners 2005**

Miners AH, Garau M, Fidan D, Fischer AJ. Comparing estimates of cost effectiveness submitted to the National Institute for Clinical Excellence (NICE) by different organisations: retrospective study. *BMJ* 2005; 330: 65.

**Napper 2005**

Napper M, Varney J. Etext on Health Technology Assessment (HTA) Information Resources. Chapter 11: Health Economics Information. Available from: http://www.nlm.nih.gov/archive//2060905/nichsr/ehta/chapter11.html (accessed 1 January 2008).

**Neumann 2005**

Neumann PJ, Greenberg D, Olchanski NV, Stone PW, Rosen AB. Growth and quality of the cost-utility literature, 1976–2001. *Value in Health* 2005; 8: 3–9.

**Philips 2004**

Philips Z, Ginnelly L, Sculpher M, Claxton K, Golder S, Riemsma R, Woolacoot N, Glanville J. Review of guidelines for good practice in decision-analytic modelling in health technology assessment. *Health Technology Assessment* 2004; 8: 36.

**Rennie 2000**

Rennie D, Luft HS. Pharmacoeconomic analyses: making them transparent, making them credible. *JAMA* 2000; 283: 2158–2160.

**Rodgers 2006**

Rodgers M, Nixon J, Hempel S, Aho T, Kelly J, Neal D, Duffy S, Ritchie G, Kleijnen J, Westwood M. Diagnostic tests and algorithms used in the investigation of haematuria: systematic reviews and economic evaluation. *Health Technology Assessment* 2006; 10: 18.

**Samuelson 2005**

Samuelson PA, Nordhaus WD. *Economics*. London (UK): McGraw-Hill, 2005.

**Sculpher 2004**
Sculpher MJ, Pang FS, Manca A, Drummond MF, Golder S, Urdahl H, Davies LM, Eastwood A. Generalisability in economic evaluation studies in healthcare: a review and case studies. *Health Technology Assessment* 2004; 8: 49.

**Shemilt 2007**
Shemilt I, Mugford M, Byford S, Drummond M, Eisenstein E, Knapp M, Mallender J, McDaid D, Vale L, Walker D. Where does economics fit in? A review of economics in Cochrane Reviews. *15th Cochrane Colloquium*, Sau Paulo (Brazil), 2007.

**Song 2000**
Song F, Eastwood AJ, Gilbody S, Duley L, Sutton AJ. Publication and related biases. *Health Technology Assessment* 2000; 4: 10.

**Weinstein 2003**
Weinstein MC, O'Brien B, Hornberger J, Jackson J, Johannesson M, McCabe C, Luce BR. Principles of good practice for decision analytic modeling in health-care evaluation: report of the ISPOR Task Force on Good Research Practices – Modeling studies. *Value in Health* 2003; 6: 9–17.

**Williams 1987**
Williams A. Health economics: The cheerful face of the dismal science? In: Williams A (editor). *Health and Economics*. London (UK): Macmillan, 1987.

**Zarnke 1997**
Zarnke KB, Levine MA, O'Brien BJ. Cost-benefit analyses in the health-care literature: don't judge a study by its label. *Journal of Clinical Epidemiology* 1997; 50: 813–822.

# 16 Special topics in statistics

Edited by **Julian PT Higgins, Jonathan J Deeks and Douglas G Altman** on behalf of the Cochrane Statistical Methods Group

## Key Points

- When missing data prevent a study from being included in a meta-analysis (and attempts to obtain the data from the original investigators have been unsuccessful), any strategies for imputing them should be described and assessed in sensitivity analyses.

- Non-standard designs, such as cluster-randomized trials and cross-over trials, should be analysed using methods appropriate to the design. Even if study authors fail to account for correlations among outcome data, approximate methods can often be applied by review authors.

- To include a study with more than two intervention groups in a meta-analysis, the recommended approach is usually to combine relevant groups to create a single pair-wise comparison.

- Indirect comparisons of interventions may be misleading, but methods are available that exploit randomization, including extensions into 'multiple-treatments meta-analysis'.

- To reduce misleading conclusions resulting from multiple statistical analyses, review authors should state in the protocol which analyses they will perform, keep the number of these to a minimum, and interpret statistically significant findings in the context of how many analyses were undertaken.

- Bayesian approaches and hierarchical (or multilevel) models allow more complex meta-analyses to be performed, and can offer some technical and interpretative advantages over the standard methods implemented in RevMan.

- Studies with no events contribute no information about the risk ratio or odds ratio. For rare events, the Peto method has been observed to be less biased and more powerful than other methods.

# 16.1   Missing data

## 16.1.1   Types of missing data

There are many potential sources of missing data in a systematic review or meta-analysis (see Table 16.1.a). For example, a whole study may be missing from the review, an outcome may be missing from a study, summary data may be missing for an outcome, and individual participants may be missing from the summary data. Here we discuss a variety of potential sources of missing data, highlighting where more detailed discussions are available elsewhere in the *Handbook*.

Whole **studies** may be missing from a review because they are never published, are published in obscure places, are rarely cited, or are inappropriately indexed in databases. Thus review authors should always be aware of the possibility that they have failed to identify relevant studies. There is a strong possibility that such studies are missing because of their 'uninteresting' or 'unwelcome' findings (that is, in the presence of publication bias). This problem is discussed at length in Chapter 10. Details of comprehensive search methods are provided in Chapter 6.

Some studies might not report any information on **outcomes** of interest to the review. For example, there may be no information on quality of life, or on serious adverse effects. It is often difficult to determine whether this is because the outcome was not measured or because the outcome was not reported. Furthermore, failure to report that outcomes

**Table 16.1.a**   Types of missing data in a meta-analysis

| Type of missing data | Some possible reasons for missing data |
| --- | --- |
| Missing studies. | Publication bias;<br>Search not sufficiently comprehensive. |
| Missing outcomes. | Outcome not measured;<br>Selective reporting bias. |
| Missing summary data. | Selective reporting bias;<br>Incomplete reporting. |
| Missing individuals. | Lack of intention-to-treat analysis;<br>Attrition from the study;<br>Selective reporting bias. |
| Missing study-level characteristics (for subgroup analysis or meta-regression). | Characteristic not measured;<br>Incomplete reporting. |

were measured may be dependent on the unreported results (selective outcome reporting bias; see Chapter 8, Section 8.13). Similarly, **summary data** for an outcome, in a form that can be included in a meta-analysis, may be missing. A common example is missing standard deviations for continuous outcomes. This is often a problem when change-from-baseline outcomes are sought. We discuss imputation of missing standard deviations in Section 16.1.3. Other examples of missing summary data are missing sample sizes (particularly those for each intervention group separately), numbers of events, standard errors, follow-up times for calculating rates, and sufficient details of time-to-event outcomes. Inappropriate analyses of studies, for example of cluster-randomized and cross-over trials, can lead to missing summary data. It is sometimes possible to approximate the correct analyses of such studies, for example by imputing correlation coefficients or standard deviations, as discussed in Section 16.3 for cluster-randomized studies and Section 16.4 for cross-over trials. As a general rule, most methodologists believe that missing summary data (e.g. "no usable data") should not be used as a reason to exclude a study from a systematic review. It is more appropriate to include the study in the review, and to discuss the potential implications of its absence from a meta-analysis.

It is likely that in some, if not all, included studies, there will be **individuals** missing from the reported results. Analyses of randomized trials that do not include all randomized participants are not intention-to-treat (ITT) analyses. It is sometimes possible to perform ITT analyses, even if the original investigators did not. We provide a detailed discussion of ITT issues in Section 16.2.

Missing data can also affect subgroup analyses. If subgroup analyses or meta-regressions are planned (see Chapter 9, Section 9.6), they require details of the **study-level characteristics** that distinguish studies from one another. If these are not available for all studies, review authors should consider asking the study authors for more information.

## 16.1.2    General principles for dealing with missing data

There is a large literature of statistical methods for dealing with missing data. Here we briefly review some key concepts and make some general recommendations for Cochrane review authors. It is important to think *why* data may be missing. Statisticians often use the terms 'missing at random' and 'not missing at random' to represent different scenarios.

Data are said to be 'missing at random' if the fact that they are missing is unrelated to actual values of the missing data. For instance, if some quality-of-life questionnaires were lost in the postal system, this would be unlikely to be related to the quality of life of the trial participants who completed the forms. In some circumstances, statisticians distinguish between data 'missing at random' and data 'missing completely at random', although in the context of a systematic review the distinction is unlikely to be important. Data that are missing at random may not be important. Analyses based on the available data will tend to be unbiased, although based on a smaller sample size than the original data set.

Data are said to be 'not missing at random' if the fact that they are missing is related to the actual missing data. For instance, in a depression trial, participants who had a relapse of depression might be less likely to attend the final follow-up interview, and more likely to have missing outcome data. Such data are 'non-ignorable' in the sense that an analysis of the available data alone will typically be biased. Publication bias and selective reporting bias lead by definition to data that are 'not missing at random', and attrition and exclusions of individuals within studies often do as well.

The principal options for dealing with missing data are:

1. analysing only the available data (i.e. ignoring the missing data);

2. imputing the missing data with replacement values, and treating these as if they were observed (e.g. last observation carried forward, imputing an assumed outcome such as assuming all were poor outcomes, imputing the mean, imputing based on predicted values from a regression analysis);

3. imputing the missing data and accounting for the fact that these were imputed with uncertainty (e.g. multiple imputation, simple imputation methods (as point 2) with adjustment to the standard error); and

4. using statistical models to allow for missing data, making assumptions about their relationships with the available data.

Option 1 may be appropriate when data can be assumed to be missing at random. Options 2 to 4 are attempts to address data not missing at random. Option 2 is practical in most circumstances and very commonly used in systematic reviews. However, it fails to acknowledge uncertainty in the imputed values and results, typically, in confidence intervals that are too narrow. Options 3 and 4 would require involvement of a knowledgeable statistician.

Four general recommendations for dealing with missing data in Cochrane reviews are as follows:

• Whenever possible, contact the original investigators to request missing data.

• Make explicit the assumptions of any methods used to cope with missing data: for example, that the data are assumed missing at random, or that missing values were assumed to have a particular value such as a poor outcome.

• Perform sensitivity analyses to assess how sensitive results are to reasonable changes in the assumptions that are made (see Chapter 9, Section 9.7).

• Address the potential impact of missing data on the findings of the review in the Discussion section.

### 16.1.3   Missing standard deviations

#### 16.1.3.1   Imputing standard deviations

Missing standard deviations are a common feature of meta-analyses of continuous out-come data. One approach to this problem is to impute standard deviations. Before imputing missing standard deviations however, authors should look carefully for statistics that allow calculation or estimation of the standard deviation (e.g. confidence intervals, standard errors, t values, P values, F values), as discussed in Chapter 7 (Section 7.7.3).

The simplest imputation is of a particular value borrowed from one or more other studies. Furukawa et al. found that imputing standard deviations either from other studies in the same meta-analysis, or from studies in another meta-analysis, yielded approximately correct results in two case studies (Furukawa 2006). If several candidate standard deviations are available, review authors would have to decide whether to use their average, the highest, a 'reasonably high' value, or some other strategy. For meta-analyses of mean differences, choosing a higher standard deviation down-weights a study and yields a wider confidence interval. However, for standardized mean difference meta-analyses, choice of an overly large standard deviation will bias the result towards a lack of effect. More complicated alternatives are available for making use of multiple candidate standard deviations. For example, Marinho et al. implemented a linear regression of log(standard deviation) on log(mean), because of a strong linear relationship between the two (Marinho 2003).

All imputation techniques involve making assumptions about unknown statistics, and it is best to avoid using them wherever possible. If the majority of studies in a meta-analysis have missing standard deviations, these values should not be imputed. However, imputation may be reasonable for a small proportion of studies comprising a small proportion of the data if it enables them to be combined with other studies for which full data are available. Sensitivity analyses should be used to assess the impact of changing the assumptions made.

#### 16.1.3.2   Imputing standard deviations for changes from baseline

A special case of missing standard deviations is for changes from baseline. Often, only the following information is available:

|  | Baseline | Final | Change |
| --- | --- | --- | --- |
| Experimental intervention (sample size) | mean, SD | mean, SD | mean |
| Control intervention (sample size) | mean, SD | mean, SD | mean |

Note that the mean change in each group can always be obtained by subtracting the final mean from the baseline mean even if it is not presented explicitly. However, the information in this table does *not* allow us to calculate the standard deviation of the changes. We cannot know whether the changes were very consistent or very variable. Some other information in a paper may help us determine the standard deviation of the changes. If statistical analyses comparing the changes themselves are presented (e.g. confidence intervals, standard errors, t values, P values, F values) then the techniques described in Chapter 7 (Section 7.7.3) may be used.

When there is not enough information available to calculate the standard deviations for the changes, they can be imputed. When change-from-baseline standard deviations for the same outcome measure are available from other studies in the review, it may be reasonable to use these in place of the missing standard deviations. However, the appropriateness of using a standard deviation from another study relies on whether the studies used the same measurement scale, had the same degree of measurement error and had the same time periods (between baseline and final value measurement).

The following alternative technique may be used for imputing missing standard deviations for changes from baseline (Follmann 1992, Abrams 2005). A typically unreported number known as the correlation coefficient describes how similar the baseline and final measurements were across participants. Here we describe (1) how to calculate the correlation coefficient from a study that is reported in considerable detail and (2) how to impute a change-from-baseline standard deviation in another study, making use of an imputed correlation coefficient. Note that the methods in (2) are applicable both to correlation coefficients obtained using (1) and to correlation coefficients obtained in other ways (for example, by reasoned argument). These methods should be used sparingly, because one can never be sure that an imputed correlation is appropriate (correlations between baseline and final values will, for example, decrease with increasing time between baseline and final measurements, as well as depending on the outcomes and characteristics of the participants). An alternative to these methods is simply to use a comparison of final measurements, which in a randomized trial in theory estimates the same quantity as the comparison of changes from baseline.

### Calculating a correlation coefficient from a study reported in considerable detail

Suppose a study is available that presents means and standard deviations for change as well as for baseline and final measurements, for example:

|  | Baseline | Final | Change |
| --- | --- | --- | --- |
| Experimental intervention (sample size 129) | mean=15.2 SD=6.4 | mean=16.2 SD=7.1 | mean=1.0 SD=4.5 |
| Control intervention (sample size 135) | mean=15.7 SD=7.0 | mean=17.2 SD=6.9 | mean=1.5 SD=4.2 |

An analysis of change from baseline is available from this study, using only the data in the final column. However, we can use the other data from the study to calculate two correlation coefficients, one for each intervention group. Let us use the following notation:

|  | Baseline | Final | Change |
|---|---|---|---|
| Experimental intervention (sample size $N_E$) | $M_{E,baseline}$, $SD_{E,baseline}$ | $M_{E,final}$, $SD_{E,final}$ | $M_{E,change}$, $SD_{E,change}$ |
| Control intervention (sample size $N_C$) | $M_{C,baseline}$, $SD_{C,baseline}$ | $M_{C,final}$, $SD_{C,final}$ | $M_{C,change}$, $SD_{C,change}$ |

The correlation coefficient in the experimental group, $Corr_E$, can be calculated as:

$$Corr_E = \frac{SD_{E,baseline}^2 + SD_{E,final}^2 - SD_{E,change}^2}{2 \times SD_{E,baseline} \times SD_{E,final}};$$

and similarly for the control intervention, to obtain $Corr_C$. In the example, these turn out to be

$$Corr_E = \frac{6.4^2 + 7.1^2 - 4.5^2}{2 \times 6.4 \times 7.1} = 0.78,$$

$$Corr_C = \frac{7.0^2 + 6.9^2 - 4.2^2}{2 \times 7.0 \times 6.9} = 0.82.$$

Where either the baseline or final standard deviation is unavailable, then it may be substituted by the other, providing it is reasonable to assume that the intervention does not alter the variability of the outcome measure. Correlation coefficients lie between $-1$ and $1$. If a value less than 0.5 is obtained, then there is no value in using change from baseline and an analysis of final values will be more precise. Assuming the correlation coefficients from the two intervention groups are similar, a simple average will provide a reasonable measure of the similarity of baseline and final measurements across all individuals in the study (the average of 0.78 and 0.82 for the example is 0.80). If the correlation coefficients differ, then either the sample sizes are too small for reliable estimation, the intervention is affecting the variability in outcome measures, or the intervention effect depends on baseline level, and the use of imputation is best avoided. Before imputation is undertaken it is recommended that correlation coefficients are computed for many (if not all) studies in the meta-analysis and it is noted whether or not they are consistent. Imputation should be done only as a very tentative analysis if correlations are inconsistent.

*Imputing a change-from-baseline standard deviation using a correlation coefficient*    Now consider a study for which the standard deviation of changes from baseline is missing. When baseline and final standard deviations are known, we can impute the missing standard deviation using an imputed value, Corr, for the correlation coefficient. The value Corr might be imputed from another study in the meta-analysis (using the method in (1) above), it might be imputed from elsewhere, or it might be hypothesized based on reasoned argument. In all of these situations, a sensitivity analysis should be undertaken, trying different values of Corr, to determine whether the overall result of the analysis is robust to the use of imputed correlation coefficients.

To impute a standard deviation of the change from baseline for the experimental intervention, use

$$SD_{E,change} = \sqrt{SD_{E,baseline}^2 + SD_{E,final}^2 - (2 \times Corr \times SD_{E,baseline} \times SD_{E,final})},$$

and similarly for the control intervention. Again, if either of the standard deviations (at baseline and final) are unavailable, then one may be substituted by the other if it is reasonable to assume that the intervention does not alter the variability of the outcome measure.

As an example, given the following data:

|  | Baseline | Final | Change |
|---|---|---|---|
| Experimental intervention (sample size 35) | mean=12.4 SD=4.2 | mean=15.2 SD=3.8 | mean=2.8 |
| Control intervention (sample size 38) | mean=10.7 SD=4.0 | mean=13.8 SD=4.4 | mean=3.1 |

and using an imputed correlation coefficient of 0.80, we can impute the change-from-baseline standard deviation in the control group as:

$$SD_{C,change} = \sqrt{4.0^2 + 4.4^2 - (2 \times 0.80 \times 4.0 \times 4.4)} = 2.68.$$

## 16.2    Intention-to-treat issues

### 16.2.1    Introduction

Often some participants are excluded from analyses of randomized trials, either because they were lost to follow-up and no outcome was obtained, or because there was some deviation from the protocol, such as receiving the wrong (or no) treatment, lack of compliance, or ineligibility. Alternatively, it may be impossible to measure certain outcomes for all participants because their availability depends on another outcome (see Section 16.2.4). As discussed in detail in Chapter 8 (Section 8.12), an estimated intervention effect may be biased if some randomized participants are excluded from the analysis. Intention-to-treat (ITT) analysis aims to include all participants randomized into a trial irrespective of what happened subsequently (Newell 1992, Lewis 1993). ITT analyses are generally preferred as they are unbiased, and also because they address a more pragmatic and clinically relevant question.

The following principles of ITT analyses are described in Chapter 8 (Section 8.12).

1. Keep participants in the intervention groups to which they were randomized, regardless of the intervention they actually received.

2. Measure outcome data on all participants.

3. Include all randomized participants in the analysis.

There is no clear consensus on whether all criteria should be applied (Hollis 1999). While the first is widely agreed, the second is often impossible and the third is contentious, since to include participants whose outcomes are unknown (mainly through loss to follow-up) involves imputing ('filling-in') the missing data (see Section 16.1.2).

An analysis in which data are analysed for every participant for whom the outcome was obtained is often described as an **available case analysis**. Some trial reports present analyses of the results of only those participants who completed the trial *and* who complied with (or received some of) their allocated intervention. Some authors incorrectly call this an ITT analysis, but it is in fact a **per-protocol analysis**. Furthermore, some authors analyse participants only according to the actual interventions received, irrespective of the randomized allocations (**treatment-received analysis**). It is generally unwise to accept study authors' description of an analysis as ITT; such a judgement should be based on the detailed information provided.

Many (but not all) people consider that available case and ITT analyses are not appropriate when assessing unintended (adverse) effects, as it is wrong to attribute these to a treatment that somebody did not receive. As ITT analyses tend to bias the results towards no difference they may not be the most appropriate when attempting to establish equivalence or non-inferiority of a treatment.

In most situations, authors should attempt to extract from papers the data to enable at least an **available case analysis**. Avoidable exclusions should be 're-included' if possible. In some rare situations it is possible to create a genuine ITT analysis from information presented in the text and tables of the paper, or by obtaining extra information from the author about participants who were followed up but excluded from the trial report. If this is possible without imputing study results, it should be done.

Otherwise, it may appear that an intention-to-treat analysis can be produced by using imputation. This involves making assumptions about the outcomes of participants for whom no outcome was recorded. However, many imputation analyses differ from available case analyses only in having an unwarranted inflation in apparent precision.

Assessing the results of studies in the presence of more than minimal amounts of missing data is ultimately a matter of judgement, as discussed in Chapter 8 (Section 8.12). Statistical analysis cannot reliably compensate for missing data (Unnebrink 2001). No assumption is likely adequately to reflect the truth, and the impact of any assumption should be assessed by trying more than one method as a sensitivity analysis (see Chapter 9, Section 9.7).

In the next two sections we consider some ways to take account of missing observations for dichotomous or continuous outcomes. Although imputation is possible, at present a sensible decision in most cases is to include data for only those participants whose results are known, and address the potential impact of the missing data in the assessment of risk of bias (Chapter 8, Section 8.12). Where imputation is used the methods and assumptions for imputing data for drop-outs should be described in the Methods section of the protocol and review.

If individual participant data are available, then detailed sensitivity analyses can be considered. Review authors in this position are referred to the extensive literature on dealing with missing data in clinical trials (Little 2004). Participants excluded from analyses in published reports should typically be re-included when possible, as is the case when individual participant data are available (Stewart 1995). Information should be requested from the trial authors when sufficient details are not available in published reports to re-include exclude participants in analyses.

## 16.2.2   Intention-to-treat issues for dichotomous data

Proportions of participants for whom no outcome data were obtained should always be collected and reported in a 'Risk of bias' table; note that the proportions may vary by outcome and by randomized group. However, there is no consensus on the best way to handle these participants in an analysis. There are two basic options, and a plausible option should be used both as a main analysis and as a basis for sensitivity analysis (see below and Chapter 9, Section 9.7).

- Available case analysis: Include data on only those whose results are known, using as a denominator the total number of people who had data recorded for the particular outcome in question. Variation in the degree of missing data across studies may be considered as a potential source of heterogeneity.

- ITT analysis using imputation: Base an analysis on the total number of randomized participants, irrespective of how the original study authors analysed the data. This will involve imputing outcomes for the missing participants. There are several approaches to imputing dichotomous outcome data. One common approach is to assume either that all missing participants experienced the event, or that all missing participants did not experience the event. An alternative approach is to impute data according to the event rate observed in the control group, or according to event rates among completers in the separate groups (the latter provides the same estimate of intervention effect but results in unwarranted inflation of the precision of effect estimates).

The choice among these assumptions should be based on clinical judgement. Studies with imputed data may be given more weight than they warrant if entered as dichotomous data into RevMan. It is possible to determine more appropriate weights (Higgins 2008); consultation with a statistician is recommended. However, none of these assumptions is likely to reflect the truth, except for imputing 'failures' in some settings such as smoking cessation trials, so an imputation approach is generally not recommended.

The potential impact of the missing data on the results should be considered in the interpretation of the results of the review. This will depend on the degree of 'missingness', the frequency of the events and the size of the pooled effect estimate. Gamble and Hollis suggest a sensitivity analysis for dichotomous outcomes based on consideration of 'best-case' and 'worst-case' scenarios (Gamble 2005). The 'best-case' scenario is that all participants with missing outcomes in the experimental intervention group had good outcomes, and all those with missing outcomes in the control intervention group had poor outcomes; the 'worst-case' scenario is the converse. The sensitivity analysis down-weights studies in which the discrepancy between 'best-case' and 'worst-case' scenarios is high, although the down-weighting may be too extreme.

A more plausible sensitivity analysis explicitly considers what the event rates might have been in the missing data. For example, suppose an available case analysis has been used, and a particular study has 20% risk in the intervention arm and 15% risk in the control arm. An available case analysis implicitly assumes that the same fractions apply in the missing data, so three suitable sensitivity analyses to compare with this analysis might consider the risk in the missing data to be 15% in both arms, or 15% and 10% in the experimental and control arms respectively, or 20% and 10% respectively. Alternatively, suppose that in the main analysis, all missing values have been imputed as events. A sensitivity analysis to compare with this analysis could consider the case that, say, 10% of missing participants experienced the event, or 10% in the intervention arm and 5% in the control arm. Graphical approaches to sensitivity analysis have been considered (Hollis 2002).

Higgins et al. suggest an alternative approach that can incorporate specific reasons for missing data, which considers plausible event risks among missing participants in relation to risks among those observed (Higgins 2008). Bayesian approaches, which automatically down-weight studies with more missing data, are considered by White et al. (White 2008a, White 2008b).

## 16.2.3 Intention-to-treat issues for continuous data

In full ITT analyses, all participants who did not receive the assigned intervention according to the protocol as well as those who were lost to follow-up are included in the analysis. Inclusion of these in an analysis requires that means and standard deviations of the outcome for all randomized participants are available. As for dichotomous data, dropout rates should always be collected and reported in a 'Risk of bias' table. Again, there are two basic options, and in either case a sensitivity analysis should be performed (see Chapter 9, Section 9.7).

- Available case analysis: Include data only on those whose results are known. The potential impact of the missing data on the results should be considered in the interpretation of the results of the review. This will depend on the degree of 'missingness', the pooled estimate of the treatment effect and the variability of the outcomes. Variation in the degree of missing data may also be considered as a potential source of heterogeneity.

- ITT analysis using imputation: Base an analysis on the total number of randomized participants, irrespective of how the original study authors analysed the data. This will involve imputing outcomes for the missing participants. Approaches to imputing missing continuous data in the context of a meta-analysis have received little attention in the methodological literature. In some situations it may be possible to exploit standard (although often questionable) approaches such as 'last observation carried forward', or, for change from baseline outcomes, to assume that no change took place, but such approaches generally require access to the raw participant data. Inflating the sample size of the available data up to the total numbers of randomized participants is not recommended as it will artificially inflate the precision of the effect estimate.

A simple way to conduct a sensitivity analysis for continuous data is to assume a fixed difference between the actual mean for the missing data and the mean assumed by the analysis. For example, after an analysis of available cases, one could consider how the results would have differed if the missing data in the intervention arm had averaged 2 units *greater* than the observed data in the intervention arm, and the missing data in the control arm had averaged 2 units *less* than the observed data in the control arm. A Bayesian approach, which automatically down-weights studies with more missing data, has been considered (White 2007).

### 16.2.4   Conditional outcomes only available for subsets of participants

Some study outcomes may only be applicable to a proportion of participants. For example, in subfertility trials the proportion of clinical pregnancies that miscarry following treatment is often reported. By definition this outcome excludes participants who do not achieve an interim state (clinical pregnancy), so the comparison is not of all participants randomized. As a general rule it is better to re-define such outcomes so that the analysis includes all randomized participants. In this example, the outcome could be whether the woman has a 'successful pregnancy' (becoming pregnant and reaching, say, 24 weeks or term). Another example is provided by a morbidity outcome measured in the medium or long term (e.g. development of chronic lung disease), when there is a distinct possibility of a death preventing assessment of the morbidity. A convenient way to deal with such situations is to combine the outcomes, for example as 'death or chronic lung disease'.

Some intractable problems arise when a continuous outcome (say a measure of functional ability or quality of life following stroke) is measured only on those who survive to the end of follow-up. Two unsatisfactory alternatives exist: (a) imputing zero functional ability scores for those who die (which may not appropriately represent the death state and will make the outcome severely skewed), and (b) analysing the available data (which must be interpreted as a non-randomized comparison applicable only to survivors). The results of the analysis must be interpreted taking into account any disparity in the proportion of deaths between the two intervention groups.

# 16.3 Cluster-randomized trials

## 16.3.1 Introduction

In **cluster-randomized trials**, groups of individuals rather than individuals are randomized to different interventions. Cluster-randomized trials are also known as group-randomized trials. We say the 'unit of allocation' is the cluster, or the group. The groups may be, for example, schools, villages, medical practices or families. Such trials may be done for one of several reasons. It may be to evaluate the group effect of an intervention, for example herd-immunity of a vaccine. It may be to avoid 'contamination' across interventions when trial participants are managed within the same setting, for example in a trial evaluating a dietary intervention, families rather than individuals may be randomized. A cluster-randomized design may be used simply for convenience.

One of the main consequences of a cluster design is that participants within any one cluster often tend to respond in a similar manner, and thus their data can no longer be assumed to be independent of one another. Many of these studies, however, are incorrectly analysed as though the unit of allocation had been the individual participants. This is often referred to as a 'unit-of-analysis error' (Whiting-O'Keefe 1984) because the unit of analysis is different from the unit of allocation. If the clustering is ignored and cluster trials are analysed as if individuals had been randomized, resulting P values will be artificially small. This can result in false positive conclusions that the intervention had an effect. In the context of a meta-analysis, studies in which clustering has been ignored will have overly narrow confidence intervals and will receive more weight than is appropriate in a meta-analysis. This situation can also arise if participants are allocated to interventions that are then applied to parts of them (for example, to both eyes or to several teeth), or if repeated observations are made on a participant. If the analysis is by the individual units (for example, each tooth or each observation) without taking into account that the data are clustered within participants, then a unit-of-analysis error can occur.

There are several useful sources of information on cluster-randomized trials (Murray 1995, Donner 2000). A detailed discussion of incorporating cluster-randomized trials in a meta-analysis is available (Donner 2002), as is a more technical treatment of the problem (Donner 2001). Special considerations for analysis of standardized mean differences from cluster-randomized trials are discussed by White and Thomas (White 2005).

## 16.3.2    Assessing risk of bias in cluster-randomized trials

In cluster-randomized trials, particular biases to consider include: (i) recruitment bias; (ii) baseline imbalance; (iii) loss of clusters; (iv) incorrect analysis; and (v) comparability with individually randomized trials.

(i) Recruitment bias can occur when individuals are recruited to the trial after the clusters have been randomized, as the knowledge of whether each cluster is an 'intervention' or 'control' cluster could affect the types of participants recruited. Farrin et al. showed differential participant recruitment in a trial of low back pain randomized by primary care practice; a greater number of less severe participants were recruited to the 'active management' practices (Farrin 2005). Puffer et al. reviewed 36 cluster-randomized trials, and found possible recruitment bias in 14 (39%) (Puffer 2003).

(ii) Cluster-randomized trials often randomize all clusters at once, so lack of concealment of an allocation sequence should not usually be an issue. However, because small numbers of clusters are randomized, there is a possibility of chance baseline imbalance between the randomized groups, in terms of either the clusters or the individuals. Although not a form of bias as such, the risk of baseline differences can be reduced by using stratified or pair-matched randomization of clusters. Reporting of the baseline comparability of clusters, or statistical adjustment for baseline characteristics, can help reduce concern about the effects of baseline imbalance.

(iii) Occasionally complete clusters are lost from a trial, and have to be omitted from the analysis. Just as for missing outcome data in individually randomized trials, this may lead to bias. In addition, missing outcomes for individuals within clusters may also lead to a risk of bias in cluster-randomized trials.

(iv) Many cluster-randomized trials are analysed by incorrect statistical methods, not taking the clustering into account. For example, Eldridge et al. reviewed 152 cluster-randomized trials in primary care of which 41% did not account for clustering in their analyses (Eldridge 2004). Such analyses create a 'unit of analysis error' and produce over-precise results (the standard error of the estimated intervention effect is too small) and P values that are too small. They do not lead to biased estimates of effect. However, if they remain uncorrected, they will receive too much weight in a meta-analysis. Approximate methods of correcting trial results that do not allow for clustering are suggested in Section 16.3.6. Some of these can be implemented by review authors.

(v) In a meta-analysis including both cluster and individually randomized trials, or including cluster-randomized trials with different types of clusters, possible differences between the intervention effects being estimated need to be considered. For example, in a vaccine trial of infectious diseases, a vaccine applied to all individuals in a community would be expected to be more effective than if the vaccine was applied to only half of the people. Another example is provided by Hahn et al., who discussed a Cochrane review of hip protectors (Hahn 2005). The cluster trials showed large positive effect whereas individually randomized trials did not show any clear benefit. One possibility is that there was a 'herd effect' in the cluster-randomized trials (which were often performed in nursing homes, where compliance with using the protectors may have been enhanced). In general, such 'contamination' would lead to underestimates of effect. Thus, if an intervention effect is still demonstrated despite contamination in those trials that were not cluster-randomized, a confident conclusion about the presence of an effect can be drawn. However, the size of the effect is likely to be underestimated. Contamination and 'herd effects' may be different for different types of cluster.

## 16.3.3 Methods of analysis for cluster-randomized trials

One way to avoid unit-of-analysis errors in cluster-randomized trials is to conduct the analysis at the same level as the allocation, using a summary measurement from each cluster. Then the sample size is the number of clusters and analysis proceeds as if the trial was individually randomized (though the clusters become the individuals). However, this might considerably, and unnecessarily, reduce the power of the study, depending on the number and size of the clusters.

Alternatively, statistical methods now exist that allow analysis at the level of the individual while accounting for the clustering in the data. The ideal information to extract from a cluster-randomized trial is a direct estimate of the required effect measure (for example, an odds ratio with its confidence interval) from an analysis that properly accounts for the cluster design. Such an analysis might be based on a 'multilevel model', a 'variance components analysis' or may use 'generalized estimating equations (GEEs)', among other techniques. Statistical advice is recommended to determine whether the method used is appropriate. Effect estimates and their standard errors from correct analyses of cluster-randomized trials may be meta-analysed using the generic inverse-variance method in RevMan.

## 16.3.4 Approximate analyses of cluster-randomized trials for a meta-analysis: effective sample sizes

Unfortunately, many cluster-randomized trials have in the past failed to report appropriate analyses. They are commonly analysed as if the randomization was performed on the individuals rather than the clusters. If this is the situation, approximately correct analyses may be performed if the following information can be extracted:

* the number of clusters (or groups) randomized to each intervention group; or the average (mean) size of each cluster;

- the outcome data ignoring the cluster design for the total number of individuals (for example, number or proportion of individuals with events, or means and standard deviations); and

- an estimate of the intracluster (or intraclass) correlation coefficient (ICC).

The ICC is an estimate of the relative variability within and between clusters (Donner 1980). It describes the 'similarity' of individuals within the same cluster. In fact this is seldom available in published reports. A common approach is to use external estimates obtained from similar studies, and several resources are available that provide examples of ICCs (Ukoumunne 1999, Campbell 2000, Health Services Research Unit 2004). ICCs may appear small compared with other types of correlations: values lower than 0.05 are typical. However, even small values can have a substantial impact on confidence interval widths (and hence weights in a meta-analysis), particularly if cluster sizes are large. Empirical research has observed that larger cluster sizes are associated with smaller ICCs (Ukoumunne 1999).

An approximately correct analysis proceeds as follows. The idea is to reduce the size of each trial to its 'effective sample size' (Rao 1992). The effective sample size of a single intervention group in a cluster-randomized trial is its original sample size divided by a quantity called the 'design effect'. The design effect is

$$1 + (M - 1)\,\text{ICC},$$

where M is the average cluster size and ICC is the intracluster correlation coefficient. A common design effect is usually assumed across intervention groups. For dichotomous data both the number of participants and the number experiencing the event should be divided by the same design effect. Since the resulting data must be rounded to whole numbers for entry into RevMan this approach may be unsuitable for small trials. For continuous data only the sample size need be reduced; means and standard deviations should remain unchanged.

## 16.3.5   Example of incorporating a cluster-randomized trial

As an example, consider a cluster-randomized trial that randomized 10 school classrooms with 295 children into an intervention group and 11 classrooms with 330 children into a control group. The numbers of successes among the children, ignoring the clustering, are

Intervention: 63/295

Control: 84/330.

Imagine an intracluster correlation coefficient of 0.02 has been obtained from a reliable external source. The average cluster size in the trial is $(295+330)/(10+11) = 29.8$. The design effect for the trial as a whole is then $1 + (M-1)\,\text{ICC} = 1 + (29.8-1)\times0.02 = 1.576$. The effective sample size in the intervention group is $295 / 1.576 = 187.2$ and for the control group is $330 / 1.576 = 209.4$.

Applying the design effects also to the numbers of events produces the following results:

Intervention: 40.0/187.2

Control: 53.3/209.4.

Once trials have been reduced to their effective sample size, the data may be entered into RevMan as, for example, dichotomous outcomes or continuous outcomes. Results from the example trial may be entered as

Intervention: 40/187

Control: 53/209.

## 16.3.6 Approximate analyses of cluster-randomized trials for a meta-analysis: inflating standard errors

A clear disadvantage of the method described in Section 16.3.4 is the need to round the effective sample sizes to whole numbers. A slightly more flexible approach, which is equivalent to calculating effective sample sizes, is to multiply the standard error of the effect estimate (from an analysis ignoring clustering) by the square root of the design effect. The standard error may be calculated from a confidence interval (see Chapter 7, Section 7.7.7). Standard analyses of dichotomous or continuous outcomes may be used to obtain these confidence intervals using RevMan. The meta-analysis using the inflated variances may be performed using RevMan and the generic inverse-variance method.

As an example, the odds ratio (OR) from a study with the results

Intervention: 63/295

Control: 84/330

is OR $= 0.795$ (95% CI 0.548 to 1.154). Using methods described in Chapter 7 (Section 7.7.7.3), we can determine from these results that the log odds ratio is lnOR $= -0.23$ with standard error 0.19. Using the same design effect of 1.576 as in Section 16.3.5, an inflated standard error that accounts for clustering is given by $0.19 \times \sqrt{1.576} = 0.24$. The log odds ratio $(-0.23)$ and this inflated standard error $(0.24)$ may be entered into RevMan under a generic inverse-variance outcome.

### 16.3.7   Issues in the incorporation of cluster-randomized trials

Cluster-randomized trials may, in principle, be combined with individually randomized trials in the same meta-analysis. Consideration should be given to the possibility of important differences in the effects being evaluated between the different types of trial. There are often good reasons for performing cluster-randomized trials and these should be examined. For example, in the treatment of infectious diseases an intervention applied to all individuals in a community may be more effective than treatment applied to select (randomized) individuals within the community since it may reduce the possibility of re-infection.

Authors should always identify any cluster-randomized trials in a review and explicitly state how they have dealt with the data. They should conduct sensitivity analyses to investigate the robustness of their conclusions, especially when ICCs have been borrowed from external sources (see Chapter 9, Section 9.7). Statistical support is recommended.

### 16.3.8   Individually randomized trials with clustering

Issues related to clustering can also occur in individually randomized trials. This can happen when the same health professional (for example doctor, surgeon, nurse or therapist) delivers the intervention to a number of participants in the intervention group. This type of clustering is discussed by Lee and Thompson, and raises issues similar to those in cluster-randomized trials (Lee 2005a).

## 16.4   Cross-over trials

### 16.4.1   Introduction

Parallel group trials allocate each participant to a single intervention for comparison with one or more alternative interventions. In contrast, **cross-over trials** allocate each participant to a sequence of interventions. A simple randomized cross-over design is an 'AB/BA' design in which participants are randomized initially to intervention A or intervention B, and then 'cross over' to intervention B or intervention A, respectively. It can be seen that data from the first period of a cross-over trial represent a parallel group trial, a feature referred to in Section 16.4.5. In keeping with the rest of the *Handbook*, we will use E and C to refer to interventions, rather than A and B.

Cross-over designs offer a number of possible advantages over parallel group trials. Among these are (i) that each participant acts as his or her own control, eliminating among-participant variation; (ii) that, consequently, fewer participants are required to obtain the same power; and (iii) that every participant receives every intervention, which allows the determination of the best intervention or preference for an individual participant. A readable introduction to cross-over trials is given by Senn (Senn 2002).

More detailed discussion of meta-analyses involving cross-over trials is provided by Elbourne et al. (Elbourne 2002), and some empirical evidence on their inclusion in systematic reviews by Lathyris et al. (Lathyris 2007).

## 16.4.2 Assessing suitability of cross-over trials

Cross-over trials are suitable for evaluating interventions with a temporary effect in the treatment of stable, chronic conditions. They are employed, for example, in the study of interventions to relieve asthma and epilepsy. They are not appropriate when an intervention can have a lasting effect that compromises entry to subsequent periods of the trial, or when a disease has a rapid evolution. The advantages of cross-over trials must be weighed against their disadvantages. The principal problem associated with cross-over trials is that of carry-over (a type of period-by-intervention interaction). Carry-over is the situation in which the effects of an intervention given in one period persist into a subsequent period, thus interfering with the effects of a different subsequent intervention. Many cross-over trials include a period between interventions known as a washout period as a means of reducing carry-over. If a primary outcome is irreversible (for example mortality, or pregnancy in a subfertility study) then a cross-over study is generally considered to be inappropriate. Another problem with cross-over trials is the risk of drop-out due to their longer duration compared with comparable parallel group trials. The analysis techniques for cross-over trials with missing observations are limited. The assessment of the risk of bias in cross-over trials is discussed in Section 16.4.3.

In considering the inclusion of cross-over trials in meta-analysis, authors should first address the question of whether a cross-over trial is a suitable method for the condition and intervention in question. For example, although they are frequently employed in the field, one group of authors decided cross-over trials were inappropriate for studies in Alzheimer's disease due to the degenerative nature of the condition, and included only data from the first period (Qizilbash 1998). The second question to be addressed is whether there is a likelihood of serious carry-over, which relies largely on judgement since the statistical techniques to demonstrate carry-over are far from satisfactory. The nature of the interventions and the length of any washout period are important considerations.

It is only justifiable to exclude cross-over trials from a systematic review if the design is inappropriate to the clinical context. Very often, however, it is difficult or impossible to extract suitable data from a cross-over trial. In Section 16.4.5 we outline some considerations and suggestions for including cross-over trials in a meta-analysis. First we discuss how the 'Risk of bias' tool described in Chapter 8 can be extended to address questions specific to cross-over trials.

## 16.4.3 Assessing risk of bias in cross-over trials

The main concerns over risk of bias in cross-over trials are: (i) whether the cross-over design is suitable; (ii) whether there is a carry-over effect; (iii) whether only first period data are available; (iv) incorrect analysis; and (v) comparability of results with those from parallel-group trials.

(i) The cross-over design is suitable to study a condition that is (reasonably) stable (e.g. asthma), and where long-term follow-up is not required. The first issue to consider therefore is whether the cross-over design is suitable for the condition being studied.

(ii) Of particular concern is the possibility of a 'carry over' of treatment effect from one period to the next. A carry-over effect means that the observed difference between the treatments depends upon the order in which they were received; hence the estimated overall treatment effect will be affected (usually underestimated, leading to a bias towards the null).

   The use of the cross-over design should thus be restricted to situations in which there is unlikely to be carry-over of treatment effect across periods. Support for this notion may not be available, however, before the trial is done. Review authors should seek information in trial reports about the evaluation of the carry-over effect. However, in an unpublished review of 116 published cross-over trials from 2000 (Mills 2005), 30% of the studies discussed carry-over but only 12% reported the analysis.

(iii) In the presence of carry-over, a common strategy is to base the analysis on only the first period. Although the first period of a cross-over trial is in effect a parallel group comparison, use of data from only the first period will be biased if, as is likely, the decision to do so is based on a test of carry-over. Such a 'two stage analysis' has been discredited (Freeman 1989) but is still used. Also, use of the first period only removes the main strength of the cross-over design, the ability to compare treatments within individuals.

   Cross-over trials for which only first period data are available should be considered to be at risk of bias, especially when the investigators explicitly used the two-stage strategy.

(iv) The analysis of a cross-over trial should take advantage of the within-person design, and use some form of paired analysis (Elbourne 2002). Although trial authors may have analysed paired data, poor presentation may make it impossible for review authors to extract paired data. Unpaired data may be available and will generally be unrelated to the estimated treatment effect or statistical significance. So it is not a source of bias, but rather will usually lead to a trial getting (much) less than its due weight in a meta-analysis.

   In the review above (Mills 2005), only 38% of 116 cross-over trials performed an analysis of paired data.

(v) In the absence of carry-over, cross-over trials should estimate the same treatment effect as parallel group trials. Although one study reported a difference in the treatment effect found in cross-over trials compared with parallel group trials

(Khan 1996), they had looked at treatments for infertility, an area notorious for the inappropriateness of the cross-over design, and a careful re-analysis did not support the original findings (te Velde 1998).

Other issues to consider for risk of bias in cross-over trials include the following.

- Participants may drop out after the first treatment, and not receive the second treatment. Such participants are usually dropped from the analysis.

- There may be a systematic difference between the two periods of the trial. A period effect is not too serious, as it applies equally to both treatments, although it may suggest that the condition being studied is not stable.

- It may not be clear how many treatments or periods were used. Lee could not identify the design for 12/64 published cross-over trials (Lee 2005b).

- It should not be assumed that the order of treatments was randomized in a cross-over trial. Occasionally a study may be encountered in which it is clear that all participants had the treatments in the same order. Such a trial does not provide a valid comparison of the treatments, since there may be a trend in outcomes over time in addition to the change in treatments.

- Reporting of drop-outs may be poor, especially for those participants who completed one treatment period. The number of participants who dropped out was specified in only nine of the 64 trials in Lee's review (Lee 2005b).

Some suggested questions for assessing risk of bias in cross-over trials are as follows:

- Was use of a cross-over design appropriate?

- Is it clear that the order of receiving treatments was randomized?

- Can it be assumed that the trial was not biased from carry-over effects?

- Are unbiased data available?

### 16.4.4   Methods of analysis for cross-over trials

If neither carry-over nor period effects are thought to be a problem, then an appropriate analysis of continuous data from a two-period, two-intervention cross-over trial is a paired t-test. This evaluates the value of 'measurement on experimental intervention (E)' minus 'measurement on control intervention (C)' separately for each participant. The mean and standard error of these difference measures are the building blocks of an effect estimate and a statistical test. The effect estimate may be included in a meta-analysis using the generic inverse-variance method in RevMan.

A paired analysis is possible if the data in any one of the following bullet points is available:

- individual participant data from the paper or by correspondence with the trialist;

- the mean and standard deviation (or standard error) of the participant-specific differences between experimental intervention (E) and control intervention (C) measurements;

- the mean difference and one of the following: (i) a t-statistic from a paired t-test; (ii) a P value from a paired t-test; (iii) a confidence interval from a paired analysis;

- a graph of measurements on experimental intervention (E) and control intervention (C) from which individual data values can be extracted, as long as matched measurements for each individual can be identified as such.

For details see Elbourne et al. (Elbourne 2002).

If results are available broken by the particular sequence each participant received, then analyses that adjust for period effects are straightforward (e.g. as outlined in Chapter 3 of Senn (Senn 2002)).

## 16.4.5    Methods for incorporating cross-over trials into a meta-analysis

Unfortunately, the reporting of cross-over trials has been very variable, and the data required to include a paired analysis in a meta-analysis are often not published. A common situation is that means and standard deviations (or standard errors) are available only for measurements on E and C separately. A simple approach to incorporating cross-over trials in a meta-analysis is thus to take all measurements from intervention E periods and all measurements from intervention C periods and analyse these as if the trial were a parallel group trial of E versus C. This approach gives rise to a unit-of-analysis error (see Chapter 9, Section 9.3) and should be avoided unless it can be demonstrated that the results approximate those from a paired analysis, as described in Section 16.4.4. The reason for this is that confidence intervals are likely to be too wide, and the trial will receive too little weight, with the possible consequence of disguising clinically important heterogeneity. Nevertheless, this incorrect analysis is conservative, in that studies are under-weighted rather than over-weighted. While some argue against the inclusion of cross-over trials in this way, the unit-of-analysis error might be regarded as less serious than some other types of unit-of-analysis error.

A second approach to incorporating cross-over trials is to include only data from the first period. This might be appropriate if carry-over is thought to be a problem, or if a cross-over design is considered inappropriate for other reasons. However, it is possible that available data from first periods constitute a biased subset of all first period data. This is because reporting of first period data may be dependent on the trialists having found statistically significant carry-over.

A third approach to incorporating inappropriately reported cross-over trials is to attempt to approximate a paired analysis, by imputing missing standard deviations. We address this approach in detail in Section 16.4.6.

Cross-over trials with dichotomous outcomes require more complicated methods and consultation with a statistician is recommended (Elbourne 2002).

## 16.4.6 Approximate analyses of cross-over trials for a meta-analysis

Table 16.4.a presents some results that might be available from a report of a cross-over trial, and presents the notation we will use in the subsequent sections. We review straight-forward methods for approximating appropriate analyses of cross-over trials to obtain mean differences or standardized mean differences for use in meta-analysis. Review authors should consider whether imputing missing data is preferable to excluding cross-over trials completely from a meta-analysis. The trade-off will depend on the confidence that can be placed on the imputed numbers, and in the robustness of the meta-analysis result to a range of plausible imputed results.

### 16.4.6.1  Mean differences

The point estimate of mean difference for a paired analysis is usually available, since it is the same as for a parallel group analysis (the mean of the differences is equal to the difference in means):

$$MD = M_E - M_C.$$

**Table 16.4.a**  Some possible data available from the report of a cross-over trial

| Data relate to | Core statistics | Related, commonly-reported statistics |
| --- | --- | --- |
| Intervention E | N, $M_E$, $SD_E$ | Standard error of $M_E$. |
| Intervention C | N, $M_C$, $SD_C$ | Standard error of $M_C$. |
| Difference between E and C | N, MD, $SD_{diff}$ | Standard error of MD; Confidence interval for MD; Paired t-statistic; P value from paired t-test. |

The standard error of the mean difference is obtained as

$$SE\,(MD) = \frac{SD_{diff}}{\sqrt{N}}.$$

where N is the number of participants in the trial, and $SD_{diff}$ is the standard deviation of *within-participant differences between E and C measurements*. As indicated in Section 16.4.4, the standard error can also be obtained directly from a confidence interval for MD, from a paired t-statistic, or from the P value from a paired t-test. The quantities MD and SE(MD) may be entered into RevMan under the generic inverse-variance outcome type.

When the standard error is not available directly and the standard deviation of the differences is not presented, a simple approach is to impute the standard deviation, as is commonly done for other missing standard deviations (see Section 16.1.3). Other studies in the meta-analysis may present standard deviations of differences, and as long as the studies use the same measurement scale, it may be reasonable to borrow these from one study to another. As with all imputations, sensitivity analyses should be undertaken to assess the impact of the imputed data on the findings of the meta-analysis (see Section 16.1 and Chapter 9, Section 9.7).

If no information is available from any study on the standard deviations of the differences, imputation of standard deviations can be achieved by assuming a particular correlation coefficient. The correlation coefficient describes how similar the measurements on interventions E and C are within a participant, and is a number between −1 and 1. It may be expected to lie between 0 and 1 in the context of a cross-over trial, since a higher than average outcome for a participant while on E will tend to be associated with a higher than average outcome while on C. If the correlation coefficient is zero or negative, then there is no statistical benefit of using a cross-over design over using a parallel group design.

A common way of presenting results of a cross-over trial is as if the trial had been a parallel group trial, with standard deviations for each intervention separately ($SD_E$ and $SD_C$; see Table 16.4.a). The desired standard deviation of the differences can be estimated using these intervention-specific standard deviations and an imputed correlation coefficient (Corr):

$$SD_{diff} = \sqrt{SD_E^2 + SD_C^2 - (2 \times Corr \times SD_E \times SD_C)}.$$

### 16.4.6.2  *Standardized mean difference*

The most appropriate standardized mean difference (SMD) from a cross-over trial divides the mean difference by the standard deviation of measurements (and not by the standard deviation of the differences). A SMD can be calculated by pooled intervention-specific standard deviations as follows:

$$SMD = \frac{MD}{SD_{pooled}},$$

where

$$SD_{pooled} = \sqrt{\frac{SD_E^2 + SD_C^2}{2}}.$$

A correlation coefficient is required for the standard error of the SMD:

$$SE(SMD) = \sqrt{\frac{1}{N} + \frac{SMD^2}{2N}} \times \sqrt{2(1 - Corr)}.$$

Alternatively, the SMD can be calculated from the MD and its standard error, using an imputed correlation:

$$SMD = \frac{MD}{SE(MD) \times \sqrt{\frac{N}{2(1 - Corr)}}}$$

In this case, the imputed correlation impacts on the magnitude of the SMD effect estimate itself (rather than just on the standard error, as is the case for MD analyses in Section 16.4.6.1). Imputed correlations should therefore be used with great caution for estimation of SMDs.

### 16.4.6.3 Imputing correlation coefficients

The value for a correlation coefficient might be imputed from another study in the meta-analysis (see below), it might be imputed from a source outside of the meta-analysis, or it might be hypothesized based on reasoned argument. In all of these situations, a sensitivity analysis should be undertaken, trying different values of Corr, to determine whether the overall result of the analysis is robust to the use of imputed correlation coefficients.

Estimation of a correlation coefficient is possible from another study in the meta-analysis if that study presents all three standard deviations in Table 16.4.a. The calculation assumes that the mean and standard deviation of measurements for intervention E is the same when it is given in the first period as when it is given in the second period (and similarly for intervention C).

$$\text{Corr} = \frac{SD_E^2 + SD_C^2 - SD_{diff}^2}{2 \times SD_E \times SD_C}.$$

Before imputation is undertaken it is recommended that correlation coefficients are computed for as many studies as possible and compared. If these correlations vary substantially then sensitivity analyses are particularly important.

### 16.4.6.4 *Example*

As an example, suppose a cross-over trial reports the following data:

| Intervention E (sample size 10) | $M_E = 7.0$, $SD_E = 2.38$ |
|---|---|
| Intervention C (sample size 10) | $M_C = 6.5$, $SD_C = 2.21$ |

*Mean difference, imputing SD of differences (SD$_{diff}$)*    The estimate of the mean difference is MD = 7.0 − 6.5 = 0.5. Suppose that a typical standard deviation of differences had been observed from other trials to be 2. Then we can estimate the standard error of MD as

$$SE\,(MD) = \frac{SD_{diff}}{\sqrt{N}} = \frac{2}{\sqrt{10}} = 0.632.$$

The numbers 0.5 and 0.632 may be entered into RevMan as the estimate and standard error of a mean difference, under a generic inverse-variance outcome.

*Mean difference, imputing correlation coefficient (Corr)*    The estimate of the mean difference is again MD = 0.5. Suppose that a correlation coefficient of 0.68 has been imputed. Then we can impute the standard deviation of the differences as:

$$SD_{diff} = \sqrt{SD_E^2 + SD_C^2 - (2 \times \text{Corr} \times SD_E \times SD_C)}$$

$$= \sqrt{2.38^2 + 2.21^2 - (2 \times 0.68 \times 2.38 \times 2.21)} = 1.8426$$

The standard error of MD is then

$$SE\,(MD) = \frac{SD_{diff}}{\sqrt{N}} = \frac{1.8426}{\sqrt{10}} = 0.583.$$

The numbers 0.5 and 0.583 may be entered into RevMan as the estimate and standard error of a mean difference, under a generic inverse-variance outcome. Correlation coefficients other than 0.68 should be used as part of a sensitivity analysis.

***Standardized mean difference, imputing correlation coefficient (Corr)*** The standardized mean difference can be estimated directly from the data:

$$\text{SMD} = \frac{\text{MD}}{\text{SD}_{\text{pooled}}} = \frac{\text{MD}}{\sqrt{\dfrac{\text{SD}_E^2 + \text{SD}_C^2}{2}}} = \frac{0.5}{\sqrt{\dfrac{2.38^2 + 2.21^2}{2}}} = 0.218.$$

The standard error is obtained thus:

$$\text{SE}(\text{SMD}) = \sqrt{\frac{1}{N} + \frac{\text{SMD}^2}{2N}} \times \sqrt{2(1 - \text{Corr})}$$

$$= \sqrt{\frac{1}{10} + \frac{0.218^2}{20}} \times \sqrt{2(1 - 0.68)} = 0.256.$$

The numbers 0.218 and 0.256 may be entered into RevMan as the estimate and standard error of a standardized mean difference, under a generic inverse-variance outcome.

We could also have obtained the SMD from the MD and its standard error:

$$\text{SMD} = \frac{\text{MD}}{\text{SE}(\text{MD}) \times \sqrt{\dfrac{N}{2(1 - \text{Corr})}}} = \frac{0.5}{0.583 \times \sqrt{\dfrac{10}{2(1 - 0.68)}}} = 0.217$$

The minor discrepancy arises due to the slightly different ways in which the two formulae calculate a pooled standard deviation for the standardizing.

## 16.4.7 Issues in the incorporation of cross-over trials

Cross-over trials may, in principle, be combined with parallel group trials in the same meta-analysis. Consideration should be given to the possibility of important differences in other characteristics between the different types of trial. For example, cross-over trials may have shorter intervention periods or may include participants with less severe illness. It is generally advisable to meta-analyse parallel-group and cross-over trials separately irrespective of whether they are also combined together.

Authors should explicitly state how they have dealt with data from cross-over trials and should conduct sensitivity analyses to investigate the robustness of their conclusions, especially when correlation coefficients have been borrowed from external sources (see Chapter 9, Section 9.7). Statistical support is recommended.

## 16.5 Studies with more than two intervention groups

### 16.5.1 Introduction

It is not uncommon for clinical trials to randomize participants to one of several intervention groups. A review of randomized trials published in December 2000 found that a quarter had more than two intervention groups (Chan 2005). For example, there may be two or more experimental intervention groups with a common control group, or two control intervention groups such as a placebo group and a standard treatment group. We refer to these studies as 'multi-arm' studies. A special case is a factorial trial, which addresses two or more simultaneous intervention comparisons using four or more intervention groups (see Section 16.5.6).

Although a systematic review may include several intervention comparisons (and hence several meta-analyses), almost all meta-analyses address pair-wise comparisons. There are three separate issues to consider when faced with a study with more than two intervention groups.

1. Determine which intervention groups are relevant to the systematic review.

2. Determine which intervention groups are relevant to a particular meta-analysis.

3. Determine how the study will be included in the meta-analysis if more than two groups are relevant.

### 16.5.2 Determining which intervention groups are relevant

For a particular multi-arm study, the intervention groups of relevance to a *systematic review* are all those that could be included in a pair-wise comparison of intervention groups that, if investigated alone, would meet the criteria for including studies in the review. For example, a review addressing only a comparison of 'nicotine replacement therapy versus placebo' for smoking cessation might identify a study comparing 'nicotine gum versus behavioural therapy versus placebo gum'. Of the three possible pair-wise comparisons of interventions, only one ('nicotine gum versus placebo gum') addresses the review objective, and no comparison involving behavioural therapy does. Thus, the behavioural therapy group is not relevant to the review. However, if the study had compared 'nicotine gum plus behavioural therapy versus behavioural therapy plus placebo gum versus placebo gum alone', then a comparison of the first two interventions might be considered relevant and the placebo gum group not.

As an example of multiple control groups, a review addressing the comparison 'acupuncture versus no acupuncture' might identify a study comparing 'acupuncture versus sham acupuncture versus no intervention'. The review authors would ask whether, on the one hand, a study of 'acupuncture versus sham acupuncture' would be included in the review and, on the other hand, a study of 'acupuncture versus no intervention' would be included. If both of them would, then all three intervention groups of the study are relevant to the review.

As a general rule, and to avoid any confusion for the reader over the identity and nature of each study, it is recommended that all intervention groups of a multi-intervention study be mentioned in the table of 'Characteristics of included studies', either in the 'Interventions' cell or the 'Notes' cell. However, it is necessary to provide detailed descriptions of only the intervention groups relevant to the review, and only these groups should be used in analyses.

The same considerations of relevance apply when determining which intervention groups of a study should be included in a particular *meta-analysis*. Each meta-analysis addresses only a single pair-wise comparison, so review authors should consider whether a study of each possible pair-wise comparison of interventions in the study would be eligible for the meta-analysis. To draw the distinction between the review-level decision and the meta-analysis-level decision consider a review of 'nicotine therapy versus placebo or other comparators'. All intervention groups of a study of 'nicotine gum versus behavioural therapy versus placebo gum' might be relevant to the review. However, the presence of multiple interventions may not pose any problem for meta-analyses, since it is likely that 'nicotine gum versus placebo gum', and 'nicotine gum versus behavioural therapy' would be addressed in different meta-analyses. Conversely, all groups of the study of 'acupuncture versus sham acupuncture versus no intervention' might be considered eligible for the same meta-analysis, if the meta-analysis would include a study of 'acupuncture versus sham acupuncture' and a study of 'acupuncture versus no intervention'. We describe methods for dealing with the latter situation in Section 16.5.4.

## 16.5.3 Assessing risk of bias in studies with more than two groups

Bias may be introduced in a multiple-intervention study if the decisions regarding data analysis are made after seeing the data. For example, groups receiving different doses of the same intervention may be combined only after seeing the results, including P values. Also, different outcomes may be presented when comparing different pairs of groups, again potentially in relation to the findings.

Juszczak et al. reviewed 60 multiple-intervention randomized trials, of which over a third had at least four intervention arms (Juszczak 2003). They found that only 64% reported the same comparisons of groups for all outcomes, suggesting selective reporting analogous to selective outcome reporting in a two-arm trial. Also, 20% reported combining groups in an analysis. However, if the summary data are provided for each intervention group, it does not matter how the groups had been combined in reported analyses; review authors do not need to analyse the data in the same way as the study authors.

Some suggested questions for assessing risk of bias in multiple-intervention studies are as follows:

- Are data presented for each of the groups to which participants were randomized?

- Are reports of the study free of suggestion of selective reporting of comparisons of intervention arms for some outcomes?

If the answer to the first question is 'yes', then the second question is unimportant (so could be answered also with a 'yes').

## 16.5.4   How to include multiple groups from one study

There are several possible approaches to including a study with multiple intervention groups in a particular meta-analysis. One approach that must be avoided is simply to enter several comparisons into the meta-analysis when these have one or more intervention groups in common. This 'double-counts' the participants in the 'shared' intervention group(s), and creates a unit-of-analysis error due to the unaddressed correlation between the estimated intervention effects from multiple comparisons (see Chapter 9, Section 9.3). An important distinction to make is between situations in which a study can contribute several *independent* comparisons (i.e. with no intervention group in common) and when several comparisons are *correlated* because they have intervention groups, and hence participants, in common. For example, consider a study that randomized participants to four groups: 'nicotine gum' versus 'placebo gum' versus 'nicotine patch' versus 'placebo patch'. A meta-analysis that addresses the broad question of whether nicotine replacement therapy is effective might include the comparison 'nicotine gum versus placebo gum' as well as the independent comparison 'nicotine patch versus placebo patch'. It is usually reasonable to include independent comparisons in a meta-analysis as if they were from different studies, although there are subtle complications with regard to random-effects analyses (see Section 16.5.5).

Approaches to overcoming a unit-of-analysis error for a study that could contribute multiple, correlated, comparisons include the following.

- Combine groups to create a single pair-wise comparison (recommended).

- Select one pair of interventions and exclude the others.

- Split the 'shared' group into two or more groups with smaller sample size, and include two or more (reasonably independent) comparisons.

- Include two or more correlated comparisons and account for the correlation.

- Undertake a *multiple-treatments meta-analysis* (see Section 16.6).

The recommended method in most situations is to combine all relevant experimental intervention groups of the study into a single group, and to combine all relevant control intervention groups into a single control group. As an example, suppose that a meta-analysis of 'acupuncture versus no acupuncture' would consider studies of either 'acupuncture versus sham acupuncture' or studies of 'acupuncture versus no intervention' to be eligible for inclusion. Then a study comparing 'acupuncture versus sham acupuncture versus no intervention' would be included in the meta-analysis by combining the participants in the 'sham acupuncture' group with participants in the 'no intervention' group. This combined control group would be compared with the 'acupuncture' group in the usual way. For dichotomous outcomes, both the sample sizes and the numbers of people with events can be summed across groups. For continuous outcomes, means and standard deviations can be combined using methods described in Chapter 7 (Section 7.7.3.8).

The alternative strategy of selecting a single pair of interventions (e.g. choosing either 'sham acupuncture' or 'no intervention' as the control) results in a loss of information and is open to results-related choices, so is not generally recommended.

A further possibility is to include each pair-wise comparison separately, but with shared intervention groups divided out approximately evenly among the comparisons. For example, if a trial compares 121 patients receiving acupuncture with 124 patients receiving sham acupuncture and 117 patients receiving no acupuncture, then two comparisons (of, say, 61 'acupuncture' against 124 'sham acupuncture', and of 60 'acupuncture' against 117 'no intervention') might be entered into the meta-analysis. For dichotomous outcomes, both the number of events and the total number of patients would be divided up. For continuous outcomes, only the total number of participants would be divided up and the means and standard deviations left unchanged. This method only partially overcomes the unit-of-analysis error (because the resulting comparisons remain correlated) so is not generally recommended. A potential advantage of this approach, however, would be that approximate investigations of heterogeneity across intervention arms are possible (for example, in the case of the example here, the difference between using sham acupuncture and no intervention as a control group).

Two final options, which would require statistical support, are to account for the correlation between correlated comparisons from the same study in the analysis, and to perform a multiple-treatments meta-analysis. The former involves calculating an average (or weighted average) of the relevant pair-wise comparisons from the study, and calculating a variance (and hence a weight) for the study, taking into account the correlation between the comparisons. It will typically yield a similar result to the recommended method of combining across experimental and control intervention groups. Multiple-treatments meta-analysis is discussed in more detail in Section 16.6.

### 16.5.5 Heterogeneity considerations with multiple-intervention studies

Two possibilities for addressing heterogeneity between studies are to allow for it in a random-effects meta-analysis, and to investigate it through subgroup analyses or meta-regression (Chapter 9, Section 9.6). Some complications arise when including multiple-intervention studies in such analyses. First, it will not be possible to investigate certain intervention-related sources of heterogeneity if intervention groups are combined as in the recommended approach in Section 16.5.4. For example, subgrouping according to 'sham acupuncture' or 'no intervention' as a control group is not possible if these two groups are combined prior to the meta-analysis. The simplest method for allowing an investigation of this difference, across studies, is to create two or more comparisons from the study (e.g. 'acupuncture versus sham acupuncture' and 'acupuncture versus no intervention'). However, if these contain a common intervention group (here, acupuncture), then they are not independent and a unit-of-analysis error will occur, even if the sample size is reduced for the shared intervention group(s). Nevertheless, splitting up the sample size for the shared intervention group remains a practical means of performing approximate investigations of heterogeneity.

A more subtle problem occurs in random-effects meta-analyses if multiple comparisons are included from the same study. A random-effects meta-analysis allows for variation by assuming that the effects underlying the studies in the meta-analysis follow a distribution across studies. The intention is to allow for study-to-study variation. However, if two or more estimates come from the same study then the same variation is assumed across comparisons within the study and across studies. This is true whether the comparisons are independent or correlated (see Section 16.5.4). One way to overcome this is to perform a fixed-effect meta-analysis across comparisons within a study, and a random-effects meta-analysis across studies. Statistical support is recommended; in practice the difference between different analyses is likely to be trivial.

## 16.5.6   Factorial trials

In a factorial trial, two (or more) intervention comparisons are carried out simultaneously. Thus, for example, participants may be randomized to receive aspirin or placebo, and also randomized to receive a behavioural intervention or standard care. Most factorial trials have two 'factors' in this way, each of which has two levels; these are called $2 \times 2$ factorial trials. Occasionally $3 \times 2$ trials may be encountered, or trials that investigate three, four, or more interventions simultaneously. Often only one of the comparisons will be of relevance to any particular review. The following remarks focus on the $2 \times 2$ case but the principles extend to more complex designs.

In most factorial trials the intention is to achieve 'two trials for the price of one', and the assumption is made that the effects of the different active interventions are independent, that is, there is no interaction (synergy). Occasionally a trial may be carried out specifically to investigate whether there is an interaction between two treatments. That aspect may more often be explored in a trial comparing each of two active treatments on its own with both combined, without a placebo group. Such trials are not factorial trials.

The $2 \times 2$ factorial design can be displayed as a $2 \times 2$ table, with the rows indicating one comparison (e.g. aspirin versus placebo) and the columns the other (e.g. behavioural intervention versus standard care):

|  | | **Randomization of B** | |
|---|---|---|---|
|  | | **Behavioural intervention (B)** | **Standard care (not B)** |
| **Randomization of A** | **Aspirin (A)** | A and B | A, not B |
|  | **Placebo (not A)** | B, not A | Not A, not B |

A 2 × 2 factorial trial can be seen as two trials addressing different questions. It is important that both parts of the trial are reported as if they were just a two-arm parallel group trial. Thus we expect to see the results for aspirin versus placebo, including all participants regardless of whether they had behavioural intervention or standard care, and likewise for the behavioural intervention. These results may be seen as relating to the margins of the 2 × 2 table. We would also wish to evaluate whether there may have been some interaction between the treatments (i.e. effect of A depends on whether B or 'not B' was received), for which we need to see the four cells within the table (McAlister 2003). It follows that the practice of publishing two separate reports, possibly in different journals, does not allow the full results to be seen.

McAlister et al. reviewed 44 published reports of factorial trials (McAlister 2003). They found that only 34% reported results for each cell of the factorial structure. However, it will usually be possible to derive the marginal results from the results for the four cells in the 2 × 2 structure. In the same review, 59% of the trial reports included the results of a test of interaction. On re-analysis, 2/44 trials (6%) had $P<0.05$, which is close to expectation by chance (McAlister 2003). Thus, despite concerns about unrecognized interactions, it seems that investigators are appropriately restricting the use of the factorial design to those situations in which two (or more) treatments do not have the potential for substantive interaction. Unfortunately, many review authors do not take advantage of this fact and include only half of the available data in their meta-analysis (e.g. including only A versus not A among those that were *not* receiving B, and excluding the valid investigation of A among those that *were* receiving B).

A suggested question for assessing risk of bias in factorial trials is as follows:

- Are reports of the study free of suggestion of an important interaction between the effects of the different interventions?

## 16.6 Indirect comparisons and multiple-treatments meta-analysis

### 16.6.1 Introduction

Head-to-head comparisons of alternative interventions may be the focus of a Cochrane Intervention review, a secondary aim of a Cochrane Intervention review, or a key feature of a Cochrane Overview of reviews. Cochrane Overviews summarize multiple Cochrane Intervention reviews, typically of different interventions for the same condition (see Chapter 22). Ideally, direct head-to-head comparisons of alternative interventions would be made within randomized studies, but such studies are often not available. Indirect comparisons are comparisons that are made between competing interventions that have not been compared directly with each other: see Section 16.6.2. Multiple-treatments meta-analysis (MTM) is an extension to indirect comparisons that allows the combination of direct with indirect comparisons, and also the simultaneous analysis of the comparative effects of many interventions: see Section 16.6.3.

## 16.6.2   Indirect comparisons

Indirect comparisons are made between interventions in the absence of head-to-head randomized studies. For example, suppose that some trials have compared the effectiveness of 'dietician versus doctor' in providing dietary advice, and others have compared the effectiveness of 'dietician versus nurse', but no trials have compared the effectiveness of 'doctor versus nurse'. We might then wish to learn about the relative effectiveness of 'doctor versus nurse' by making indirect comparisons. In fact, doctors and nurses can be compared indirectly by contrasting trials of 'dietician versus doctor' with trials of 'dietician versus nurse'.

One approach that should never be used is the direct comparison of the relevant single arms of the trials. For example, patients receiving advice from a nurse (in the 'dietician versus nurse' trials) should not be compared directly with patients receiving advice from a doctor (in the 'dietician versus doctor' trials). This comparison ignores the potential benefits of randomization and suffers from the same (usually extreme) biases as a comparison of independent cohort studies.

More appropriate methods for indirect comparisons are available, but the assumptions underlying the methods need to be considered carefully. A relatively simple method is to perform subgroup analyses, the different subgroups being defined by the different comparisons being made. For the particular case of two subgroups (two comparisons; three interventions) the difference between the subgroups can be estimated, and the statistical significance determined, using a simple procedure described by Bucher (Bucher 1997). In the previous example, one subgroup would be the 'dietician versus doctor' trials, and the other subgroup the 'dietician versus nurse' trials. The difference between the summary effects in the two subgroups will provide an estimate of the desired comparison, 'doctor versus nurse'. The test can be performed using the test for differences between subgroups, as implemented in RevMan (see Chapter 9, Section 9.6.3.1). The validity of an indirect comparison relies on the different subgroups of trials being similar, on average, in all other factors that may affect outcome. More extensive discussions of indirect comparisons are available (Song 2003, Glenny 2005).

Indirect comparisons are not randomized comparisons, and cannot be interpreted as such. They are essentially observational findings across trials, and may suffer the biases of observational studies, for example due to confounding (see Chapter 9, Section 9.6.6). In situations when both direct and indirect comparisons are available in a review, then unless there are design flaws in the head-to-head trials, the two approaches should be considered separately and the direct comparisons should take precedence as a basis for forming conclusions.

### 16.6.3 Multiple-treatments meta-analysis

Methods are available for analysing, simultaneously, three or more different interventions in one meta-analysis. These are usually referred to as 'multiple-treatments meta-analysis' ('MTM'), 'network meta-analysis', or 'mixed treatment comparisons' ('MTC') meta-analysis. Multiple-treatments meta-analyses can be used to analyse studies with multiple intervention groups, and to synthesize studies making different comparisons of interventions. Caldwell et al. provide a readable introduction (Caldwell 2005); a more comprehensive discussion is provided by Salanti et al. (Salanti 2008). Note that multiple-treatments meta-analyses retain the identity of each intervention, allowing multiple intervention comparisons to be made. This is in contrast to the methods for dealing with a single study with multiple intervention groups that are described in Section 16.5, which focus on reducing the multiple groups to a single pair-wise comparison.

The simplest example of a multiple-treatments meta-analysis is the indirect comparison described in Section 16.6.2. With three interventions (e.g. advice from dietician, advice from doctor, advice from nurse), any two can be compared indirectly through comparisons with the third. For example, doctors and nurses can be compared indirectly by contrasting trials of 'dietician versus doctor' with trials of 'dietician versus nurse'. This analysis may be extended in various ways. For example, if there are also trials of the direct comparison 'doctor versus nurse', then these might be combined with the results of the indirect comparison. If there are more than three interventions, then there will be several direct and indirect comparisons, and it will be more convenient to analyse them simultaneously.

If each study compares exactly two interventions, then multiple-treatments meta-analysis can be performed using subgroup analyses, and the test for subgroup differences used as described in Chapter 9 (Section 9.6.3.1). However, it is preferable to use a random-effects model to allow for heterogeneity within each subgroup, and this can be achieved by using meta-regression instead (see Chapter 9, Section 9.6.4). When some studies include more than two intervention groups, the synthesis requires multivariate meta-analysis methods. Standard subgroup analysis and meta-regression methods can no longer be used, although the analysis can be performed in a Bayesian framework using WinBUGS: see Section 16.8.1. A particular advantage of using a Bayesian framework is that all interventions in the analysis can be ranked, using probabilistic, rather than crude, methods.

Multiple treatment meta-analyses are particularly suited to problems addressed by Overviews of reviews (Chapter 22). However, they rely on a strong assumption that studies of different comparisons are similar in all ways other than the interventions being compared. The indirect comparisons involved are not randomized comparisons, and may suffer the biases of observational studies, for example due to confounding (see Chapter 9, Section 9.6.6). In situations when both direct and indirect comparisons are available in a review, any use of multiple-treatments meta-analyses should be to supplement, rather than to replace, the direct comparisons. Expert statistical support, as well as subject expertise, is required for a multiple-treatments meta-analysis.

# 16.7  Multiplicity and the play of chance

## 16.7.1  Introduction

A Cochrane review might include multiple analyses because of a choice of several outcome measures, outcomes measured at multiple time points, a desire to explore subgroup analyses, the inclusion of multiple intervention comparisons, or other reasons. The more analyses that are done, the more likely it is that some of them will be found to be 'statistically significant' by chance alone. Using the conventional significance level of 5%, it is expected that one in 20 tests will be statistically significant even when there is truly no difference between the interventions being compared. However, after 14 independent tests, it is more likely than not (probability greater than 0.5) that at least one test will be significant, even when there is no true effect. The probability of finding at least one statistically significant result increases with the number of tests performed. The likelihood of a spurious finding by chance is higher when the analyses are independent. For example, multiple analyses of different subgroups are usually more problematic in this regard than multiple analyses of various outcomes, since the latter involve the same participants so are not independent.

The problem of multiple significance tests occurs in clinical trials, epidemiology and public health research (Bauer 1991, Ottenbacher 1998) as well as in systematic reviews (Bender 2008). There is an extensive statistical literature about the multiplicity issue. Many statistical approaches have been developed to adjust for multiple testing in various situations (Bender 2001, Cook 2005, Dmitrienko 2006). However, there is no consensus about when multiplicity should be taken into account, or about which statistical approach should be used if an adjustment for multiple testing is made. For example, the use of adjustments appropriate for independent tests will lead to P values that are too large when the multiple tests are not independent. Adjustments for multiple testing are used in confirmatory clinical trials to protect against spuriously significant conclusions when multiple hypothesis tests are used (Koch 1996) and have been incorporated in corresponding statistical guidelines (CPMP Working Party on Efficacy of Medicinal Products 1995). In exploratory studies, in which there is no pre-specified key hypothesis, adjustments for multiple testing might not be required and are often not feasible (Bender 2001). Statistically significant results from exploratory studies should be thought of as 'hypothesis generating', regardless of whether adjustments for multiple testing have been performed.

## 16.7.2  Multiplicity in systematic reviews

Adjustments for multiple tests are not routinely used in systematic reviews, and we do not recommend their use in general. Nevertheless, issues of multiplicity apply just as much to systematic reviews as to other types of research. Review authors should remember that in a Cochrane review the emphasis should generally be on estimating intervention effects rather than testing for them. However, the general problem of multiple comparisons affects interval estimation just as much as hypothesis testing (Chen 2005, Bender 2008).

Some additional problems associated with multiplicity occur in systematic reviews. For instance, when the results of a study are presented, it is not always possible to know how many tests or analyses were done. It is likely that in some studies interesting findings were selected for presentation or publication in relation to statistical significance, and other 'uninteresting' findings omitted, leading to misleading results and spurious conclusions. Such selective reporting is discussed in more detail in Chapter 8 (Section 8.13).

Adequate planning of the statistical testing of hypotheses (including any adjustments for multiple testing) should ideally be done at the design stage. Unfortunately, this can be difficult for systematic reviews when it might not be known, at the outset, which outcomes and which effect measures will be available from the included studies. This makes the *a priori* planning of multiple test procedures for systematic reviews more difficult or even impossible. Moreover, only some of the multiple comparison procedures developed for single studies can be used in meta-analyses of summary data. More research is required to develop adequate multiple comparison procedures for use in systematic reviews (Bender 2008).

In summary, there is no simple or completely satisfactory solution to the problem of multiple testing and multiple interval estimation in systematic reviews. However, the following general advice can be offered. More detailed advice can be found elsewhere (Bender 2008).

- In the protocol for the review, state which analyses and outcomes are of particular interest (the fewer the better). Outcomes should be classified in advance as primary and secondary outcomes, and main outcomes to appear in the 'Summary of findings' table should be pre-specified. If there is a clear key hypothesis, which could be tested by means of multiple significance tests, performing an adequate adjustment for multiple testing will lead to stronger confidence in any conclusions that are drawn.

- Although it is recommended that Cochrane reviews should seek to include all outcomes that are likely to be important to users of the review, overall conclusions are more difficult to draw if there are multiple analyses. Bear in mind, when drawing conclusions, that approximately one in 20 independent statistical tests will be statistically significant (at a 5% significance level) due to chance alone when there is no real difference between the groups.

- Do not select results for emphasis (e.g. in the abstract) on the basis of a statistically significant P value.

- If there is a choice of time-points for an outcome, attempts should be made to present a summary effect over all time-points, or to choose one time-point that is the most appropriate one (although availability of suitable data from all trials may be a problem). Multiple testing of the effect at each of the time-points should be avoided.

- Keep subgroup analyses to a minimum and interpret them cautiously.

- Interpret cautiously any findings that were not hypothesized in advance, even when they are 'statistically significant'. Such findings should only be used to generate hypotheses, not to prove them.

# 16.8   Bayesian and hierarchical approaches to meta-analysis

## 16.8.1   Bayesian methods

Bayesian statistics is an approach to statistics based on a different philosophy from that which underlies significance tests and confidence intervals. It is essentially about updating of evidence. In a Bayesian analysis, initial uncertainty is expressed through a **prior distribution** about the quantities of interest. Current data and assumptions concerning how they were generated are summarized in the **likelihood**. The **posterior distribution** for the quantities of interest can then be obtained by combining the prior distribution and the likelihood. The posterior distribution may be summarized by point estimates and credible intervals, which look much like classical estimates and confidence intervals. Bayesian analysis cannot be carried out in RevMan, but may be performed using WinBUGS software (Smith 1995, Lunn 2000).

In the context of a meta-analysis, the prior distribution will describe uncertainty regarding the particular effect measure being analysed, such as the odds ratio or the mean difference. This may be an expression of subjective belief about the size of the effect, or it may be from sources of evidence not included in the meta-analysis, such as information from non-randomized studies. The width of the prior distribution reflects the degree of uncertainty about the quantity. When there is little or no information, a 'non-informative' prior can be used, in which all values across the possible range are equally likely. The likelihood summarizes both the data from studies included in the meta-analysis (for example, $2 \times 2$ tables from randomized trials) and the meta-analysis model (for example, assuming a fixed effect or random effects).

The choice of prior distribution is a source of controversy in Bayesian statistics. Although it is possible to represent beliefs about effects as a prior distribution, it may seem strange to combine objective trial data with subjective opinion. A common practice in meta-analysis is therefore to use non-informative prior distributions to reflect a position of prior ignorance. This is particularly true for the main comparison. However, prior distributions may also be placed on other quantities in a meta-analysis, such as the extent of among-study variation in a random-effects analysis. It may be useful to bring in judgement, or external evidence, on some of these other parameters, particularly when there are few studies in the meta-analysis. It is important to carry out sensitivity analyses to investigate how the results depend on any assumptions made.

A difference between Bayesian analysis and classical meta-analysis is that the interpretation is directly in terms of belief: a 95% credible interval for an odds ratio is that region in which we believe the odds ratio to lie with probability 95%. This is how many practitioners actually interpret a classical confidence interval, but strictly in the classical framework the 95% refers to the long-term frequency with which 95% intervals contain the true value. The Bayesian framework also allows a review author to calculate the probability that the odds ratio has a particular range of values, which cannot be done in the classical framework. For example, we can determine the probability that the odds ratio is less than 1 (which might indicate a beneficial effect of an experimental intervention), or that it is no larger than 0.8 (which might indicate a clinically important effect). It should be noted that these probabilities are specific to the choice of the prior distribution. Different meta-analysts may analyse the same data using different prior distributions and obtain different results.

Bayesian methods offer some potential advantages over many classical methods for meta-analyses. For example, they can be used to:

- incorporate external evidence, such as on the effects of interventions or the likely extent of among-study variation;

- extend a meta-analysis to decision-making contexts, by incorporating the notion of the *utility* of various clinical outcome states;

- allow naturally for the imprecision in the estimated between-study variance estimate (see Chapter 9, Section 9.5.4);

- investigate the relationship between underlying risk and treatment benefit (see Chapter 9, Section 9.6.7);

- perform complex analyses (e.g. multiple-treatments meta-analysis), due to the flexibility of the WinBUGS software; and

- examine the extent to which data would change people's beliefs (Higgins 2002).

Statistical expertise is strongly recommended for review authors wishing to carry out Bayesian analyses. There are several good texts (Sutton 2000, Sutton 2001, Spiegelhalter 2004).

## 16.8.2 Hierarchical models

Some sophisticated techniques for meta-analysis exploit a statistical framework called hierarchical models, or multilevel models (Thompson 2001). This is because the information in a meta-analysis usually stems from two levels: studies at the higher level, and participants within studies at the lower level. Sometimes additional levels may be relevant, for example centres in a multicentre trial, or clusters in a cluster-randomized trial. A hierarchical framework is appropriate whether meta-analysis is of summary statistic information (for example, log odds ratios and their variances) or individual patient data (Turner 2000). Such a framework is particularly relevant when random effects are used to represent unexplained variation in effect estimates among studies (see Chapter 9, Section 9.5.4).

Hierarchical models rather than simpler methods of meta-analysis are useful in a number of contexts. For example, they can be used to:

- allow for the imprecision of the variance estimates of treatment effects within studies;

- allow for the imprecision in the estimated between-study variance estimate, tau-squared (see Chapter 9, Section 9.5.4);

- provide methods that explicitly model binary outcome data (rather than summary statistics);

- investigate the relationship between underlying risk and treatment benefit (see Chapter 9, Section 9.6.7); and

- extend methods to incorporate either study-level characteristics (see Chapter 9, Section 9.6.4) or individual-level characteristics (see Chapter 18).

Hierarchical models are particularly relevant where individual patient data (IPD) on both outcomes and covariates are available (Higgins 2001). However even using such methods, care still needs to be exercised to ensure that within- and between-study relationships are not confused.

Implementing hierarchical models needs sophisticated software, either using a classical statistical approach (e.g. SAS proc mixed, or MlwiN) or a Bayesian approach (e.g. WinBUGS). Much current methodological research in meta-analysis uses hierarchical model methods, often in a Bayesian implementation.

# 16.9　Rare events (including zero frequencies)

## 16.9.1　Meta-analysis of rare events

For rare outcomes, meta-analysis may be the only way to obtain reliable evidence of the effects of healthcare interventions. Individual studies are usually underpowered to detect differences in rare outcomes, but a meta-analysis of many studies may have adequate power to investigate whether interventions do impact on the incidence of the rare event. However, many methods of meta-analysis are based on large sample approximations, and are unsuitable when events are rare. Thus authors must take care when selecting a method of meta-analysis.

There is no single risk at which events are classified as 'rare'. Certainly risks of 1 in 1000 constitute rare events, and many would classify risks of 1 in 100 the same way. However, the performance of methods when risks are as high as 1 in 10 may also be affected by the issues discussed in this section. What is typical is that a high proportion of the studies in the meta-analysis observe no events in one or more study arm.

## 16.9.2 Studies with zero-cell counts

Computational problems can occur when no events are observed in one or both groups in an individual study. Inverse variance meta-analytical methods (both the inverse-variance fixed effect and DerSimonian and Laird random-effects methods) involve computing an intervention effect estimate and its standard error for each study. For studies where no events were observed in one or both arms, these computations often involve dividing by a zero count, which yields a computational error. Most meta-analytical software (including RevMan) automatically check for problematic zero counts, and add a fixed value (typically 0.5) to all cells of study results tables where the problems occur. The Mantel-Haenszel methods only require zero-cell corrections if the same cell is zero in all the included studies, and hence need to use the correction less often. However, in many software applications the same correction rules are applied for Mantel-Haenszel methods as for the inverse-variance methods. Odds ratio and risk ratio methods require zero-cell corrections more often than difference methods, except for the Peto odds ratio method, which only encounters computation problems in the extreme situation of no events occurring in all arms of all studies.

Whilst the fixed correction meets the objective of avoiding computational errors, it usually has the undesirable effect of biasing study estimates towards no difference and overestimating variances of study estimates (consequently down-weighting inappropriately their contribution to the meta-analysis). Where the sizes of the study arms are unequal (which occurs more commonly in non-randomized studies than randomized trials), they will introduce a directional bias in the treatment effect. Alternative non-fixed zero-cell corrections have been explored by Sweeting et al., including a correction proportional to the reciprocal of the size of the contrasting study arm, which they found preferable to the fixed 0.5 correction when arm sizes were not balanced (Sweeting 2004).

## 16.9.3 Studies with no events

The standard practice in meta-analysis of odds ratios and risk ratios is to exclude studies from the meta-analysis where there are no events in both arms. This is because such studies do not provide any indication of either the direction or magnitude of the relative treatment effect. Whilst it may be clear that events are very rare on both the experimental intervention and the control intervention, no information is provided as to which group is likely to have the higher risk, or on whether the risks are of the same or different orders of magnitude (when risks are very low, they are compatible with very large or very small ratio measures). Whilst one might be tempted to infer that the risk would be lowest in the group with the larger sample size (as the upper limit of the confidence interval would be lower), this is not justified as the sample size allocation was determined by the study investigators and is not a measure of the incidence of the event.

Risk difference methods superficially appear to have an advantage over odds ratio methods in that the RD is defined (as zero) when no events occur in either arm. Such studies are therefore included in the estimation process. Bradburn et al. undertook simulation studies which revealed that all risk difference methods yield confidence intervals that are too wide when events are rare, and have associated poor statistical power, which make them unsuitable for meta-analysis of rare events (Bradburn 2007). This is especially relevant when outcomes that focus on treatment safety are being studied, as the ability to identify correctly (or attempt to refute) serious adverse events is a key issue in drug development.

It is likely that outcomes for which no events occur in either arm may not be mentioned in reports of many randomized trials, precluding their inclusion in a meta-analysis. It is unclear, though, when working with published results, whether failure to mention a particular adverse event means there *were* no such events, or simply that such events were not included as a measured endpoint. Whilst the results of risk difference meta-analyses will be affected by non-reporting of outcomes with no events, odds and risk ratio based methods naturally exclude these data whether or not they are published, and are therefore unaffected.

## 16.9.4 Confidence intervals when no events are observed

It is possible to put upper confidence bounds on event risks when no events are observed, which may be useful when trying to ascertain possible risks for serious adverse events. A simple rule termed the 'rule of threes' has been proposed such that if no events are observed in a group, then the upper confidence interval limit for the number of events is three, and for the risk (in a sample of size N) is 3/N (Hanley 1983). The application of this rule has not directly been proposed or evaluated for systematic reviews. However, when looking at the incidence of a rare event that is not observed in any of the intervention groups in a series of studies (which randomized trials, non-randomized comparison or case series), it seems reasonable to apply it, taking N as the sum of the sample sizes of the arms receiving intervention. However, it will not provide any information about the relative incidence of the event between two groups.

The value 3 coincides with the upper limit of a one-tailed 95% confidence interval from the Poisson distribution (equivalent to a two-tailed 90% confidence interval). For the risk to be for a more standard one-tailed 97.5% confidence interval (equivalent to a two-tailed 95% confidence interval) then 3.7 should be used in all calculations in place of 3 (Newcombe 2000). An alternative recommendation which gives similar values is the 'rule of fours' which takes the upper limit of the risk to be 4/(N+4). Either of these options is recommended for use in Cochrane reviews. For example, if no events were observed out of 10, the upper limit of the confidence interval for the number of events is 3.7, and for the risk is 3.7 out of 10 (i.e. 0.37). If no events were observed out of 100, the upper limit on the number of events is still 3.7, but for the risk is 3.7 out of 100 (i.e. 0.037).

## 16.9.5  Validity of methods of meta-analysis for rare events

Simulation studies have revealed that many meta-analytical methods can give misleading results for rare events, which is unsurprising given their reliance on asymptotic statistical theory. Their performance has been judged suboptimal either through results being biased, confidence intervals being inappropriately wide, or statistical power being too low to detect substantial differences.

Below we consider the choice of statistical method for meta-analyses of odds ratios. Appropriate choices appear to depend on the control group risk, the likely size of the treatment effect and consideration of balance in the numbers of treated and control participants in the constituent studies. No research has evaluated risk ratio measures directly, but their performance is likely to be very similar to corresponding odds ratio measurement. When events are rare, estimates of odds and risks are near identical, and results of both can be interpreted as ratios of probabilities.

Bradburn et al. found that many of the most commonly used meta-analytical methods were biased when events were rare (Bradburn 2007). The bias was greatest in inverse variance and DerSimonian and Laird odds ratio and risk difference methods, and the Mantel-Haenszel odds ratio method using a 0.5 zero-cell correction. As already noted, risk difference meta-analytical methods tended to show conservative confidence interval coverage and low statistical power when risks of events were low.

At event rates below 1% the Peto one-step odds ratio method was found to be the least biased and most powerful method, and provided the best confidence interval coverage, provided there was no substantial imbalance between treatment and control group sizes within studies, and treatment effects were not exceptionally large. This finding was consistently observed across three different meta-analytical scenarios, and was also observed by Sweeting et al. (Sweeting 2004).

This finding was noted despite the method producing only an approximation to the odds ratio. For very large effects (e.g. risk ratio = 0.2) when the approximation is known to be poor, treatment effects were underestimated, but the Peto method still had the best performance of all the methods considered for event risks of 1 in 1000, and the bias was never more than 6% of the control group risk.

In other circumstances (i.e. event risks above 1%, very large effects at event risks around 1%, and meta-analyses where many studies were substantially imbalanced) the best performing methods were the Mantel-Haenszel OR without zero-cell corrections, logistic regression and an exact method. None of these methods is available in RevMan.

Methods that should be avoided with rare events are the inverse-variance methods (including the DerSimonian and Laird random-effects method). These directly incorporate the study's variance in the estimation of its contribution to the meta-analysis, but these are usually based on a large-sample variance approximation, which was not intended for use with rare events. The DerSimonian and Laird method is the only random-effects method commonly available in meta-analytic software. We would suggest that incorporation of heterogeneity into an estimate of a treatment effect should be a secondary consideration when attempting to produce estimates of effects from sparse data – the primary concern is to discern whether there is any signal of an effect in the data.

## 16.10    Chapter information

**Editors**: Julian PT Higgins, Jonathan J Deeks and Douglas G Altman on behalf of the
Cochrane Statistical Methods Group.

**This chapter should be cited as**: Higgins JPT, Deeks JJ, Altman DG (editors). Chapter
16: Special topics in statistics. In: Higgins JPT, Green S (editors), *Cochrane Handbook
for Systematic Reviews of Interventions*. Chichester (UK): John Wiley & Sons, 2008.

**Contributing authors**: Doug Altman, Deborah Ashby, Ralf Bender, Catey Bunce,
Marion Campbell, Mike Clarke, Jon Deeks, Simon Gates, Julian Higgins, Nathan Pace
and Simon Thompson.

**Acknowledgements**: We particularly thank Joseph Beyene, Peter Gøtzsche, Steff
Lewis, Georgia Salanti, Stephen Senn and Ian White for helpful comments on earlier
drafts. For details of the Cochrane Statistical Methods Group, see Chapter 9 (Box 9.8.a).

## 16.11    References

**Abrams 2005**
Abrams KR, Gillies CL, Lambert PC. Meta-analysis of heterogeneously reported trials as-
sessing change from baseline. *Statistics in Medicine* 2005; 24: 3823–3844.
**Bauer 1991**
Bauer P. Multiple testing in clinical trials. *Statistics in Medicine* 1991; 10: 871–889.
**Bender 2001**
Bender R, Lange S. Adjusting for multiple testing – when and how? *Journal of Clinical
Epidemiology* 2001; 54: 343–349.
**Bender 2008**
Bender R, Bunce C, Clarke M, Gates S, Lange S, Pace NL, Thorlund K. Attention should be
given to multiplicity issues in systematic reviews. *Journal of Clinical Epidemiology* 2008;
61: 857–865.
**Bradburn 2007**
Bradburn MJ, Deeks JJ, Berlin JA, Russell LA. Much ado about nothing: a comparison of
the performance of meta-analytical methods with rare events. *Statistics in Medicine* 2007;
26: 53–77.
**Bucher 1997**
Bucher HC, Guyatt GH, Griffith LE, Walter SD. The results of direct and indirect treatment
comparisons in meta- analysis of randomized controlled trials. *Journal of Clinical Epidemi-
ology* 1997; 50: 683–691.
**Caldwell 2005**
Caldwell DM, Ades AE, Higgins JPT. Simultaneous comparison of multiple treatments:
combining direct and indirect evidence. *BMJ* 2005; 331: 897–900.
**Campbell 2000**
Campbell M, Grimshaw J, Steen N. Sample size calculations for cluster randomised trials.
Changing Professional Practice in Europe Group (EU BIOMED II Concerted Action). *Journal
of Health Services Research and Policy* 2000; 5: 12–16.

**Chan 2005**
Chan AW, Altman DG. Epidemiology and reporting of randomised trials published in PubMed journals. *The Lancet* 2005; 365: 1159–1162.

**Chen 2005**
Chen T, Hoppe FM. Simultaneous confidence intervals. In: Armitage P, Colton T (editors). *Encyclopedia of Biostatistics* (2nd edition). Chichester (UK): John Wiley & Sons, 2005.

**Cook 2005**
Cook RJ, Dunnett CW. Multiple comparisons. In: Armitage P, Colton T (editors). *Encyclopedia of Biostatistics* (2nd edition). Chichester (UK): John Wiley & Sons, 2005.

**CPMP Working Party on Efficacy of Medicinal Products 1995**
CPMP Working Party on Efficacy of Medicinal Products. Biostatistical methodology in clinical trials in applications for marketing authorizations for medicinal products. *Statistics in Medicine* 1995; 14: 1659–1682.

**Dmitrienko 2006**
Dmitrienko A, Hsu JC. Multiple testing in clinical trials. In: Kotz S, Balakrishnan N, Read CB, Vidakovic B (editors). *Encyclopedia of Statistical Sciences* (2nd edition). Hoboken (NJ): John Wiley & Sons, 2006.

**Donner 1980**
Donner A, Koval JJ. The estimation of intraclass correlation in the analysis of family data. *Biometrics* 1980; 36: 19–25.

**Donner 2000**
Donner A, Klar N. *Design and Analysis of Cluster Randomization Trials in Health Research.* London (UK): Arnold, 2000.

**Donner 2001**
Donner A, Piaggio G, Villar J. Statistical methods for the meta-analysis of cluster randomized trials. *Statistical Methods in Medical Research* 2001; 10: 325–338.

**Donner 2002**
Donner A, Klar N. Issues in the meta-analysis of cluster randomized trials. *Statistics in Medicine* 2002; 21: 2971–2980.

**Elbourne 2002**
Elbourne DR, Altman DG, Higgins JPT, Curtin F, Worthington HV, Vaillancourt JM. Meta-analyses involving cross-over trials: methodological issues. *International Journal of Epidemiology* 2002; 31: 140–149.

**Eldridge 2004**
Eldridge SM, Ashby D, Feder GS, Rudnicka AR, Ukoumunne OC. Lessons for cluster randomized trials in the twenty-first century: a systematic review of trials in primary care. *Clinical Trials* 2004; 1: 80–90.

**Farrin 2005**
Farrin A, Russell I, Torgerson D, Underwood M, UK BEAM Trial Team. Differential recruitment in a cluster randomized trial in primary care: the experience of the UK back pain, exercise, active management and manipulation (UK BEAM) feasibility study. *Clinical Trials* 2005; 2: 119–124.

**Follmann 1992**
Follmann D, Elliott P, Suh I, Cutler J. Variance imputation for overviews of clinical trials with continuous response. *Journal of Clinical Epidemiology* 1992; 45: 769–773.

**Freeman 1989**
Freeman PR. The performance of the two-stage analysis of two-treatment, two-period cross-over trials. *Statistics in Medicine* 1989; 8: 1421–1432.

**Furukawa 2006**

Furukawa TA, Barbui C, Cipriani A, Brambilla P, Watanabe N. Imputing missing standard deviations in meta-analyses can provide accurate results. *Journal of Clinical Epidemiology* 2006; 59: 7–10.

**Gamble 2005**

Gamble C, Hollis S. Uncertainty method improved on best-worst case analysis in a binary meta-analysis. *Journal of Clinical Epidemiology* 2005; 58: 579–588.

**Glenny 2005**

Glenny AM, Altman DG, Sakarovitch C, Deeks JJ, D'Amico R, Bradburn M, Eastwood AJ. Indirect comparisons of competing interventions. *Health Technology Assessment* 2005; 9: 26.

**Hahn 2005**

Hahn S, Puffer S, Torgerson DJ, Watson J. Methodological bias in cluster randomised trials. *BMC Medical Research Methodology* 2005; 5: 10.

**Hanley 1983**

Hanley JA, Lippman-Hand A. If nothing goes wrong, is everything all right? Interpreting zero numerators. *JAMA* 1983; 249: 1743–1745.

**Health Services Research Unit 2004**

Health Services Research Unit. Database of ICCs: Spreadsheet (Empirical estimates of ICCs from changing professional practice studies) [page last modified 11 Aug 2004]. Available from: http://www.abdn.ac.uk/hsru/epp/cluster.shtml (accessed 1 January 2008).

**Higgins 2001**

Higgins JPT, Whitehead A, Turner RM, Omar RZ, Thompson SG. Meta-analysis of continuous outcome data from individual patients. *Statistics in Medicine* 2001; 20: 2219–2241.

**Higgins 2002**

Higgins JPT, Spiegelhalter DJ. Being sceptical about meta-analyses: a Bayesian perspective on magnesium trials in myocardial infarction. *International Journal of Epidemiology* 2002; 31: 96–104.

**Higgins 2008**

Higgins, JPT, White, IR, Wood, AM. Imputation methods for missing outcome data in meta-analysis of clinical trials. *Clinical Trials* 2008; 5: 225–239.

**Hollis 1999**

Hollis S, Campbell F. What is meant by intention to treat analysis? Survey of published randomised controlled trials. *BMJ* 1999; 319: 670–4.

**Hollis 2002**

Hollis S. A graphical sensitivity analysis for clinical trials with non-ignorable missing binary outcome. *Statistics in Medicine* 2002; 21: 3823–3834.

**Juszczak 2003**

Juszczak E, Altman D, Chan AW. A review of the methodology and reporting of multi-arm, parallel group, randomised clinical trials (RCTs). *3rd Joint Meeting of the International Society for Clinical Biostatistics and Society for Clinical Trials*, London (UK), 2003.

**Khan 1996**

Khan KS, Daya S, Collins JA, Walter SD. Empirical evidence of bias in infertility research: overestimation of treatment effect in crossover trials using pregnancy as the outcome measure. *Fertility and Sterility* 1996; 65: 939–945.

**Koch 1996**

Koch GG, Gansky SA. Statistical considerations for multiplicity in confirmatory protocols. *Drug Information Journal* 1996; 30: 523–534.

**Lathyris 2007**

Lathyris DN, Trikalinos TA, Ioannidis JP. Evidence from crossover trials: empirical evaluation and comparison against parallel arm trials. *International Journal of Epidemiology* 2007; 36: 422–430.

**Lee 2005a**

Lee LJ, Thompson SG. Clustering by health professional in individually randomised trials. *BMJ* 2005; 330: 142–144.

**Lee 2005b**

Lee SHH. *Use of the two-stage procedure for analysis of cross-over trials in four aspects of medical statistics* (PhD thesis). University of London, 2005.

**Lewis 1993**

Lewis JA, Machin D. Intention to treat – who should use ITT? *British Journal of Cancer* 1993; 68: 647–650.

**Little 2004**

Little RJA, Rubin DB. *Statistical Analysis with Missing Data* (2nd edition). Hoboken (NJ): John Wiley & Sons, 2004.

**Lunn 2000**

Lunn DJ, Thomas A, Best N, Spiegelhalter D. WinBUGS – a Bayesian modelling framework: concepts, structure, and extensibility. *Statistics and Computing* 2000; 10: 325–337.

**Marinho 2003**

Marinho VCC, Higgins JPT, Logan S, Sheiham A. Fluoride toothpaste for preventing dental caries in children and adolescents. *Cochrane Database of Systematic Reviews* 2003, Issue 1. Art No: CD002278.

**McAlister 2003**

McAlister FA, Straus SE, Sackett DL, Altman DG. Analysis and reporting of factorial trials: a systematic review. *JAMA* 2003; 289: 2545–2553.

**Mills 2005**

Mills EJ, Chan AW, Guyatt GH, Altman DG. Design, analysis, and presentation of cross-over trials. *5th Peer Review Congress*, Chicago (IL), 2005.

**Murray 1995**

Murray DM, Short B. Intraclass correlation among measures related to alcohol-use by young-adults-estimates, correlates and applications in intervention studies. *Journal of Studies on Alcohol* 1995; 56: 681–694.

**Newcombe 2000**

Newcombe RN, Altman DG. Proportions and their differences. In: Altman DG, Machin D, Bryant TN, Gardner MJ (editors). *Statistics with Confidence* (2nd edition). London (UK): BMJ Books, 2000.

**Newell 1992**

Newell DJ. Intention-to-treat analysis: implications for quantitative and qualitative research. *International Journal of Epidemiology* 1992; 21: 837–841.

**Ottenbacher 1998**

Ottenbacher KJ. Quantitative evaluation of multiplicity in epidemiology and public health research. *American Journal of Epidemiology* 1998; 147: 615–619.

**Puffer 2003**

Puffer S, Torgerson D, Watson J. Evidence for risk of bias in cluster randomised trials: review of recent trials published in three general medical journals. *BMJ* 2003; 327: 785–789.

**Qizilbash 1998**

Qizilbash N, Whitehead A, Higgins J, Wilcock G, Schneider L, Farlow M. Cholinesterase inhibition for Alzheimer disease: a meta-analysis of the tacrine trials. *JAMA* 1998; 280: 1777–1782.

**Rao 1992**

Rao JNK, Scott AJ. A simple method for the analysis of clustered binary data. *Biometrics* 1992; 48: 577–585.

**Salanti 2008**

Salanti G, Higgins J, Ades AE, Ioannidis JP. Evaluation of networks of randomized trials. *Statistical Methods in Medical Research* 2008; 17: 279–301.

**Senn 2002**

Senn S. *Cross-over Trials in Clinical Research* (2nd edition). Chichester (UK): John Wiley & Sons, 2002.

**Smith 1995**

Smith TC, Spiegelhalter DJ, Thomas A. Bayesian approaches to random-effects meta-analysis: A comparative study. *Statistics in Medicine* 1995; 14: 2685–2699.

**Song 2003**

Song F, Altman DG, Glenny AM, Deeks JJ. Validity of indirect comparison for estimating efficacy of competing interventions: empirical evidence from published meta-analyses. *BMJ* 2003; 325: 472–475.

**Spiegelhalter 2004**

Spiegelhalter DJ, Abrams KR, Myles JP. *Bayesian Approaches to Clinical Trials and Health-Care Evaluation*. Chichester (UK): John Wiley & Sons, 2004.

**Stewart 1995**

Stewart LA, Clarke MJ. Practical methodology of meta-analyses (overviews) using updated individual patient data. *Statistics in Medicine* 1995; 14: 2057–2079.

**Sutton 2000**

Sutton AJ, Abrams KR, Jones DR, Sheldon TA, Song F. *Methods for Meta-analysis in Medical Research*. Chichester (UK): John Wiley & Sons, 2000.

**Sutton 2001**

Sutton AJ, Abrams KR. Bayesian methods in meta-analysis and evidence synthesis. *Statistical Methods in Medical Research* 2001; 10: 277–303.

**Sweeting 2004**

Sweeting MJ, Sutton AJ, Lambert PC. What to add to nothing? Use and avoidance of continuity corrections in meta-analysis of sparse data. *Statistics in Medicine* 2004; 23: 1351–1375.

**te Velde 1998**

te Velde ER, Cohlen BJ, Looman CW, Habbema JD. Crossover designs versus parallel studies in infertility research. *Fertility and Sterility* 1998; 69: 357–358.

**Thompson 2001**

Thompson SG, Turner RM, Warn DE. Multilevel models for meta-analysis, and their application to absolute risk differences. *Statistical Methods in Medical Research* 2001; 10: 375–392.

**Turner 2000**

Turner RM, Omar RZ, Yang M, Goldstein H, Thompson SG. A multilevel model framework for meta-analysis of clinical trials with binary outcomes. *Statistics in Medicine* 2000; 19: 3417–3432.

**Ukoumunne 1999**

Ukoumunne OC, Gulliford MC, Chinn S, Sterne JA, Burney PG. Methods for evaluating area-wide and organisation-based interventions in health and health care: a systematic review. *Health Technology Assessment* 1999; 3: 5.

**Unnebrink 2001**

Unnebrink K, Windeler J. Intention-to-treat: methods for dealing with missing values in clinical trials of progressively deteriorating diseases. *Statistics in Medicine* 2001; 20: 3931–3946.

**White 2005**

White IR, Thomas J. Standardized mean differences in individually-randomized and cluster-randomized trials, with applications to meta-analysis. *Clinical Trials* 2005; 2: 141–151.

**White 2007**

White IR, Carpenter J, Evans S, Schroter S. Eliciting and using expert opinions about dropout bias in randomized controlled trials. *Clinical Trials* 2007; 4: 125–139.

**White 2008a**

White IR, Higgins JPT, Wood A. Allowing for uncertainty due to missing data in meta-analysis. Part 1: Two-stage methods. *Statistics in Medicine* 2008; 27: 711–727.

**White 2008b**

White IR, Welton N, Wood A, Ades AE, Higgins JPT. Allowing for uncertainty due to missing data in meta-analysis. Part 2: Hierarchical models. *Statistics in Medicine* 2008; 27: 728–745.

**Whiting-O'Keefe 1984**

Whiting-O'Keefe QE, Henke C, Simborg DW. Choosing the correct unit of analysis in medical care experiments. *Medical Care* 1984; 22: 1101–1114.

# 17 Patient-reported outcomes

Donald L Patrick, Gordon H Guyatt and Catherine
Acquadro on behalf of the Cochrane Patient Reported
Outcomes Methods Group

## Key Points

- Patient-reported outcomes (PROs) are reports coming directly from patients about how they feel or function in relation to a health condition and its therapy without interpretation by healthcare professionals or anyone else.

- PROs can relate to symptoms, signs, functional status, perceptions, or other aspects such as convenience and tolerability.

- Items reflecting the concepts included in a PRO questionnaire are elicited from the target population; patient involvement in questionnaire generation is essential for content validity.

- A glossary is provided on the PRO Methods Group web site (www.cochrane-pro-mg.org) for finding definitions of terms unfamiliar to authors.

- PROs are not only important when more objective measures of disease outcome are not available but also to represent what is most important to patients about a condition and its treatment.

- PROs can be continuous or categorical. Techniques are available to pool both kinds of measures.

- Review authors may need to do background reading about PROs to ensure they understand those chosen for inclusion into trials, in particular their validity and ability to detect change.

- A checklist is provided in this chapter on issues relating to PROs that authors should consider before incorporating PROs into their reviews and 'Summary of findings' tables.

- If completed reviews fail to record PROs when they were chosen as important outcomes in the review protocol, then they should be highlighted in the review as a deficiency in the current research on efficacy of treatment.

## 17.1  What are patient-reported outcomes?

Patient-reported outcomes (PROs) are any reports coming directly from patients about how they function or feel in relation to a health condition and its therapy, without interpretation of the patient's responses by a clinician, or anyone else. PROs include any treatment or outcome evaluation obtained directly from patients through interviews, self-completed questionnaires, diaries or other data collection tools such as hand-held devices and web-based forms (US Food and Drug Administration 2006). Proxy reports from caregivers, health professionals, or parents and guardians (necessary in some conditions such as advanced cancer and cognitive impairment) cannot be considered PROs and should be considered as a separate category of outcomes.

PROs provide patients' perspective on treatment benefit; directly measure treatment benefit beyond survival, disease, and physiologic markers; and are often the outcomes of greatest importance to patients. Reports from patients may include the signs and symptoms reported in diaries, the evaluation of sensations (most commonly classified as symptoms), reports of behaviours and abilities (most commonly classified as functional status), general perceptions or feelings of well-being, and other reports including satisfaction with treatment, general or health-related quality of life, and adherence to treatments. Reports may also include adverse or side effects (see Chapter 14).

PROs are sometimes used as primary outcomes in clinical trials, particularly when no surrogate measure of direct benefit is available to capture the patient's well-being. More often, PROs complement primary outcomes such as survival, disease indicators, clinician ratings and physiologic or laboratory-based measures. Figure 17.1.a shows those outcomes that are considered most often as important to patients within a classification of all outcomes.

PROs may be collected using a measure (or instrument) that is disease-specific, condition-specific or generic. Disease-specific measures describe severity, symptoms, or functional limitations specific to a particular disease state, condition or diagnostic grouping (e.g. arthritis or diabetes). Condition-specific measures describe patient symptoms or experiences related to a specific condition or problem (e.g. low-back pain) or related to particular interventions or treatments (e.g. knee-replacement or coronary artery bypass graft surgery). Generic measures are designed for use with any illness group or population sample.

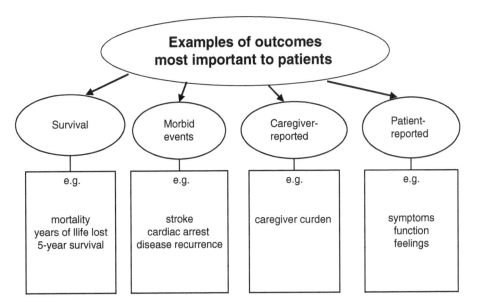

**Figure 17.1.a** Classification of clinical trial outcomes with illustration of those most important to patients

A glossary on PROs is available from the Cochrane Patient Reported Outcomes Methods Group web site (see Box 17.9.a).

## 17.2 Patient-reported outcomes and Cochrane reviews

Systematic review authors will select PROs for inclusion depending on the scope and aims of their review. PROs are most important when externally observable patient-important outcomes are unavailable, or rare. For many conditions, including pain, functional disorders, sexual dysfunction and insomnia, no satisfactory biological measures are available. Conditions in which outcomes are known only to the patients themselves, such as pain intensity and emotions, demand PROs as primary outcomes. PROs are also important when observable outcomes are available, because they reflect directly what is important to patients.

An important early part of the systematic review process is to define and list all patient-important outcomes that are relevant to their question (Guyatt 2004) (see Chapter 5, Section 5.4.1). This step is highly germane to the measurement of PROs. Many primary studies fail to measure aspects of perceived health and quality of life that are very important to patients. When this is the case, evidence regarding impact of interventions on PROs may be much weaker than evidence regarding impact on disease indicators such as morbidity or mortality. In the extreme, there may be a line in a 'Summary of findings' table that is blank, that is, for instance, a line specifying health-related quality of life (HRQL) that is blank because no study addressed this issue directly. The careful prior consideration of all patient-important outcomes and inclusion as a blank row in a 'Summary of findings' table will highlight what is missing in outcome measurement in the eligible randomized trials and other studies.

It is important that review authors understand the nature of the PROs used in the studies included in their review, and communicate this information to the reader. In clinical trials, investigators use many instruments to capture PROs, and methods for developing, validating, and analysing PRO data are diverse.

# 17.3    Health status and quality of life as PRO outcomes

Health status and quality of life outcomes are an important category of PROs. Published papers often use the terms 'quality of life' (QOL), 'health status', 'functional status', 'health-related quality of life' (HRQOL) and 'well-being' loosely and interchangeably, despite clear definitions of terms (see Table 17.3.a).

Different types of instruments are available for measuring health status and quality of life (see Table 17.3.b). These may yield an overall score or **indicator number** (representing impact of the intervention on physical or emotional function, for instance), an **index number** (again an overall score, but weighted in terms of anchors of death and full health), a **profile** (individual scores of dimensions or domains), or a **battery** of tests (multiple outcome assessing different concepts): see Table 17.3.b.

HRQOL can be measured using generic or specific instruments, or a combination of both. If investigators were interested in going beyond the specific illness and possibly making comparisons between the impact of treatments on HRQOL across diseases or

**Table 17.3.a**  Definitions of selected terms related to quality of life

| Term | Definition |
| --- | --- |
| Functional status | An individual's effective performance of or ability to perform those roles, tasks, or activities that are valued (e.g. going to work, playing sports, or maintaining the house). |
| Health-related quality of life (HRQOL) | Personal health status. HRQOL usually refers to aspects of our lives that are dominated or significantly influenced by our mental or physical well-being. |
| Quality of life (QOL) | An evaluation of all aspects of our lives, including, for example, where we live, how we live, and how we play. It encompasses such life factors as family circumstances, finances, housing and job satisfaction. (See also health-related quality of life). |
| Well-being | Subjective bodily and emotional states; how an individual feels; a state of mind distinct from functioning that pertains to behaviours and activities. |

**Table 17.3.b** A taxonomy of health status and quality-of-life measures adapted from Patrick and Erickson (Patrick 1993)

| Measure | Strengths | Weaknesses |
|---|---|---|
| **Types of Scores Produced** | | |
| Single indicator number. | Global evaluation; Useful for population. | May be difficult to interpret. |
| Single index number. | Represents net impact; Useful for cost-effectiveness. | Sometimes not possible to disaggregate contribution of domains to the overall score. |
| Profile of interrelated scores. | Single instrument; Contribution of domains to overall score possible. | Length may be a problem; May not have overall score. |
| Battery of independent scores. | Wide range of relevant outcomes possible. | Cannot relate different outcomes to common measurement scale; May need to adjust for multiple comparisons; May need to identify major outcome. |
| **Range of Populations and Concepts** | | |
| Generic: applied across diseases, conditions, populations, and concepts. | Broadly applicable; Summarizes range of concepts; Detection of unanticipated effects possible. | May not be responsive to change; May not have focus of patient interest; Length may be a problem; Effects may be difficult to interpret. |
| Specific: applied to individuals, diseases, conditions, populations, or concepts/domains. | More acceptable to respondents; May be more responsive to change. | Cannot compare across conditions or populations; Cannot detect unanticipated effects. |
| **Weighting System** | | |
| Utility: preference weights from patients, providers, or community. | Interval scale; Patient or consumer view incorporated. | May have difficulty obtaining weights; May not differ from equal weighting, which is easier to obtain. |
| Equal weighting: items weighted equally or from frequency or responses. | More familiar techniques; Appears easier to use. | May be influenced by prevalence; Cannot incorporate tradeoffs. |

conditions, they may have chosen generic HRQOL measures that cover all relevant areas of HRQOL (including, for example, mobility, self-care, and physical, emotional, and social function), and are designed for administration to people with any kind of underlying health problems (or no problem at all). These instruments are sometimes called health profiles; the most commonly used health profiles are short forms of the instruments used in the Medical Outcomes Study (Tarlov 1989, Ware 1995). Alternatively (or in addition) randomized trials and other studies may have relied on instruments that are specific to function (e.g. sleep or sexual function), a problem (e.g. pain), or a disease (e.g. heart failure, asthma, or irritable bowel syndrome).

Elicitation of concepts and items for a PRO questionnaire should come from qualitative research with patients, family members, clinical experts, and the literature. For a guide to using qualitative methods, see Chapter 20. Involvement of patients in PRO questionnaire development is essential to ensure content validity. The concepts that are included and measured in an included study can only be determined by examining the actual content of items or questions included in an instrument claiming to measure quality of life or health-related quality of life. The *concept* is the 'thing' being measured. Concepts may relate to an individual item or to a subset of items that refer to the same concept, often referred to as domains. For example, an item measuring pain, a sensation known only to the patient, would be a symptom and the symptom concept that is being measured can be labelled as pain. An item assessing difficulty walking up stairs would be a concept related to physical functioning and might be labelled walking up stairs or as part of physical function. The labelling of concepts varies widely among researchers and there is no agreed-upon classification of concepts. Nonetheless, each item, subdomain, domain, or overall score addresses one or more concepts, which authors can identify from the content, e.g. language, used in the label for an item, domain, or overall score.

Review authors may gain considerable insight from what the authors of the original PRO development studies write about the nature or sources of items chosen for inclusion in a specific instrument. Unfortunately review authors will often find themselves reading between the lines of published clinical trial results to try and get a precise notion of the concepts or constructs under consideration. They may, to gain a full understanding, have to make at least a brief foray into the articles that describe the development and prior use of the PRO instruments included in the primary studies.

For example, authors of a Cochrane review of cognitive behavioural therapy (CBT) for tinnitus included quality of life as an outcome (Martinez-Devesa 2007). Quality of life was assessed in four trials using the Tinnitus Handicap Questionnaire, in one trial the Tinnitus Questionnaire, and in one trial the Tinnitus Reaction Questionnaire. The original sources are cited in the review. Citations to articles on the psychometric properties are also available in MEDLINE for all three instruments and could easily be identified with a search using the Google search engine. Information on the items and the concepts measured are contained in these articles, and review authors were able to compare the content of the instruments.

Another issue to consider in understanding what is being measured is how the PRO instruments are weighted. Many specific instruments weight items equally when producing an overall score. Utility instruments designed primarily for economic analysis put great stress on item weighting, attempting to present HRQOL as a continuum anchored between death and full health. Readers interested the issues we have laid out in the previous paragraph can look to an old, but still useful summary (Guyatt 1993).

# 17.4   Issues in the measurement of patient-reported outcomes

## 17.4.1   Validity of instruments

Validity has to do with whether the instrument is measuring what it is intended to measure. Empirical evidence that PROs measure the domains of interest allows strong inferences regarding validity. To provide such evidence, investigators have borrowed validation strategies from psychologists who for many years have struggled with determining whether questionnaires assessing intelligence and attitudes really measure what is intended.

Validation strategies include:

- content-related: evidence that the items and domains of an instrument are appropriate and comprehensive relative to its intended measurement concept(s), population and use;

- construct-related: evidence that relationships among items, domains, and concepts conform to *a priori* hypotheses concerning logical relationships that should exist with other measures or characteristics of patients and patient groups;

- criterion-related (for a PRO instrument used as diagnostic tool): the extent to which the scores of a PRO instrument are related to a criterion measure.

Establishing validity involves examining the logical relationships that should exist between assessment measures. For example, we would expect that patients with lower treadmill exercise capacity generally will have more shortness of breath in daily life than those with higher exercise capacity, and we would expect to see substantial correlations between a new measure of emotional function and existing emotional function questionnaires.

When we are interested in evaluating change over time, we examine correlations of change scores. For example, patients who deteriorate in their treadmill exercise capacity should, in general, show increases in dyspnoea, whereas those whose exercise capacity improves should experience less dyspnoea. Similarly, a new emotional function measure should show improvement in patients who improve on existing measures of emotional function. The technical term for this process is testing an instrument's construct validity.

Review authors should look for, and evaluate the evidence of, the validity of PROs used in their included studies. Unfortunately, reports of randomized trials and other studies using PROs seldom review evidence of the validity of the instruments they use, but review authors can gain some reassurance from statements (backed by citations) that the questionnaires have been validated previously.

A final concern about validity arises if the measurement instrument is used with a different population, or in a culturally and linguistically different environment, than the one in which it was developed (typically, use of a non-English version of an English-language questionnaire). Ideally, one would have evidence of validity in the population enrolled in the randomized trial. Ideally PRO measures should be re-validated in each study using whatever data are available for the validation, for instance, other endpoints measured. Authors should note, in evaluating evidence of validity, when the population assessed in the trial is different from that used in validation studies.

### 17.4.2    Ability of an instrument to measure change

When we use instruments to evaluate treatment effects, they must be able to measure differences between groups, if differences do in fact exist. Randomization should ensure that participants in experimental and control intervention groups begin studies with the same status on whatever concept or construct the PRO is designed to measure. PROs must be able to detect what is important to patients and distinguish among participants who remain the same, improve, or deteriorate over the course of the trial. This is sometimes referred to as responsiveness, or sensitivity to change.

An instrument with a poor ability to measure change can result in false-negative results in which the experimental intervention improves how patients feel, yet the instrument fails to detect the improvement. This problem may be particularly salient for generic questionnaires that have the advantage of covering all relevant areas of HRQOL, but the disadvantage of covering each area superficially. In studies that show no difference in PROs between experimental and control intervention, lack of instrument responsiveness is one possible reason.

## 17.5    Locating and selecting studies with patient-reported outcomes

Searching methods for PROs are the same as for other outcomes (see Chapter 6). Usually all reports retrieved by the review's search strategy will be examined to identify those that include the PROs of interest. Sometimes a separate, additional, PRO search might be used to supplement the standard strategy. For example, if a review of randomized trials and other studies in the area of asthma did not yield studies using PROs, a separate search could be performed to include search terms specific to PROs used in asthma, such as 'asthma-specific quality of life'. However, this relies on there being mention of the PROs in the electronic record within the databases searched.

Index terms for PROs differ between the major bibliographic databases. Review authors cannot rely on a single index or subheading search term to identify studies addressing PROs. Multiple search terms are usually necessary. For example, Maciejewski et al. used the following MEDLINE index terms in their systematic review to estimate the effect of weight-loss interventions on health-related quality of life in randomized trials (Maciejewski 2005): 'Contingent valuation'; 'Health status'; 'Health-related Quality of Life'; 'Psychological aspects'; 'Psychosocial'; 'Quality of life'; 'Self-efficacy';

'SF-36'; 'Utility'; 'Well-being'; 'Willingness to pay'. Free-text searches should also include as many relevant synonyms as possible. The search needs to combine index terms and free-text terms and is likely to take several iterations.

Review authors may find it useful to design and use a separate section of the data collection form used in the systematic review to include review of PRO methods and results. An example of such a form can be found on our web site: www.cochrane-pro-mg.org/documents.html. Review authors should attend to alternative ways of collecting data from instruments: in particular, whether they can collect data in forms that facilitate analysis of data both in the form of continuous variables and dichotomous outcomes.

# 17.6   Assessing and describing patient-reported outcomes

Table 17.6.a presents selected issues specific to PROs that review authors should consider in incorporating PROs into their reviews. Authors may want to consider describing PROs in detail, according to this checklist, in the 'Characteristics of included studies' table or as an Additional table.

**Table 17.6.a**   A checklist for describing and assessing PROs in clinical trials

Based on Chapter 7 of Patrick and Erickson, a Users' Guide to the Medical Literature, CDC guidance for evaluation of community preventive services, and criteria used by the Medical Outcomes Trust (Patrick 1993, Guyatt 1997, Zaza 2000, Lohr 2002).

1. What were PROs measuring?
   a. What concepts were the PROs used in the study measuring?
   b. What rationale (if any) for selection of concepts or constructs did the authors provide?
   c. Were patients involved in the selection of outcomes measured by the PROs?
2. Omissions
   a. Were there any important aspects of health (e.g., symptoms, function, perceptions) or quality of life (e.g. overall evaluation, satisfaction with life) that were omitted in this study from the perspectives of the patient, clinician, significant others, payers, or other administrators and decision makers?
3. If randomized trials and other studies measured PROs, what were the instruments' measurement strategies?
   a. Did investigators use instruments that yield a single indicator or index number, a profile, or a battery of instruments?
   b. If investigators measure PROs, did they use specific or generic measures, or both?
   c. Who exactly completed the instruments?
4. Did the instruments work in the way they were supposed to work – validity?
   a. Had the instruments used been validated previously (provide reference)? Was evidence of prior validation for use in this population presented?
   b. Were the instruments re-validated in this study?
5. Did the instruments work in the way they were supposed to work – ability to measure change?
   a. Are the PROs able to detect change in patient status, even if those changes are small?
6. Can you make the magnitude of effect (if any) understandable to readers? (You must!)
   a. Can you provide an estimate of the difference in patients achieving a threshold of function or improvement, and the associated number needed to treat (NNT).

## 17.7 Comparability of different patient-reported outcome measures

Investigators may choose different instruments to measure PROs, either because they use different definitions of a particular PRO or because they choose different instruments to measure the same PRO. For example, an investigator may choose to use a generic instrument to measure functional status or a different disease-specific instrument to measure functional status. The definition of the outcome may or may not differ. Review authors must decide how to categorize PROs across studies, and when to pool results. These decisions will be based in the characteristics of the PRO, which will need to be extracted and reported in the review.

On many occasions, studies using PROs will make baseline and follow-up measurements and the outcome of interest will thus be the difference in change from baseline to follow-up between intervention and control groups. Ideally then, to pool data across two PROs that are conceptually related, one will have evidence of strong longitudinal correlations of change in the two measures in individual patient data, and evidence of similar responsiveness of the instruments. Further supportive evidence could come from correlations of differences between treatment and control, or difference between before and after measurements, across studies. If one cannot find any of these data, one could fall back on cross-sectional correlations in individual patients at a point in time.

For example, the two major instruments used to measure health-related quality of life in patients with chronic obstructive disease are the Chronic Respiratory Questionnaire (CRQ) and the St. George's Respiratory Questionnaire (SGRQ). Correlations between the two questionnaires in individual studies have varied from 0.3 to 0.6 in both cross-sectional (correlations at a point in time) and longitudinal (correlations of change) comparisons (Rutten-van Mölken 1999, Singh 2001, Schünemann 2003, Schünemann 2005).

In a subsequent investigation, investigators examined the correlations between mean changes in the CRQ and SGRQ in 15 studies including 23 patient groups and found a correlation of 0.88 (Puhan 2006). Despite this extremely strong correlation, the CRQ proved more responsive than the SGRQ: standardized response means of the CRQ (median of the standardized response means 0.51, IQR 0.19 to 0.98) were significantly higher ($P < 0.001$) than those associated with the SGRQ (median of the standardized response means 0.26, IQR $-0.03$ to 0.40). That is, in situations when both instruments were used together in the same study, the CRQ yielded systematically larger treatment effects. As a result, pooling results from trials using these two instruments could lead to underestimates of treatment effect in studies using the SGRQ.

Most of the time, unfortunately, detailed data such as those described in the previous paragraph will be unavailable. Investigators must then fall back on intuitive decisions about the extent to which different instruments are measuring the same underlying construct. For example, the authors of a meta-analysis of psychosocial interventions in the treatment of pre-menstrual syndrome faced a profusion of outcome measures, with 25 PROs reported in their nine eligible studies. They dealt with this problem by having two investigators independently examine each instrument – including all domains – and group them into six discrete conceptual categories; discrepancies were resolved by discussion to achieve consensus. The pooled analysis of each category included between two and six studies.

Meta-analyses of studies using different measurement scales will usually be undertaken using standardized mean differences (SMDs; see Chapter 9, Section 9.2.3). However, SMDs are highly problematic when the focus is on comparing change from baseline in intervention and control groups, because standard deviations of change do not measure between-patient variation (they depend also on the correlation between baseline and final measurements; see Chapter 9, Section 9.4.5.2).

Similar principles apply to studies in which review authors choose to focus on available data that are presented in dichotomous fashion, or from which review authors can extract dichotomous outcome data with relative ease. For example, investigators studying the impact of flavanoids on symptoms of haemorrhoids found that eligible randomized trials did not consistently use similar symptom measures; all but one of 14 trials, however, recorded the proportion of patients either free of symptoms, with symptom improvement, still symptomatic, or worse (Alonso-Coello 2006). In the primary analysis investigators considered outcomes of patients free of symptoms and patients with symptomatic/some improvement as equivalent, and pooled each outcome of interest based on the *a priori* expectation of a similar magnitude and direction of treatment effect.

This left a question of how to deal with studies that reported that patients experienced 'some improvement'. The investigators undertook analyses comparing the approach of dichotomizing including 'some improvement' as a positive outcome and as a negative outcome (similar to no improvement). Dichotomizing outcomes is often very useful, particularly for making results easily interpretable for clinicians and patients. Imaginative and yet rigorous ways of dichotomizing will result in summary statistics that provide useful guides to clinical practice.

The use of multiple instruments for measuring a particular PRO, and experimentation with multiple methods for analysis, can lead to selective reporting of the most interesting findings and introduce serious bias into a systematic review. Review authors focusing on PROs should be alert to this problem. When only a small number of eligible studies have reported a particular outcome, particularly if it is a salient outcome that one would expect conscientious investigators to measure, authors should note the possibility of reporting bias (see Chapter 10).

# 17.8   Interpreting results

## 17.8.1   Study summaries focusing on a single patient-reported outcome

When a meta-analysis includes studies reporting only a single PRO, presented as a continuous variable, a pooled result will generate a mean difference. The problem with this mean difference is that clinicians may have difficulty with its interpretation. For example, if told that the mean difference between rehabilitation and standard care in a series of randomized trials using the Chronic Respiratory Questionnaire was 1.0 (95%

CI 0.6–1.5), many readers would have no idea if this represents a trivial, small but important, moderate, or large effect.

The systematic review author can aid interpretation by reporting the range of possible results and the range of mean results in treatment and control groups in the studies. Most useful, however – if it is available – is an estimate of the smallest difference that patients are likely to consider important (the minimally important difference or MID). There are a variety of methods for generating estimates of the MID, including use of global ratings of change (Guyatt 2002). Ideally, review authors will present estimates of the MID in the abstract. For example, investigators examining the impact of respiratory rehabilitation in patients with chronic lung disease on health-related quality of life reported, in their abstract, that "for two important features of HRQL, dyspnea and mastery, the overall effect was larger than the MCID: 1.0 (95% CI 0.6–1.5) and 0.8 (0.5–1.2), respectively, compared with an MCID of 0.5." (Lacasse 1996).

While this is very helpful, it potentially tempts clinicians to make inappropriate inferences. If the MID is 0.5 and the mean difference between treatments is 0.4, clinicians may infer that nobody benefits from the intervention. If the mean difference is 0.6, they may conclude that everyone benefits. Both inferences may be misguided. First, they ignore the uncertainty (confidence intervals) around the point estimate. More importantly, they ignore the variation (standard deviation) in responses across individuals.

It is also possible for investigators to provide a 'responder' definition to help interpret outcomes (see Chapter 12, Section 12.6.1). It is useful to know the definition that characterizes an individual patient as a responder to treatment. Such a responder definition is based upon pre-specified criteria backed by empirically derived evidence supporting the responder definition as a measure of benefit. Methods for defining a responder include: (1) a pre-specified change from baseline on one or more scales; (2) a change in score of a certain size or greater (e.g. a 2-point change on an 8-point scale); and (3) a percentage change from baseline.

## 17.8.2 Study summaries using more than one patient-reported outcome

As the discussion in Section 17.8.1 pointed out, when pooling across PROs the mean difference is no longer a possible measure of effect and we therefore replace it with the standardized mean difference (SMD) (see Chapter 9, Section 9.2.3). Unfortunately, there are no fully satisfactory ways of providing a sense of the magnitude of effect in a PRO when one has had to resort to SMD to generate a summary. One can offer readers standard rules of thumb in interpretation of effect sizes (for instance 0.2 represents a small effect, 0.5 a moderate effect, and 0.8 a large effect (Cohen 1988) or some variation ($<0.41$ = small, 0.40 to 0.70 = moderate, $>0.70$ = large). Another, perhaps even less satisfactory, approach suggests that a standardized mean difference of 0.5 approximates, in many cases, to a minimal important difference (Norman 2003).

General methods of reporting and interpreting PROs, and other clinical outcomes, with respect to drawing inferences and conclusions are discussed in Chapter 12 (Section 12.6).

### 17.8.3 When studies do not address patient-reported outcomes

Many primary studies fail to measure aspects of perceived health and quality of life that are very important to patients. When this is the case, evidence regarding interventions' impact on PROs may be much weaker than evidence regarding impact on disease indicators morbidity or mortality. In the extreme, no study may address PROs directly. The careful prior consideration of all patient-important outcomes will highlight what is missing in outcome measurement in the eligible randomized trials and other studies. This omission should be highlighted in the reviews authors' conclusions as an implication for future research.

## 17.9 Chapter information

**Authors:** Donald L Patrick, Gordon H Guyatt and Catherine Acquadro on behalf of the Cochrane Patient Reported Outcomes Methods Group.

---

**Box 17.9.a The Cochrane Patient Reported Outcomes Methods Group**

The main objective of the Patient Reported Outcomes Methods Group (PRO MG) is to advise Cochrane authors about when and how to incorporate health status and quality-of-life data into systematic reviews. Some Cochrane Review Groups have encountered difficulties when incorporating PRO data in reviews. Examples of such difficulties include pooling and interpreting data and evaluating the validity of PRO scales.

The PRO MG aims to:

• refine methods of literature search on PRO studies;
• develop methods for systematically reviewing HRQL studies;
• refine methods for meta-analysis of PRO studies (in collaboration with the Statistical Methods Group);
• refine methods for use of PRO measures in economic evaluations in collaboration with the Campbell-Cochrane Economics Methods Group; and
• advise on software development.

The group gives advice to the Cochrane Collaboration Steering Group upon request, convenes workshops on health and patient-reported outcomes issues and methods, in response to the needs of the Collaboration, and prepares recommendations for this *Handbook*. Members of the group will take part in the preparation of Cochrane reviews and will give advice to authors through written material and training workshops. Members of the group will help review authors to develop protocols and reviews where it has been decided to include PRO outcomes.

*Web site*: www.cochrane-pro-mg.org/

---

**This chapter should be cited as:** Patrick D, Guyatt GH, Acquadro C. Chapter 17: Patient-reported outcomes. In: Higgins JPT, Green S (editors), *Cochrane Handbook for Systematic Reviews of Interventions*. Chichester (UK): John Wiley & Sons, 2008.

**Acknowledgements:** Jason Busse, Peter Fayers, Toshi Furukawa, Madeleine King and Milo Puhan provided comments on drafts.

## 17.10  References

**Alonso-Coello 2006**
Alonso-Coello P, Zhou Q, Martinez-Zapata MJ, Mills E, Heels-Ansdell D, Johanson JF, Guyatt G. Meta-analysis of flavonoids for the treatment of haemorrhoids. *British Journal of Surgery* 2006; 93: 909–920.

**Cohen 1988**
Cohen J. *Statistical Power Analysis in the Behavioral Sciences* (2nd edition). Hillsdale (NJ): Lawrence Erlbaum Associates, Inc., 1988.

**Guyatt 1993**
Guyatt GH, Feeny DH, Patrick DL. Measuring health-related quality of life. *Annals of Internal Medicine* 1993; 118: 622–629.

**Guyatt 1997**
Guyatt GH, Naylor CD, Juniper E, Heyland DK, Jaeschke R, Cook DJ. Users' guides to the medical literature. XII. How to use articles about health-related quality of life. Evidence-Based Medicine Working Group. *JAMA* 1997; 277: 1232–1237.

**Guyatt 2002**
Guyatt GH, Osoba D, Wu AW, Wyrwich KW, Norman GR, Clinical Significance Consensus Meeting Group. Methods to explain the clinical significance of health status measures. *Mayo Clinic Proceedings* 2002; 77: 371–383.

**Guyatt 2004**
Guyatt G, Montori V, Devereaux PJ, Schünemann H, Bhandari M. Patients at the center: in our practice, and in our use of language. *ACP Journal Club* 2004; 140: A11–A12.

**Lacasse 1996**
Lacasse Y, Wong E, Guyatt GH, King D, Cook DJ, Goldstein RS. Meta-analysis of respiratory rehabilitation in chronic obstructive pulmonary disease. *The Lancet* 1996; 348: 1115–1119.

**Lohr 2002**
Lohr K. Assessing health status and quality-of-life instruments: attributes and review criteria. *Quality of Life Research* 2002; 11: 193–205.

**Maciejewski 2005**
Maciejewski ML, Patrick DL, Williamson DF. A structured review of randomized controlled trials of weight loss showed little improvement in health-related quality of life. *Journal of Clinical Epidemiology* 2005; 58: 568–578.

**Martinez-Devesa 2007**
Martinez-Devesa P, Waddell A, Perera R, Theodoulou M. Cognitive behavioural therapy for tinnitus. *Cochrane Database of Systematic Reviews* 2007, Issue 1. Art No: CD005233.

**Norman 2003**
Norman GR, Sloan JA, Wyrwich KW. Interpretation of changes in health-related quality of life: the remarkable universality of half a standard deviation. *Medical Care* 2003; 41: 582–592.

**Patrick 1993**
Patrick DL, Erickson P. *Health Status and Health Policy: Quality of Life in Health Care Evaluation and Resource Allocation.* New York (NY): Oxford University Press, 1993.

**Puhan 2006**
Puhan M, Soesilo I, Guyatt GH, Schünemann HJ. Combining scores from different patient reported outcome measures in meta-analyses: when is it justified? *Health and Quality of Life Outcomes* 2006; 4: 94.

**Rutten-van Mölken 1999**
Rutten-van Mölken M, Roos B, Van Noord JA. An empirical comparison of the St George's Respiratory Questionnaire (SGRQ) and the Chronic Respiratory Disease Questionnaire (CRQ) in a clinical trial setting. *Thorax* 1999; 54: 995–1003.

**Schünemann 2003**
Schünemann HJ, Griffith L, Jaeschke R, Goldstein R, Stubbing D, Guyatt GH. Evaluation of the minimal important difference for the feeling thermometer and the St. George's Respiratory Questionnaire in patients with chronic airflow obstruction. *Journal of Clinical Epidemiology* 2003; 56: 1170–1176.

**Schünemann 2005**
Schünemann HJ, Goldstein R, Mador MJ, McKim D, Stahl E, Puhan MA, Griffith LE, Grant B, Austin P, Collins R, Guyatt GH. A randomised trial to evaluate the self-administered standardised chronic respiratory questionnaire. *European Respiratory Journal* 2005; 25: 31–40.

**Singh 2001**
Singh SJ, Sodergren SC, Hyland ME, Williams J, Morgan MD. A comparison of three disease-specific and two generic health-status measures to evaluate the outcome of pulmonary rehabilitation in COPD. *Respiratory Medicine* 2001; 95: 71–77.

**Tarlov 1989**
Tarlov AR, Ware JE, Jr., Greenfield S, Nelson EC, Perrin E, Zubkoff M. The Medical Outcomes Study. An application of methods for monitoring the results of medical care. *JAMA* 1989; 262: 925–930.

**US Food and Drug Administration 2006**
US Food and Drug Administration. Guidance for Industry. Patient-Reported Outcome Measures: Use in Medical Product Development to Support Labeling Claims [February 2006]. Available from: http://www.fda.gov/cber/gdlns/prolbl.htm (accessed 1 January 2008).

**Ware 1995**
Ware JE, Kosinski M, Bayliss MS, McHorney CA, Rogers WH, Raczek A. Comparison of methods for the scoring and statistical analysis of SF-36 health profile and summary measures: summary of results from the Medical Outcomes Study. *Medical Care* 1995; 33: AS264–AS279.

**Zaza 2000**
Zaza S, Wright-De Agüero LK, Briss PA, Truman BI, Hopkins DP, Hennessy MH, Sosin DM, Anderson L, Carande-Kulis VG, Teutsch SM, Pappaioanou M, Task Force on Community Preventive Services. Data collection instrument and procedure for systematic reviews in the Guide to Community Preventive Services. *American Journal of Preventive Medicine* 2000; 18 (Suppl 1): 44–74.

# 18 Reviews of individual patient data

**Lesley A Stewart, Jayne F Tierney and Mike Clarke on behalf of the Cochrane Individual Patient Data Meta-analysis Methods Group**

## Key Points

- In an individual patient data (IPD) meta-analysis, the original research data for each participant in each study are sought directly from the researchers responsible for that study.

- Having access to the 'raw' data for each study enables data checking, thorough exploration, and re-analysis of the data in a consistent way.

- IPD meta-analysis has particular benefits when the published information does not permit a good quality review, or where particular types of analyses are required that are not feasible using summary data.

- Most IPD meta-analyses are carried out and published by a collaborative group, comprising a project team or secretariat, the researchers who contribute their study data, and often also an advisory group.

- An IPD approach usually takes longer and costs more than a conventional systematic review relying on published or aggregate data.

- There may be circumstances where the benefits of obtaining IPD are marginal; others where it could be vital.

# 18.1    Introduction

### 18.1.1    What is an IPD review?

Individual patient data (IPD) meta-analysis is a specific type of systematic review. Instead of extracting data from study publications, the original research data for each participant in an included study are sought directly from the researchers responsible for that study. These data can then be re-analysed centrally and, if appropriate, combined in meta-analyses. Cochrane reviews can be undertaken as IPD reviews, but IPD reviews usually require dedicated staff and would be difficult to conduct in 'free time'. The approach requires particular skills and usually takes longer and costs more than a conventional systematic review relying on published or aggregate data. However, IPD reviews offer benefits related particularly to the quality of data and the type of analyses that can be done (Stewart 1995, Stewart 2002). For this reason they are considered to be a 'gold standard' of systematic review. This chapter aims to provide an overview of the IPD approach to systematic review, to help authors decide whether collecting IPD might be useful and feasible in their review. It does not provide detailed methodology, and anyone contemplating carrying out their first IPD review should seek appropriate advice and guidance from experienced researchers through the IPD Meta-analysis Methods Group (see Box 18.6.a).

### 18.1.2    When should an IPD review be done?

IPD reviews should be considered in circumstances where the published information does not permit a good quality review, or where particular types of analyses are required that are not feasible using standard approaches. There are situations where the IPD approach will not be feasible, because data have been destroyed or lost or, despite every effort, researchers do not wish to collaborate. There may also be circumstances where it may not be necessary, for example if all the required data are readily available in a suitable format within publications. Further details of when IPD many be beneficial are given in Box 18.1.a.

### 18.1.3    How are IPD review methods different?

The general approach to IPD meta-analysis is the same as for any other systematic review, and the methods used should differ substantially only in the data collection, checking and analysis stages. Just as for any Cochrane review, a detailed protocol should be prepared, setting out the objective for the review, the specific questions to be addressed, study inclusion and exclusion criteria, the reasons why IPD are sought, the methods to be used and the analyses that are planned. Similarly, the methods used to identify and screen studies for eligibility should be the same irrespective of whether IPD will be sought, although the close involvement of the original researchers in the project might make it easier to find other studies done by them or known to them. The

---

**Box 18.1.a    Potential benefits of IPD**

**IPD may be beneficial in the following situations.**

- Many studies are unpublished or published only in the grey literature.
- There is poor reporting of studies (e.g. information presented is inadequate, selective or ambiguous).
- A high proportion of individuals has been excluded from published analyses.
- Obtaining additional longer-term outcome data beyond that reported may provide useful insights (e.g. for mortality or child development outcomes).
- Outcome measures have been defined differently across studies.
- Time-to-event outcome measures are required.
- Multivariate or other complex analyses are required.
- Exploration of interactions between interventions and patient-level characteristics is important.

---

project should culminate in the preparation and dissemination of a structured report. An IPD review might also include a meeting at which results are presented and discussed with the collaborating researchers.

## 18.1.4    How are IPD reviews organized?

IPD reviews are usually carried out as collaborative projects whereby all researchers contributing information from their studies, together with those managing the project, become part of an active collaboration. The projects are managed by a small local project group or secretariat, which may be aided in important and strategic decision-making by a larger advisory group. Results are usually published in the name of the collaborative group. The secretariat may also be responsible for organizing meetings of collaborators, to bring individuals together to discuss the preliminary results.

## 18.1.5    What healthcare areas have used the IPD approach?

IPD meta-analyses have an established history in cardiovascular disease and cancer, where the methodology has been developing steadily since the late 1980s. In cancer, for example, there are now more than 50 IPD meta-analyses of screening and treatment across a wide range of solid tumour sites and haematological malignancies (Clarke 1998). IPD have also been used in systematic reviews in many other fields (Simmonds 2005), including HIV infection, dementia, epilepsy, depression, malaria, hernia and asthma. The Cochrane Collaboration Individual Patient Data Meta-analysis Methods Group web site includes a database of ongoing and completed IPD reviews where further information can be found (see Box 18.6.a).

### 18.1.6   If I am thinking about doing an IPD review, what should I do first?

Before embarking on an IPD review, the skills and funding required for the success of the project should be considered carefully and training and advice should be sought. The Cochrane Collaboration Individual Patient Data Meta-analysis Methods Group is a good first point of contact (Box 18.6.a).

## 18.2   The collaborative nature of IPD meta-analyses

### 18.2.1   Collaborative groups

Most IPD meta-analyses are carried out and published by collaborative groups. These groups comprise the project team or secretariat managing the IPD review, members of the advisory group (if there is one) and the researchers who contribute their study data for re-analysis.

### 18.2.2   Negotiating collaboration

Establishing collaboration takes considerable time and effort. It can be difficult to trace the people responsible for eligible studies and they may be initially reluctant to participate in the meta-analysis. Often the first approach will be by letter, inviting collaboration, explaining the project, describing what participation will entail and how the meta-analysis will be managed and published. The letter is often from the project team and might be sent on behalf of the advisory group for the review. A protocol is generally supplied at this stage to provide further information, but data are not usually sought in the first correspondence. It may also be necessary to establish separate contact with the data centre or research organization who are (or have been) responsible for management of the study data, and to whom data queries will need to be sent. In encouraging the original investigators to take part in the IPD review, it is important to be as supportive and flexible as possible, to take the time required to build relationships and to keep all collaborators involved and informed of progress. Regular newsletters and e-mail updates can be useful ways of keeping the collaborative group up to date and involved, especially if the project will take place over a prolonged period.

### 18.2.3   Confidentiality

Researchers naturally require safeguards on the use of their study data and wish to ensure that it will be stored securely and used appropriately. For this reason, a signed confidentiality agreement is often used as a 'contract' between the original investigators and the IPD review team. The details of such agreements will vary, but most will state that data will be held securely, be accessed only by authorized members of the project team and will not be copied or distributed elsewhere. It is also good practice to request that individual participants are de-identified in supplied data, such that individuals are identified only by a study identifier code and not by name. This seems to be an increasing requirement for obtaining IPD from some countries where data protection legislation requires that a participant cannot be identified from the data supplied. Data sent by email should be encrypted wherever possible.

## 18.3　Dealing with data

### 18.3.1　Deciding what data to collect

The protocol should specify what outcomes and patient characteristics are to be analysed. However, before embarking on data collection it is sensible to ask the original investigators about what data are actually available. When deciding which variables to collect, it is often sensible to start by considering carefully what analyses are planned and what data will be needed to do them. This minimizes the possibility that essential information will not be sought or that unnecessary data will be collected. Understandably, investigators can get upset or suspicious if they have gone to the trouble of providing data that are not subsequently analysed and reported.

Although in many cases it will be possible to collect specific variables for outcomes and characteristics as defined in the individual studies, it may be necessary to consider whether there are any data items for which further or constituent variables may be required. For instance, if studies have used different definitions of outcomes it may be desirable to redefine these for each patient in a consistent way across studies, and additional variables may be needed. For example, to redefine pre-eclampsia, data on systolic and diastolic blood pressure and proteinurea would need to be collected.

### 18.3.2　Data format

Once original investigators have agreed to collaborate, the next step is to provide clear instructions on what data they need to supply and on any preferred data format. The project team should be prepared to accept data in whatever format is most convenient for those supplying it, whether that is electronically, as printouts, or on paper forms, and should be prepared to recode information as necessary. However, although the early IPD meta-analyses in the 1980s relied heavily on data being supplied on paper, most information is now supplied by email or on disk, and investigators are often willing to transform or code their data according to the specified format.

### 18.3.3　Re-coding and re-defining supplied variables

Collecting data at the level of the individual participant enables translation between different staging, grading, ranking or other scoring systems, and may therefore allow pooling of data from studies that would not otherwise be possible, because of differences between the data collection tools. To allow this, it is important that the appropriate data are sought (see Section 18.3.1) and that the data supplied are recoded or transformed to reflect common definitions. For example, if the outcome of interest is pre-eclampsia, data on blood pressure and proteinurea would need to be collected and considered together to define whether the pre-eclampsia (according to the review protocol definition) had been observed.

## 18.3.4  Checking data supplied

The aims of checking data are to increase the probability that data supplied are accurate, to confirm that trials are appropriately randomized, and where appropriate to make sure that, as far as possible, the data are up to date. The exact checking procedures to be carried out will depend on the healthcare area and question addressed, as well as the nature of the data supplied, but four main areas are typical:

### 18.3.4.1  Checking for missing or duplicated data

When data are received, it is important to check these as soon as possible to ensure that they can be read and loaded into the central analysis system. For example, if the data arrive as email attachments, it should be checked that the files can be opened and that the information is for the correct study. At this stage it is useful to confirm that data have been received for all appropriate (usually all randomized) individuals, checking that the numbers supplied are consistent with any publications or other information and that, for example, there are no obvious omissions or duplicates in the sequence of patient record or study identifier numbers.

### 18.3.4.2  Checking plausibility

Plausibility checks should include range checks on variables supplied, asking the original investigators to confirm any extreme outliers or unusual values: for example, confirming that records of unusually old or young patients or those with abnormally high or low cholesterol levels are indeed correct. Information supplied should also be checked against any relevant study publications, for example by confirming that the distribution of baseline characteristics, the number of participants and outcome results are consistent (bearing in mind that continued enrolment or additional follow-up may have altered information subsequent to publication).

### 18.3.4.3  Checking randomization

It is often helpful to check that randomization appears to have been done appropriately. Where dates of randomization are available, this can be explored by looking at plots of cumulative accrual over time; one would expect numbers enrolled to each intervention to be similar and for enrolment curves to cross frequently. It can also be informative to look at the distribution of randomizations by day of the week. Here, provided that reasonable numbers of individuals have been randomized, one would expect to see roughly the same numbers randomized to each intervention on any given weekday, and that trials randomizing during normal clinic hours have few, if any, participants enrolled on unexpected days. It is also useful to check that the intervention groups are balanced for important baseline characteristics and within important participant subgroups, but bearing in mind that statistically significant imbalances can occur by chance.

### 18.3.4.4 Checking information is up to date

For outcomes where events are observed over a prolonged period, for example survival in cancer trials, it is important to check that follow-up is as up to date as possible and that it is consistent for each of the intervention groups. Producing a 'reverse' Kaplan Meier curve, based on just those patients who have not experienced the event of interest, with censoring then used as the event, can provide a useful check on the balance of follow-up across the groups.

For any individual study, the results of all these checks should be considered together to build up an overall picture of the study and the quality of the data that have been supplied, and any potential problems. Any concerns should be brought diplomatically to the attention of the researchers responsible. Usually, problems turn out to be simple errors or misunderstandings, which can be resolved through discussion. Major problems that cannot be resolved are rare.

A copy of the data as supplied should be archived before carrying out conversions or modifications to the data. Throughout the data checking processes, it is important that any changes and alterations made to the supplied data are properly logged.

## 18.4 Analysis

### 18.4.1 Analysis advantages

Having access to the 'raw' data for each study enables checking, thorough exploration, and re-analysis of the data in a consistent way. Thus, one does not have to rely on interpreting information and analyses presented in published reports, be constrained by summary data provided in tabular format, or be forced to consider combining the summary statistics from studies that have been calculated in different ways. It also avoids problems with the original analyses; for example it might be possible to carry out analyses according to intention-to-treat principles, even if the original trial analyses did not do this.

### 18.4.2 General approach

Most IPD meta-analyses to date have used a two-stage approach to analysis. In the first stage, each individual study is analysed in the same way, as set out in the meta-analysis protocol or analysis plan. In the second step, the results, or summary statistics, of each of these individual study analyses are combined to provide a pooled estimate of effect in the same way as for a conventional systematic review (Simmonds 2005). More complex approaches using multilevel modelling have been described for binary data (Turner 2000), continuous data (Higgins 2001), ordinal data (Whitehead 2001) and time-to-event data (Tudor Smith 2005b) but, currently, their application is less common. When there is no heterogeneity between trials, a stratified log-rank two-stage approach for time-to-event data may be best avoided for estimating larger intervention effects (Tudor Smith 2005a).

### 18.4.3    Time-to-event analyses

Collecting IPD that include the time interval between the randomization and the event of interest enables time-to-event analyses to be conducted. These include, for example, time to recovery, time free of seizures, time to conception and time to death. Indeed, one of the main reasons that IPD meta-analyses have been so important in the cancer field is that time-to-event analysis of survival is vital in evaluating therapies. Most interventions are more likely to lead to a prolongation of survival rather than a cure. Therefore, it is important to measure not only whether a death happens, but also the time at which it takes place. To allow this type of analysis one needs to know the time that each individual spends 'event-free'. This is usually collected as the date of randomization, the event status (i.e. whether the event was observed or not) and the date of last evaluation for the event. Sometimes, it will be collected as the interval in days between randomization and the most recent evaluation for the event. Time-to-event analyses are performed for each trial to calculate hazard ratios, which are then pooled in the meta-analysis (see Section 9.4.9).

### 18.4.4    Bringing analyses up to date: long-term outcomes

For outcomes such as survival, where events can continue to take place over time, IPD meta-analyses can provide an important opportunity to examine the effects of interventions over a prolonged period. They can also provide an opportunity for researchers to provide more up-to-date data for relevant outcomes such as mortality than they have published for their study.

### 18.4.5    Subgroup analysis

Collecting IPD is also the most practical way to carry out analyses to investigate whether any observed effect of an intervention is consistent across well-defined types of participants, for example whether women gain a smaller or larger benefit from treatment than men. In conventional analyses using aggregate data from publications, it is usually very difficult to extract sufficient compatible data to undertake meaningful subgroup analyses, and especially difficult to characterize individuals by more than one factor at a time. In contrast, IPD permit straightforward categorization of individuals for subgroup analysis (stratified by study) defined by single or multiple factors. The collection of IPD will also allow more complex analyses, such as multilevel modelling, to explore associations between intervention effects and patient characteristics.

### 18.4.6 Additional analyses

Access to the IPD also permits an in-depth exploration of patient characteristics themselves, irrespective of the intervention. For example, the large datasets collected can be used in the construction of prognostic indices that may be able to predict outcome based on patient characteristics. (International Germ Cell Cancer Collaborative Group 1997).

### 18.4.7 Software

IPD cannot be analysed directly in RevMan. The data need to be first analysed outside of this software, and summary statistics for each study may be entered into RevMan if a two-stage approach is used. For dichotomous and continuous outcomes, data may be entered in the usual way. For time-to-event outcomes, the observed-minus-expected number of events and variance may be entered using the 'O − E and Variance' option. Alternatively the generic inverse-variance option may be used to analyse effect estimates such as hazard ratios, rate ratios or adjusted estimates.

Although many standard statistical packages can perform the necessary analyses of IPD from the individual studies, it can be unwieldy and time-consuming to have to analyse each outcome in each study one at a time, and commercially available software is not currently available that supports the direct analysis, pooling and plotting of IPD in a meta-analysis. A non-commercial analysis package, 'SCHARP', which analyses each study, pools results and outputs tabulated results and forest plots for dichotomous, continuous and time-to-event IPD, is available free of charge to not-for-profit organizations. This SAS-based package has been developed by the Meta-analysis Group of the UK Medical Research Council Clinical Trials Unit. It is available from the authors, who can be contacted through the IPD Meta-analysis Methods Group (see Box 18.6.a).

## 18.5 Limitations and caveats

### 18.5.1 What an IPD review cannot fix

Although the IPD approach can help avoid problems associated with the analyses and reporting of studies, it cannot, generally, help avoid bias associated with study design or conduct. If there are such problems (which would also be reflected in study publications and any systematic reviews based upon them), the study may need to be excluded from the meta-analysis.

## 18.5.2 Unavailable studies

Obtaining IPD often enables inclusion of studies that could not be included in a standard systematic review because they are either unpublished or do not report sufficient information to allow them to be included in the analyses. This may help avoid many types of publication bias (Stewart 2002). However, one must ensure that by restricting analyses to those studies that can supply IPD, bias is not introduced through selective availability of study data.

The success and validity of the IPD approach requires that data from all or nearly all studies will be available. If unavailability is related to the study results, for example if investigators are keen to supply data from studies with promising results but reluctant to provide data from those that were less encouraging, then ignoring the unavailable studies could bias the results of the IPD review. If a large proportion of the data have been obtained, perhaps 90% or more of individuals randomized, we can be relatively confident of the results. However, with less information we need to be suitably circumspect in drawing conclusions. Sensitivity analysis combining the results of any unavailable studies (as extracted from publications or obtained in tabular form) and comparing these with the main IPD results are a useful aid to interpreting the data. Reports of IPD reviews that were unable to obtain IPD from all studies should state reasons why IPD were not available, and the likelihood of ensuing bias.

As for other types of Cochrane review, IPD meta-analyses should clearly state what studies were not included and the reasons why. If only a limited number of studies are able to provide IPD for analysis, then the value of the approach is questionable. Experiences in cancer have been good and in most cases perseverance has led to data being available from a high proportion of eligible trials. This can make it especially important to explore the ability and willingness of the primary investigators to supply IPD at an early stage in the project.

## 18.5.3 Deciding when an IPD review is appropriate

When initiating any systematic review it is useful to consider carefully which approach and which type of data will be most appropriate at the outset. Particular thought should be given to factors that are likely to introduce bias to the review. There may be cases where the benefits of obtaining IPD turn out to be marginal, and others where it could be vital.

## 18.6 Chapter information

**Authors**: Lesley A Stewart, Jayne F Tierney and Mike Clarke on behalf of the Cochrane Individual Patient Data Meta-analysis Methods Group.

**This chapter should be cited as**: Stewart LA, Tierney JF, Clarke M. Chapter 19: Reviews of individual patient data. In: Higgins JPT, Green S (editors), *Cochrane Handbook for Systematic Reviews of Interventions*. Chichester (UK): John Wiley & Sons, 2008.

**Acknowledgements**: We thank Paula Williamson for helpful comments on an earlier draft.

---

**Box 18.6.a  The Cochrane Individual Patient Data Meta-analysis Methods Group**

The Individual Patient Data Meta-analysis Methods Group (IPD MA MG) comprises individuals who are involved or interested in the conduct of systematic reviews that include IPD and related methodological research. The Group aims to provide guidance to those undertaking IPD meta-analyses within Cochrane reviews.

Activities of IPD MA MG members include the following:

- Undertaking IPD meta-analyses.
- Undertaking empirical research, for example in the relative benefits of IPD meta-analyses compared with other forms of systematic review. and using information collected for IPD meta-analyses to explore whether aspects of design, analysis and reporting of randomized trials and systematic reviews may be sources of bias and heterogeneity.
- Helping authors of Cochrane reviews decide whether it would be appropriate for their systematic review to be conducted using IPD and, if so, to offer advice on how to do so.
- Offering training workshops at Cochrane Colloquia and disseminating training materials from these.
- Maintaining a register of reviews that have used (or will use) IPD and a database of methodological research projects and meta-analyses.

*Web site*: www.ctu.mrc.ac.uk/cochrane/ipdmg

---

# 18.7  References

**Clarke 1998**
Clarke M, Stewart L, Pignon JP, Bijnens L. Individual patient data meta-analysis in cancer. *British Journal of Cancer* 1998; 77: 2036–2044.

**Higgins 2001**
Higgins JPT, Whitehead A, Turner RM, Omar RZ, Thompson SG. Meta-analysis of continuous outcome data from individual patients. *Statistics in Medicine* 2001; 20: 2219–2241.

**International Germ Cell Cancer Collaborative Group 1997**
International Germ Cell Cancer Collaborative Group. International Germ Cell Consensus Classification: a prognostic factor-based staging system for metastatic germ cell cancers. *Journal of Clinical Oncology* 1997; 15: 594–603.

**Simmonds 2005**
Simmonds MC, Higgins JPT, Stewart LA, Tierney JF, Clarke MJ, Thompson SG. Meta-analysis of individual patient data from randomized trials: a review of methods used in practice. *Clinical Trials* 2005; 2: 209–217.

**Stewart 1995**

Stewart LA, Clarke MJ. Practical methodology of meta-analyses (overviews) using updated individual patient data. *Statistics in Medicine* 1995; 14: 2057–2079.

**Stewart 2002**

Stewart LA, Tierney JF. To IPD or not to IPD? Advantages and disadvantages of systematic reviews using individual patient data. *Evaluation in the Health Professions* 2002; 25: 76–97.

**Tudor Smith 2005a**

Tudor Smith C, Williamson PR. Meta-analysis of individual patient data with time to event outcomes. *International Conference of the Royal Statistical Society*, Cardiff (UK), 2005.

**Tudor Smith 2005b**

Tudor Smith C, Williamson PR, Marson AG. Investigating heterogeneity in an individual patient data meta-analysis of time to event outcomes. *Statistics in Medicine* 2005; 24: 1307–1319.

**Turner 2000**

Turner RM, Omar RZ, Yang M, Goldstein H, Thompson SG. A multilevel model framework for meta-analysis of clinical trials with binary outcomes. *Statistics in Medicine* 2000; 19: 3417–3432.

**Whitehead 2001**

Whitehead A, Omar RZ, Higgins JPT, Savaluny E, Turner RM, Thompson SG. Meta-analysis of ordinal outcomes using individual patient data. *Statistics in Medicine* 2001; 20: 2243–2260.

# 19 Prospective meta-analysis

Davina Ghersi, Jesse Berlin and Lisa Askie on behalf of
the Cochrane Prospective Meta-analysis Methods Group

## Key Points

- A prospective meta-analysis is a meta-analysis of studies (usually randomized trials) that were identified, evaluated and determined to be eligible for the meta-analysis before the results of any of those studies became known.

- Prospective meta-analyses enable hypotheses to be specified in advance of the results of individual trials; enable prospective application of study selection criteria; and enable *a priori* statements of intended analyses. As meta-analyses rather than multi-centre trials, they allow variation in the protocols of the included studies, while maximizing power in the pre-planned meta-analyses.

- Prospective meta-analyses are usually undertaken by a collaborative group, and they usually collect and analyse individual patient data.

- Protocols are important for prospective meta-analyses, and they may be published as protocols for Cochrane reviews. The Cochrane Prospective Meta-analysis Methods Group maintains a registry of prospective meta-analysis projects and is able to provide advice on their conduct.

## 19.1 Introduction

### 19.1.1 What is a prospective meta-analysis?

A properly conducted systematic review defines the question to be addressed in advance of the identification of potentially eligible trials. Systematic reviews are by nature, however, retrospective because the trials included are usually identified after the trials have been completed and the results reported (Pogue 1998, Zanchetti 1998). Knowledge of the results of individual randomized trials may introduce bias into a retrospective systematic review if the selection of the key components of the review question is based on reports of one or more positive trials. This might include influencing:

- the criteria for study selection (i.e. the types of trial considered eligible);
- the selection of the target population;
- the nature of the intervention;
- the choice of comparator; and
- the outcomes to be assessed and their measures.

Take, for example, a systematic review in which the results of one study are in the opposite direction to those of the other studies in the review. The authors of the review discuss possible explanations for this apparent heterogeneity and decide that there is a clinical explanation. On this basis, the authors subsequently decide to exclude the study. This may be a reasonable decision; however, it is one made after the effect of the study's results on the overall summary estimate is known, and hence is intrinsically problematic.

As described in detail in Chapter 10 (Section 10.2), awareness of the results of a trial may also influence the decision to publish those results. Even within a published trial, results may be selectively reported, thereby introducing a more subtle form of publication bias into the review (Chan 2004).

A prospective meta-analysis (PMA) is a meta-analysis of studies (usually randomized trials) that were identified, evaluated and determined to be eligible for the meta-analysis before the results of any of those studies became known. They have features in common with both cumulative meta-analyses and those involving individual patient data (Egger 1997). PMA can help to overcome some of the recognized problems of retrospective meta-analyses (see also Chapter 18, Section 18.5) by:

- Enabling hypotheses to be specified a priori ignorant of the results of individual trials;

- Enabling prospective application of study selection criteria;

- Enabling *a priori* statements of intended analyses, including subgroup analyses, to be made before the results of individual trials are known. This avoids potential difficulties in interpretation related to the data-dependent emphasis on particular subgroups.

Systematic reviews also depend on the ability of the review authors to obtain data on all randomized patients for the relevant outcomes, which can be difficult if full information is not reported in the trial publications. As most PMAs will collect and analyse individual patient data (IPD) they will be able to overcome this problem, with the additional advantage of being able to conduct time-to-event analyses if appropriate. Planned subgroup analyses based on patient-level factors can give misleading results if relying only on aggregate-level data, highlighting another advantage of IPD. PMA also provides a unique opportunity for trial design, data collection and other clinical trial processes to be standardized across trials. For example, the investigators may agree to use the same instrument to measure a particular outcome, and to measure the outcome at the same time-points in each trial. In a Cochrane review of interventions for preventing obesity in children, for example, the heterogeneity and unreliability of the some of the outcome measures made it difficult to pool data across trials (Summerbell 2005). A prospective meta-analysis of this question has proposed a set of commonly shared standards, so that some of the issues raised by lack of standardization can be addressed (Steinbeck 2006).

## 19.1.2 What is the difference between a prospective meta-analysis and a large multi-centre trial?

Prospective meta-analyses are an attractive option to clinical trialists who, although appreciating the benefits of single, adequately sized trials, are unable to undertake them (Simes 1987, Probstfield 1998). It can be a useful methodology, for example, when large sample sizes are required to ensure adequate power, but single, large-scale trials are not feasible. This could be due to local interests preventing participation in a trial when information is perceived to be 'lost overseas'. This can also be a particular problem in rare diseases where gaining access to large numbers of trial participants in a timely manner may be difficult.

Hence, an alternative is for investigators to conduct their own study locally, and to collaborate with the investigators of similar studies, arranging for the results to be combined at the completion of each trial. This enables individual investigators to maintain a certain amount of autonomy, and at the same time to plan appropriately for the meta-analysis. Another situation where it may be beneficial, particularly in the absence of mandatory prospective registration of randomized trials, is when two or more trials addressing the same question commence and the investigators are ignorant of the existence of the other trial(s). Once similar trials are identified, investigators can collaborate (adapting data collection if necessary) and plan prospectively to combine their results in a meta-analysis.

What also distinguishes a PMA from a multicentre trial is that there is no requirement in a PMA for the protocols to be identical across studies. Variety in the design of the studies may be viewed by some as a desirable feature of PMA, and thus a degree of expected variation in populations or in aspects of the interventions is considered acceptable. FICSIT (Frailty and Injuries: Cooperative Studies of Intervention Techniques) is an example of a pre-planned meta-analysis of eight studies of exercise-based interventions in a frail elderly population (Schechtman 2001). The eight FICSIT sites defined their own interventions using site-specific endpoints and evaluations and differing entry criteria (except that all participants were elderly). This deliberate introduction of *systematic* variability in design, known as a 'meta-experimental design', is a possible approach to PMA (Cholesterol Treatment Trialists' (CTT) Collaborators 2005).

### 19.1.3    What healthcare areas have used the prospective meta-analysis approach?

Prospective meta-analysis is a method that has been utilized in recent years by trialists in cardiovascular disease (Simes 1995, WHO–ISI Blood Pressure Lowering Treatment Trialists' Collaboration 1998), childhood leukaemia (Shuster 1996, Valsecchi 1996) and childhood and adolescent obesity (Steinbeck 2006). In addition, some have identified areas, such as infectious diseases, where the opportunity to use PMA has largely been missed (Ioannidis 1999). The Cochrane Prospective Meta-analysis Methods Group web site includes a list of ongoing and completed PMA where further information can be found (Ghersi 2005).

### 19.1.4    What resources do I need?

PMAs are significant undertakings and should not be embarked on lightly. They are likely to take many years to complete and require a committed, ongoing, appropriately staffed and adequately funded Secretariat. Once the PMA collaborative group is formed (see Section 19.2) resources are needed to ensure the ongoing commitment of the group over many years, usually a much longer time period than is required for a retrospective IPD review (see Chapter 18). The Secretariat will be required to organize regular teleconferences, face-to-face meetings (at least annually), newsletters, update contact details and implement other mechanisms to keep the collaborative group together. This type of activity is akin to that undertaken by the co-ordinating centre of a multicentre randomized trial. A benefit of these Secretariat activities is that they often help facilitate adherence to the PMA protocol and encourage complete follow-up within individual participating trials.

## 19.2    The collaborative nature of prospective meta-analyses

### 19.2.1    Collaborative groups

As with IPD meta-analyses (see Chapter 18, Section 18.2.1) most PMA are carried out and published by collaborative groups. The collaborative group should include representatives from each of the participating trials and will usually have a steering group or Secretariat who manages the project on a day-to-day basis. The collaborative group may choose to create small, *ad hoc* groups to address specific issues as they arise, and to provide advice to the steering group or Secretariat on clinical, technical or other issues that may impact on the project.

## 19.2.2 Negotiating collaboration

As with IPD meta-analyses (see Chapter 18, Section 18.2.2) negotiating and establishing a strong collaboration with the participating trialists is essential for the success of a PMA. The focus of a PMA, however, is not primarily about locating and obtaining data from individual trials. As the collaboration needs to be formed prior to the results of any trial being known, the focus of a PMA's collaborative efforts, at least initially, is on reaching agreement regarding study population, design and data collection methods for each of the participating studies. When members of a PMA collaborative group agree to participate in the project, they need to agree to a core common protocol and core common data items that will be collected across all trials. Individual trials can include local protocol amendments or additional data items but they need to ensure that these will not compromise the core common protocol elements.

In a PMA, efforts are made to identify *all* ongoing trials, both to maximize precision and to avoid bias that might be introduced by excluding studies based (at least in part) on knowledge of the results of those studies. To certify that an individual study is eligible for inclusion in the PMA there should be evidence to support the claim that, at the time of the agreement to be part of the PMA, trial results were not known outside the trial's own data monitoring committee. This should ideally be in the form of evidence that the trial was prospectively registered (Laine 2007). It is also advisable for the collaborative group to obtain an explicit (and signed) agreement from each of the trial groups to collaborate. The idea is to encourage substantive contributions by the individual investigators and to get 'buy-in' to the concept of the PMA and the details of the protocol.

## 19.2.3 Confidentiality

Confidentiality issues regarding data anonymity and security are similar to those described for IPD meta-analyses in Chapter 18 (Section 18.2.3). Specific issues for PMA include adequate planning regarding how to deal with trials within the PMA that reach completion and will publish their results, and how to manage issues relating to data and safety monitoring, including the impact of interim analyses of individual trials in the PMA, or possibly a pooled interim analysis of the PMA (see also Section 19.5.2).

# 19.3 The prospective meta-analysis protocol

## 19.3.1 What should the protocol contain?

All PMAs should have a publicly available protocol. Developing a protocol for a PMA is similar, conceptually, to doing so for a single trial. The essential elements of a PMA are detailed as follows and summarized in Box 19.3.a.

---

### Box 19.3.a    Elements of a prospective meta-analysis protocol

**Objectives:**
- Define the specific hypotheses/objectives.

**Methods: Criteria for considering studies for this review:**
- Eligibility criteria for trial design (e.g. requirements for randomization, minimum follow-up);
- Eligibility criteria for the patient population;
- Eligibility criteria for each intervention and comparator;
- Outcomes information: specification of primary and secondary endpoints, definitions, measurement instruments, timing;
- Details of subgroups.

**Methods: Search methods for identification of studies:**
- Describe efforts made to identify ongoing trials.

**Methods: Data collection and analysis:**
- Trial details:
  - List details of trials identified for inclusion;
  - A statement outlining if, at the time of submission for registration of the PMA, any trial results were known (to anyone outside the trial's own data monitoring committee). Trials should be included only if their results were unknown at the time they were identified and added to the PMA;
  - Whether a signed agreement to collaborate has been obtained from the appropriate representative of each trial (e.g. the Sponsor or Principal Investigator).
- Analysis Plan:
  - Details of sample size and power calculation (for the PMA), interim analyses, subgroup analyses etc.
- Management and Co-ordination:
  - Details of management structure and committees;
  - Data management (data to be collected, format required, when required, quality assurance procedures, etc);
  - Responsibility for statistical analyses.
- Publication Policy:
  - Policy regarding authorship (e.g. publication in 'group' name);
  - Writing Committee (membership, responsibilities);
  - Policy regarding manuscript (e.g. circulated to all trialists for comment).

---

*Objectives, eligibility and outcomes*    As in any protocol, the first important step is to define the hypotheses and then to establish eligibility criteria for studies. For example, studies to be included in the PMA may be required to use random assignment of participants to interventions, although it is possible to include other study designs in a PMA. If randomized, the individual trials may choose to share a common randomization method, or at least to use the same stratification factors. The required attributes of the participating population need to be specified, as do the minimum requirements for each of the interventions and the comparator arms. The protocol should also specify what outcomes need to be measured, when and how they should be measured, and which are primary and which are secondary, as well as other features of study design as necessary. If a PMA is established de novo, it may be possible for each trial in the PMA to share exactly the same trial protocol.

*Search methods*   The protocol should describe in detail the efforts made to identify ongoing trials, including how potential collaborators have been (or will be) located and approached to participate.

*Trial details*   Details of trials already identified for inclusion (if relevant) should be listed in the protocol. The listing might include the anticipated number of participants and timelines for each participating trial. The protocol should include a statement outlining if, at the time of submission for registration, any trial results were known (to anyone outside the trial's own data monitoring committee). Trials should be included only if their results were unknown at the time they were identified and added to the PMA. If eligible trials are identified but not included in the PMA because their results are already known, the PMA protocol should outline how these data will be dealt with. For example, secondary sensitivity analyses using aggregate or individual patient data from these trials might be undertaken. The protocol should describe actions to be taken if subsequent trials are located while the PMA is in progress.

*Analysis plan*   The protocol should outline the plans for the collection and analyses of data in a similar manner to that of an IPD meta-analyses (see Chapter 18). This would include details of sample size and power calculation (for the PMA), any interim analyses to be undertaken, and details of planned subgroup analyses. Strategies for addressing additional questions beyond the main hypothesis of interest can also be incorporated in a PMA. These additional questions can be added as long as the results of studies to be included in the analysis are not known, i.e. they not 'data-driven' research questions. Of note, there may be analyses that are unique to the PMA, that are *not* done within the individual trials, such as subgroup analyses.

The investigators of trials to be included in a PMA should generally be asked to agree to provide individual patient data. The protocol should describe what will occur if the investigators of some studies within the PMA are unable (or unwilling) to provide patient-level data, perhaps because of concerns about confidentiality or informed consent. Would the PMA Secretariat, for example, accept appropriate summary data? (A two-stage analysis could be performed, in which the effect estimate of interest is calculated separately within each study, using the patient-level data, and those within-study estimates are then combined across studies using standard meta-analytic methods.) The protocol should specify whether it is intended to update the PMA data at regular intervals via ongoing cycles of data collection (e.g. 5 yearly), and hence when trialists would be expected to supply updated, long-term outcome data.

*Management and co-ordination*    The PMA protocol should outline details of project management structure (including any committees, see Section 19.2.1), the procedures for data management (how data are to be collected, the format required, when data will be required to be submitted, quality assurance procedures, etc; see Chapter 18, Section 18.3), and who will be responsible for the statistical analyses.

*Publication policy*    A key element of the PMA protocol is the publication policy. It is essential to have a policy regarding authorship (e.g. specifying that publication will be in the group name, but also include a list of individual authors). A policy regarding manuscript preparation is also important. For example, it might be specified that drafts of papers be circulated to all trialists for comment, prior to submission for publication. There might be a writing committee, like those that are often formed within cooperative study groups.

A unique issue that arises in the context of the PMA (which would generally not arise for a multicentre study or an IPD meta-analysis) is whether or not individual studies should publish on their own and the timing of those publications. Most investigators would want to publish their own studies individually in addition to contributing to the PMA, and it is likely that the investigators would want these publications to appear before the PMA is published, so as to avoid issues related to duplicate publication of the same data. In a similar spirit, though, any PMA publication(s) should clearly indicate the sources of the included data and refer to prior publications of the same data. The PMA protocol should also state what will occur if any of the participating trials fail to publish their individual results within a specified timeframe. This may occur if a trial is not completed due to insufficient funds, is terminated prematurely or the trial simply remains unpublished after a pre-specified date. The protocol should also address how to deal with trials that renege on their agreement to participate in the PMA.

### 19.3.2    Publication of the protocol

If prepared as a Cochrane review, the PMA protocol should be submitted to the appropriate Cochrane Review Group to appear in the *Cochrane Database of Systematic Reviews*. Otherwise, a protocol should be published elsewhere (for example, the CTT/PPP Protocol (Cholesterol Treatment Trialists' (CTT) Collaborators 2005)). It is also desirable that PMA projects are registered on the Cochrane Prospective Meta-analysis Methods Group web site (see Box 19.6.a) and information about the project should be updated at least annually. Each trial within the PMA should be registered on a publicly accessible, WHO recognized, Primary Registry (www.who.int/ictrp/network/list_registers) prior to enrolment of the first participant, in accordance with international requirements (Sim 2006, Laine 2007).

## 19.4    Data collection in prospective meta-analysis

Participating trials in a PMA usually supply individual patient data once their individual trial is completed and published. The advantage of the PMA design is that trialists prospectively decide what data they will collect and in what format, making the need to redefine and recode supplied data less problematic than is often the case with a retrospective IPD. The PMA should develop a data transfer protocol that may incorporate current data interchange standards, such as those developed by the Clinical Data Interchange Standard Consortium (CDISC; www.cdisc.org).

Once data are received by the PMA Secretariat, they should be rigorously checked using the same procedures as for IPD meta-analyses, including checking for missing or duplicated data, running data plausibility checks, assessing patterns of randomization and ensuring the information supplied is up to date (see Chapter 18, Section 18.4.4). Data queries will be resolved by direct consultation with the individual trialists before being included in the final dataset for analysis.

# 19.5 Analysis issues in prospective meta-analysis

## 19.5.1 General approach

Most PMAs will use similar general analysis techniques to that of retrospective IPD meta-analyses. These techniques are outlined in detail in Chapter 18 (Section 18.4) and include the general approach to these analyses and the ability to undertake time-to-event analyses (if appropriate). The use of patient-level data also permits more statistically powerful subgroup analyses and multilevel modelling to explore associations between intervention effects and patient characteristics, as well as prognostic modelling in some cases. Chapter 18 (Section 18.4.7) describes some of the potential software packages that can be used to analyse these types of data.

## 19.5.2 Interim analysis and data monitoring

It is increasingly common practice for individual clinical trials to include a plan for interim analyses of the data, and to monitor safety. PMA offers a unique opportunity to perform these interim looks using the data contributed by all trials. The data may be pooled for this analysis, or looked at separately for each trial and the results then shared amongst the data monitoring committees of the participating trials.

The ability to perform interim analyses raises a number of ethical issues. Is it, for example, appropriate to continue randomization to ongoing studies after an overall benefit (in terms of the primary outcome, for example) of an intervention has been demonstrated? When results are not known in the subgroups of clinical interest, or for less common endpoints, should the investigators proceed with the study to obtain further information on overall net clinical benefit, for example, evidence of benefit for one outcome but not another, or evidence of harm.

If each trial has its own data monitoring committee, then communication among committees might be beneficial in this regard, as recommended by Hillman and Louis (Hillman 2003). The various committees would need to be aware of the other trials included within the PMA and their results, because these external considerations might influence the decisions made by a given monitoring committee: for example, whether or not to close a study early because of evidence of efficacy. Conversely, it might be argued that knowledge of emerging safety data from all participating trials might reduce the chances of spurious early stopping of an individual trial due to concerns about interim safety outcomes. It would be helpful, thus, for the various trial data safety monitoring committees to adopt a common understanding that individual trials should not be stopped until the goals of the PMA, with respect to subgroups and uncommon endpoints (or 'net clinical benefit'), are achieved.

Another possible option might be to consider limiting enrolment in the continuing trials to patients in the subgroup(s) of interest if such a decision makes clinical and statistical sense. In any case, it might be appropriate to apply the concepts of sequential clinical trials methodology, such as the approach described by Whitehead (Whitehead 1997), to derive rigorous and stringent stopping rules for the PMA as individual trial results become available.

---

### Box 19.5.a  The Cochrane Prospective Meta-analysis Methods Group

The role of the Prospective Meta-analysis Methods Group (PMA MG) is:

- To provide a mechanism to enable the registration of prospective meta-analyses:
  - cochrane (via Cochrane Review Groups); and
  - non-Cochrane (via PMA MG).
- To provide a mechanism for evaluating protocols submitted for registration to ensure they are indeed prospective meta-analyses. This may be achieved by:
  - providing training for members of Cochrane Review Groups (e.g. editors and peer-reviewers);
  - members of the PMA MG peer reviewing protocols; and
  - a checklist for investigators performing or peer-reviewing a PMA.
- To develop appropriate methodological standards for prospective meta-analyses.
- To provide advice and support to those embarking on (or contemplating) prospective meta-analyses.

Membership of the group is open to anyone who is conducting, has conducted, or is interested in conducting a prospective meta-analysis, regardless of the area of health care investigated. To join, individuals are asked to detail their level of commitment on a Prospective Meta-analysis Methods Group Questionnaire (available on the PMA web site, below). Members will be asked to update this information annually.

*Web site*: www.cochrane.org/docs/pma.htm

## 19.6   Chapter information

**Authors**: Davina Ghersi, Jesse Berlin and Lisa Askie on behalf of the Cochrane Prospective Meta-analysis Methods Group.

**This chapter should be cited as**: Ghersi D, Berlin J, Askie L. Chapter 19: Prospective meta-analysis. In: Higgins JPT, Green S (editors), *Cochrane Handbook for Systematic Reviews of Interventions*. Chichester (UK): John Wiley & Sons, 2008.

## 19.7   References

**Chan 2004**
Chan AW, Hróbjartsson A, Haahr MT, Gøtzsche PC, Altman DG. Empirical evidence for selective reporting of outcomes in randomized trials: comparison of protocols to published articles. *JAMA* 2004; 291: 2457–2465.

**Cholesterol Treatment Trialists' (CTT) Collaborators 2005**
Cholesterol Treatment Trialists' (CTT) Collaborators. Efficacy and safety of cholesterol-lowering treatment: prospective meta-analysis of data from 90 056 participants in 14 randomised trials of statins. *The Lancet* 2005; 366: 1267–1278.

**Egger 1997**
Egger M, Davey Smith G. Meta-analysis: potentials and promise. *BMJ* 1997; 315: 1371–1374.

**Ghersi 2005**
Ghersi D. Cochrane Prospective Meta-analysis Methods Group. *About the Cochrane Collaboration (Methods Groups)* 2005, Issue 2. Art No: CE000132.

**Hillman 2003**
Hillman DW, Louis TA. DSMB case study: decision making when a similar clinical trial is stopped early. *Controlled Clinical Trials* 2003; 24: 85–91.

**Ioannidis 1999**
Ioannidis JPA, Lau J. State of the evidence: current status and prospects of meta-analysis in infectious diseases. *Clinical Infectious Diseases* 1999; 29: 1178–1185.

**Laine 2007**
Laine C, Horton R, DeAngelis CD, Drazen JM, Frizelle FA, Godlee F, Haug C, Hebert PC, Kotzin S, Marusic A, Sahni P, Schroeder TV, Sox HC, Van der Weyden MB, Verheugt FW. Clinical trial registration: looking back and moving ahead. *Canadian Medical Association Journal* 2007; 177: 57–58.

**Pogue 1998**
Pogue J, Yusuf S. Overcoming the limitations of current meta-analysis of randomissed controlled trials. *The Lancet* 1998; 351: 47–52.

**Probstfield 1998**
Probstfield J, Applegate WB. Prospective meta-analysis: Ahoy! A clinical trial? *Journal of the American Geriatrics Society* 1988; 43: 452–453.

**Schechtman 2001**
Schechtman K, Ory M. The effects of exercise on the quality of life of frail older adults: a preplanned meta-analysis of the FICSIT trials. *Annals of Behavioural Medicine* 2001; 23: 186–197.

**Shuster 1996**
Shuster JJ, Gieser PW. Meta-analysis and prospective meta-analysis in childhood leukemia clinical research. *Annals of Oncology* 1996; 7: 1009–1014.

**Sim 2006**
Sim I, Chan AW, Gulmezoglu M, Evans T, Pang T. Clinical trial registration: transparency is the watchword. *The Lancet* 2006; 367: 1631–1633.

**Simes 1987**
Simes RJ. Confronting publication bias: a cohort design for meta-analysis. *Statistics in Medicine* 1987; 6: 11–29.

**Simes 1995**
Simes RJ. Prospective meta-analysis of cholesterol-lowering studies: the Prospective Pravastatin Pooling (PPP) Project and the Cholesterol Treatment Trialists' (CTT) Collaboration. *American Journal of Cardiology* 1995; 76: 122c–126c.

**Steinbeck 2006**
Steinbeck KS, Baur LA, Morris AM, Ghersi D. A proposed protocol for the development of a register of trials of weight management of childhood overweight and obesity. *International Journal of Obesity* 2006; 30: 2–5.

**Summerbell 2005**
Summerbell CD, Waters E, Edmunds LD, Kelly S, Brown T, Campbell KJ. Interventions for preventing obesity in children. *Cochrane Database of Systematic Reviews* 2005, Issue 3. Art No: CD001871.

**Valsecchi 1996**
Valsecchi MG, Masera G. A new challenge in clinical research in childhood ALL: the prospective meta-analysis strategy for intergroup collaboration. *Annals of Oncology* 1996; 7: 1005–1008.

**Whitehead 1997**
Whitehead A. A prospectively planned cumulative meta-analysis applied to a series of concurrent clinical trials. *Statistics in Medicine* 1997; 16: 2901–2913.

**WHO – ISI Blood Pressure Lowering Treatment Trialists' Collaboration 1998**
WHO – ISI Blood Pressure Lowering Treatment Trialists' Collaboration. Protocol for prospective collaborative overviews of major randomised trials of blood-pressure-lowering treatments. *Journal of Hypertension* 1998; 16: 127–137.

**Zanchetti 1998**
Zanchetti A, Mancia G. Searching for information from unreported trials – amnesty for the past and prospective meta-analysis for the future. *Journal of Hypertension* 1998; 16: 125.

# 20 Qualitative research and Cochrane reviews

Jane Noyes, Jennie Popay, Alan Pearson, Karin Hannes
and Andrew Booth on behalf of the Cochrane Qualitative
Research Methods Group

## Key Points

- Evidence from qualitative studies can play an important role in adding value to systematic reviews for policy, practice and consumer decision-making.

- It is likely that outcome studies included in Cochrane reviews will have qualitative research embedded within, or associated with, them.

- Qualitative research can contribute to Cochrane Intervention reviews in four ways:

  ○ informing reviews by using evidence from qualitative research to help define and refine the question, and to ensure the review includes appropriate studies and addresses important outcomes;

  ○ enhancing reviews by synthesizing evidence from qualitative research identified whilst looking for evidence of effectiveness;

  ○ extending reviews by undertaking a search to specifically seek out evidence from qualitative studies to address questions directly related to the effectiveness review; and

  ○ supplementing reviews by synthesizing qualitative evidence within a stand-alone, but complementary, qualitative review to address questions on aspects other than effectiveness.

- There are many methods of qualitative evidence synthesis that are appropriate to the aims and scope of Cochrane Intervention reviews.

- The synthesis of qualitative research is an area of debate and evolution. The Cochrane Qualitative Methods Group provides a forum for discussion and further development of methodology in this area.


## 20.1    Introduction

The purpose of this chapter is to outline ways in which qualitative research might be used to inform, enhance, extend and supplement Cochrane reviews. Qualitative evidence is not intended to contribute to the measures of effect of interventions, but rather to help explain, interpret and apply the results of a Cochrane review. In this way, evidence derived from qualitative studies complements systematic reviews of quantitative studies.

This chapter aims to enable authors to:

1. consider the types of reviews and review questions for which a synthesis of qualitative evidence could enhance or extend a Cochrane review;

2. consider the resource and methodological issues when deciding to synthesize qualitative evidence to complement a Cochrane review;

3. signpost some of the approaches and methods available for the synthesis of qualitative evidence; and

4. access further information, advice and resources if required.

The chapter is divided into two parts. The first part (Section 20.2) provides some considerations and guidance for the incorporation of evidence from qualitative research in Cochrane reviews, including resource implications. The second part (Section 20.3) provides a more general discussion of methodological issues, key reading and the role and details for the Cochrane Qualitative Research Methods Group. We provide an exemplar showing how a synthesis of qualitative evidence has been used to complement an existing Cochrane review of effects.


## 20.2    Incorporating evidence from qualitative research in Cochrane Intervention reviews: concepts and issues

### 20.2.1    Definition of qualitative research

Qualitative researchers study things in their natural settings, attempting to make sense of, or to interpret, phenomena in terms of the meanings people bring to them (Denzin

1994). Qualitative research is intended to penetrate to the deeper significance that the subject of the research ascribes to the topic being researched. It involves an interpretive, naturalistic approach to its subject matter and gives priority to what the data contribute to important research questions or existing information.

Within health care an understanding of the value of evidence from qualitative research to systematic reviews must consider the varied and diffuse nature of evidence (Popay 1998b, Pearson 2005). Qualitative research encompasses a range of philosophies, research designs and specific techniques including in-depth qualitative interviews; participant and non-participant observation; focus groups; document analyses; and a number of other methods of data collection (Pope 2006). Given this range of data types, there are also diverse methodological and theoretical approaches to study design and data analysis such as phenomenology; ethnography; grounded theory; action research; case studies; and a number of others. Theory and the researchers' perspective also play a key role in qualitative data analysis and in the bases on which generalizations to other contexts may be made.

Within the empirical sciences, the standing of a given theory or hypothesis is entirely dependent upon the quantity and character of the evidence in its favour. It is the relative weight of supporting evidence that allows us to choose between competing theories. Within the natural sciences, knowledge generation involves testing a hypothesis or a set of hypotheses by deriving consequences from it and then testing whether those consequences hold true by experiment and observation.

Health professionals seek evidence to substantiate the worth of a very wide range of activities and interventions and thus the type of evidence needed depends on the nature of the activity and its purpose. For many research questions, for example, those about parental beliefs and childhood vaccination (Mills 2005a, Mills 2005b), qualitative research is an appropriate and desirable methodology.

## 20.2.2   Using evidence from qualitative research in Cochrane reviews

Cochrane Intervention reviews aim primarily to determine whether an intervention is effective compared with a control and, if so, to estimate the size of the effect. High quality randomized trials are central to the endeavours of The Cochrane Collaboration in this respect. It is neither appropriate nor possible to include evidence from qualitative research in all Cochrane reviews.

However, it is increasingly being recognized that evidence from qualitative studies that explore the experience of those involved in providing and receiving interventions, and studies evaluating factors that shape the implementation of interventions, have an important role in ensuring that systematic reviews are of maximum value to policy, practice and consumer decision-making (Mays 2005, Arai 2005, Popay 2005).

The relevance of qualitative evidence to the assessment of interventions has only recently received recognition in the health field, but it is now more common for qualitative components to be built into the evaluation of health interventions (Pope 2006) and for the evaluation of complex interventions such as differing models of health service delivery to use a 'mixed methods' approach. It is therefore increasingly likely that outcome studies included in Cochrane reviews will have qualitative research embedded within, or associated with, them. Authors of Cochrane reviews are therefore increasingly asking how to utilize evidence from qualitative research to enhance the relevance and utility of their review to potential users.

A synthesis of evidence from qualitative research can explore questions such as how do people experience illness, why does an intervention work (or not), for whom and in what circumstances? In some reviews, particularly those addressing healthcare delivery, it may be desirable to draw on qualitative evidence to address questions such as what are the barriers and facilitators to accessing health care, or what impact do specific barriers and facilitators have on people, their experiences and behaviours? These may be generated, for example, through ethnographies and interview studies of help-seeking behaviour. Evidence from qualitative research can help with interpretation of systematic review results by aiding understanding of the way in which an intervention is experienced by all of those involved in developing, delivering or receiving it; what aspects of the intervention they value, or not; and why this is so. These types of qualitative evidence can provide insight into factors that are external to an intervention including, for example, the impact of other policy developments, factors which facilitate or hinder successful implementation of a programme, service or treatment and how a particular intervention may need to be adapted for large-scale roll-out (Roen 2006).

We identify four ways in which qualitative research can contribute to Cochrane Intervention reviews for health policy and practice (Popay 2006a).

1. **Informing** reviews by using evidence from qualitative research to help define and refine the question. This ensures the review includes appropriate studies and addresses important outcomes, allowing the review to be of maximum relevance to potential users.

2. **Enhancing** reviews by synthesizing evidence from qualitative research identified whilst looking for evidence of effectiveness. Qualitative evidence associated with trials can be used to explore issues of implementation of the intervention. We consider qualitative research performed alongside randomized trials in more detail in Section 20.2.3.

3. **Extending** reviews by undertaking a search and synthesis specifically of evidence from qualitative studies to address questions directly related to the effectiveness review.

4. **Supplementing** reviews by synthesizing qualitative evidence to address questions on aspects other than effectiveness.

Qualitative syntheses for extending and supplementing reviews take either a multi-level or a parallel synthesis approach, as discussed in Section 20.3.2.5. No template is currently in place to allow a Cochrane review solely of qualitative evidence.

The Cochrane Public Health and Health Promotion field have produced additional guidance on the types of reviews and questions where qualitative research can add value (see Chapter 21). Such reviews are designed to answer the following questions: 1) does the intervention work (effectiveness), 2) why does it work or not work – including how does it work (feasibility, appropriateness and meaningfulness), and 3) how do participants experience the intervention?

Where qualitative research is used to enhance or extend a Cochrane Intervention review, methods for the specification, identification, critical appraisal and synthesis of qualitative research should be described under a separate heading under 'Data collection and analysis' in the Methods of the review.

## 20.2.3 Considering qualitative studies that are identified within, or alongside, randomized controlled trials

As 'mixed methods' evolve to evaluate the effects of complex interventions such as health service delivery strategies, it is increasingly likely that studies included in Cochrane Intervention reviews will have qualitative research embedded within or associated with them, although the evidence resulting from the qualitative studies may not be reported in the same publication as that of the trial. For example, in an exemplar review we summarize in Box 20.3.a, five out of six trials included in the Cochrane Intervention review had a qualitative component or associated study, although not all qualitative data had been analysed or published. Importantly, this qualitative component was not always referenced in the trial report. Indeed some studies only came to light after making contact with the trial principal investigator.

When considering qualitative research identified within or alongside randomized trials, the following issues need to be considered:

1. Identification of qualitative evidence: Qualitative evidence retrieved using a topic-based search strategy designed to identify trials cannot be viewed as being either comprehensive or representative. Such a search strategy is not designed for the purpose of identifying qualitative studies and indeed achieves a measure of specificity by purposefully excluding many qualitative research types.

2. Qualitative evidence synthesis to explore the experience of having the disease: If the experience of the disease is the focus of interest then qualitative sources identified from the trial search strategy will not necessarily provide a holistic or comprehensive view. In these cases a multilevel or parallel synthesis should be considered or facilitated (see Section 20.3.2.5). Ideally an author would work with a qualitative researcher and information specialist to develop a qualitative search strategy to identify other relevant studies.

3. Qualitative synthesis to explore issues of implementation of the intervention: If issues surrounding implementation are the focus of interest then qualitative evidence embedded within or associated with the trials would be most relevant. Such implementation evidence is most likely to be generated by mixed methods research and to include both qualitative and quantitative evidence. Steps need to be taken to

identify all qualitative sources associated with the trials, such as undertaking additional targeted searching and contacting the trial principal investigator.

4. Considering qualitative evidence within studies excluded from Cochrane Intervention reviews: There may be occasions when a trial does not meet the eligibility criteria for a Cochrane Intervention review (for example due to unacceptable risk of bias) but the qualitative research embedded within or accompanying the trial is considered high quality. The guiding principle follows that if the qualitative evidence appears robust, the qualitative evidence can be incorporated into the review.

### 20.2.4    Resource considerations

The prospect of incorporating evidence from qualitative research in a Cochrane review inevitably has many consequences for authors and Cochrane Review Groups (CRGs). Resource limitations may dictate the extent to which supplementary qualitative syntheses can be undertaken to accompany reviews. Authors will need to consider the following when contemplating the incorporation of evidence from qualitative research into a Cochrane review:

- Does the team have the appropriate expertise or access to advice from experienced qualitative syntheses researchers?

- Will additional training be required?

- Will the budget cover the additional time and resources needed?

- Does the team have access to appropriate databases and journals?

- Does the team have access to an information specialist who is familiar with the particular challenges of retrieving qualitative research?

- Does the CRG responsible for the review support the incorporation of qualitative evidence and have the resources to support the review through the editorial process?

## 20.3    Qualitative evidence synthesis

### 20.3.1    Exemplar of synthesizing qualitative evidence to supplement a Cochrane Intervention review: directly observed therapy and tuberculosis (TB)

Before considering methodology for qualitative evidence synthesis, we provide an exemplar, summarized in Box 20.3.a. The full review is published in the *Journal of*

## Box 20.3.a  Directly observed therapy and tuberculosis: a synthesis of qualitative evidence – summary

**Background:** DOT is part of a World Health Organization (WHO)-branded package of interventions to improve the management of TB and adherence with treatment (Maher 1999). DOT involves asking people with TB to visit a health worker, or other appointed person, to receive and be observed taking a dose of medication. A Cochrane Intervention review of trials of DOT showed conflicting evidence as to the effects of DOT when compared with self-administration of therapy. To supplement this review, we conducted a synthesis of qualitative evidence concerning people with, or at risk of, TB, service providers and policy makers, to explore their experience and perceptions of TB and treatment. Findings were used to help explain and interpret the Cochrane Intervention review and to consider implications for research, policy and practice.

**Review questions:** Two broad research questions were addressed:
1. What are the facilitators and barriers to accessing and complying with tuberculosis treatment?
2. Can exploration of qualitative studies and/or qualitative components of the studies included in the intervention review explain the heterogeneity of findings?

**Method:**

**Search methods:** A systematic search of the wider English-language literature was undertaken: The following terms were used: DOT; DOTS; Directly observed therapy; Directly observed treatment; supervised swallowing; self-supervis*; in combination with TB and tuberculosis. We experimented with using methodological filters by including terms such as 'qualitative', but found this approach unhelpful as the Medline MeSH heading 'Qualitative Research' was only introduced in 2003, and even after 2003 many papers were not identified appropriately as qualitative. We searched MEDLINE, CINAHL, HMIC, Embase, British Nursing Index, International Bibliography of the Social Sciences, Sociological Abstracts, SIGLE, ASSIA, Psych Info, Econ lit, Ovid, Pubmed, the London School of Hygiene and Tropical Medicine database of TB studies (courtesy of Dr Simon Lewin), and Google Scholar. Reference lists contained within published papers were also scrutinized. A network of personal contacts was also used to identify papers. All principal researchers involved in the six randomized trials included in the Cochrane Intervention review were contacted and relevant qualitative studies obtained.

**Selection and appraisal of studies:** The following definition was used to select studies: 'papers whose primary focus was the experiences and/or perceptions of TB and its treatment amongst people with, or at risk of, TB and service providers'. The study had to use qualitative methods of data collection and analysis, as either a stand-alone study or a discrete part of a larger mixed-method study. To appraise methodological and theoretical dimensions of study quality, two contrasting frameworks were used independently by JN and JP (Popay 1998a, Critical Appraisal Skills Programme 2006). Studies were not excluded on quality grounds, but lower quality studies were reviewed to see if they altered the outcome of the synthesis – which they did not.

**Analysis:** Thematic analysis techniques were used to synthesize data from 1990–2002, and an update of literature to December 2005. Themes were identified by bringing together components of ideas, experiences and views embedded in the data – themes were constructed to form a comprehensive picture of participants' collective experiences. A narrative summary technique was used to aid interpretation of trial results.

**Findings:** Fifty-eight papers derived from 53 studies were included. Five themes emerged from the 1990–2002 synthesis, including: socio-economic circumstances, material resources and individual agency; explanatory models and knowledge systems in relation to tuberculosis and its treatment; the experience of stigma and public discourses around tuberculosis; sanctions, incentives and support, and the social organization and social relationships of care. Two additional themes emerged from the 2005 update: the barriers created by programme implementation, and the challenge to the model that culturally determined factors are the central cause of treatment failure.

**Conclusions:** The Cochrane Intervention review did not show statistically significant differences between DOT and self-supervision, thereby suggesting that it was not DOT per se that led to an improvement in treatment outcomes. The six randomized trials tested eight variations of DOT compared with self-supervision and varied enormously in the degree to which they were tailored around the needs of people with TB. The variants of DOT differed in important ways in terms of who was being observed, where the observation took place and how often observation occurred. The synthesis of qualitative research suggests that these elements of DOT will be crucial in determining how effective a particular type of DOT will be in terms of increased cure rates. The qualitative review also highlighted the key role of social and economic factors and physical side effects of medication in shaping behaviour in relation to seeking diagnosis and adhering to treatment. More specifically, a predominantly inspectorial approach to observation is not likely to increase uptake of service or adherence with medication. Inspectorial elements may be needed in treatment packages, but when the primary focus of direct observation was inspectorial rather than supportive in nature, observation was least effective. Direct observation of an inspectorial nature had the most negative impact on those who had the most to fear from disclosure, such as disadvantaged women who experienced gender-related discrimination. In contrast, treatment packages in which the emphasis is on person-centred support are more likely to increase uptake and adherence. Qualitative evidence also provided some insights into the type of support that people with TB find most helpful. Primarily, the ability of the observer to add value depended on the observer and the service being able to adapt to the widely-varying individual circumstances of the person being observed (age, gender, agency, location, income, etc.). Given the heterogeneity amongst those with TB, findings support the need for locally tailored, patient-centred programmes rather than a single worldwide intervention.

*Advanced Nursing* (Noyes 2007). This parallel qualitative evidence synthesis both extends and supplements a Cochrane Intervention review of directly observed therapy (supervised swallowing of medication) as an intervention to improve peoples' adherence to TB regimens (Volmink 2007), which included six randomized trials but found no statistically significant effect of directly observed therapy (DOT) when compared with people treating themselves at home. The accompanying synthesis of qualitative evidence focuses on lay experiences and perceptions of TB treatment to consider whether evidence from these studies could help explain the results of the randomized trials and contribute to the development of policy for the treatment of TB. In doing so the qualitative evidence synthesis addressed questions beyond those of the Cochrane Intervention review such as the appropriateness of DOT and the way it was facilitated in practice.

## 20.3.2 Methodological issues

The main methodological challenges of qualitative evidence syntheses relate to the design and conduct of search strategies, the appraisal of study quality and the appropriate methods for synthesis.

### *20.3.2.1 Search strategies*

Significant progress has been made in analysing indexing systems of databases for qualitative studies. The Hedges Project at McMaster University has expanded its coverage of empirically-tested methodological filters to include qualitative research filters for MEDLINE (Wong 2004), CINAHL (Wilczynski 2007), PsycINFO (McKibbon 2006) and EMBASE (Walters 2006). Nevertheless evidence from qualitative studies collected and reported within randomized trials or as part of linked studies are difficult to retrieve (Evans 2002). MEDLINE introduced the MeSH term 'qualitative research' only in 2003. CINAHL introduced 'Qualitative Studies' in 1988, reflecting particular interest in qualitative studies for nursing researchers, with a corresponding focus on 'quality of life' issues (see Chapter 17, Section 17.3). However, locating qualitative studies remains problematic because of the varied use of the term 'qualitative' (Grant 2004).

In addition, current strategies for indexing terms related to qualitative study designs and protocol-driven search strategies are only of limited value (Evans 2002, Barroso 2003, Greenhalgh 2005). Review authors must be aware that limiting a search to well-known databases may result in missing much useful information. An audit of sources for a review of complex interventions (including qualitative evidence) found that only 30% were identified from databases and hand searches. About half of studies were identified by 'snowballing' and another 24% by personal knowledge or personal contact (Greenhalgh 2005). Search strategies to identify qualitative studies using a range of different qualitative methods need to be further developed.

While there is general agreement on the need for search strategies aiming to identify qualitative research to be systematic and explicit, there is recent debate on whether qualitative evidence syntheses share the need for comprehensive, exhaustive searches. It has been argued that a more purposive sampling approach, aiming to provide a holistic interpretation of a phenomenon, where the extent of searching is driven by the need to reach theoretical saturation and the identification of the 'disconfirming case' may be more appropriate (Dixon-Woods 2006). Nevertheless this places an even greater imperative to improve quality of reporting standards of search methods (Booth 2006).

### 20.3.2.2   *Critical appraisal*

Assessment of study quality (critical appraisal) is a particularly contested issue in relation to qualitative evidence synthesis. At present, opinion on the value of formal quality assessment is divided and there is insufficient evidence to inform a judgement on the rigour or added value of various approaches.

This is an evolving field and Cochrane Qualitative Research Methods Group members are actively involved in contributing to knowledge and practice in this area. We, however, feel that it is important to consider and debate the arguments for and against critical appraisal in qualitative evidence synthesis.

Over one hundred tools and frameworks are available to aid the appraisal of qualitative research, mirroring those available for the appraisal of methodological quality in randomized trials and other forms of quantitative research (Vermeire 2002, Cote 2005). However, it is important to recognize that questions about 'quality' are very different in the context of qualitative research. Formal appraisal processes and standards of evidence presented as rigid checklists informing an 'in or out' decision can be argued to be inappropriate for qualitative research (Popay 1998a, Barbour 2001, Spencer 2003). Rather, such tools are perhaps best utilized as part of a process of exploration and interpretation. Studies rated of low methodological quality on the basis of a rigid formulaic method can generate new insights, grounded in the data, while methodologically sound studies may suffer from poor interpretation, leading to insufficient insight into the phenomenon under study. Dixon-Woods et al. compared three structured appraisal approaches and concluded that structured approaches may not produce greater consistency of judgements about whether to include qualitative papers in a systematic review (Dixon-Woods 2007).

A further issue relates to the timing of quality assessment and when outcomes from the process should be taken into account – should critical appraisal be viewed as a hurdle for establishing a quality threshold or as a filter for mediating the differing strength of the resultant messages from included research?

If authors decide to incorporate quality appraisal as part of the systematic review process then they may use the framework that is integral to the particular method (such as the Evidence for Policy and Practice Information (EPPI) approach or Joanna Briggs Institute (JBI) approach), or select any published qualitative appraisal tool, framework or checklist. Spencer et al. have undertaken a review of many of the current appraisal frameworks and checklists, which authors may find helpful in deciding which approach to apply (Spencer 2003). Expert judgement is also an important factor when appraising the quality of studies.

Key references reflecting this debate are included in Section 20.6.6: Further Reading.

### 20.3.2.3 *Synthesizing evidence from qualitative research*

Qualitative evidence synthesis is a process of combining evidence from individual qualitative studies to create new understanding by comparing and analysing concepts and findings from different sources of evidence with a focus on the same topic of interest. Therefore, qualitative evidence synthesis can be considered a complete study in itself, comparable to any meta-analysis within a systematic review on effects of interventions or diagnostic tests. It can be an aggregative or interpretive process but requires transparency of process and requires authors to identify and extract evidence from studies included in the review; to categorize the evidence; and to combine these categories to develop synthesized findings. In undertaking this methodological work, however, it is important to recognize that the real prize from the synthesis of qualitative evidence is not just a description of how people feel about an issue or treatment but an understanding of 'why' they feel and behave the way they do (Popay 2005).

For example, primary qualitative research on the experience of chronic illness presents people's accounts of the onset of their illness. But this body of work also moves beyond description to seek to explain the social purpose of these accounts – showing how through these narratives people 'reconstruct' a sense of worth in a social context in which all illness has moral overtones (Williams 1984). Similarly, a recent systematic review of qualitative research on medicine taking (Campbell 2003, Pound 2005) utilizing meta-ethnography as a method for synthesis moves beyond providing a summary of recurring 'themes' across studies to build an explanation of why people use medication (or not) in the way they do.

### 20.3.2.4 *Choosing an appropriate method*

The choice of method for inclusion of qualitative evidence in a qualitative evidence synthesis will depend on a number of factors, including the:

- type and scope of the review and review question(s);
- pool of available evidence;
- expertise of the team; and
- available resources.

There are a number of evolving methods for the synthesis of qualitative and mixed-method evidence. Along with other interested individuals and systematic review organizations, Cochrane Qualitative Research Methods Group members are actively involved in developing and more recently beginning to evaluate the range of methods available. Members have contributed to two core texts on synthesizing qualitative and quantitative health evidence, which provide more detailed information and guidance on methods and processes (Petticrew 2006, Pope 2007).

We recommend that any high quality method of qualitative evidence synthesis may be used that is best suited to the type of Intervention review.

It is beyond the scope of the chapter to include detailed description of the range of methods available for qualitative and mixed method evidence synthesis. A variety of methods have been used in published reviews. Examples include: Bayesian meta-analysis, critical interpretive synthesis, Evidence for Policy and Practice Information (EPPI) Coordinating Centre approach, Joanna Briggs Institute (JBI) approach, meta-ethnography, meta-synthesis, meta-study, meta-summary, narrative synthesis, qualitative evidence synthesis drawing on grounded theory, realist synthesis, and secondary thematic analysis.

Most methods have associated detailed guidance (see for example Noblit and Hare on meta-ethnography and Popay et al. on narrative synthesis (Noblit 1988, Popay 2006b)), which should be referred to. Dixon-Woods et al. provide a detailed overview of the potential of several methods and associated challenges (Dixon-Woods 2005, Dixon-Woods 2006). As yet, little evaluation has been undertaken to determine the robustness of different methods. Further reading can be found in Section 20.6.

### 20.3.2.5    *Approaches to integrating qualitative and quantitative evidence syntheses*

There are two broad approaches that can be used to integrate qualitative and quantitative findings:

1. Multilevel syntheses: Qualitative evidence (synthesis 1) and quantitative evidence (synthesis 2) can be conducted as separate streams or separate, but linking, reviews and the product of each synthesis is then combined (synthesis 3) (see, for example, Thomas et al. (Thomas 2004)).

2. Parallel syntheses: Qualitative evidence (synthesis 1) and quantitative evidence (synthesis 2) can be conducted as separate streams or separate but linked reviews. The qualitative synthesis (1) can then be used in parallel and juxtaposed alongside to aid the interpretation of synthesized trials (synthesis 2) (see, for example, Noyes and Popay (Noyes 2007)).

Multilevel and parallel syntheses both require a separate systematic review of evidence, which at a later stage is synthesized with, or juxtaposed alongside, the synthesis of trials. Guidance on the conduct of narrative synthesis (Popay 2006b) contains a toolkit for bringing together findings from different study designs within different methods and approaches. Further methodological work is required on the processes by which evidence from studies using different qualitative methods and generating a range of types of evidence can be synthesized and combined with quantitative findings on effect without compromising the need to minimize bias (Lucas 2007).

### 20.3.2.6 Conclusion

Interest in systematically reviewing broader forms of evidence and in particular evidence from qualitative research is being driven by a growing recognition that qualitative research can improve the relevance and utility of a review. However, research evidence that is rigorously generated, regardless of design, demands due consideration of its quality before it can be used in the clinical environment. To be considered for a Cochrane Intervention review, evidence from qualitative research must be subjected to equally rigorous methods of review. Methods for appraising and analysing evidence from qualitative research are now emerging and will continue to evolve over time. Further evidence is required to establish the rigour and added value of the various approaches to quality appraisal in the systematic review process.

## 20.4 Chapter information

**Authors:** Jane Noyes, Jennie Popay, Alan Pearson, Karin Hannes and Andrew Booth on behalf of the Cochrane Qualitative Research Methods Group.

**This chapter should be cited as:** Noyes J, Popay J, Pearson A, Hannes K, Booth A. Chapter 20: Qualitative research and Cochrane reviews. In: Higgins JPT, Green S (editors), *Cochrane Handbook for Systematic Reviews of Interventions*. Chichester (UK): John Wiley & Sons, 2008.

---

**Box 20.4.a   The Cochrane Qualitative Research Methods Group**

The Cochrane Qualitative Research Methods Group (QRMG) develops and supports methodological work on the inclusion in systematic reviews of evidence from research using qualitative methods and disseminates this work within and beyond the Collaboration's CRGs.

The QRMG is attempting to fulfil its role by:

- identifying appropriate roles for evidence from qualitative research within the context of Cochrane systematic reviews;
- collating, developing and disseminating appropriate methodological standards for:
  - Searching for qualitative research relevant to Cochrane reviews;
  - Critically appraising qualitative studies;

- ○ Combining evidence from qualitative research with other data within the context of a systematic review;
- ○ Dissemination of these methodological standards through various routes including contributing to the guidance for authors in the *Handbook*;
- providing a forum for discussion and debate about the role of qualitative evidence within the systematic review process and the development of rigorous and systematic methods to promote this role to:
  - ○ Encourage transparency of, and learning about, method developments;
  - ○ Encourage and facilitate liaison and sharing with other methods groups;
- providing links for Cochrane Review Groups to people with expertise and experience of qualitative research to:
  - ○ Provide advice and support for people aiming to incorporate qualitative research into a review;
  - ○ Provide a mechanism for evaluating and developing review protocols;
- providing training for members of Cochrane Review Groups and Campbell Coordinating Groups;
- maintaining a register/database of relevant methodological papers;
- maintaining a register/database of systematic review protocols that include qualitative evidence synthesis or are solely focused on the systematic review of qualitative evidence;
- maintaining a register/database of completed systematic reviews that include qualitative evidence synthesis; and of reviews that are solely focused on the systematic review of qualitative evidence; and
- surveying members on an annual basis to identify developing interests and ongoing contributions.

Members of the Group have contributed to the guidance on the commissioning and conduct of systematic reviews produced by the Centre for Reviews and Dissemination at the University of York and have supported the development of guidance produced by the Cochrane Health Promotion and Public Health Field.

*Web site:* www.joannabriggs.edu.au/cqrmg

## 20.5 References

**Arai 2005**

Arai L, Roen K, Roberts H, Popay J. It might work in Oklahoma but will it work in Oakhampton? Context and implementation in the effectiveness literature on domestic smoke detectors. *Injury Prevention* 2005; 11: 148–151.

**Barbour 2001**

Barbour RS. Checklists for improving rigour in qualitative research: a case of the tail wagging the dog? *BMJ* 2001; 322: 1115–1117.

**Barroso 2003**

Barroso J, Gollop CJ, Sandelowski M, Meynell J, Pearce PF, Collins LJ. The challenges of searching for and retrieving qualitative studies. *Western Journal of Nursing Research* 2003; 25: 153–178.

**Booth 2006**

Booth A. "Brimful of STARLITE": toward standards for reporting literature searches. *Journal of the Medical Library Association* 2006; 94: 421–429.

**Campbell 2003**

Campbell R, Pound P, Pope C, Britten N, Pill R, Morgan M, Donovan J. Evaluating meta-ethnography: a synthesis of qualitative research on lay experiences of diabetes and diabetes care. *Social Science and Medicine* 2003; 56: 671–684.

**Cote 2005**

Cote L, Turgeon J. Appraising qualitative research articles in medicine and medical education. *Medical Teacher* 2005; 27: 71–75.

**Critical Appraisal Skills Programme 2006**

Critical Appraisal Skills Programme. 10 questions to help you make sense of qualitative research [2006]. Available from: http://www.phru.nhs.uk/Pages/PHD/resources.htm (accessed 1 January 2008).

**Denzin 1994**

Denzin NK, Lincoln YS. Introduction. Entering the field of qualitative research. In: Denzin NK, Lincoln YS (editors). *Handbook of Qualitative Research*. Thousand Oaks (CA): Sage Publications, 1994.

**Dixon-Woods 2005**

Dixon-Woods M, Agarwal S, Jones D, Young B, Sutton A. Synthesising qualitative and quantitative evidence: a review of possible methods. *Journal of Health Services Research and Policy* 2005; 10: 45–53.

**Dixon-Woods 2006**

Dixon-Woods M, Bonas S, Booth A, Jones DR, Miller T, Sutton AJ, Shaw RL, Smith JA, Young B. How can systematic reviews incorporate qualitative research? A critical perspective. *Qualitative Research* 2006; 6: 27–44.

**Dixon-Woods 2007**

Dixon-Woods M, Sutton A, Shaw R, Miller T, Smith J, Young B, Bonas S, Booth A, Jones D. Appraising qualitative research for inclusion in systematic reviews: a quantitative and qualitative comparison of three methods. *Journal of Health Services Research and Policy* 2007; 12: 42–47.

**Evans 2002**

Evans D. Database searches for qualitative research. *Journal of the Medical Library Association* 2002; 90: 290–293.

**Grant 2004**

Grant MJ. How does your searching grow? A survey of search preferences and the use of optimal search strategies in the identification of qualitative research. *Health Information and Libraries Journal* 2004; 21: 21–32.

**Greenhalgh 2005**

Greenhalgh T, Peacock R. Effectiveness and efficiency of search methods in systematic reviews of complex evidence: audit of primary sources. *BMJ* 2005; 331: 1064–1065.

**Lucas 2007**

Lucas PJ, Baird J, Arai L, Law C, Roberts HM. Worked examples of alternative methods for the synthesis of qualitative and quantitative research in systematic reviews. *BMC Medical Research Methodology* 2007; 7: 4.

**Maher 1999**

Maher D, Mikulencak M. *What is DOTS? A Guide to Understanding the WHO-recommended TB Control Strategy Known as DOTS*. Geneva (Switzerland): World Health Organization, 1999.

**Mays 2005**

Mays N, Pope C, Popay J. Systematically reviewing qualitative and quantitative evidence to inform management and policy-making in the health field. *Journal of Health Services Research and Policy* 2005; 10 (Suppl 1): 6–20.

**McKibbon 2006**

McKibbon KA, Wilczynski NL, Haynes RB. Developing optimal search strategies for retrieving qualitative studies in PsycINFO. *Evaluation and the Health Professions* 2006; 29: 440–454.

**Mills 2005a**

Mills E, Jadad AR, Ross C, Wilson K. Systematic review of qualitative studies exploring parental beliefs and attitudes toward childhood vaccination identifies common barriers to vaccination. *Journal of Clinical Epidemiology* 2005; 58: 1081–1088.

**Mills 2005b**

Mills EJ, Montori VM, Ross CP, Shea B, Wilson K, Guyatt GH. Systematically reviewing qualitative studies complements survey design: an exploratory study of barriers to paediatric immunisations. *Journal of Clinical Epidemiology* 2005; 58: 1101–1108.

**Noblit 1988**

Noblit GW, Hare RD. *Meta-ethnography: Synthesising Qualitative Studies* (Qualitative Research Methods). London: Sage Publications, 1988.

**Noyes 2007**

Noyes J, Popay J. Directly observed therapy and tuberculosis: how can a systematic review of qualitative research contribute to improving services? A qualitative meta-synthesis. *Journal of Advanced Nursing* 2007; 57: 227–243.

**Pearson 2005**

Pearson A, Wiechula R, Court A, Lockwood C. The JBI model of evidence-based healthcare. *JBI Reports* 2005; 3: 207–216.

**Petticrew 2006**

Petticrew M, Roberts H. *Systematic Reviews in the Social Sciences: A Practical Guide*. Oxford (UK): Blackwell, 2006.

**Popay 1998a**

Popay J, Rogers A, Williams G. Rationale and standards for the systematic review of qualitative literature in health services research. *Qualitative Health Research* 1009; 8: 341–351.

**Popay 1998b**

Popay J, Williams G. Qualitative research and evidence-based healthcare. *Journal of the Royal Society of Medicine* 1998; 91 (Suppl 35): 32–37.

**Popay 2005**

Popay J. Moving beyond floccinaucinihilipilification: enhancing the utility of systematic reviews. *Journal of Clinical Epidemiology* 2005; 58: 1079–1080.

**Popay 2006a**

Popay J. Incorporating qualitative information in systematic reviews. *14th Cochrane Colloquium*, Dublin (Ireland), 2006.

**Popay 2006b**

Popay, J, Roberts, H, Sowden, A, Petticrew, M, Arai, L, Rodgers, M, Britten, N, Roen, K, Duffy, S. Guidance on the conduct of narrative synthesis in systematic reviews. Results of an ESRC funded research project. Unpublished report, University of Lancaster, UK, 2006.

**Pope 2006**

Pope C, Mays N. Qualiative methods in health research. In: Pope C, Mays N (editors). *Qualitative Research in Health Care* (3rd edition). Malden (MA): Blackwell Publications/BMJ Books, 2006.

**Pope 2007**

Pope C, Mays N, Popay J. *Synthesising Qualitative and Quantitative Health Research: A Guide to Methods.* Maidenhead (UK): Open University Press, 2007.

**Pound 2005**

Pound P, Britten N, Morgan M, Yardley L, Pope C, Daker-White G, Campbell R. Resisting medicines: a synthesis of qualitative studies of medicine taking. *Social Science and Medicine* 2005; 61: 133–155.

**Roen 2006**

Roen K, Arai L, Roberts H, Popay J. Extending systematic reviews to include evidence on implementation: methodological work on a review of community-based initiatives to prevent injuries. *Social Science and Medicine* 2006; 63: 1060–1071.

**Spencer 2003**

Spencer L. *Quality in Qualitative Evaluation: A Framework for Assessing Research Evidence.* London (UK): Government Chief Social Researcher's Office, Cabinet Office, 2003. Available from www.gsr.gov.uk/downloads/evaluating_policy/a_quality_framework.pdf.

**Thomas 2004**

Thomas J, Harden A, Oakley A, Oliver S, Sutcliffe K, Rees R, Brunton G, Kavanagh J. Integrating qualitative research with trials in systematic reviews. *BMJ* 2004; 328: 1010–1012.

**Vermeire 2002**

Vermeire E, Van Royen P, Griffiths F, Coenen S, Peremans L, Hendrickx K. The critical appraisal of focus group research articles. *European Journal of General Practice* 2002; 8: 104–108.

**Volmink 2007**

Volmink J, Garner P. Directly observed therapy for treating tuberculosis. *Cochrane Database of Systematic Reviews* 2006, Issue 4. Art No: CD003343.

**Walters 2006**

Walters LA, Wilczynski NL, Haynes RB. Developing optimal search strategies for retrieving clinically relevant qualitative studies in EMBASE. *Qualitative Health Research* 2006; 16: 162–168.

**Wilczynski 2007**

Wilczynski NL, Marks S, Haynes RB. Search strategies for identifying qualitative studies in CINAHL. *Qualitative Health Research* 2007; 17: 705–710.

**Williams 1984**

Williams G. The genesis of chronic illness: narrative re-construction. *Sociology of Health and Illness* 1984; 6: 175–200.

**Wong 2004**

Wong SS, Wilczynski NL, Haynes RB, Hedges Team. Developing optimal search strategies for detecting clinically relevant qualitative studies in MEDLINE. *Medinfo* 2004; 11: 311–316.

## 20.6 Further selected reading

### 20.6.1 Qualitative research, general

Boulton M, Fitzpatrick R. Qualitative methods for assessing health care. *Quality in Health Care* 1994; 3: 107–113.

Britten N, Jones R, Murphy E, Stacey R. Qualitative research methods in general practice and primary care. *Family Practice* 1995; 12:104–114.

Esterberg KG. *Qualitative Methods in Social Research*. Boston (US): McGraw-Hill, 2002.

Giacomini MK. The rocky road: qualitative research as evidence. *Evidence-Based Medicine* 2001; 6: 4–5

Grbich C. *Qualitative Research in Health: An Introduction*. London (UK): Sage Publications, 1999.

Green J, Britten N. Qualitative research and evidence-based medicine. *BMJ* 1998; 316:1230–2.

Guba RG, Lincoln YS. Competing paradigms in qualitative research. In: Denzin NK, Lincoln YS (Eds) *Handbook of Qualitative Research*. Thousand Oaks (CA): Sage Publications, 1994.

Miller S, Fredericks M. The nature of "evidence" in qualitative research methods. *International Journal of Qualitative Methods* 2003; 2: Article 4. Retrieved 1 January 2008 from http://www.ualberta.ca/~ijqm.

Murphy E, Dingwall R, Greatbach D, Parker S, Watson P. Qualitative research methods in health technology assessment: a review of the literature. *Health Technology Assessment* 1998; 2: 1–274.

Popay J, Williams G. Qualitative research and evidence based healthcare. *Journal of the Royal Society of Medicine* 1998; 91(Suppl 35): 32–37.

Pope C, Mays N. Qualitative research: reaching the parts other methods cannot reach: an introduction to qualitative methods in health and health service research. *BMJ* 1995; 311: 42–45.

Pope C, Van Royen P, Baker R. Qualitative methods in research on healthcare quality. *Quality and Safety in Health Care* 2002; 11:148–152.

## 20.6.2  Qualitative methods

Fetterman DM. *Ethnography. Step by Step*. Newbury Park (CA): Sage Publications, 1989.

Glaser BG, Strauss AL. *The Discovery of Grounded Theory: Strategies for Qualitative Research*. Chicago (IL): Aldine, 1967.

Hammersley M. *Reading Ethnographic Research*. New York (NY): Langman, 1990.

Hammersley M, Atkinson P. *Ethnography: Principles in Practice*. London (UK): Routledge, 1995.

Lambert H, McKevitt C. Anthropology in health research: from qualitative methods to multi-disciplinarity. *BMJ* 2002; 325: 210–213.

Maggs-Rapport F. Combining methodological approaches in research: ethnography and interpretive phenomenology. *Journal of Advanced Nursing* 2000; 31: 219–225.

Meyer J. Using qualitative methods in health related action research. In: Pope C, Mays N (Eds). *Qualitative Research in Health Care*. London (UK): BMJ Books, 1999.

Savage J. Ethnography and health care. *BMJ* 2000; 321:1400–1402.

Strauss A, Corbin J. *Grounded Theory in Practice*. Thousand Oaks (CA): Sage Publications, 1997.

Strauss A, Corbin J. *Basics of Qualitative Research Techniques and Procedures for Developing Grounded Theory*. Thousand Oaks (CA): Sage Publications, 1998.

Taylor SJ, Bogdan R. *Introduction to Qualitative Research Methods: A Guidebook and Resource*. New York (NY), John Wiley & Sons, 1998.

Yin RK. *Case Study Research: Designs and Methods*. Newbury Park (CA): Sage Publications, 1989.

## 20.6.3    Qualitative literature searching

Flemming K, Briggs M. Electronic searching to locate qualitative research: evaluation of three strategies. *Journal of Advanced Nursing* 2007; 57: 95–100.

Shaw RL, Booth A, Sutton AJ, Miller T, Smith JA, Young B, Jones DR, Dixon-Woods M. Finding qualitative research: an evaluation of search strategies. *BMC Medical Research Methodology* 2004; 4: 5

InterTASC Information Subgroup, University of York web site:

• http://www.york.ac.uk/inst/crd/intertasc/

## 20.6.4    Synthesizing qualitative evidence

Jensen LA, Allen MN. Meta-synthesis of qualitative findings. *Qualitative Health Research* 1996; 6: 553–560.

Noblit GW, Hare RD. *Meta-Ethnography: Synthesising Qualitative Studies*. Newbury Park (CA): Sage Publications, 1988.

Paterson BL, Thorne SE, Canam C, Jillings C. *Meta-Study of Qualitative Health Research. A Practical Guide to Meta-Analysis and Meta-Synthesis*. Thousand Oaks (CA): Sage Publications, 2001.

Pearson A. Balancing the evidence: incorporating the synthesis of qualitative data into systematic reviews. *JBI Reports* 2004; 2 :45–64.

Sandelowski M, Barroso. Creating metasummaries of qualitative findings. *Nursing Research* 2003; 52: 226–33.

Sandelowski M, Barroso J. *Handbook for Synthesising Qualitative Research*. New York (NY): Springer, 2007.

Sandelowski M, Docherty S, Emden C. Focus on qualitative methods. Qualitative meta-synthesis: issues and techniques. *Research in Nursing and Health* 1997; 20: 365–371.

Thorne S, Jensen L, Kearney MH, Noblit G, Sandelowski M. Qualitative metasynthesis: reflections on methodological orientation and ideological agenda. *Qualitative Health Research* 2004; 14: 1342–1365.

Zhao S. Metatheory, metamethod, qualitative meta-analysis: what, why and how? *Sociological Perspectives* 1991; 34: 377–390.

## 20.6.5    Synthesizing qualitative and quantitative evidence

Dixon-Woods M, Cavers D, Agarwal S, Annandale E, Arthur A, Harvey J, Hsu R, Katbamna S, Olsen R, Smith L, Riley R, Sutton AJ. Conducting a critical interpretive synthesis of the literature on access to healthcare by vulnerable groups. *BMC Medical Research Methodology* 2006; 6: 35.

Dixon-Woods M, Fitzpatrick R. Qualitative research in systematic reviews. *BMJ* 2001; 323: 765–766

Dixon-Woods M, Fitzpatrick R, Roberts K. Including qualitative research in systematic reviews; opportunities and problems. *Journal of Evaluation in Clinical Practice* 2001; 7: 125–133.

Greenhalgh T, Robert G, Macfarlane F, Bate P, Kyriakidou O, Peacock R. Storylines of research in diffusion of innovation: a meta-narrative approach to systematic review. *Social Science and Medicine* 2005; 61: 417–430.

Harden A, Garcia J, Oliver S, Rees R, Shepherd J, Brunton G, Oakley A. Applying systematic review methods to studies of people's views: an example from public health research. *Journal of Epidemiology and Community Health* 2004; 58: 794–800.

Pawson, R. Evidence-based policy: the promise of 'realist synthesis'. *Evaluation* 2002; 8: 340–358.

Pawson R. *Evidence Based Policy: A Realist Perspective.* London (UK): Sage Publications, 2006.

Pearson, A, Field, J, Jordan, Z. *Evidence-based Clinical Practice in Nursing and Healthcare: Assimilating Research, Experience and Expertise.* Oxford (UK): Blackwell, 2007.

Petticrew M, Roberts H. *Systematic Reviews in the Social Sciences: A Practical Guide.* Oxford (UK): Blackwell, 2006.

Pope C, Mays N, Popay J. *Synthesising Qualitative and Quantitative Health Research: A Guide to Methods.* Maidenhead (UK): Open University Press, 2007.

Popay J (Ed) Moving beyond Effectiveness in Evidence Synthesis: Methodological Issues in the Synthesis of Diverse Sources of Evidence. London (UK): NICE, 2006.

Roberts K, Dixon-Woods M, Fitzpatrick R, Abrams K, Jones D. Factors affecting uptake of childhood immunisation: a Bayesian synthesis of qualitative and quantitative evidence. *The Lancet* 2002; 360: 1596–1599.

Webb C, Roe B (Eds). *Reviewing Research Evidence for Nursing Practice.* Oxford (UK): Blackwell, 2007.

## 20.6.6 Critical appraisal of qualitative studies

Blaxter M. Criteria for evaluation of qualitative research. *Medical Sociology News* 1996; 22: 68–71.

CASP (Critical Appraisal Skills Programme). 10 Questions to make sense of qualitative research [2006]. Available from: http://www.phru.nhs.uk/pages/phd/resources.htm (accessed 1 January 2008).

Dixon-Woods M, Shaw RL, Agarwal S, Smith JA. The problem of appraising qualitative research. *Quality and Safety in Healthcare* 2004; 13: 223–225.

Elder NC, Miller WL. Reading and evaluation qualitative research studies. *Journal of Family Practice* 1995; 41: 279–285

Forchuk C, Roberts J. How to critique qualitative research articles. *Canadian Journal of Nursing Research* 1993; 25: 47–55.

Horsburgh D. Evaluation of qualitative research. *Journal of Clinical Nursing* 2003; 12: 307–312.

Malterud K Qualitative research: standards, challenges, and guidelines. *The Lancet* 2001; 358: 483–488.

Popay J, Rogers A, Williams G. Rationale and standards for the systematic review of qualitative literature in health service research. *Qualitative Health Research* 1998; 8: 341–351.

Secker J, Wimbush E, Watson J, Milburn K. Qualitative methods in health promotion research: some criteria for quality. *Health Education Journal* 1995; 54: 74–87.

Spencer L, Ritchie J, Lewis J, Dillon L. *Quality in Qualitative Evaluation: A Framework for Assessing Research Evidence*. London (UK): Government Chief Social Researcher's Office, 2003.

Vermeire E, Van Royen P, Griffiths F, Coenen S, Peremans L, Hendrickx K. The critical appraisal of focus group research articles. *European Journal of General Practice* 2002; 8: 104–108.

## 20.6.7   Web sites

(Accessed 1 January 2008)

**Campbell Collaboration**
A Campbell Review can include evidence from studies of the implementation of an intervention.

- www.campbellcollaboration.org

**Centre for Reviews and Dissemination (CRD), University of York, UK**
In addition to a handbook, CRD has an online resource centre.

- www.york.ac.uk/inst/crd

**Evidence for Policy and Practice Information and Coordinating (EPPI) Centre**
The EPPI Centre provides links to methods, tools and databases.

- eppi.ioe.ac.uk/cms

**Joanna Briggs Institute (JBI)**
JBI offers a variety of evidence-based health care resources concerning the synthesis of evidence.

- www.joannabriggs.edu.au

**National Institute for Health and Clinical Excellence (NICE)**
NICE has produced guidance on methods for development of NICE public health guidance which incorporate diverse study designs.

- www.nice.org.uk

**Social Care Institute for Excellence (SCIE)**
SCIE has produced guidance on the conduct of knowledge reviews which incorporate diverse study designs.

- www.scie.org.uk

# 21 Reviews in public health and health promotion

**Edited by Rebecca Armstrong, Elizabeth Waters and Jodie Doyle**

## Key Points

- Public health and health promotion (PHHP) interventions are broadly-defined activities that are evaluated using a wide variety of approaches and study designs, including cluster-randomized trials. For some questions, the best available evidence may be from non-randomized studies.

- Searching for public health and health promotion literature can be a very complex task, and requires authors to use methods other than database searching to retrieve studies.

- Systematic reviews of public health and health promotion interventions have the potential to investigate differential outcomes for groups with varying levels of disadvantage. However, addressing inequalities is complicated not only by limited collection of information about differences between groups, but also by the fact that there is limited participation of disadvantaged groups in research.

- A further problem in reviewing public health and health promotion interventions is how to disentangle intervention effects from the influence of the context in which the intervention is implemented.

- Information should be sought on contextual factors and on intervention characteristics that may explain the extent to which the intervention or outcomes are sustained.

## 21.1 Introduction

Guidelines specific to conducting reviews public health and health promotion interventions were developed by the Cochrane Health Promotion and Public Health (HPPH)

Field (now transitioned to the Cochrane Public Health Review Group) in 2005 and up-dated in 2007. This chapter provides an overview of issues specific to health promotion and public health not discussed elsewhere in the *Handbook*. The complete version of the *Guidelines for Health Promotion and Public Health Systematic Reviews* can be accessed at the Cochrane Public Health Review Group's web site: www.ph.cochrane.org..

## 21.2   Study designs to include

Public health and health promotion are broadly-defined activities that are evaluated using a wide variety of approaches and designs. No single method can be used to answer all relevant questions about all public health and health promotion problems and interventions. If the review question has been specified clearly then types of study designs needed to answer it should automatically follow (Petticrew 2003). A preliminary scoping search will also help to identify the types of study designs that may have been used to study the intervention. The criteria used to select studies should primarily reflect the question or questions being answered in the review, rather than any predetermined hierarchy (Glasziou 2004). The decisions about which type(s) of study design to include will influence subsequent phases of the review, particularly searching, assessment of risk of bias, and analysis (especially for meta-analyses).

Randomized trials provide a useful source of evidence of effectiveness, although their results may have limited generalizability (Black 1996). For many health promotion and public health interventions randomized trials may not be available, due to issues including feasibility and ethics. Cluster-randomized trials are increasingly adopted within the field of public health; some interventions require their application at the cluster level (Donner 2004). These trials can contribute valuable evidence if a sufficient number of units are randomized to ensure even distribution of potential confounders among groups: see Chapter 16 (Section 16.3).

For some questions, non-randomized studies may represent the best available evidence (of effectiveness). Reviewing non-randomized evidence can give an estimate of the nature, direction and size of effects. Demonstrating the patterns of evidence drawn from different study designs may lead to the development of subsequent study designs (including randomized trials) to test the intervention. Studies generating qualitative data may also be relevant to other kinds of questions beyond effectiveness questions. For example, data may be gathered on the preferences of the likely recipients of the interventions and the factors that constrain or facilitate the successful outcome of particular interventions. Research is ongoing into the differences between randomized and non-randomized studies of public health and health promotion interventions (for example the UK Methodology Programme). Chapter 13 discusses general issues on the inclusion of non-randomized studies in Cochrane reviews, and Chapter 20 addresses qualitative studies.

## 21.3   Searching

Finding studies on public health and health promotion interventions is much more complicated than retrieving medical studies due to literature being widely scattered

(Peersman 2001). The multidisciplinary nature of public health and health promotion means that studies can be found in a number of different areas and through a wide range of electronic databases (Beahler 2000, Grayson 2003). Difficulties also arise because terminology is imprecise and constantly changing (Grayson 2003). Therefore, searching for public health and health promotion literature can be a very complex task, and requires authors to use retrieval methods other than database searching to retrieve studies.

To overcome some of the difficulties in identifying the qualitative research, current best practice requires the researcher to conduct comprehensive searches (e.g. sensitive searches of multiple sources). However, this approach, which attempts to maximize the number of relevant records identified, results in the retrieval of high numbers of records, many of which will not be relevant (Shaw 2004). Due to inadequate indexing terms for qualitative research in bibliographic databases, we do not currently recommend that study design filters be applied. We recognize that often pragmatic decisions may need to be taken when balancing the time and other resources required in conducting comprehensive searches against the ratio of relevant to non-relevant studies identified. Researchers may decide that they need to apply study design filters and, if so, they need to report this when describing their search strategies to make the potential limitations of the searches clear. Table 21.3.a lists some electronic databases relevant to a variety of public health and health promotion topics.

## 21.4 Assessment of study quality and risk of bias

Assessing the quality of public health and health promotion studies, and their resulting risk of bias, may be difficult, partly due to the wide variety of study designs used. Authors need to consider the criteria to be used to assess quality at the planning stage of the review. Appraisal criteria will depend on the type of study included in the review. Authors should be guided by the Cochrane Review Group (CRG) editing their review and the appraisal tools they use. However the following describes tools which may be useful for assessing studies of public health and health promotion interventions.

- The risk of bias in randomized trials should be assessed using the Collaboration's 'Risk of bias' tool described in Chapter 8 (Section 8.5).

- Issues for cluster-randomized trials are discussed in Chapter 16 (Section 16.3.2).

- For risk of bias in non-randomized studies, authors should consult Chapter 13 (Section 13.5).

- Authors may choose to use the Quality Assessment Tool for Quantitative Studies (Effective Public Health Practice Project 2007). This tool was developed by the Effective Public Health Practice Project, Canada, and covers any quantitative study design. The tool takes between 10–15 minutes to complete. A comprehensive dictionary for the assessment tool is also published on their web site (http://www.myhamilton .ca/myhamilton/CityandGovernment/HealthandSocialServices/Research/EPHPP/). This tool includes components of intervention integrity and was judged to be suitable

**Table 21.3.a**   Electronic databases relevant to public health and health promotion (web sites listed for databases freely available via the internet)

| Field | Resources |
|---|---|
| Psychology | PsycINFO/PscyLIT |
| Biomedical | CINAHL, LILACS (Latin American Caribbean Health Sciences Literature, www.bireme.br/bvs/I/ibd.htm), Web of Science, Medline, EMBASE, CENTRAL, SCOPUS |
| Sociology | Sociofile, Sociological Abstracts, Social Science Citation Index, Social Policy and Practice. |
| Education | ERIC (Educational Resources Information Center), C2-SPECTR (Campbell Collaboration Social, Psychological, Educational and Criminological Trials Register, www.campbellcollaboration.org), REEL (Research Evidence in Education Library, EPPI-Centre, eppi.ioe.ac.uk). |
| Transport | NTIS (National Technical Information Service), TRIS (Transport Research Information Service, ntl.bts.gov/tris), IRRD (International Road Research Documentation), TRANSDOC (from ECMT, European Conference of Ministers of Transport). |
| Physical activity | SportsDiscus |
| HP/PH | BiblioMap, TRoPHI (Trials Register of Promoting Health Interventions) and DoPHER (Database of Promoting Health Effectiveness Reviews) (EPPI-Centre, eppi.ioe.ac.uk), Public Health Electronic Library (National Institute for Health and Clinical Excellence, www.nice.org.uk/guidance) |
| | Database of abstracts of reviews of effectiveness (DARE) |
| Other | Popline (population health, family planning) db.jhuccp.org/popinform/basic.html, Enviroline (environmental health) – available on Dialog, Toxfile (toxicology) – available on Dialog, Econlit (economics), NGC (National Guideline Clearinghouse, www.guideline.gov). |
| Qualitative | ESRC Qualitative Data Archival Resource Centre (QUALIDATA, www.qualidata.essex.ac.uk), Database of Interviews on Patient Experience (DIPEX, www.dipex.org) |

to use in systematic reviews of effectiveness in the review by Deeks et al. (Deeks 2003).

- Guidance is available from the Cochrane Effective Practice and Organisation of Care Group on interrupted time series and controlled before-and-after studies (Cochrane EPOC Group 2008).

- The results of uncontrolled studies (also called before-and-after studies without a control group) should be treated with caution. The absence of a comparison group makes it impossible to know what would have happened without the intervention. Some of the particular problems with interpreting data from uncontrolled studies include susceptibility to problems with confounding (including seasonality) and regression to the mean.

## 21.5   Ethics and inequalities

Public health and health promotion interventions have the potential to improve the health of populations. Systematic reviews can determine the effectiveness of these interventions in achieving their desired outcomes. There are some specific ethical considerations that should be taken into account in reviewing the effectiveness of public health and health promotion interventions. Effectiveness is typically measured in terms of the total number (population) who benefit from the intervention. This consequentialist approach takes no account of the distribution of benefits (Hawe 1995), and therefore does not address issues of health equity. Overall improvements in health behaviours or health outcomes may actually mask the differences in health outcomes between groups (Macintyre 2003). Interventions that work for those in the middle and upper socio-economic positions may not be as effective for those who are disadvantaged. Even well-intentioned interventions may actually increase inequalities. Health differentials that exist between groups may be due to complex interactions between many of the factors relating to disadvantage (Jackson 2003).

Systematic reviews of public health and health promotion interventions have the potential to investigate differential outcomes for groups with varying levels of disadvantage. This is important as identifying the effect of interventions on disadvantaged groups can inform strategies aimed at reducing health inequalities and health inequities. Health inequalities are "differences, variations, and disparities in the health achievements of individuals and groups" (Kawachi 2002). Health equity is an ethical concept referring to the fairness or unfairness of particular health inequalities. The International Society for Equity in Health defines equity in health as: "the absence of potentially remediable, systematic differences in one or more aspects of health status across socially, economically, demographically, or geographically defined populations or subgroups" (Macinko 2002). Turning this around, health inequities are those health inequalities that are unfair or unjust, or stem from some kind of injustice (Kawachi 2002). Reviews of effectiveness of public health and health promotion interventions can provide information about the effects of interventions on health inequalities. This information can then be used to address health inequities.

Disadvantage may be considered in terms of place of residence, race or ethnicity, occupation, gender, religion, education, socio-economic position (SES) and social capital, known by the PROGRESS acronym (Evans 2003). Authors should carefully consider which of these are relevant to their population of interest; data will then be extracted by these factors. The Cochrane Health Equity Field and Campbell Equity Methods Group are working on definitions of equity as relevant to Cochrane reviews: www.equity. cochrane.irg.au/en/index.html.

Systematic reviews rely upon there being sufficient detail in study data to allow for identification of relevant subgroups for analysis in relation to health inequalities. This requires attention not only to levels of benefit or harm, but also to the distributions of these: who is benefiting, who is harmed, who is excluded?

Reviews of the effectiveness of interventions in relation to health inequalities require three components for calculation:

- a valid measure of health status (or change in health status);

- a measure of socio-economic position (or disadvantage); and

- a statistical method for summarizing the magnitude of health differences between people in different groups.

Review authors should decide which indicator(s) of disadvantage or status are relevant to the review topic. There are many factors that relate to disadvantage (acronym PROGRESS) and authors will need to collect data on any of the factors likely to be relevant to their population of interest (PROGRESS = residence, race or ethnicity, occupation, gender, religion, education, socio-economic position (SES) and social capital).

Conducting reviews addressing inequalities is complicated not only by limited collection of information about differences between groups, but also by the fact that there is limited participation of disadvantaged groups in research. Despite these barriers, systematic reviews can play an important role in raising awareness of health inequalities. The Cochrane Health Equity Field and Campbell Equity Methods Group have identified a number of equity-relevant reviews that may provide additional guidance for authors.

To locate studies that examine inequalities, review authors will need to cast the net broadly when performing searches and contact authors for further information regarding socio-economic data. This latter task may be necessary because primary studies often fail to present information on the socio-economic composition of participants (Oakley 1998, Jackson 2003, Ogilvie 2004). Once studies have been appraised and data have been extracted, studies need to be classified as to whether they are effective for reducing health inequalities. An effective intervention to reduce inequity is generally one that is more effective for disadvantaged groups or individuals. A potentially effective intervention for reducing inequities is one that is equally effective across the socio-economic spectrum (may reduce health inequalities due to the prevalence of health problems among the disadvantaged being greater). The judgement becomes more difficult when the intervention is targeted only at disadvantaged individuals or groups. In a Cochrane review of school feeding problems, effective interventions aimed solely at disadvantaged children were labelled as 'potentially' effective in reducing socio-economic inequalities in health (Kristjansson 2007). It is impossible to determine differential effectiveness if studies comprise mixed levels of advantage and disadvantage but do not include results that can be broken down by socio-economic (or similar) grouping.

## 21.6 Context

The type of interventions implemented and their subsequent success or failure are highly dependent on the social, economic and political context in which they are developed and implemented (see example in Figure 21.6.a). A problem in reviewing public health and health promotion interventions is how to disentangle 'intervention' effects from effects that should be more appropriately called 'program by context interactions' (Hawe 2004). Traditionally, outcomes have been attributed to the intervention. However, the outcomes noted in studies may in fact be due to pre-existing factors of the context into which the intervention was introduced. Hence, context should be considered and measured as an effect modifier in studies (Eccles 2003, Hawe 2004). Such contextual factors might relate to aspects of the program's 'host organization'. Broader aspects of context might include aspects of the *system within which the host organization operates*. Some investigators would also argue that context factors also pertain to the *characteristics of the target group or population.* For many years these aspects have been acknowledged (but not clearly specified) when decision makers have argued that results of evidence reviews from other countries do not apply in their own country.

Use of the term 'context evaluation' became more prevalent in health promotion after the review by Israel and colleagues (Israel 1995). However the systematic investigation of context-level interactions as part of the design of randomized trials of community or organizational-level interventions is almost unknown (Eccles 2003, Hawe 2004). Instead, aspects of context have been explored as part of the more developed field of sustainability research or research on program institutionalization: see Section 21.7. A related and growing multidisciplinary research field is the implementation and integration sciences that are leading researchers more into the complexity of the change processes that interventions represent (Ottoson 1987, Bauman 1991, Scheirer 1994). At the present time, quantitative studies lag behind qualitative analyses of context.

Systematically disentangling context effects from intervention effects in anything other than a study set up for this purpose is extremely difficult. Whilst some programs have been transferred from one context to another and benefits have been observed (Resnicow 1993), others have not (Lumley 2004). Cluster-randomized designs may be expected (in theory) to even out important aspects of context, provided that the sample size is sufficient. However, few investigators at present measure or report on any aspect of context that might be important to our assessment. We also note recent calls for a greater focus on external validity (Glasgow 2006, Green 2006). Working together,

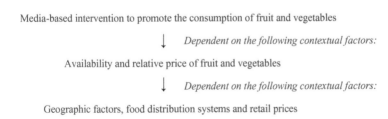

Media-based intervention to promote the consumption of fruit and vegetables

↓  *Dependent on the following contextual factors:*

Availability and relative price of fruit and vegetables

↓  *Dependent on the following contextual factors:*

Geographic factors, food distribution systems and retail prices

**Figure 21.6.a**  Example of intervention success as dependent on the context in which it is implemented (Frommer 2003)

journal editors and researchers are encouraging more examination of, and reporting on, aspects of intervention context (Armstrong 2008). This should be reflected in the content of future Cochrane reviews.

## 21.7  Sustainability

Sustainability refers to the general phenomenon of the continuation of an intervention or its effects (Shediac-Rizkallah 1998, Swerissen 2004). Sustainability of interventions should be an important consideration in systematic reviews. Attention to the long-term viability of health interventions is likely to increase as policy makers, practitioners and funders become increasingly concerned with allocating scarce resources effectively and efficiently (Shediac-Rizkallah 1998). Users of reviews are interested in knowing whether the health benefits, such as reductions in specific diseases or improvements in health, are going to be sustained beyond the life of the interventions.

Unfortunately, collecting data on the extent to which the intervention and outcomes are sustained is often not carried out, which limits the extent to which long-term impacts can be assessed. Careful consideration in Cochrane reviews of how previous studies have (or have not) addressed issues of sustainability will increase our understanding in this area and hopefully also stimulate improved design for assessment of sustainability in future studies.

A sustained or sustainable program does not necessarily result in sustained outcomes and not all interventions need to be sustained in order to be useful or effective (Shediac-Rizkallah 1998). Also, review authors should consider whether the sustainability of the outcomes is relevant to the objectives of the intervention. If this is the case, authors should consider what outcomes have (or should have) been measured, over what period, and what the pattern of outcomes is over time.

Information should be sought on both contextual factors and intervention characteristics that may explain the extent to which the interventions or outcomes are sustained. Where sustainability of outcomes has not been measured, authors should explore the *potential* of the intervention outcomes to be sustained. Four frameworks may be useful to assist in determining sustainability:

1. Bossert lists the following five factors influencing sustainability (Bossert 1990):

   - the economic and political variables surrounding the implementation and evaluation of the intervention;

   - the strength of the institution implementing the intervention;

   - the full integration of activities into existing programs/services/curriculum/etc;

   - whether the program includes a strong training component (capacity building); and

   - community involvement/participation in the program;

2. The framework developed by Swerissen and Crisp (Swerissen 2004) guides decisions about the likely sustainability of interventions and effects at different levels of social organization. This framework outlines the relationships between intervention level, strategies and the likely sustainability of interventions and effects.

3. Shediac-Rizkallah and Bone present a useful framework for conceptualizing sustainability (Shediac-Rizkallah 1998). In this framework key aspects of program sustainability are defined as 1) maintenance of health benefits from the program; 2) institutionalization of a program within an organization; and 3) capacity building in the recipient community. Key factors influencing sustainability are defined as 1) factors in the broader environment; 2) factors within the organizational setting; and 3) project design and implementation factors.

4. The Centre for Health Promotion, University of Toronto, has also produced a document outlining four integrated components of sustainability (Health Communication Unit 2001).

## 21.8 Applicability and transferability

Applicability needs to be considered when deciding how to translate the findings of a given study or review to a specific population, intervention, or setting (see Chapter 12, Section 12.3). *Transferability* or the *potential for translation* are similar and appropriate terms. Applicability is closely related to integrity, context, and sustainability as discussed in previous sections of this chapter.

Systematic reviews of public health and health promotion interventions encompass several issues that make the process of determining applicability even more complex than in the clinical trials literature. First, a number of public health interventions do not involve randomization. Although not an inherent characteristic of non-randomized designs, these studies may have less well-defined eligibility criteria, settings, and interventions, making determinations of applicability more difficult. Then again, results from randomized trials may be less generalizable due to unrepresentative providers of the intervention or study participants not being typical of the target group (Black 1996). Second, public health and health promotion interventions tend to have multiple components. This makes it difficult to 1) determine what specific intervention component had the noted effect, and 2) assess the synergy between components. Third, in community interventions, implementation and adherence may be much more difficult to achieve and to measure. This also makes it harder to interpret and apply the findings. Fourth, in public health and health promotion interventions the underlying socio-cultural characteristics of communities are complex and difficult to measure. Thus it is difficult to define to whom and to what degree the intervention was applied, complicating determinations of applicability. On the other hand, this heterogeneity may increase applicability, as the original populations, settings, and interventions may be quite diverse, increasing the likelihood that the evidence can be applied broadly.

Review authors are ideally positioned to summarize the various aspects of the evidence that are relevant to potential users. This enables users to compare their situation or setting to that presented in the review and note the similarities and differences. Users can then be explicit about the relationship between the body of evidence and their specific situation.

The following questions may assist authors to consider issues of applicability and transferability relevant to health promotion and public health (Wang 2006).

*Applicability*

- Does the **political environment** of the local society allow this intervention to be implemented?

- Is there any political barrier to implementing this intervention?

- Would the general public and the targeted (sub) population accept this intervention? Does any aspect of the intervention go against local **social norms**? Is it ethically acceptable?

- Can the contents of the intervention be tailored to suit the local culture?

- Are the essential **resources** for implementing this intervention available in the local setting? (a list of essential resources may help to answer this question);

- Does the target population in the local setting have a sufficient **educational** level to comprehend the contents of the intervention?

- Which organization will be responsible for the provision of this intervention in the local setting?

- Is there any possible barrier to implementing this intervention due to the **structure of that organization**?

- Does the provider of the intervention in the local setting have the **skill** to deliver this intervention? If not-will training be available?

*Transferability*

- What is the **baseline prevalence** of the health problem of interest in the local setting? What us the difference in prevalence between the study setting and the local setting?

- Are the **characteristics of the target population** comparable between the study setting and the local setting? With regard to the particular aspects that will be addressed in the intervention is it possible that the characteristics of the target population, such as ethnicity, socio-economic status, educational level etc. will have an impact on the effectiveness of the intervention?

- Is the **capacity to implement** the intervention comparable between the study setting in such matters as political environment, social acceptability, resources, organizational structure and the skills of the local providers?

## 21.9 Chapter information

**Editors:** Rebecca Armstrong, Elizabeth Waters and Jodie Doyle.

**This chapter should be cited as:** Armstrong R, Waters E, Doyle J (editors). Chapter 21: Reviews in health promotion and public health. In Higgins JPT, Green S (editors). *Cochrane Handbook for Systematic Reviews of Interventions*. Chichester (UK): John Wiley & Sons, 2008.

**Contributing Authors**: Rebecca Armstrong, Elizabeth Waters, Nicki Jackson, Sandy Oliver, Jennie Popay, Jonathan Shepherd, Mark Petticrew, Laurie Anderson, Ross Bailie, Ginny Brunton, Penny Hawe, Elizabeth Kristjansson, Lucio Naccarella, Susan Norris, Elizabeth Pienaar, Helen Roberts, Wendy Rogers, Amanda Sowden and Helen Thomas.

## 21.10 References

**Armstrong 2008**
Armstrong R, Waters E, Moore L, Riggs E, Cuervo LG, Lumbiganon P, Hawe P. Improving the reporting of public health intervention research: advancing TREND and CONSORT. *Journal of Public Health* (Oxford) (in press, 2008).

**Bauman 1991**
Bauman LJ, Stein RE, Ireys HT. Reinventing fidelity: the transfer of social technology among settings. *American Journal of Community Psychology* 1991; 19: 619–639.

**Beahler 2000**
Beahler CC, Sundheim JJ, Trapp NI. Information retrieval in systematic reviews: challenges in the public health arena. *American Journal of Preventive Medicine* 2000; 18: 6–10.

**Black 1996**
Black N. Why we need observational studies to evaluate the effectiveness of health care. *BMJ* 1996; 312: 1215-1218.

**Bossert 1990**
Bossert TJ. Can they get along without us? Sustainability of donor-supported health projects in Central America and Africa. *Social Science and Medicine* 1990; 30: 1015–1023.

**Cochrane EPOC Group 2008**
Cochrane EPOC Group. Cochrane Effective Practice and Organisation of Care Group. Available from: http://www.epoc.cochrane.org (accessed 1 January 2008).

**Deeks 2003**

Deeks JJ, Dinnes J, D'Amico R, Sowden AJ, Sakarovitch C, Song F, Petticrew M, Altman DG. Evaluating non-randomised intervention studies. *Health Technology Assessment* 2003; 7: 27.

**Donner 2004**

Donner A, Klar N. Pitfalls of and controversies in cluster randomization trials. *American Journal of Public Health* 2004; 94: 416–422.

**Eccles 2003**

Eccles M, Grimshaw J, Campbell M, Ramsay C. Research designs for studies evaluating the effectiveness of change and improvement strategies. *Quality and Safety in Health Care* 2003; 12: 47-52.

**Effective Public Health Practice Project 2007**

Effective Public Health Practice Project. Effective Public Health Practice Project [Updated 25 October 2007]. Available from: http://www.city.hamilton.on.ca/PHCS/EPHPP (accessed 1 January 2008).

**Evans 2003**

Evans T, Brown H. Road traffic crashes: operationalizing equity in the context of health sector reform. *Injury Control and Safety Promotion* 2003; 10: 11–12.

**Frommer 2003**

Frommer M, Rychetnik L. From evidence-based medicine to evidence-based public health. In: Lin V, Gibson B (editors). *Evidence-based Health Policy: Problems and Possibilities.* Melbourne (Australia): Oxford University Press, 2003.

**Glasgow 2006**

Glasgow RE, Green LW, Klesges LM, Abrams DB, Fisher EB, Goldstein MG, Hayman LL, Ockene JK, Orleans CT. External validity: we need to do more. *Annals of Behavioral Medicine* 2006; 31: 105-108.

**Glasziou 2004**

Glasziou P, Vandenbroucke JP, Chalmers I. Assessing the quality of research. *BMJ* 2004; 328: 39–41.

**Grayson 2003**

Grayson L, Gomersall A. *A Difficult Business: Finding the Evidence for Social Science Reviews.* London (UK): ESRC UK Centre for Evidence Based Policy and Practice, 2003.

**Green 2006**

Green LW, Glasgow RE. Evaluating the relevance, generalization, and applicability of research: issues in external validation and translation methodology. *Evaluation and the Health Professions* 2006; 29: 126–153.

**Hawe 1995**

Hawe P, Shiell A. Preserving innovation under increasing accountability pressures: the health promotion investment portfolio approach. *Health Promotion Journal of Australia* 1995; 5: 4–9.

**Hawe 2004**

Hawe P, Shiell A, Riley T, Gold L. Methods for exploring implementation variation and local context within a cluster randomised community intervention trial. *Journal of Epidemiology and Community Health* 2004; 58: 788–793.

**Health Communication Unit 2001**

Health Communication Unit. Overview of Sustainability [Version 8.2, 30 April 2001]. Available from: http://www.thcu.ca/infoandresources/sustainability.htm (accessed 1 January 2008).

**Israel 1995**

Israel BA, Cummings KM, Dignan MB, Heaney CA, Perales DP, Simons-Morton BG, Zimmerman MA. Evaluation of health education programs: current assessment and future directions. *Health Education Quarterly* 1995; 22: 364–389.

**Jackson 2003**

Jackson T, Aldrich R, Dixon J, Furler J, Turrell G, Wilson A, Duell N, Robertson L, Leonard J. *Using Socioeconomic Evidence in Clinical Practice Guidelines.* Canberra (Australia): National Health and Medical Research Council, 2003.

**Kawachi 2002**

Kawachi I, Subramanian SV, Almeida-Filho N. A glossary for health inequalities. *Journal of Epidemiology and Community Health* 2002; 56: 647–652.

**Kristjansson 2007**

Kristjansson EA, Robinson V, Petticrew M, MacDonald B, Krasevec J, Janzen L, Greenhalgh T, Wells G, MacGowan J, Farmer A, Shea BJ, Mayhew A, Tugwell P. School feeding for improving the physical and psychosocial health of disadvantaged elementary school children. *Cochrane Database of Systematic Reviews* 2007, Issue 1. Art No: CD004676.

**Lumley 2004**

Lumley J, Oliver SS, Chamberlain C, Oakley L. Interventions for promoting smoking cessation during pregnancy. *Cochrane Database of Systematic Reviews* 2004, Issue 4. Art No: CD001055.

**Macinko 2002**

Macinko JA, Starfield B. Annotated Bibliography on Equity in Health, 1980–2001. *International Journal for Equity in Health* 2002; 1: 1.

**Macintyre 2003**

Macintyre S. Evaluating the evidence on measures to reduce inequalities in health. In: Oliver A, Exworthy M (editors). *Health Inequalities: Evidence, Policy and Implementation. Proceedings from a meeting of the Health Equity Network.* London (UK): The Nuffield Trust, 2003.

**Oakley 1998**

Oakley A, Peersman G, Oliver S. Social characteristics of participants in health promotion effectiveness research; trial and error? *Education for Health* 1998; 11: 305–317.

**Ogilvie 2004**

Ogilvie D, Petticrew M. Reducing social inequalities in smoking: can evidence inform policy? A pilot study. *Tobacco Control* 2004; 13: 129–131.

**Ottoson 1987**

Ottoson JM, Green LW. Reconciling concept and context: theory of implementation. In: Ward WB (editors). *Advances in Health Education and Promotion Volume 2.* Greenwich (CT): JAI Press, 1987.

**Peersman 2001**

Peersman G, Oakley A. Learning from research. In: Oliver S, Peersman G (editors). *Using Research for Effective Health Promotion.* Buckingham (UK): Open University Press, 2001.

**Petticrew 2003**

Petticrew M, Roberts H. Evidence, hierarchies, and typologies: horses for courses. *Journal of Epidemiology and Community Health* 2003; 57: 527–529.

**Resnicow 1993**

Resnicow K, Cross D, Wynder E. The Know Your Body program: a review of evaluation studies. *Bulletin of the New York Academy of Medicine* 1993; 70: 188–207.

**Scheirer 1994**

Scheirer MA. Designing and using process evaluations. In: Wholey JS, Hatry HP, Newcomer KE (editors). *Handbook of Practical Program Evaluation*. San Francisco: Jossey Bass, 1994.

**Shaw 2004**

Shaw RL, Booth A, Sutton AJ, Miller T, Smith JA, Young B, Jones DR, xon-Woods M. Finding qualitative research: an evaluation of search strategies. *BMC Medical Research Methodology* 2004; 4: 5.

**Shediac-Rizkallah 1998**

Shediac-Rizkallah MC, Bone LR. Planning for the sustainability of community-based health programs: conceptual frameworks and future directions for research, practice and policy. *Health Education Research* 1998; 13: 87–108.

**Swerissen 2004**

Swerissen H, Crisp BR. The sustainability of health promotion interventions for different levels of social organization. *Health Promotion International* 2004; 19: 123–130.

**Wang 2006**

Wang S, Moss JR, Hiller JE. Applicability and transferability of interventions in evidence-based public health. *Health Promotion International* 2006; 21: 76–83.

# 22 Overviews of reviews

## Lorne A Becker and Andrew D Oxman

## Key Points

- Cochrane Overviews of reviews (Overviews) are intended primarily to summarize multiple Cochrane Intervention reviews addressing the effects of two or more potential interventions for a single condition or health problem.

- In the absence of a relevant Cochrane Intervention review, Cochrane Overviews may additionally include systematic reviews published elsewhere.

- Overviews should be conducted in priority areas where a number of Cochrane Intervention reviews exist.

- Overviews have a similar structure to Intervention reviews, but include reviews rather than primary studies.

- Overviews include an 'Overviews of reviews' table designed to reflect the 'Summary of findings' tables in Cochrane Intervention reviews.

- Overviews should be updated when the included reviews are updated.

## 22.1 Introduction

### 22.1.1 Definition of Cochrane Overviews of reviews

**Cochrane Overviews of reviews** (Cochrane Overviews) are Cochrane reviews designed to compile evidence from multiple systematic reviews of interventions into one accessible and usable document. This chapter outlines the rationale for Cochrane Overviews and details the methods that authors and Cochrane Review Groups (CRGs) should follow in completing these reviews.

## 22.1.2   Rationale for Cochrane Overviews

Cochrane Overviews are intended primarily to overview multiple Cochrane Intervention reviews addressing the effects of two or more potential interventions for a single condition or health problem. Cochrane Overviews highlight the Cochrane reviews that address these potential interventions and summarize their results for important outcomes.

It is important to note that there are other reasons for undertaking overviews of reviews. Cochrane Overviews of reviews can accommodate some, but not all of these objectives. Table 22.1.a outlines different reasons for overviewing systematic reviews and indicates which of these are suitable for publication as a Cochrane Overview. Before registering or publishing a Cochrane Overview, CRGs should ensure that a planned Overview is suitable for publication.

As can be surmised from Table 22.1.a, a central aim of Cochrane Overviews is to serve as a 'friendly front end' to *The Cochrane Library,* allowing the reader a quick overview (and an exhaustive list) of Cochrane Intervention reviews relevant to a specific decision. The primary audiences envisioned are decision makers (such as a clinicians, policy makers, or informed consumers) who are accessing *The Cochrane Library* for evidence on a specific problem. Once completed, Cochrane Overviews will be published as part of the *Cochrane Database of Systematic Reviews* in a format that allows readers to readily distinguish them from Cochrane Intervention reviews, Diagnostic test accuracy reviews and Methodology reviews.

# 22.2   Preparing a Cochrane Overview of reviews

## 22.2.1   Organizational issues

The impetus for initiation of a Cochrane Overview should be an area of priority where a number of Cochrane Intervention reviews exist. The identification of a need for an Overview could come from a team of interested authors, a CRG, or a grouping of CRGs. Fields or Centres might also set priority areas for Cochrane Overviews and attempt to find authors to undertake them. Authors of Cochrane Intervention reviews may take on the role of Overview author if they wish, but are not automatically required to do so. Authors of Overviews should be familiar with the methodology of Cochrane Intervention reviews, ideally having co-authored one.

One CRG will have editorial control over each Overview of reviews; titles and protocols should be submitted in the same way as for Intervention reviews. In most cases, all of the Cochrane reviews to be included in the Overview will be expected to come from a single CRG, and that CRG would have editorial responsibility. If it is anticipated that Cochrane reviews from more than one CRG will be included, for example in Overviews of reviews addressing an intervention used in the management of several conditions, the editorial process would be discussed among the relevant CRGs,

**Table 22.1.a** Reasons for overviewing reviews and their suitability for publication as a Cochrane Overview

| Objective | Selection criteria | Examples of overviews | Suitable for inclusion as a Cochrane Overview of reviews | Comments |
|---|---|---|---|---|
| To summarize evidence from more than one systematic review of **different interventions** for the same condition or problem. | Cochrane Intervention reviews. | A Cochrane Overview of interventions for nocturnal enuresis (Russell 2006) | Yes. | This is the primary purpose of Cochrane Overviews (and should be referred to as an Overview of Cochrane reviews in the objectives section of the abstract and the text). |
| | Cochrane Intervention reviews and non-Cochrane systematic reviews. | Some *BMJ Clinical Evidence* chapters and an increasing number of health technology assessment (HTA) reports. | Possibly. | It may sometimes be appropriate to include non-Cochrane systematic reviews as well as Cochrane reviews, for example, if there are important interventions for which good quality systematic reviews have been published and a Cochrane review is not available. However, CRGs are encouraged to focus primarily on Overviews of Cochrane reviews as: <br>• searching for and including non-Cochrane reviews in Overviews entails additional work and challenges <br>• non-Cochrane reviews may not be accessible to users of *The Cochrane Library* <br>• the primary aim of Cochrane Overviews is to summarize Cochrane reviews and to provide a user-friendly front end. |

*- (Continued)*

**Table 22.1.a** *(Continued)*

| Objective | Selection criteria | Examples of overviews | Suitable for inclusion as a Cochrane Overview of reviews | Comments |
|---|---|---|---|---|
| To summarize evidence from more than one systematic review of the same condition or problem where **different outcomes** are addressed in different systematic reviews. | Cochrane Intervention reviews. | An overview of Cochrane reviews of hormone replacement therapy (HRT) for menopause where outcomes may include bone density, menopausal symptoms, cardiovascular risk/ events, cognitive function etc. | Occasionally. | As a rule, individual Cochrane reviews should include all outcomes that are important to people making decisions about an intervention. However, occasionally, as with HRT, different outcomes have to a large extent been considered in different systematic reviews. |
| | Cochrane Intervention reviews and non-Cochrane reviews. | Some *BMJ Clinical Evidence* chapters and some HTA reports. | Rarely. | The considerations for including non-Cochrane systematic reviews are the same as those noted above. |
| To summarize evidence from more than one systematic review of the same intervention for **different conditions, problems or populations.** | Cochrane Intervention reviews. | An overview of Cochrane reviews of vitamin A for different populations and conditions. | Occasionally. | The same or similar interventions may sometimes be used for different conditions or different studies and reviews may focus on different populations. While an overview of these reviews is unlikely to be of interest to clinicians and patients deciding how best to address a specific problem, an overview may be relevant to policy makers or to addressing questions that cut across the different reviews. |

| | | | | |
|---|---|---|---|---|
| | Cochrane Intervention reviews and non-Cochrane reviews. | | Rarely. | The considerations for including non-Cochrane systematic reviews are the same as those noted above. |
| To summarize evidence about **adverse effects** of an intervention from more than one systematic review of use of the intervention for one or more conditions. | Cochrane Intervention reviews only or Cochrane Intervention reviews and non-Cochrane systematic reviews. | An overview of adverse effects of NSAIDs when used for osteoarthritis or rheumatoid arthritis or menorraghia. | Rarely. | While many Cochrane reviews report on adverse effects, few if any are designed primarily to assess rates of adverse effects. Many important adverse effects occur so rarely that their true prevalence cannot be accurately assessed from results of controlled trials. For these reasons, an overview based solely on Cochrane or other systematic reviews of controlled trials may not give an accurate picture of the adverse effect profile of a specific intervention – unless the systematic reviews it summarizes have been specifically designed to address the rates of adverse effects (see Chapter 14 for further information on the reporting of adverse effects in Cochrane reviews. |

(*Continued*)

**Table 22.1**  (*Continued*)

| Objective | Selection criteria | Examples of overviews | Suitable for inclusion as a Cochrane Overview of reviews | Comments |
|---|---|---|---|---|
| To provide a comprehensive overview of an area, including **studies not included in systematic reviews.** | Systematic reviews and studies not included in systematic reviews. | Some *BMJ Clinical Evidence* chapters, an increasing number of HTA reports or a synoptic review article for a journal. | No. | Including studies that have not previously been included in a systematic review may be appropriate in a number of circumstances, for example when undertaking a HTA report, developing a clinical practice guideline, or for resources such as *BMJ Clinical Evidence*. However, this is beyond the scope of what should be done in a Cochrane Overview. Authors of Cochrane Overviews should note when included reviews are out of date, particularly if new relevant studies have been published, and if there are relevant interventions for which a systematic review has not yet been published. However, they should not undertake an update of a systematic review or a new systematic review within the Overview. |

and a decision made about which CRG(s) would take the editorial role, as currently happens for some reviews when more than one CRG is involved.

Authors of an Overview who identify studies not included in existing Cochrane Intervention reviews may consider approaching the relevant CRG to plan a new Cochrane review with a broader scope, to update an existing Cochrane review or to undertake a new Cochrane review for an intervention not already included in an existing review.

### 22.2.2 Methodological issues

Cochrane Overviews use different methods from Cochrane Intervention reviews; they summarize existing Intervention reviews rather than find and summarize or synthesize original studies. Key differences in methods between Cochrane Intervention reviews and Cochrane Overviews are summarized in Table 22.2.a.

Cochrane Overviews of reviews do not aim to repeat the searches, assessment of eligibility, assessment of risk of bias or meta-analyses from the included Intervention reviews. In addition, they do not typically aim to identify systematically any additional studies or to extract additional outcomes from studies. They do include assessment of limitations of included systematic reviews, and may include meta-analyses across reviews to provide indirect comparisons of the effects of different interventions on a given outcome. This is not to imply that overviews of systematic reviews that undertake a more detailed analysis including critical appraisal, new searches and new analyses are inappropriate, but they are not what is envisaged for Cochrane Overviews.

### 22.2.3 Updating Cochrane Overviews

Regular updating of Cochrane Overviews is very important and follows the usual process for the updating of Cochrane reviews (see Chapter 3). A Cochrane Overview will require updating whenever any of the included reviews are updated. In many cases, only minor changes to the Cochrane Overview will be required. For example, if no new studies were found in the update of a Cochrane Intervention review, only the information on the date of last update for that review would need to be changed in the Overview. However, whenever an update results in a change to the results and conclusions of an included Intervention review, the Overview will require more extensive revisions.

## 22.3 Format of a Cochrane Overview

### 22.3.1 Title and review information (or protocol information)

The title of an Overview should have the form: [Interventions or comparisons] for [health problem] in OR for [types of people, disease or problem and setting if specified].

**Table 22.2.a** Comparison of methods between Cochrane Intervention reviews and Cochrane Overviews of reviews

|  | Cochrane Intervention reviews | Cochrane Overviews of reviews | Comments regarding Cochrane Overviews of reviews |
|---|---|---|---|
| Objectives. | To summarize evidence from studies of the effects of interventions. | To summarize evidence from systematic reviews of the effects of interventions. | Appropriate when there are two or more interventions for the same condition or problem presented in separate Cochrane Intervention reviews. |
| Selection criteria. | Describe inclusion and exclusion criteria for studies. | Describe inclusion and exclusion criteria for reviews. | Primarily only Cochrane Intervention reviews are included. Sometimes Cochrane Intervention reviews and other reviews found in *The Cochrane Library* (*Database of Abstracts of Reviews of Effects* or *Health Technology Assessment Database*) may be included. Occasionally other systematic reviews may be included. |
| Search. | Comprehensive search for relevant studies. | Typically search for only relevant Cochrane Intervention reviews. | May occasionally search for non-Cochrane systematic reviews. |
| Data collection. | From included studies. | From included systematic reviews. | If necessary, authors of Overviews may seek additional information from the authors of included systematic reviews or occasionally from the primary studies included in systematic reviews. |
| Assessment of limitations. | For included studies; i.e. risk of bias. | For included systematic reviews. | Authors of Cochrane Overviews should critically appraise included reviews using explicit criteria. Both general limitations (e.g. whether the review is up to date) and specific limitations should be considered (i.e. if a systematic review has limitations relative to the specific objectives of the Overview). |
| Quality of evidence. | Across studies for each important outcome. | So far as possible should be based on assessments reported in the included systematic reviews. | It is recommended that each Overview should include an assessment of the quality of evidence for each important outcome. If such an assessment was not done in included systematic reviews, authors of Overviews should try to do it. If it was done in included systematic reviews, authors of Overviews should critically appraise the judgements that were made and try to ensure that these judgements were made consistently across included reviews. |

**Table 22.2.a**   *(Continued)*

| | Cochrane Intervention reviews | Cochrane Overviews of reviews | Comments regarding Cochrane Overviews of reviews |
|---|---|---|---|
| Analysis. | Syntheses of results across included studies for each important outcome. | Summary of review results; additional analyses may be undertaken for comparisons across reviews, typically indirect comparisons of multiple interventions. | So far as possible authors of Cochrane Overviews should rely on analyses reported in the included reviews. Occasionally data may need to be reanalysed, for example if different populations or subgroups are analysed in different reviews and it is possible to undertake comparable analyses across reviews. |

The 'Interventions or comparisons' part of the title can take various formats, depending on the scope of the review. If all potential interventions with systematic review evidence are to be considered, this section should simply read 'Interventions for'. If the Overview is to be restricted to a subset of potential interventions, the title should indicate the subset, for example 'Surgical interventions for '. If two types of intervention are to be compared, the comparator should be included in the title, for example 'Surgical or pharmacological interventions for'.

All other review information is the same as for Intervention reviews, as described in Chapter 4 (Section 4.2).

## 22.3.2   Abstract

The content under each heading in the abstract should be as follows:

**Background:** This should be one or two sentences to explain the context or elaborate on the purpose and rationale of the Overview.
**Objectives:** This should be a precise statement of the primary objective of the Overview, ideally in a single sentence. Where possible the style should be of the form 'To summarize Cochrane reviews that assess the effects of *[interventions or comparisons]* for *[health problem]* for/in *[types of people, disease or problem and setting if specified]*'.
**Methods:** This section should succinctly address the search strategy used to identify systematic reviews for inclusion in the Overview and the methods used for data collection and analysis. The latter should be restricted to description of the guidelines used for extracting data and assessing data quality and validity and not include details of what data were extracted. The method by which the guidelines were applied should be stated (for example, independent extraction by multiple review authors).
**Main results:** This section should begin with the total number of systematic reviews included in the Overview, and brief details pertinent to the interpretation of the results

(for example, the quality of the included systematic reviews or a comment on the comparability of the reviews, if appropriate). It should address the primary objective and be restricted to the main qualitative and quantitative results (generally including not more than seven key results). The outcomes included should be selected based on their expected value in helping someone to make a decision about whether or not to use a particular intervention. If relevant, the number of studies and participants contributing to the separate outcomes should be noted, along with the quality of evidence specific to these outcomes. The results should be expressed in narrative as well as quantitatively if the numerical results are not clear or intuitive (such as those from standardized mean differences analyses). The summary statistics in the abstract should be the same as those highlighted in the text of the Overview, and should be presented in a standard way, such as 'risk ratio 2.31 (95% confidence interval 1.13 to 3.45)'. Both absolute and relative effects should be reported, if possible. However, review authors should be cautious about reporting absolute effects when control group risk for an outcome varies across studies or reviews (see Chapter 11, Section 11.5.5). If overall results are not calculated in an included review, a qualitative assessment or a description of the range and pattern of the results can be given. However, 'vote counts' in which the numbers of 'positive' and 'negative' studies (or reviews) are reported should be avoided.

**Authors' conclusions:** The primary purpose of the Overview should be to present information, rather than to offer advice. The Authors' conclusions should be succinct and drawn directly from the findings of the Overview so that they directly reflect the main results. Authors should be careful not to confuse a lack of evidence with a lack of effect. Assumptions should not be made about practice circumstances, values, preferences, tradeoffs; and the giving of advice or recommendations should generally be avoided. Any important limitations of data and analyses should be noted. Important conclusions about specific implications for research, including systematic reviews, should be included if relevant. Authors should not make general statements that 'more research is needed'.

## 22.3.3 Plain language summary

The plain language summary (formerly called the 'synopsis') aims to summarize the Overview in a straightforward style that can be understood by consumers of health care: see Chapter 4 (Section 4.4).

## 22.3.4 Text of a Cochrane Overview

The target audience for a Cochrane Overview is people who make decisions about health care (e.g. clinicians, informed consumers and policy makers) who already have some basic understanding of the underlying disease or problem and wish to discover the extent to which the potential interventions for the problem have been addressed in *The Cochrane Library*. The Overview should provide an overview of the findings of relevant Cochrane reviews, and direct the reader to the individual reviews for additional detail.

The text of a Cochrane Overview contains a number of fixed headings. Subheadings may be added by the author at any point. Certain specific headings are designated as 'recommended'. The content of recommended sections should be included in all Overviews, but the use of the actual subheading is not mandatory and should be avoided if they make individual sections needlessly short. Additional subheadings that may or may not be relevant to a particular review are also provided. In the rest of this section, the relevant category (fixed, recommended, optional) is noted for each of the headings described.

# Background

This section should address the already-formed body of knowledge that comprises the context of the Cochrane reviews summarized in the Overview. The background helps set the rationale for the Overview. It should specify the research question(s) being addressed by the Overview, including a clear description of the condition of interest, the interventions, comparisons, and the outcomes considered. Furthermore, it should explain why the questions being asked are important. It should be presented in a fashion that is understandable to the users of the health care under investigation, and should be concise (generally around one page when printed). The background section should contain the following components. Although subheadings are not mandatory, they are recommended.

## Description of the condition

The review should begin with a brief description of the condition being addressed and its significance. It may include information about the biology, diagnosis, prognosis and public health importance (including prevalence or incidence).

## Description of the interventions

This section should mention all of the interventions currently available for the condition, whether or not the interventions have been evaluated in a Cochrane Intervention review. Where reasonable, grouping interventions will simplify the text (e.g. listing non-steroidal anti-inflammatory drugs rather than providing an exhaustive list of all such drugs by name). The possibility of concurrent use of different interventions (e.g. radiation plus chemotherapy) should be addressed, if applicable. The relative status of the various potential interventions in current clinical practice may be mentioned (if feasible).

## How the interventions might work

Systematic reviews gather evidence to assess whether the expected effect of an intervention does indeed occur. This section might describe the theoretical reasoning why the interventions under review might have an impact on potential recipients of health care, for example, by relating a drug intervention to the biology of the condition. Authors may refer to a body of empirical evidence such as similar interventions having an impact or identical interventions having an impact on other populations. Authors may also refer to a body of literature that justifies the possibility of effectiveness. References to existing literature should not include any discussion of the results of the systematic reviews contained in the Overview or the studies addressed in those reviews; this material should be covered in the Results section.

### Why it is important to do this overview

The background helps set the rationale for the Overview, and should explain why the questions being asked are important. It should make clear why this Overview was undertaken, who the target audience is, and what decisions it is intended to help inform.

## Objectives

This should begin with a precise statement of the primary aim of the review, including the intervention(s) reviewed and the targeted problem. This might be followed by a series of specific objectives relating to different participant groups, different comparisons of interventions or different outcome measures.

## Methods

The Methods section in a protocol should be written in the future tense. The Methods section of the review should describe what was done to obtain the results and conclusions of the current version of the Overview. It should not discuss the methods of the underlying systematic reviews that are being summarized. Comments on the methods of these reviews should be addressed in the section 'Description of included reviews'. The Methods section should have a number of component subsections.

### Criteria for considering reviews for inclusion

The Overview research question should guide selection of reviews for inclusion, including a clear description of the participants (condition or health problem), the interventions, comparison groups and outcomes of interest. In general, Overviews should include all Cochrane reviews that address one or more of the interventions available for the condition or health problem that is the topic of the Overview. However, in some cases the authors of the Overview may wish to restrict this focus in some way. For example, Overview authors may wish to restrict their scope to certain types of interventions (e.g. all drug therapies, excluding non-drug therapies). Restrictions would be particularly appropriate if the existing Cochrane reviews address varied clinical populations (e.g. groups that differ by age, ethnicity, sex, stage of disease or types of co-morbidity). In making decisions to lump or split, it will be helpful to keep in mind the perspective of the decision maker reading the overview and to focus on the information that would be required to make an individual decision. For example, Cochrane Intervention reviews addressing prevention of a given condition should probably not be grouped in a single Overview with Intervention reviews addressing treatment of the same condition – since prevention decisions and treatment decisions are made for different populations. If such considerations are involved in the selection of reviews for inclusion in the Overview, they should be clearly spelled out in this section.

If non-Cochrane systematic reviews are included, this section should specify the criteria that will be used to determine whether non-Cochrane reviews are systematic reviews, and the criteria that will be used to determine which systematic reviews will be included when there are two or more reviews that address the same question.

## Search methods for identification of reviews

This should address the methods used in the Overview to find Cochrane reviews or other systematic reviews. The search involved will be much simpler than the search strategies within a Cochrane Intervention review, because the basic search for underlying articles will have already been performed. If only Cochrane reviews are to be included in the overview, the search can be performed within the *Cochrane Database of Systematic Reviews* without the need to search other databases. If systematic reviews from other sources are included, this section should clearly outline the databases searched (e.g. *Database of Abstracts of Reviews of Effects* (Petticrew 1999)) and the search strategies and retrieval methods used.

## Data collection and analysis

This section should present a brief description of the methods used in the Overview. The following issues should be addressed:

### *Selection of reviews*

The method used to apply the selection criteria to reviews identified in the search and whether the criteria are applied independently by more than one review author should be stated, along with how any disagreements are resolved.

### *Data extraction and management*

The method used to extract or obtain data from the included reviews (for example, using a data collection form) should be described in this section. Whether data are extracted independently by more than one author should be stated, along with how any disagreements are resolved. If relevant, methods for processing data in preparation for analysis should be clearly described. Authors should also describe what, if anything, is done to collect data that are missing from the included reviews.

### Assessment of methodological quality of included reviews

Two different quality assessments must be addressed by the Overview authors in each Overview: the methodological quality of the reviews summarized in the Overview, and the quality of the evidence in these reviews, as described below.

The methods used in performing both types of assessment should be described in this section. For both assessments it is recommended that more than one review author should apply the criteria independently. This should be stated, along with how any disagreements are resolved. The tools used (e.g. GRADE) should be described or referenced, with an indication of how these assessments are incorporated into the interpretation of the results of the Overview.

***Quality of included reviews***    The methods used to assess the methodological quality of the reviews included in the Overview should be described. There has been limited research on the assessment of quality, or risk of bias, in systematic reviews, and we are unable to recommend a specific instrument for reaching judgements about the quality of included reviews. However, some questionnaires and checklists are available (Oxman 1994, Shea 2006).

***Quality of evidence in included reviews***    Cochrane Intervention reviews that use excellent methods may summarize evidence with important limitations, because of potential biases within and across the included studies, conflicting results across individual studies, sparse evidence or a lack of relevance (directness) to the review question (see Chapter 12, Section 12.2). The methods used in the Overview to determine the quality of the evidence in support of each of the Overview's conclusions should be summarized. Ideally, the information on which to base such assessments should be available in the 'Characteristics of included studies', 'Risk of bias' and 'Summary of findings' tables provided in the included reviews. It is now recommended that assessments of the risk of bias should be reported in a standardized way in Cochrane reviews (see Chapter 8) and that the GRADE approach should be used to assess the quality of evidence across studies for each important outcome for both Cochrane Intervention reviews and Overviews of Cochrane reviews (see Chapter 11, Section 11.5, and Chapter 12, Section 12.2).

### Data synthesis

Many Overviews will simply extract data from the underlying systematic reviews and reformat them in tables or figures. However, in some cases Overviews may include indirect comparisons based on formal statistical analyses, especially if there is no evidence on direct comparisons (Glenny 2005). Statistical methods for undertaking indirect comparisons, and for simultaneous meta-analyses of multiple interventions, are highly relevant to Overviews, and are discussed in Chapter 16 (Section 16.6). Evidence from indirect comparisons may be less reliable than evidence from direct (head to head) comparisons. If no included reviews have investigated direct comparisons, but studies of direct comparisons are known or believed to have been performed, then authors of Overviews should not attempt indirect comparisons. Authors who wish to undertake indirect comparisons or multiple-treatments meta-analyses should seek appropriate statistical and methodological support.

When more qualitative or narrative approaches are used, review authors should state what, if any, methods are used to standardize reporting of results across included reviews, including converting summary statistics and any standardization for different control group risks. Authors should be cautious when comparing absolute effects across reviews if there are differences in control group risks (see Chapter 11, Section 11.5.5).

# Results

## Description of included reviews

The description of included reviews should be concise, but provide sufficient detail to allow the reader to get an idea of the characteristics of participants included in the summarized reviews: the dose, duration, or other characteristics of the interventions. If there are important differences between these component reviews (e.g. differences in the review criteria for inclusion or exclusion of studies, different comparators, or the use of different outcome measures) these should be clearly noted. In addition, any discrepancies between the objectives and eligibility criteria of the included reviews and the objectives of the Overview should be noted. For example, the review authors may have omitted analyses of a specific subgroup or of a key outcome that was of particular interest to the Overview authors. If some reviews have been updated more recently than others, this should also be noted. Much of the material in this section can be summarized in a 'Characteristics of included reviews' table (see Section 22.3.6 for details).

## Methodological quality of included reviews

### Quality of included reviews

The general quality of the systematic reviews included in the Overview should be summarized, including any variability across reviews and any important flaws in individual reviews. The criteria that were used to assess review quality should be described or referenced under 'Methods' and not here. If it is felt to be important to provide details on how each included review was rated against each criterion, this should be reported in an Additional table and not described in detail in the text.

*Quality of evidence in included reviews*

The general quality of the evidence in the included reviews should be summarized, for example using GRADE for the most important outcomes (see also Chapter 13, Section 13.2).

## Effect of interventions

The main findings on the effects of the interventions studied in the included reviews should be summarized here. The section should be organized around clinically mean-ingful categories rather than simply listing the findings of each included review in turn. These categories could include things such as types of interventions (drug treat-ments, surgical interventions, behavioural interventions, etc); stages of disease (pre-symptomatic, early disease, advanced disease); participant characteristics (age, sex, ethnicity); or types of outcomes (survival, functional status, adverse effects). Subhead-ings are encouraged if they make reading easier. The findings of individual reviews, and any statistical summary of these, should be included in summary tables or figures.

Note should be made in this section of any outcomes that the Overview authors consider important but for which the review authors could not find evidence (either because no studies were found or because the studies identified did not report on the important outcome). In addition, this section should include a narrative summary of important results that can not easily be summarized using numerical data, and will not likely be included in the results tables of the Overview.

Authors should avoid making inferences in this section. A common mistake to avoid (both in describing the results and in drawing conclusions) is the confusion of 'no evidence of an effect' with 'evidence of no effect'. When there is inconclusive evidence, it is wrong to claim that the Overview shows that an intervention has 'no effect' or is 'no different' from the control intervention. In this situation it is more appropriate to report the data, with a confidence interval, as being compatible with either a reduction or an increase in the outcome.

# Discussion

## Summary of main results

Provide a concise summary here of the main findings, the balance between important benefits and important harms and highlight any outstanding uncertainties.

## Overall completeness and applicability of evidence

Are the reviews included sufficient to address all of the objectives of the Overview? If not, what gaps are present? Have all relevant types of participants, interventions and outcomes been investigated? Describe the relevance of the evidence to the Overview question. This should lead to an overall judgement of the external validity of the Overview. Comments on how the results of the Overview fit into the context of current practice might be included here, although authors should bear in mind that current practice might vary internationally and between populations.

## Quality of the evidence

Do the reviews included in the Overview allow a robust conclusion regarding the objective(s) addressed in the Overview? The discussion might include whether all relevant studies were identified in the original review, whether all relevant data could be obtained, or whether the methods used (for example, searching, study selection, data collection and analysis) could have introduced bias. This may vary for different interventions, outcomes or clinical subgroups. If so, the discussion should clearly identify the quality of evidence for each of the key areas of interest.

## Potential biases in the overview process

State the strengths and limitations of the Overview with regard to preventing bias. These may be factors within, or outside, the control of the Overview authors. The discussion might include whether all relevant reviews were identified and included in the Overview, whether all relevant data could be obtained, or whether the methods used (for example, searching, study selection, data collection and analysis) could have introduced bias.

## Agreements and disagreements with other studies or reviews

Comments on how the included reviews fit into the context of other evidence might be included here, stating clearly whether the other evidence was systematically reviewed.

# Authors' conclusions

This section should present the conclusions of the authors of the overview, not simply restate the varying conclusions of the authors of the included/underlying reviews. The primary purpose of this section should be to present information rather than to offer advice. Conclusions of the authors are divided into two sections as follows.

## Implications for practice

The implications for practice should be as practical and unambiguous as possible. They should not go beyond the evidence that was reviewed and should be justifiable by the data presented in the review. 'No evidence of effect' should not be confused with 'evidence of no effect'.

## Implications for research

This section should address the key clinical issues that remain unresolved after review of the evidence presented in the included/underlying reviews. If there are important potential interventions for the condition under consideration that have not been addressed in a Cochrane Intervention review, this gap should be clearly noted in this section. In addition to providing an agenda for future research, this section can be useful to clinical decision makers by clearly indicating the remaining areas of uncertainty.

# Acknowledgements

This section should be used to acknowledge any people or organizations that the authors wish to acknowledge, including people who are not listed among the authors: see Chapter 4 (Section 4.5).

# Contributions of authors

The contributions of the current co-authors should be described in this section: see Chapter 4 (Section 4.5).

# Declarations of interest

Authors should report any present or past affiliations or other involvement in any organization or entity with an interest in the review that might lead to a real or perceived conflict of interest: see Chapter 4 (Section 4.5). Authors must state if they have been involved in a study included in a component review, or in authoring a systematic review included in the Overview.

# Differences between protocol and review

It is sometimes necessary to use different methods from those described in the original protocol: see Chapter 4 (Section 4.5).

# Published notes

See Chapter 4 (Section 4.5).

## 22.3.5 Reviews and references

Authors should check all references for accuracy.

### 22.3.5.1 References to reviews

A 'Reference ID' should be created for each included review, and used throughout the Overview. This would usually comprise the last name of the first author and the year of the most recent citation version for the review (e.g. Efron 2006). Where two or more reviews share the same first author and year, a letter may be added (e.g. Efron 2007a, Efron 2007b). Reviews are organized under two fixed headings as follows.

**Included reviews**   Reviews that specifically meet the eligibility criteria and are included in the overview.

**Excluded reviews**   Reviews (if any) that do not specifically meet the eligibility criteria and are not included in the overview.

### 22.3.5.2 Other references

Other references cited in the text, including those cited in the background and methods sections, should be listed.

## 22.3.6 Tables

Several types of tables should be considered for Overviews; all can be created as Additional tables in RevMan.

### 22.3.6.1 'Characteristics of included reviews' table

Each Overview should contain one or more tables using the format shown in Figure 22.3.a to allow readers to rapidly review the essential features of the Cochrane reviews included in the Overview.

**Notes on completing columns**

*Review*   The 'Reference ID' for each included review (see Section 22.3.5.1).

*Date assessed as up to date*   This column should list the date on which the included review was last assessed as up to date (see Chapter 3, Section 3.3.2). This date should

| Review | Date assessed as up to date | Population | Interventions | Comparison interventions | Outcomes for which data were reported | Review limitations |
|---|---|---|---|---|---|---|
| | | | | | | |
| | | | | | | |
| | | | | | | |

**Figure 22.3.a**   Template for a 'Characteristics of included reviews' table

be within approximately six months of a search for studies, and the results of this search should have been incorporated into the review.

*Population*    Use this column to note any specific features of the population covered in the Cochrane review, i.e. any restrictions in age, sex, ethnicity, stage of disease, co-morbidity, etc should be noted here.

*Interventions*    List the specific interventions covered within the scope of the review, whether or not studies with data concerning those interventions were identified and included in the Cochrane review.

*Comparison interventions*    List the types of comparison interventions that were used (e.g. placebo, no-treatment or alternative intervention control groups).

*Outcomes for which data were reported*    Include important outcomes for which the review presented data, whether or not the outcomes are included in the summary data presented in the Overview.

*Review limitations*    In this column, provide a brief description of any important limitations of methods used in the Cochrane (or other) review. Do not use this column to summarize the quality of studies identified in the review – that information can be included in the 'Overview of reviews' table (see Section 22.3.6.2).

### 22.3.6.2 'Overview of reviews' table

Each Overview should contain one or more tables using the format shown in Figure 22.3.b to summarize its results. This format has been designed to reflect (as much as possible) the format of 'Summary of findings' tables: see Chapter 11 (Section 11.5) for additional guidance. If the Overview addresses more than one clinical population (e.g. groups that differ by stage or severity of disease, co-morbidities, or other factors likely to affect the outcomes under study) then separate tables should be used for the different clinical populations. Clearly the exact form may vary with review topics but each table should include both beneficial and harmful outcomes, the frequency or severity of these outcomes in the control groups, estimates of the relative and absolute

| Interventions for [Condition] in [Population] | | | | | | | |
|---|---|---|---|---|---|---|---|
| Outcome | Intervention and Comparison intervention | Illustrative comparative risks (95% CI) | | Relative effect (95% CI) | Number of participants (studies) | Quality of the evidence (GRADE) | Comments |
| | | Assumed risk | Corresponding risk | | | | |
| | | With comparator | With intervention | | | | |
| Outcome #1 | | | | | | | |
| | Intervention/Comparison #1 | | | | | | |
| | Intervention/Comparison #2 | | | | | | |
| | Etc... | | | | | | |
| Outcome #2 | | | | | | | |
| | Intervention/Comparison #1 | | | | | | |
| | Intervention/Comparison #2 | | | | | | |
| | Etc... | | | | | | |
| Outcome #3 | | | | | | | |
| | Intervention/Comparison #1 | | | | | | |
| | Intervention/Comparison #2 | | | | | | |
| | Etc... | | | | | | |

**Figure 22.3.b** Template for an 'Overview of reviews' table

effects of the interventions, indications of the risk of bias (which may vary by outcome and comparison), and any comments.

## Template for an 'Overview of reviews' table

Figure 22.3.b provides a template for an 'Overview of reviews' table. The intention is to make the format for this table as similar as possible to that used for 'Summary of findings' tables. If the recommended format for 'Summary of findings' tables changes, the recommended format for this table will change as well.

*The row headings* The rows should be organized by outcome, beginning with the primary outcome of interest. Within each outcome a series of rows should provide the results from the various intervention or comparison pairs for which data are available. Generally, one or more rows for adverse outcomes should be included, even if the included reviews did not report results for these.

## *Notes on completing columns*

*1. Outcomes*   The main beneficial and harmful outcomes should be listed (those most relevant to participants, preferably determined prior to completing the results of the Overview to avoid the potential of selection of reported outcomes based on significance and not clinical importance). The number of outcomes should not exceed seven. Important outcomes for which no data are available may be listed in the table as well.

   If there are multiple interventions being compared, the table should be primarily organized by outcome, with rows included in each outcome subsection that present data comparing the results of two interventions regarding that outcome.

*2. Assumed risk (With comparator)*   Representative comparator group risks should be provided for each row. These might be obtained from control group risks as reported in the included Cochrane reviews. If there is important variation in control group risks, two or three representative rates should be included for each row of the table – representing a low risk, moderate risk and high risk population. Whenever possible, indicate the types of participants to which a given control group risk may apply in this column, in the comments column or in a footnote.

*3. Corresponding risk (With intervention)*   This column is intended to show the expected absolute risk upon intervention at the one, two or three assumed comparator risks cited in the previous column. The numbers can be calculated by applying the relative effect to each assumed risk for the same row (see Chapter 11, Section 11.5.4).

*4. Relative effect*   For dichotomous outcomes, the risk ratio or odds ratio should generally be used. So far as possible the summary statistic that is used should be standardized across included reviews even if different reviews used different summary statistics in their analyses. The 95% confidence interval should be included to provide a measure of uncertainty. This may be calculated using either a fixed or random-effects model; however, the same model should be used for all results relative to a given outcome.

*5. Number of participants and studies*   In many cases, the number of studies and participants for whom data are available for a specific outcome and treatment comparison will be less than the total number of studies and participants reported in the Cochrane review from which the data are extracted (because the Cochrane review may include studies that did not report on a specific outcome or a specific comparison). If so, the number of studies and participants reported in this column should reflect only the subset providing data for the comparison and outcome of interest.

*6. Quality*   Comment on the quality of the evidence for each row of the table (note that, because different rows may contain data extracted from different Cochrane reviews or from different studies within an individual Cochrane review, the quality of evidence may vary from row to row). Use of the specific evidence grading system developed by the GRADE group (GRADE Working Group 2004) is recommended and is incorporated in the software available to authors of Cochrane reviews for preparing 'Summary of findings' tables. The system and methods employed to grade quality of evidence should be described in the Methods section of the Overview.

*7. Comments*   The aim of this field is to provide additional comments to help interpret the information or data identified in the row. For example this may be on the validity of the outcome measure or effect modification. Important caveats about the results should be flagged here. Not all rows will need comments, so it is best to leave a blank if there is nothing of importance to comment on.

***Continuous Outcome Measures***   Continuous outcome measures can be shown in the Overview table, but should be clinically meaningful. This requires that the units are clear and that these units are readily interpretable, for example days of pain or frequency of headache are readily interpretable. However, many scales are not readily interpretable by non-specialist clinicians or patients, for example points on a Beck Depression Inventory or quality-of-life score. For these, a more meaningful presentation might be to express results in terms of risks (e.g. of a 50% improvement) where possible, as discussed in Chapter 12 (Section 12.6).

The labelling of the outcomes should also be kept simple. For example, 'ability to perform everyday functions' would be preferred to 'functional status'. If specific details of outcome definitions are required, these might be added as footnotes.

***Heterogeneity***   A detailed discussion of heterogeneity generally should not be part of the summary table. However, if either (i) heterogeneity made important changes to the clinical or statistical significance; or (ii) there were important effect modifiers, then these should be reported in the Comments column. Occasionally an important effect modification may require a separate row or separate table to describe, for instance, difference in effect of endarterectomy for different grades of stenosis.

### 22.3.6.3   *Other tables*

Other tables may be used for information that cannot be conveniently placed in the text, in 'Characteristics of included reviews' tables or in 'Overview of reviews' tables. Examples include the following:

• Information to support the background.

• Details of search methods.

• Details of quality assessments of included reviews.

• 'Summary of findings' tables for included reviews prepared by the authors of the Overview and not found in the included reviews.

## 22.3.7 Figures

The addition of one or two (at most) figures may help readers of an Overview better appreciate differences in effectiveness of the interventions being compared in the review. The preferred format for Overview figures is the 'forest top plot' where each row in the figure represents the results (summary effect and 95% confidence interval) of a meta-analysis comparing two interventions. Each figure should address a single outcome, but may include several pair-wise comparisons of interventions. Direct comparisons, calculated indirect comparisons, and calculated combinations of direct and indirect comparisons may be included in the same figure, but must be clearly labelled. The text should provide information about the methods used in such calculations. An example of a forest top plot using data from the overview on enuresis (Russell 2006) is included in Figure 22.3.c.

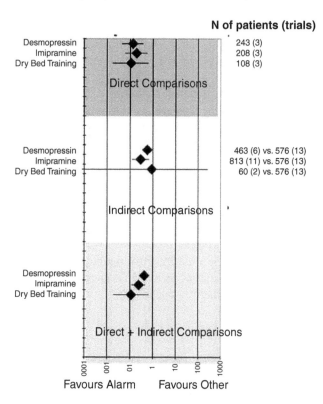

**Figure 22.3.c** Example of a 'forest top plot' comparing interventions for enuresis in children. This example was prepared using Microsoft Excel

## 22.4 Chapter information

**Authors**: Lorne A Becker and Andrew D Oxman.

**This chapter should be cited as**: Becker LA, Oxman AD. Chapter 22: Overviews of reviews. In: Higgins JPT, Green S (editors), *Cochrane Handbook for Systematic Reviews of Interventions*. Chichester (UK): John Wiley & Sons, 2008.

**Acknowledgements**: Methods for Cochrane Overviews have been developed by a working group convened by the Cochrane Collaboration Steering Group, consisting of Lorne Becker (Convenor), Jon Deeks, Paul Glasziou, Jill Hayden, Steff Lewis, Yoon Loke, Lara Maxwell, Andy Oxman, Rebecca Ryan, Denise Thomson, Peter Tugwell and Janet Wale. We thank these for their contributions, and also Lesley Gillespie, Helen Handoll and Julian Higgins for comments on previous drafts.

## 22.5 References

**Glenny 2005**
Glenny AM, Altman DG, Song F, Sakarovitch C, Deeks JJ, D'Amico R, Bradburn M, Eastwood AJ. Indirect comparisons of competing interventions. *Health Technology Assessment* 2005; 9: 26.

**GRADE Working Group 2004**
GRADE Working Group. Grading quality of evidence and strength of recommendations. *BMJ* 2004; 328: 1490–1494.

**Oxman 1994**
Oxman AD. Checklists for review articles. *BMJ* 1994; 309: 648–651.

**Petticrew 1999**
Petticrew M, Song F, Wilson P, Wright K. Quality-assessed reviews of health care interventions and the database of abstracts of reviews of effectiveness (DARE). NHS CRD Review, Dissemination, and Information Teams. *International Journal of Technology Assessment in Health Care* 1999; 15: 671–678.

**Russell 2006**
Russell K, Kiddoo D. The Cochrane Library and nocturnal enuresis; an umbrella review. *Evidence-Based Child Health* 2006; 1: 5–8.

**Shea 2006**
Shea B, Boers M, Grimshaw JM, Hamel C, Bouter LM. Does updating improve the methodological and reporting quality of systematic reviews? *BMC Medical Research Methodology* 2006; 6: 27.

# Index

*This index was prepared by Neil Manley, and edited by Julian Higgins.*